BMA

The British
Medical Association

CONCISE GUIDE TO
MEDICINES
AND DRUGS

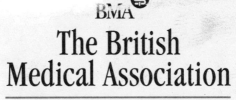

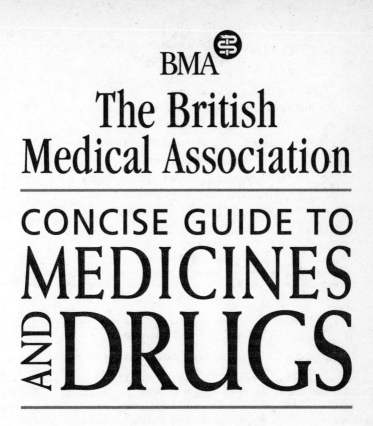

BMA

The British Medical Association

CONCISE GUIDE TO
MEDICINES
AND DRUGS

Chief Medical Editor

PROFESSOR JOHN A. HENRY MB FRCP

St Mary's Hospital, London

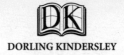

DORLING KINDERSLEY

BMA Consulting Medical Editor Dr. Michael Peters MB BS

Project Editors Teresa Pritlove, Katie John, Sunrita Sen

Senior Managing Editor Martyn Page

Managing Art Editor Marianne Markham

Senior Art Editor Ian Spick

DTP Designers Julian Dams, Pankaj Sharma

Production Controller Stuart Masheter

Publishing Director Corinne Roberts

First UK Edition 2001
Second UK Edition, 2005
The British Medical Association Concise Guide to Medicines and Drugs is based on
The British Medical Association New Guide to Medicines and Drugs (6th edition)
2 4 6 8 10 9 7 5 3 1

Published in the United Kingdom by Dorling Kindersley Limited
80 Strand, London WC2R 0RL, England

A CIP catalogue record for this book is available from the British Library
ISBN 1-4053-0694-7

Printed and bound in Great Britain by Clays Ltd. St Ives plc

see our complete catalogue at
www.dk.com

CONTENTS

INTRODUCTION

The British Medical Association Concise Guide to Medicines and Drugs provides clear information and practical advice on drugs and medicines that can be readily understood by a non-medical reader. The text reflects current medical knowledge and standard medical practice in this country. It is intended to complement and reinforce the advice of your doctor.

The book is divided into three parts. The first part covers the major groups of drugs. The second part gives detailed information about 259 individual drugs, arranged alphabetically. The third part consists of the drug finder index.

PART 1: MAJOR DRUG GROUPS

This part of the book is subdivided into sections on each body system or major disease grouping. It contains descriptions of the principal drug groups and information on the uses, actions, effects, and risks associated with each. Common drugs in each group are listed to allow cross-reference to Part 2.

A–Z OF DRUGS

This part consists of profiles of 262 key drugs. Each profile gives detailed information and practical advice and is intended to provide reference and guidance for non-medical readers taking drug treatment. It is impossible, however, to take into account every variation in individual circumstances; readers should always follow a doctor's or pharmacist's instructions where they differ from the advice in this section.

The drugs have been selected to provide representative coverage of the principal classes of drugs in medical use today. For some disorders, a number of drugs are available and the most commonly used drugs have been chosen. Emphasis has also been placed on the drugs likely to be used in the home, although in a few cases drugs administered only in hospital have been included when the drug has been judged to be of sufficient general interest.

HOW TO UNDERSTAND THE PROFILES

For ease of reference, the information on each drug is arranged in a consistent format under standard headings.

Drug name Tells you the drug's generic name, brand names under which the drug is marketed, and combined preparations that contain the drug.

Quick reference Summarizes important facts regarding the drug.

General information Gives a brief summary of the drug's important characteristics.

Information for users Practical information on how and when to take the drug, the usual recommended dosage, how soon it takes effect, how long it is active, and advice on diet, storage, and missed doses.

Overdose action Indicates the symptoms that may occur if an overdose has been taken and tells you what immediate action is required.

Possible adverse effects Indicates adverse effects that may be experienced with the drug.

Interactions Tells you how the drug may interact with other drugs or substances taken at the same time.

Special precautions Describes circumstances in which the drug should be taken with special caution or in which it might not be suitable.

Prolonged use Tells you what effects the drug may have when taken long term and what monitoring may be advised.

PART 3: DRUG FINDER INDEX

The drug finder index provides basic information on over 2,500 generic and brand-name drugs and drug groups, and also directs you to further information about them throughout the book.

PART 1

MAJOR DRUG GROUPS

Subdivided into sections dealing with each body system (such as heart and circulation) or major disease grouping (such as malignant and immune disease), this part of the book contains descriptions of the principal classes of drugs (such as corticosteroids), with information on the uses, actions, effects, and risks associated with each group of drugs. Individual drugs common to each group are listed to allow cross-reference to Part 2.

BRAIN AND NERVOUS SYSTEM

The human brain contains over 100 billion nerve cells (neurons). These nerve cells receive electro-chemical impulses from everywhere in the body. They interpret these impulses and send responsive signals back to various glands and muscles. The brain functions continuously as a switchboard for the human communications system. At the same time, it serves as the seat of emotions and mood, of memory, personality, and thought. Extending from the brain is an additional column of nerve cells that forms the spinal cord. Together, these two elements comprise the central nervous system.

Radiating from the central nervous system is the peripheral nervous system, which has three parts. One part branches off the spinal cord and extends to skin and muscles throughout the body. Another, in the head, links the brain to the eyes, ears, nose, and taste buds. The third is a semi-independent network called the autonomic, or involuntary, nervous system (see below right). This is the part of the nervous system that controls unconscious body functions such as breathing and digestion.

Signals traverse the nervous system by electrical and chemical means. Electrical impulses carry signals from one end of a neuron to the other. To cross the gap between neurons, chemical neurotransmitters are released from one cell to bind to the receptor sites of nearby cells. Excitatory transmitters stimulate action; inhibitory transmitters reduce it.

WHAT CAN GO WRONG

Disorders of the brain and nervous system may manifest themselves as physical impairments, such as epilepsy or strokes, or as mental and emotional impairments (such as schizophrenia or depression).

Illnesses causing physical impairments can result from different types of disorder of the brain and nervous system. Death of nerve cells resulting from poor circulation can result in paralysis, while electrical disturbances of certain nerve cells cause the fits of epilepsy. Temporary changes in blood circulation within and around the brain are thought to cause migraine. Parkinson's disease is caused by a lack of dopamine, a neurotransmitter produced by specialized brain cells.

The causes of disorders that trigger mental and emotional impairment are not known, but these illnesses have been linked with the defective functioning of nerve cells and neurotransmitters. The nerve cells may be under- or overactive, or poorly coordinated. Alternatively, mental and emotional disorders may be due to too much or too little neurotransmitter in one area of the brain.

WHY DRUGS ARE USED

By and large, the drugs that are described in this section do not eliminate nervous system disorders; their function is to correct or modify the communication of the signals that traverse the nervous system. By doing so, they can improve symptoms or return functioning and behaviour towards normal. In some cases, such as anxiety and insomnia, drugs are used to lower the level of activity in the brain. In other disorders – depression, for example – drugs encourage the opposite effect, increasing the level of activity.

Drugs that act on the nervous system are also used for conditions that outwardly have nothing to do with nervous system disorders. Migraine headaches, for example, are often treated with drugs that cause the autonomic nervous system to send out signals constricting the dilated blood vessels that cause the migraine.

AUTONOMIC NERVOUS SYSTEM

The autonomic, or involuntary, nervous system governs the actions of the muscles of the organs and glands. Such vital functions as heart beat and digestion continue without conscious direction, whether we are awake or asleep.

The autonomic nervous system is divided into two parts: the sympathetic and parasympathetic nervous systems. The effects of one generally balance those of the other; the sympathetic has a mainly excitatory effect, while the parasympathetic, by contrast, has an opposite effect.

Although the functional pace of most organs results from the interplay between the two systems, the muscles in the blood vessel walls respond only to the signals of the sympathetic nervous system. Whether a vessel is dilated or constricted is determined by the relative stimulation of two sets of receptor sites: alpha sites and beta sites.

Blood vessels in the skin These are constricted by stimulation of alpha receptors by the sympathetic; the parasympathetic has no effect on them.

The heart The rate and strength of the heart are increased by the sympathetic and reduced by the parasympathetic.

The pupils These are dilated by the sympathetic and constricted by the parasympathetic.

The airways The bronchial muscles are relaxed and widened by the sympathetic and contracted and narrowed by the parasympathetic.

Intestines The activity of the intestinal wall muscles is reduced by the sympathetic and increased by the parasympathetic.

NEUROTRANSMITTERS

The sympathetic nervous system relies on epinephrine (adrenaline) and norepinephrine (noradrenaline), products of the adrenal glands and neurons that act as both hormones and neurotransmitters. The parasympathetic nervous system depends on the neurotransmitter acetylcholine to transmit signals from cell to cell.

DRUGS THAT ACT ON THE SYMPATHETIC NERVOUS SYSTEM

The drugs that stimulate the sympathetic nervous system are called adrenergics (or sympathomimetics). They either promote the release of epinephrine (adrenaline) and norepinephrine (noradrenaline) or mimic their effects. Drugs that interfere with the action of the sympathetic nervous system are called sympatholytics. Alpha blockers act on alpha receptors; beta blockers act on beta receptors (see also Beta blockers, p.30).

DRUGS THAT ACT ON THE PARA-SYMPATHETIC NERVOUS SYSTEM

Drugs that stimulate the parasympathetic nervous system are called cholinergics (or parasympathomimetics); drugs that oppose its action are called anticholinergics. Many prescribed drugs have anticholinergic properties.

MAJOR DRUG GROUPS

◆ Analgesics
◆ Sleeping drugs
◆ Anti-anxiety drugs
◆ Antidepressant drugs
◆ Antipsychotic drugs
◆ Antimanic drugs
◆ Anticonvulsant drugs
◆ Drugs for parkinsonism
◆ Drugs for dementia
◆ Nervous system stimulants
◆ Drugs used for migraine
◆ Anti-emetics

Analgesics

Analgesics (painkillers) are drugs that relieve pain. Since pain is not a disease but a symptom, long-term relief depends on treatment of the underlying cause. The pain of toothache, for example, can be relieved by drugs but can be cured only by appropriate dental treatment. If the underlying disorder cannot be cured (as in some rheumatic conditions) long-term analgesic treatment may be necessary.

Damage to body tissues as a result of disease or injury is detected by nerve endings that transmit signals to the brain. Interpretation of these sensations can be affected by an individual's psychological state, so that pain is worsened by anxiety and fear, for example. Often, a reassuring explanation of the cause of discomfort can make pain easier to bear and may even relieve it. Anti-anxiety drugs (see p.13) are helpful when pain is accompanied by anxiety, and some are also used to reduce painful muscle spasms. Antidepressant drugs (see p.14) block the transmission of impulses signalling pain and are particularly useful for nerve pains (neuralgia), which do not always respond to analgesics.

TYPES OF ANALGESIC

Analgesics are divided into the opioids (with similar properties to drugs derived from opium, such as morphine) and non-opioids. Non-opioids consist of all other analgesics, including paracetamol, nefopam, and also the non-steroidal anti-inflammatory drugs (NSAIDs), the most well known of which is aspirin. In most circumstances, the non-opioids are less powerful as painkillers than the opioids. Local anaesthetics (see facing page) are also used to relieve pain.

Opioid drugs and paracetamol act directly on the brain and spinal cord to alter the perception of pain. Opioids act like the endorphins, hormones naturally produced in the brain that stop the cell-to-cell transmission of pain sensation. NSAIDs prevent stimulation of nerve endings at the site of the pain.

When pain is treated under medical supervision, it is common to start with an NSAID or paracetamol; if neither provides adequate relief, they may be combined. A mild opioid (such as codeine) may also be used. If the less powerful drugs are ineffective, a strong opioid such as morphine may be given. As there is now a wide variety of oral analgesic formulations, injections are seldom necessary to control even the most severe pain.

When using over-the-counter preparations (for example, taking aspirin for a headache), you should seek medical advice if the pain persists for longer than 48 hours, recurs, or is worse than or different from previous pain.

NON-OPIOID ANALGESICS

Paracetamol This analgesic is believed to act by reducing the production of chemicals called prostaglandins in the brain. It does not affect prostaglandin production in the rest of the body, so it does not reduce inflammation, although it can reduce fever. Paracetamol can be used for aches and pains, such as headache and joint pain. It is given as liquid to treat pain and reduce fever in children.

As well as being the most widely used analgesic, it is one of the safest when taken correctly. It does not usually irritate the stomach, and allergic reactions are rare. However, an overdose can cause severe and possibly fatal liver or kidney damage. The toxic potential of paracetamol may be increased in heavy drinkers.

Non-steroidal anti-inflammatory drugs (NSAIDs): Aspirin Used for many years to relieve pain and reduce fever, aspirin also reduces inflammation by blocking the production of prosta-glandins, which contribute to the swelling and pain in inflamed tissue. It is useful for headaches, toothache, mild rheumatic pain, sore throat, and the discomfort of feverish illnesses. Given regularly, it can also relieve the pain and inflammation of chronic rheumatoid arthritis (see Antirheumatic drugs, p.52).

Aspirin is found in combination with other substances in a variety of medicines (see Cold cures, p.28). It is also used in the treatment of some blood disorders, since it helps to prevent abnormal clotting (see Drugs that affect blood clotting, p.38). For this reason, it is sometimes unsuitable for people whose blood does not clot normally.

Aspirin in the form of soluble tablets, dissolved in water before being taken, is absorbed into the bloodstream more quickly, thereby relieving pain faster than tablets. Soluble aspirin is not, however, less irritating to the stomach lining. Aspirin is available in many forms, all of which have a similar effect but, because the amount of aspirin in a tablet of each type varies, it is important to read the packet for the correct dosage. It is not recommended for children aged under 16 years because its use has been linked to Reye's syndrome, a rare but potentially fatal liver and brain disorder.

Other NSAIDs These drugs can relieve both pain and inflammation. NSAIDs are related to aspirin and also work by blocking the production of prostaglandins. They are most commonly used to treat muscle and joint pain and may also be prescribed for other types of pain including period pain. For further information on these drugs, see p.50.

COMBINED ANALGESICS

Mild opioids, such as codeine, are often found in combination preparations with non-opioids, such as NSAIDs or paracetamol. The prefix "co-" is used to denote a drug combination. These mixtures may combine the advantages of analgesics that act through two different pathways. Another advantage of combining analgesics is that the reductions in dose of the components may reduce the side effects of the preparation. Combinations can be helpful in reducing the number of tablets taken during long-term treatment.

OPIOID ANALGESICS

These drugs are related to opium, an extract of poppy seeds. They act directly on several sites in the central nervous system to block the transmission of pain signals. Because they act directly on the parts of the brain where pain is perceived, opioids are the strongest analgesics and are therefore used to treat the pain arising from surgery, serious injury, and cancer. These drugs are particularly valuable for relieving severe pain during terminal illnesses. In addition, their ability to produce a state of relaxation and euphoria is often of help in relieving the stress that accompanies severe pain.

Morphine is the best known opioid analgesic. Others include diamorphine (heroin) and pethidine. The use of these powerful opioids is strictly controlled because the euphoria produced can lead to abuse and addiction. When these opioids are given under medical supervision to treat severe pain, the risk of addiction is negligible.

Opioid analgesics may prevent clear thought and cloud the consciousness. Other possible adverse effects include nausea, vomiting, constipation, drowsiness, and depressed breathing. Taken in overdose, these drugs may induce a deep coma and lead to fatal breathing difficulties.

In addition to the powerful opioids, some less powerful drugs in this group, such as dihydrocodeine, dextropropoxyphene, and codeine, are used to relieve mild to moderate pain. Their normally unwanted side effects of depressing respiration and causing constipation make them useful as cough suppressants (p.27) and antidiarrhoeal drugs (p.44).

LOCAL ANAESTHETICS

These drugs are used to prevent pain, usually in minor surgical procedures (for example, dental treatment and stitching cuts). They can also be injected into the space around the spinal cord to numb the lower half of the body. This is called spinal or epidural anaesthesia and can be used for some major operations in people who are not fit for a general anaesthetic. Epidural anaesthesia is also used during childbirth.

Local anaesthetics block the passage of nerve impulses at the site of administration, deadening all feeling conveyed by the nerves with which they come into contact. They do not interfere with consciousness, however. Local anaesthetics are usually given by injection but can also be applied to the skin, mouth, and other areas lined with mucous membrane (such as the vagina), or the eye to relieve pain. Some local anaesthetics are formulated for injection together with epinephrine (adrenaline). Epinephrine constricts the blood vessels and prevents the local anaesthetic from being absorbed into the bloodstream. This action keeps the anaesthetic at the site, thus prolonging its effect.

Local anaesthetic creams are often used to numb the skin before injections in children and those people with a fear of needles.

COMMON DRUGS

Opioids Co-codamol, Co-codaprin, Codeine*, Co-dydramol, Co-proxamol*, Dipipanone, Fentanyl, Meptazinol, Methadone*, Morphine*, Pentazocine, Pethidine, Phenazocine, Tramadol*

NSAIDs (see p.50) Aspirin*, Diclofenac*, Etodolac, Fenbufen, Fenoprofen, Ibuprofen*, Indometacin, Ketoprofen*, Ketorolac, Mefenamic acid*, Naproxen*, Piroxicam*

Other non-opioids Nefopam, Paracetamol*

* See part 2

Sleeping drugs

Difficulty in getting to sleep or staying asleep (insomnia) has many causes. Most people suffer from sleepless nights from time to time, usually as a result of a temporary worry or discomfort from a minor illness. Persistent sleeplessness can be caused by psychological problems, including anxiety or depression, or the pain and discomfort of a physical disorder.

WHY THEY ARE USED

For occasional sleeplessness, simple, common remedies, such as a warm bath or a hot milk drink before bedtime, promote relaxation and are usually the best treatment. Sleeping drugs (also known as hypnotics) are normally prescribed only when self-help remedies have failed and lack of sleep is beginning to affect your general health. They are used to re-establish the habit of sleeping and should be used in the smallest dose and for the shortest possible time (not more than three weeks). It is best not to use them every night (see Risks and special precautions, below right). Do not use alcohol to help you sleep; it can cause disturbed sleep and insomnia. Long-term treatment of sleeplessness depends on resolving the underlying cause.

TYPES OF SLEEPING DRUG

Benzodiazepines are the most commonly used class of sleeping drugs because they have comparatively few adverse effects and are relatively safe in overdose. They are also used to treat anxiety (see p.13).

Barbiturates are now rarely used because of the risks of abuse, dependence, and toxicity in overdose. There is also a risk of prolonged sedation ("hangover").

Chloral derivatives effectively promote sleep but are little used now. If prescribed, triclofos causes fewer gastrointestinal side effects than chloral hydrate.

Other non-benzodiazepine sleeping drugs Zopiclone, zaleplon, and zolpidem are non-benzodiazepine sleeping drugs that work in a similar way to benzodiazepines. They are not intended for long-term use, and withdrawal symptoms have been reported.

Antihistamines are widely used to treat allergic symptoms (see p.58). Because they also cause drowsiness, they are sometimes used to promote sleep in children and the elderly.

Antidepressants may be used to promote sleep in depressed people (see p.14) and are effective in treating underlying depressive illness.

HOW THEY WORK

Most sleeping drugs promote sleep by depressing brain function. They interfere with chemical activity in the brain and nervous system by reducing communication between nerve cells. This reduces brain activity, allowing you to fall asleep more easily, but the nature of the sleep is affected. Benzodiazepines and related drugs are the most widely used class of sleeping drug.

HOW THEY AFFECT YOU

A sleeping drug rapidly produces drowsiness and slowed reactions. Some people find that that the drug makes them appear drunk, with slurred speech, especially if they delay going to bed after taking their dose. Most people find that they usually fall asleep within an hour of taking the drug.

Because drug-induced sleep is not the same as normal sleep, many people find they do not feel as well rested by it as by a night of natural sleep. This is the result of suppressed brain activity. Sleeping drugs also suppress the sleep during which dreams occur, and both dream sleep and non-dream sleep are essential components of a good night's sleep.

Some people experience a variety of "hangover" effects the following day. Some benzodiazepines may produce minor side effects such as daytime drowsiness, dizziness, and unsteadiness that can impair the ability to drive or operate machinery. Elderly people are especially likely to become confused; for them, selection of an appropriate drug is particularly important.

RISKS AND SPECIAL PRECAUTIONS

Sleeping drugs become less effective after the first few nights, and it may be tempting to increase the dose. Apart from the antihistamines, most sleeping drugs can produce psychological and physical dependence when they are taken regularly for more than a few weeks, especially if larger-than-normal doses are taken.

When sleeping drugs are suddenly withdrawn, anxiety, convulsions, and hallucinations sometimes occur. Nightmares and vivid dreams may be a problem because the time spent in dream sleep increases. Sleeplessness will recur and may lead to a temptation to use sleeping drugs again. Anyone who wishes to stop taking sleeping drugs, particularly after prolonged use, should seek his or her doctor's advice to prevent these withdrawal symptoms from occurring.

COMMON DRUGS

Benzodiazepines Flurazepam, Loprazolam, Lormetazepam, Nitrazepam, Temazepam*
Barbiturate Amobarbital
Chloral derivatives Chloral hydrate, Triclofos
Other non-benzodiazepine sleeping drugs
Clomethiazole, Promethazine*, Zaleplon, Zolpidem, Zopiclone*
* See part 2

Anti-anxiety drugs

A certain amount of stress can be beneficial, providing a stimulus to action. But too much will often result in anxiety, which might be described as fear or apprehension not caused by any real danger.

Clinically, anxiety arises when the balance of certain chemicals in the brain is disturbed. The feelings of fear or apprehension increase brain activity, stimulating the sympathetic nervous system (see Autonomic nervous system, p.8), and often trigger physical symptoms (such as breathlessness, shaking, palpitations, digestive distress, and headaches).

WHY THEY ARE USED

Anti-anxiety drugs (also known as anxiolytics or minor tranquillizers) are prescribed for short-term relief of severe anxiety and nervousness caused by psychological problems. However, these drugs cannot resolve the causes. Tackling the underlying problem through counselling and perhaps psychotherapy offer the best hope of a long-term solution. Anti-anxiety drugs are also used in hospitals to calm and relax people undergoing uncomfortable medical procedures.

There are two main classes of drugs for relieving anxiety: benzodiazepines and beta blockers. Benzodiazepines, which are the most widely used, are given as regular treatment for short periods to promote relaxation. Most benzodiazepines have a strong sedative effect, and they can help to relieve the insomnia that accompanies anxiety (see also Sleeping drugs, p.11).

Beta blockers are mainly used to reduce the physical symptoms of anxiety, such as shaking and palpitations. These drugs are commonly prescribed for people who feel excessively anxious in certain situations, such as interviews or public appearances.

Many antidepressants, including SSRIs, clomipramine, and venlafaxine, are proving useful in some anxiety disorders.

HOW THEY WORK

Benzodiazepines and related drugs depress activity in the part of the brain that controls emotion by promoting the action of the neurotransmitter gamma-aminobutyric acid (GABA) which binds to neurons, blocking transmission of electrical impulses and thus reducing communication between brain cells. Benzodiazepines increase the inhibitory effect of GABA on brain cells, preventing the excessive brain activity that causes anxiety.

Buspirone is different from other anti-anxiety drugs; it binds mainly to receptors for serotonin (another neurotransmitter), and it does not cause drowsiness. Its effect is not felt for at least two weeks after treatment has begun.

Beta blockers block the action of a chemical transmitter called norepinephrine (noradrenaline) in the body, reducing the physical symptoms of anxiety. These symptoms are produced by an increase in the activity of the sympathetic nervous system. Sympathetic nerve endings release norepinephrine, which stimulates the heart, digestive system, and other organs. For more information on beta blockers, see p.30.

HOW THEY AFFECT YOU

Benzodiazepines and related drugs reduce feelings of restlessness and agitation, slow mental activity, and often produce drowsiness. They are said to reduce motivation and, if they are taken in large doses, may lead to apathy. They also have a relaxing effect on the muscles, and some benzodiazepines are used specifically for that purpose (see Muscle relaxants, p.54).

Minor adverse effects of these drugs include dizziness and forgetfulness. People who need to drive or operate potentially dangerous machinery should be aware that their reactions may be slowed. Because the brain soon becomes tolerant to and dependent on their effects, benzodiazepines are usually effective for only a few weeks at a time.

Beta blockers reduce the physical symptoms of anxiety. This effect, in turn, may promote greater mental calmness. Because they do not cause drowsiness, they are safer for people who need to drive.

RISKS AND SPECIAL PRECAUTIONS

The benzodiazepines are safe for most people and are not likely to be fatal in overdose. The main risk is psychological and physical dependence, especially for people who take them regularly or when larger-than-average doses have been used. For this reason, they are usually given for courses of two weeks or less. If they have been used for a longer period, they should be withdrawn gradually under medical supervision. If they are stopped suddenly, withdrawal symptoms, such as excessive anxiety, nightmares, and restlessness, may occur.

Benzodiazepines have been abused for their sedative effect, and are therefore prescribed with caution for people with a history of drug or alcohol abuse.

COMMON DRUGS

Benzodiazepines Alprazolam, Chlordiazepoxide*, Diazepam*, Lorazepam, Oxazepam
Beta blockers Atenolol*, Oxprenolol, Propranolol*
Other non-benzodiazepines Buspirone, Meprobamate
* **See part 2**

Antidepressant drugs

Occasional sadness or loss of heart are normal, and they usually pass quickly. However, more severe depression that is accompanied by feelings of despair, lethargy, loss of sex drive, and often poor appetite may call for medical attention. Such depression can arise from life stresses such as the death of someone close, an illness, or sometimes from no apparent cause.

Three main types of antidepressant are used to treat depression: tricyclic antidepressants (TCAs), selective serotonin re-uptake inhibitors (SSRIs), and monoamine oxidase inhibitors (MAOIs). Treatment usually begins with either a TCA or an SSRI. Both groups of drugs are equally effective.

WHY THEY ARE USED

Minor depression does not usually require drug treatment, and support and help in coming to terms with the cause of the depression is often all that is needed. Moderate or severe depression usually requires drug treatment, which is effective in most cases. Antidepressants may have to be taken for many months. Treatment should not be stopped too soon because symptoms are likely to reappear. When treatment with some types of antidepressant is stopped, the dose should be reduced gradually over several weeks because withdrawal symptoms may occur if they are stopped suddenly.

TYPES OF ANTIDEPRESSANT

Treatment usually begins with either a TCA or an SSRI.

TCAs Some TCAs (such as amitriptyline) cause drowsiness, which is useful for sleep problems in depression. TCAs also cause anticholinergic effects (see Drugs that act on the parasympathetic nervous system, p.9), including blurred vision, dry mouth, and urinary difficulties.

SSRIs These drugs generally have fewer side effects than TCAs. The main unwanted effects are nausea and vomiting. Anxiety, headache, and restlessness may also occur at the beginning of treatment.

MAOIs These are especially effective in people who are anxious as well as depressed, or who suffer from phobias.

Lithium Salts of this metallic element are used to treat manic depression (see Antimanic drugs, p.16). They are sometimes used with an antidepressant drug for resistant depression.

Other antidepressants These drugs include venlafaxine, nefazodone, maprotiline, mianserin, and trazodone.

HOW THEY WORK

Normally, the brain cells release sufficient quantities of certain chemicals (known as neurotransmitters) in the brain to stimulate neighbouring cells. The neurotransmitters are constantly reabsorbed into the brain cells, where they are broken down by an enzyme called monoamine oxidase.

Depression is thought to be caused by a reduction in the level of neurotransmitters being released. Antidepressants bring these levels back to normal.

TCAs and venlafaxine work by blocking the reabsorption of the neurotransmitters serotonin and norepinephrine (noradrenaline), thereby increasing the level of these neurotransmitters in the brain.

SSRIs act by blocking the reabsorption of only one neurotransmitter, serotonin.

MAOIs prevent the breakdown of neurotransmitters – mainly serotonin and norepinephrine (noradrenaline) – by blocking the action of monoamine oxidase, the enzyme that breaks them down.

HOW THEY AFFECT YOU

The antidepressant effect of these drugs starts after 10 to 14 days' treatment and it may be six to eight weeks before the full effect is seen. However, side effects may occur at once. Tolerance to these side effects usually occurs and treatment should be continued.

RISKS AND SPECIAL PRECAUTIONS

Overdose can be dangerous. TCAs can produce coma, fits, and disturbed heart rhythm, which may be fatal; MAOIs can also cause muscle spasms and even death. Both types of drug are prescribed with caution for people with heart problems or epilepsy. SSRIs are safer in overdose.

MAOIs taken with certain drugs or foods rich in tyramine (such as cheese, meat, yeast extracts, and red wine) can produce a dramatic rise in blood pressure, with headache or vomiting. People taking MAOIs are given a card that lists prohibited drugs and foods. Apart from moclobemide, MAOIs are used much less frequently today because of this adverse interaction, and SSRIs or TCAs are prescribed in preference to them.

COMMON DRUGS

TCAs Amitriptyline*, Amoxapine, Clomipramine*, Dosulepin*, Doxepin, Imipramine*, Lofepramine*, Nortriptyline, Trimipramine
SSRIs Citalopram*, Escitalopram, Fluoxetine*, Fluvoxamine, Paroxetine*, Sertraline*
MAOIs Isocarboxazid, Moclobemide, Phenelzine, Tranylcypromine
Other drugs Flupentixol*, Maprotiline, Mianserin, Mirtazapine, Nefazodone, Reboxetine, Trazodone*, Tryptophan, Venlafaxine*
* **See part 2**

Antipsychotic drugs

Psychosis is a term used to describe mental disorders that prevent the sufferer from thinking clearly, acting rationally, and recognizing reality. These disorders include schizophrenia and manic depression. Their precise causes are unknown, but several factors, including stress, heredity, and brain injury, may be involved. Temporary psychosis can also arise as a result of alcohol withdrawal or the abuse of mind-altering drugs. A variety of drugs is used to treat psychotic disorders (see Common drugs, p.16), most of which have similar actions and effects. One exception is lithium, which is particularly useful for manic depression (see Antimanic drugs, p.16).

WHY THEY ARE USED

A person with a psychotic illness may recover spontaneously, so a drug will not always be prescribed. Long-term treatment is started only when normal life is seriously disrupted. Antipsychotic drugs (also called major tranquillizers or neuroleptics) do not cure the disorder, but they do help to control symptoms.

By controlling the symptoms of psychosis, antipsychotic drugs enable most sufferers to live in the community and only be admitted to hospital for acute episodes.

The drug given to a particular individual depends on the nature of his or her illness and the expected adverse effects of that drug. Drugs differ in the amount of sedation produced; the need for sedation also influences the choice of drug.

Antipsychotics may also be given to calm or sedate a highly agitated or aggressive person, whatever the cause. Some antipsychotics also have a powerful action against nausea and vomiting (see Anti-emetics, p.21) and are therefore sometimes used as premedication before surgery.

HOW THEY WORK

It is thought that some forms of mental illness are caused by increased communication between brain cells due to overactivity of dopamine, an excitatory chemical. This may disturb normal thought processes and lead to abnormal behaviour. Dopamine combines with receptors on the brain cells; antipsychotic drugs reduce the transmission of nerve signals by binding to these receptors, thereby making the brain cells less sensitive to dopamine. Some new antipsychotic drugs, such as clozapine (see p.197), risperidone (see p.374), and sertindole, also bind to receptors for the chemical serotonin.

HOW THEY AFFECT YOU

Because antipsychotics depress the action of dopamine, they can disturb its balance with acetylcholine, another chemical in the brain. If an imbalance occurs, extrapyramidal side effects (EPSE) may appear. These include restlessness, movement disorders, and parkinsonism (see Drugs for parkinsonism, p.18). In these circumstances, a change to a different type of antipsychotic may be necessary. If this is not possible, an anticholinergic drug (see Drugs that act on the parasympathetic nervous system, p.9) may be prescribed.

Antipsychotics may block the action of norepinephrine (noradrenaline), another neurotransmitter in the brain. This lowers blood pressure, especially when you stand up, causing dizziness. It may also prevent ejaculation.

RISKS AND SPECIAL PRECAUTIONS

It is important to continue taking these drugs even if all symptoms have gone, because the symptoms are controlled only by taking the prescribed dose.

Because antipsychotic drugs can have permanent as well as temporary side effects, the minimum dosage is used. This is found by starting with a low dose and increasing it until the symptoms are controlled. Sudden withdrawal after more than a few weeks can cause nausea, sweating, headache, and restlessness. Therefore, when treatment needs to be stopped, the dose is reduced gradually.

A major long-term risk of antipsychotic drug treatment is a disorder known as tardive dyskinesia, which may develop after one to five years. It consists of repeated jerking movements of the mouth, tongue, and face, and sometimes the hands and feet. The condition is less common with the newer antipsychotics (atypical antipsychotics) than the older drugs (typical antipsychotics).

HOW THEY ARE ADMINISTERED

Antipsychotics may be given by mouth as tablets, capsules, or syrup, or by injection. They can also be given in the form of a depot injection which releases the drug slowly over several weeks. This is helpful for people who might forget to take their drugs or who might take an overdose.

COMMON DRUGS

Typical antipsychotics Benperidol, Chlorpromazine*, Flupentixol*, Fluphenazine, Haloperidol*, Methotrimeprazine, Pericyazine, Perphenazine, Pimozide, Pipotiazine, Thioridazine*, Trifluoperazine, Zuclopenthixol

Atypical antipsychotics Amisulpride/Sulpiride*, Clozapine*, Olanzapine*, Quetiapine*, Risperidone*, Zotepine

* See part 2

Antimanic drugs

Changes in mood are normal, but when a person's mood swings become grossly exaggerated, with peaks of elation or mania alternating with troughs of depression, it becomes an illness known as manic depression. It is usually treated with salts of lithium (p.292), a drug that reduces the intensity of the mania, lifts the depression, and lessens the frequency of mood swings. Because it can take three weeks for lithium salts to work, an antipsychotic may be prescribed with lithium at first to give immediate relief of symptoms.

Lithium can be toxic if blood levels of the drug rise too high. Regular checks on the blood concentration of lithium should therefore be carried out during treatment. Symptoms of lithium poisoning include blurred vision, twitching, vomiting, and diarrhoea.

COMMON DRUGS

Carbamazepine*, Lithium*
* See part 2

Anticonvulsant drugs

Electrical signals from nerve cells in the brain are normally finely coordinated to produce smooth movements of the arms and legs. In some cases, however, these signals can become irregular and chaotic and trigger the disorderly muscular activity and mental changes characteristic of a seizure (also called a fit or convulsion). The most common cause of seizure is epilepsy, which often occurs as a result of brain disease or injury. In epileptics, fits may be triggered by outside stimuli, such as flashing lights. Seizures can also result from toxic effects of certain drugs and, in young children, a high temperature (febrile convulsions).

Different anticonvulsants are used both to reduce the risk of an epileptic seizure and to stop one that is in progress.

WHY THEY ARE USED

Isolated convulsions seldom require drug treatment, but anticonvulsant drugs are the usual treatment for controlling seizures caused by epilepsy. These drugs permit most people with epilepsy to lead a normal life.

Most people who have epilepsy need to take anticonvulsants on a regular basis to prevent seizures. Usually a single drug is used, and treatment may need to be lifelong.

If one drug is not effective, then a different anticonvulsant will be tried. Occasionally, it is necessary to take a combination of drugs. Even when receiving treatment, a person can suffer seizures. A prolonged fit can be halted by injection of diazepam or a similar drug.

The selection of anticonvulsant (antiepileptic) drug depends on the type of epilepsy, the age of the patient, and his or her particular response to individual drug treatment.

Generalized epilepsy In this form of epilepsy, there is widespread disturbance of electrical activity in the brain, and loss of consciousness occurs at the outset. In its simplest form, absence seizure, there is momentary loss of consciousness, during which the sufferer may stare into space. This form mainly affects children; convulsions do not occur.

Another form of generalized epilepsy causes a brief jerk of a limb (myoclonus).

The most severe type is a tonic-clonic (grand mal) seizure, which is characterized by loss of consciousness and convulsions that may last for a few minutes.

Sufferers may have one or more of these types of generalized epilepsy. Sodium valproate, lamotrigine, topiramate, levetiracetam, or the benzodiazepines are normally used for these types of epilepsy.

Partial (focal) epilepsy This type of epilepsy is caused by an electrical disturbance in only one part of the brain. The result is a disturbance

of function, such as an abnormal sensation or movement of a limb, without loss of consciousness. Known as a simple partial seizure, this may precede a more serious attack associated with loss of consciousness (complex partial seizure), which may in turn progress to a generalized convulsive seizure.

Carbamazepine, lamotrigine, or phenytoin may be prescribed for this type of epilepsy.

Status epilepticus Repeated attacks without full recovery between, or a single attack lasting more than 10 minutes, occur in this form of epilepsy. Emergency treatment is required.

HOW THEY WORK

Brain cells bring about body movement by electrical activity that passes through the nerves to the muscles. In an epileptic fit, uncontrolled electrical activity starts in one part of the brain and spreads to other parts, causing uncontrolled stimulation of brain cells. Most of the anticonvulsants have an inhibitory effect on brain cells and damp down electrical activity, preventing the excessive build-up that causes epileptic seizures.

HOW THEY AFFECT YOU

Ideally, the only effect an anticonvulsant drug should have is to reduce the frequency of or prevent epileptic seizures. Unfortunately, no drug prevents seizures without potentially affecting normal brain function, leading to poor memory, inability to concentrate, lack of coordination, and lethargy. It is important, therefore, to find a dosage sufficient to prevent seizures without causing any unacceptable side effects. The dose has to be carefully tailored to the individual. It is usual to start with a low dose of a selected drug and to increase it gradually until a balance is achieved between the effective control of seizures and the occurrence of side effects. Many of these side effects wear off after the first few weeks of treatment.

Blood tests are used to monitor the levels of some anticonvulsant drugs in the body as an aid to dose adjustment. It may be several months before the correct dose is found.

RISKS AND SPECIAL PRECAUTIONS

Each anticonvulsant drug has its own specific adverse effects and risks. In addition, some anticonvulsants affect the ability of the liver to break down other drugs and may therefore influence the action of other drugs that you are taking. Doctors try to prescribe no more than the minimum number of anticonvulsants needed to control the person's seizures in order to reduce the risk of such interactions occurring.

Some anticonvulsants pose risks for a developing baby; if you are planning pregnancy, it is important to discuss the risks, and whether your medication should be changed, with your doctor. People taking anticonvulsants need to be careful to take their medicine regularly as prescribed. If the anticonvulsant levels in the body are allowed to fall suddenly, seizures are very likely to occur. The dose should not be reduced or treatment stopped, except on the advice of a doctor.

If anticonvulsant drug treatment needs to be stopped, the dose should be reduced gradually. People on anticonvulsant therapy are advised to carry an identification tag giving full details of their condition and treatment.

COMMON DRUGS

Carbamazepine*, Clobazam, Clonazepam*, Diazepam*, Gabapentin*, Lamotrigine*, Levetiracetam, Lorazepam, Phenobarbital*, Phenytoin*, Piracetam, Primidone*, Sodium valproate*, Tiagabine, Topiramate, Vigabatrin
* See part 2

Drugs for Parkinsonism

Parkinsonism is a general term used to describe shaking of the head and limbs, muscular stiffness, an expressionless face, and inability to control or initiate movement. It is caused by an imbalance of chemicals in the brain in which the effect of acetylcholine (see Neurotransmitters, p.9) is increased by a reduction in the action of dopamine (an excitatory chemical).

Parkinsonism has a variety of causes, but the most common is Parkinson's disease, in which there is degeneration of the dopamine-producing cells in the brain. Other causes include side effects of certain drugs, notably antipsychotics (see p.15), and narrowing of blood vessels in the brain.

WHY THEY ARE USED
Drugs can relieve the symptoms of parkinsonism and can minimize symptoms for many years. Unfortunately, they cannot halt the degeneration of brain cells.

HOW THEY WORK
Drugs treat parkinsonism by restoring the balance between dopamine and acetylcholine. There are two main groups: those that reduce the effect of acetylcholine (anticholinergics) and those that boost the effect of dopamine.

Anticholinergics combine with receptors on brain cells, preventing acetylcholine from binding to them. This action reduces acetylcholine's relative overactivity and restores the balance with dopamine.

Dopamine cannot pass from the blood to the brain and cannot therefore be given to boost levels in the brain. Levodopa (L-dopa), the chemical from which it is naturally produced in the brain, is combined with carbidopa or benserazide to prevent it from being converted to dopamine before it reaches the brain. Amantadine (also used as an antiviral, see p.69) boosts levels of dopamine in the brain by stimulating its release. The action of dopamine can also be boosted by other drugs, including bromocriptine, lisuride, or apomorphine (injection only), which mimic the action of dopamine.

CHOICE OF DRUG
Anticholinergics are often effective in the early stages of Parkinson's disease and are used to treat parkinsonism due to antipsychotic drugs (which have dopamine-blocking properties). L-dopa is usually given when the disease impairs walking. Its effectiveness usually wanes after two to five years, in which case other dopamine-boosting drugs may also be prescribed.

COMMON DRUGS
Anticholinergic drugs Benzatropine, Biperiden, Orphenadrine*, Procyclidine*, Trihexyphenidyl/benzhexol
Dopamine-boosting drugs Amantadine*, Apomorphine, Bromocriptine*, Cabergoline, Entacapone, Levodopa*, Lisuride, Pergolide, Pramipexole, Ropinirole, Selegiline
* See part 2

Drugs for Dementia

Dementia is a progressive decline in mental function that is severe enough to affect normal social or occupational activities. It usually develops gradually and may be a feature of a number of disorders, including poor circulation in the brain, multiple sclerosis, and Alzheimer's disease. A great deal of research is in progress on the cause of Alzheimer's disease, which is the single most common cause of dementia.

WHY THEY ARE USED

Drugs called acetylcholinesterase inhibitors have been found to lessen the symptoms of dementia in Alzheimer's disease, but they do not prevent its long-term progression.

HOW THEY WORK

In healthy people, acetylcholinesterase (an enzyme in the brain) breaks down the neurotransmitter acetylcholine, balancing its levels and limiting its effects. In Alzheimer's disease, there is a deficiency of acetylcholine. Acetylcholinesterase inhibitors block the action of acetylcholinesterase, raising the levels of acetylcholine in the brain, thereby increasing alertness and slowing the rate of deterioration.

HOW THEY AFFECT YOU

Following assessment of mental function by a specialist, drug treatment is started at a low dose and increased gradually to minimize side effects. Any improvements should begin to appear in about 3 weeks. Assessment is repeated after 3 months to see if the treatment has been beneficial. About half of those people treated show some improvement.

RISKS AND SPECIAL PRECAUTIONS

It is important to continue taking these drugs because there is a gradual loss of improvement after they are stopped. Side effects include urinary difficulties, nausea, vomiting, and diarrhoea.

COMMON DRUGS

Acetylcholinesterase inhibitors Donepezil*, Galantamine, Rivastigmine*
* See part 2

Nervous system stimulants

A person's state of mental alertness varies throughout the day and is under the control of chemicals in the brain; some of the chemicals are depressant, causing drowsiness, and others are stimulant, heightening awareness.

Increased activity of the depressant chemicals is thought to be responsible for narcolepsy, in which there is a tendency to fall asleep during the day for no obvious reason. To increase wakefulness, nervous system stimulants, including the amfetamines (usually dexamfetamine), the related drug methylphenidate, and modafinil, are given. Amfetamines are used less often these days due to the risk of dependence. The most common home remedy to increase alertness is caffeine, a mild stimulant found in coffee, tea, and cola.

WHY THEY ARE USED

In adults with narcolepsy, some of these drugs prevent excessive daytime drowsiness. Stimulants do not cure narcolepsy and, since the disorder is lifelong, may have to be taken indefinitely. Methylphenidate or dexamfetamine are sometimes given to children with ADHD (attention deficit hyperactivity disorder). Stimulants have also been used as part of the treatment for obesity because reduced appetite is a side effect of amfetamines, but they are no longer thought appropriate for weight reduction. Diet is now the main treatment, together with orlistat or sibutramine if necessary.

Caffeine is added to some analgesics to enhance their the effects, but no clear medical justification exists for this.

Respiratory stimulants such as doxapram are related to caffeine and are used to improve breathing. They act on the the respiratory centre – the part of the brain that controls breathing. They are sometimes used in hospitals to help people who have difficulty in breathing, mainly very young babies and adults with severe lung disease.

Apart from their use in narcolepsy, nervous system stimulants are not useful in the long term because the brain soon develops tolerance to them.

HOW THEY WORK

An individual's level of wakefulness is normally controlled by a part of the brain stem known as the reticular activating system (RAS). Activity in this area depends on the balance between certain chemicals, some of which are excitatory – including norepinephrine (noradrenaline) – and some of which are inhibitory, such as gamma aminobutyric acid (GABA). Nervous system stimulants promote the release of noradrenaline, increasing activity in the RAS and other parts of the brain and thereby raising alertness.

HOW THEY AFFECT YOU

In adults, the central nervous system stimulants taken in the prescribed dose for narcolepsy increase wakefulness, thereby allowing normal concentration and thought processes to occur. They may also reduce appetite and cause tremors. In hyperactive children, they reduce the general level of activity to a more normal level and increase the attention span.

RISKS AND SPECIAL PRECAUTIONS

Some people, especially the elderly or those with previous psychiatric problems, are particularly sensitive to stimulants and may experience adverse effects, even when the drugs are given in comparatively low doses. Stimulants need to be used with caution in children because, taken for prolonged periods, they can retard growth. An excess of these drugs given to a child may depress the nervous system, producing drowsiness or even loss of consciousness. Palpitations may also occur.

These drugs reduce the level of natural stimulants in the brain, so after regular use for a few weeks a person may become physically dependent on them for normal function. If they are abruptly withdrawn, the excess of natural inhibitory chemicals in the brain depresses central nervous system activity, producing withdrawal symptoms. These may include lethargy, depression, increased appetite, and difficulty staying awake. Stimulants can produce overactivity in the brain if they are used inappropriately or in excess, resulting in extreme restlessness, sleeplessness, nervousness, or anxiety. They also stimulate the sympathetic branch of the autonomic nervous system (see p.8), causing shaking, sweating, and palpitations. More serious risks of exceeding the prescribed dose are fits and a major disturbance in mental functioning that may result in delusions and hallucinations. Because these drugs have been abused, amfetamines and methylphenidate are classified as controlled drugs.

COMMON DRUGS

Respiratory stimulants Doxapram, Theophylline/aminophylline*
Other drugs Caffeine, Dexamfetamine, Methylphenidate, Modafinil, Sibutramine*
* **See part 2**

Drugs used for Migraine

Migraine is a term applied to recurrent, severe headaches affecting only one side of the head and caused by changes in the blood vessels around the brain and scalp. The headaches may be accompanied by nausea and vomiting and preceded by warning signs, usually an impression of flashing lights or numbness and tingling in the arms. Occasionally, speech may be impaired, or the attack may be disabling. The cause of migraine is unknown, but an attack may be triggered by a blow to the head, physical exertion, certain foods and drugs, or emotional factors such as excitement, tension, or shock. A family history of migraine also increases the chance of an individual suffering from it.

WHY THEY ARE USED

Drugs are used either to relieve symptoms of migraine or to prevent attacks. Different drugs are used in each approach, but none cures the underlying disorder. However, a susceptibility to migraine headaches can clear up spontaneously and, if you are taking drugs regularly, your doctor may recommend that you stop them after a few months to see if this has happened.

For most people, migraine headaches can be relieved by a mild analgesic (painkiller), such as paracetamol or aspirin, or a stronger one, such as codeine (see Analgesics, p.9). If nausea and vomiting accompany the migraine, drugs taken as tablets may not be absorbed sufficiently from the gut. Absorption can be increased if the drugs are taken as soluble tablets in water or with an anti-emetic (see below right).

Some of the drugs used to relieve attacks of migraine can be administered by injection, inhaler, nasal spray, or suppository. Preparations that contain caffeine should be avoided because headaches may be caused by excessive use or on stopping treatment. Ergotamine or $5HT_1$ agonist drugs (such as sumatriptan) are used if analgesics are not effective. Ergotamine is used less often now because it has been superseded by newer drugs.

The factors that trigger attacks should be identified so that they can be avoided. Anti-anxiety drugs are not usually prescribed if stress is a precipitating factor because of the potential for dependence. If the attacks occur more frequently than once a month, drugs that prevent migraine from occurring may be taken every day. Drugs to prevent migraine include propranolol (a beta blocker, see p.30) and pizotifen (an antihistamine, see p.58, and serotonin blocker). Other drugs that have been used include nifedipine, amitriptyline (an antidepressant, see p.14), clonidine, verapamil, and cyproheptadine. Methysergide is no longer recommended because of serious side effects.

HOW THEY WORK

A migraine attack begins when blood vessels surrounding the brain constrict (become narrower), producing the typical migraine warning signs. The constriction is thought to be caused by certain chemicals found in food or produced by the body. The neurotransmitter serotonin causes large blood vessels in the brain to constrict. Pizotifen and propranolol block the effect of chemicals on blood vessels and thereby prevent attacks.

The next stage of a migraine attack occurs when blood vessels in the scalp and around the eyes dilate (widen). As a result, chemicals called prostaglandins are released, producing pain. Aspirin and paracetamol relieve this pain by blocking prostaglandins. Codeine acts directly on the brain, altering pain perception (see Analgesics, p.9). Ergotamine and $5HT_1$ agonists relieve pain by narrowing dilated blood vessels in the scalp.

HOW THEY AFFECT YOU

Each drug has its own adverse effects. $5HT_1$ agonists may cause drowsiness and chest tightness. Ergotamine may cause drowsiness, muscle cramps, and weakness in the legs; vomiting may be made worse. Pizotifen may cause drowsiness and weight gain. For the effects of propranolol, see p.361; for those of analgesics, see p.9.

RISKS AND SPECIAL PRECAUTIONS

$5HT_1$ agonists should not usually be used by people with high blood pressure, angina, or coronary heart disease. Ergotamine can damage blood vessels by prolonged over-constriction, so it should be used with caution by those with poor circulation. Excessive use of $5HT_1$ agonists can lead to dependence and many adverse effects, including headache. You should not take more than your doctor advises in any one week.

HOW THEY ARE ADMINISTERED

These drugs are usually taken by mouth as tablets or capsules. Sumatriptan can also be taken as an injection or a nasal spray. Ergotamine can be taken as suppositories, or as tablets that dissolve under the tongue.

COMMON DRUGS

Drugs to prevent migraine Amitriptyline*, Cyproheptadine, Nifedipine*, Pizotifen*, Propranolol*, Sodium valproate*, Verapamil*
$5HT_1$ agonists Almotriptan, Eletriptan, Naratriptan, Rizatriptan, Sumatriptan*, Zolmitriptan
Other drugs to relieve migraine Aspirin*, Codeine*, Ergotamine*, Isometheptene, Paracetamol*, Tolfenamic acid
* See part 2

Anti-emetics

Drugs used to treat or prevent vomiting or the feeling of sickness (nausea) are known as anti-emetics. Vomiting is a reflex action for getting rid of harmful substances, but it may also be a symptom of disease. Vomiting and nausea are often caused by travel sickness, a digestive tract infection, pregnancy, or vertigo (a balance disorder involving the inner ear that causes a sensation of things spinning around). They can also occur as a side effect of some drugs, especially those that are used in cancer treatment, radiation therapy, or general anaesthesia.

Commonly used anti-emetics include metoclopramide, domperidone, cyclizine, haloperidol, ondansetron, granisetron, prochlorperazine, and promethazine; the antihistamine cinnarizine is also commonly used. The phenothiazine and butyrophenone drug groups are also used as antihistamines (see p.58) and to treat some types of mental illness (see Antipsychotic drugs, p.15).

WHY THEY ARE USED

Doctors usually diagnose the cause of vomiting before prescribing an anti-emetic because the vomiting may be caused by an infection of the digestive tract or some other condition of the abdomen that might require treatment such as surgery. Treating only the vomiting and nausea might delay diagnosis, correct treatment, and recovery.

Anti-emetics may be taken to prevent travel sickness (using one of the antihistamines) and to relieve vomiting resulting from anticancer drugs (see p.96) and other drug treatments (using metoclopramide, haloperidol, domperidone, ondansetron, and prochlorperazine, for example).

The anti-emetic drug prochlorperazine, the drug betahistine, or an anti-anxiety drug (see p.13) are usually used to treat Ménière's disease, a disorder in which excess fluid builds up in the inner ear, causing vertigo, noises in the ear, and gradual deafness. A diuretic (see p.32) may also be given to reduce the excess fluid in the ear.

Anti-emetics are also used to help the nausea that occurs in vertigo and are occasionally also used to relieve cases of severe vomiting that occur during pregnancy. You should not take an anti-emetic drug during pregnancy, except on medical advice.

No anti-emetic drug should be taken for longer than a couple of days without consulting your doctor.

HOW THEY WORK

Nausea and vomiting occur when the vomiting centre in the brain is stimulated by signals from three places in the body: the digestive tract, the part of the inner ear controlling balance, and the brain itself (through thoughts and emotions and via its chemoreceptor trigger zone, which responds to harmful substances in the blood). Anti-emetic drugs may act at one or more of these places. Some help the stomach to empty its contents into the intestine. A combination may be used that works at different sites and has an additive effect.

HOW THEY AFFECT YOU

As well as treating vomiting and nausea, many anti-emetic drugs may make you feel drowsy. However, to help prevent travel sickness on long journeys, a sedating antihistamine may be an advantage.

Some anti-emetics (in particular, antihistamines and phenothiazines) can block the parasympathetic nervous system (see Autonomic nervous system, p.8), causing a dry mouth, blurred vision, or difficulty in passing urine. The phenothiazines may also lower blood pressure, leading to dizziness or fainting.

RISKS AND SPECIAL PRECAUTIONS

Because some antihistamines can make you drowsy, it may be advisable not to drive while taking them. Phenothiazines, butyrophenones, and metoclopramide can produce uncontrolled movements of the face and tongue, so they are used with caution in people with parkinsonism.

COMMON DRUGS

Antihistamines Cinnarizine *, Cyclizine, Meclozine, Promethazine *

Phenothiazines Chlorpromazine*, Levomepromazine, Perphenazine, Prochlorperazine*, Trifluoperazine

5HT₃ antagonists Granisetron, Ondansetron* Tropisetron

Butyrophenones Haloperidol*

Other drugs Betahistine*, Domperidone*, Hyoscine hydrobromide*, Metoclopramide*, Nabilone

* See part 2

RESPIRATORY SYSTEM

The respiratory system consists of the lungs and the air passages leading to them. Through the process of inhaling and exhaling air (breathing), the body obtains the oxygen necessary for survival, and expels carbon dioxide, the waste product of the basic human biological process.

Air enters the trachea (windpipe), which branches into two main bronchi, one for each lung. Within the lungs, the air passes into bronchioles, smaller tubes whose muscular walls may contract or dilate in response to drugs and nerve signals. The bronchioles open out into tiny, blood-vessel-lined air sacs (alveoli), which allow oxygen to pass into the bloodstream and carbon dioxide to pass from the bloodstream for expiration.

WHAT CAN GO WRONG

Difficulty in breathing may be due to narrowing of the air passages from spasm, as in asthma and bronchitis, or swelling of the linings of the air passages, as in bronchiolitis and bronchitis. Breathing difficulties may also be due to infection of the lung tissue, as in pneumonia and bronchitis, or damage to the alveoli from smoking or inhaled dusts or moulds, which cause emphysema, pneumoconiosis and farmer's lung. Smoking and air pollution can affect the respiratory system as irritants and toxins, leading to diseases such as lung cancer and bronchitis.

Sometimes difficulty in breathing may be due to congestion of the lungs from heart disease, an inhaled object such as a peanut, or infection or inflammation of the throat. Symptoms of breathing difficulties often include a cough and a tight feeling in the chest.

WHY DRUGS ARE USED

Drugs with a variety of actions are used to clear the air passages, soothe inflammation, and reduce the production of mucus. Some can be bought without a prescription as single- or combined-ingredient preparations, often with an analgesic (see p.9).

Decongestants (see p.27) reduce the swelling inside the nose, thereby making it possible to breathe more freely. If the cause of the congestion is an allergic response, an antihistamine (see p.58) is often recommended to relieve symptoms or to prevent attacks. Infections of the respiratory tract are usually treated with antibiotics (see p.62).

Bronchodilators (see below) are drugs that widen the bronchi. They are used to prevent and relieve asthma attacks. Corticosteroids (see p.80) reduce inflammation in the swollen inner layers of the airways. They are used to prevent asthma attacks. Other drugs, such as sodium cromoglicate, may be used for treating allergies and preventing asthma attacks but they are not effective once an asthma attack has begun.

A variety of drugs are used to relieve a cough, depending on the type of cough involved. Some drugs make it easier to eliminate phlegm; others suppress the cough by inhibiting the cough reflex.

MAJOR DRUG GROUPS

◆ Bronchodilators
◆ Drugs for asthma
◆ Decongestants
◆ Drugs to treat coughs
◆ See also sections on Allergy (p.58) and Infections (p.61)

Bronchodilators

Air entering the lungs passes through narrow tubes called bronchioles. In asthma and bronchitis the bronchioles become narrower, either because of contraction of the muscles in their walls or as a result of mucus congestion. This narrowing of the bronchioles obstructs the flow of air into and out of the lungs and causes breathlessness.

Bronchodilators are prescribed to widen the bronchioles and improve breathing. There are three main groups of bronchodilators: sympathomimetics, anticholinergics, and xanthine drugs (which are related to caffeine). They are all used for relief of symptoms, and do not affect the underlying disease process. Anticholinergics are thought to be more effective for bronchitis, and are used particularly for this condition. In asthma, they are less effective, and are usually prescribed as additional therapy when control with other drugs is inadequate. The sympathomimetics are first choice drugs in the management of asthma, and are frequently used in bronchitis. Xanthines have been used for many years, both for asthma and bronchitis. They usually need precise adjustment of dosage to be effective while avoiding side effects. This makes them more difficult to use, and they are reserved for people whose condition cannot be controlled by other bronchodilators alone.

WHY THEY ARE USED

Bronchodilators help to dilate the bronchioles of people suffering from asthma and bronchitis. However, they are of little benefit to those who are suffering from severe chronic bronchitis.

Bronchodilators can either be taken when they are needed in order to relieve an attack of breathlessness that is in progress, or on a regular basis to prevent such attacks from occurring. Some people find it helpful to take an extra dose of their bronchodilator immediately before undertaking any activity likely to provoke an attack of breathlessness. A patient who requires treatment with a sympathomimetic inhaler more than once daily should see his or her doctor about preventative treatment with an inhaled corticosteroid. Sympathomimetic drugs are mainly used for the rapid relief of breathlessness; anticholinergic and xanthine drugs are used long term.

HOW THEY WORK

Bronchodilator drugs act by relaxing the muscles surrounding the bronchioles. Sympathomimetic and anticholinergic drugs achieve this by interfering with nerve signals passed to the muscles through the autonomic nervous system (see p.8). Xanthine drugs are thought to relax the muscles in the bronchioles by a direct effect on the muscle fibres, but their precise action is not known.

Bronchodilator drugs usually improve breathing within a few minutes of administration. Corticosteroids usually start to increase the sufferer's capacity for exercise within a few days, and most people find that the frequency of their attacks of breathlessness is reduced.

Because sympathomimetic drugs stimulate a branch of the autonomic nervous system that controls heart rate, they may sometimes cause palpitations and trembling. Typical side effects of anticholinergic drugs include dry mouth, blurred vision, and difficulty in passing urine. Xanthine drugs may cause headaches and nausea.

RISKS AND SPECIAL PRECAUTIONS

Since most bronchodilators are not taken by mouth but inhaled, they do not commonly cause serious side effects. However, because of their possible effect on heart rate, xanthine and sympathomimetic drugs need to be prescribed with caution to people with heart problems, high blood pressure, or an overactive thyroid gland. Smoking tobacco and drinking alcohol increase the breakdown of xanthines or their excretion from the body, reducing their effects. Stopping smoking after being stabilized on a xanthine may produce a rise in the blood concentration and an increased risk of side effects. It is advisable to stop smoking before starting treatment. The anticholinergic drugs may not be suitable for people with urinary retention or those who have a tendency to glaucoma.

COMMON DRUGS

Sympathomimetics Bambuterol, Eformoterol, Ephedrine*, Epinephrine (Adrenaline)*, Fenoterol, Reproterol, Salbutamol*, Salmeterol*, Terbutaline*, Tulobuterol
Anticholinergics Ipratropium bromide*, Oxitropium, Tiotropium*
Xanthines Theophylline/aminophylline*
* **See Part 2**

Drugs for asthma

Asthma is a chronic lung disease characterized by episodes in which the bronchioles constrict due to over-sensitivity. The attacks are usually, but not always, reversible; asthma is also known as reversible airway obstruction. About 5 per cent of adults and 10 per cent of children have the disease. Sometimes the inflammation causing the constriction is due to an identifiable allergen in the atmosphere, such as house dust mites, but often there is no obvious trigger. Breathlessness is the main symptom, and wheezing, coughing, and chest tightness are common. Asthma sufferers often have attacks during the night and wake up with breathing difficulty. The illness varies in severity, and it can be life-threatening.

There are a number of drugs that are used in the control of asthma. Where drugs are needed only to control an occasional attack, a sympathomimetic bronchodilator will probably be used in inhaler form. When the patient needs continuous preventative treatment there are a number of choices: often an inhaled corticosteroid or sodium cromoglicate may be used (with a sympathomimetic inhaler if attacks persist). More severe cases may require higher dose corticosteroids or the addition of a long-acting sympathomimetic bronchodilator. If this is not adequate, a high dose corticosteroid will be used with an anticholinergic drug, or theophylline, or these in combination with others already tried. There are also leukotriene antagonists, which may be used alone or with corticosteroids; they are less effective in severe cases when patients are taking high doses of other drugs. Some people who suffer from very severe asthma may need such large doses of corticosteroids that tablets have to be taken. Antihistamines have been prescribed for asthma in the past but this has not proved to be a successful treatment.

WHY THEY ARE USED

In asthma, the airways (bronchioles) constrict, making it difficult to get air in or out of the lungs. Bronchodilators (sympathomimetics, anticholinergics, and theophylline) (see p.23) relax the constricted muscles around the bronchioles. Short-acting sympathomimetics act almost immediately when inhaled and are used to provide relief of symptoms during an attack, and in more severe cases the long-acting sympathomimetics may be used to help with continuous protective cover. Anticholinergic drugs do not act as rapidly as the sympathomimetics. They are used for continuous prevention.

Theophylline/aminophylline must be given by mouth or injection; the tablets are used for regular continuous dosing, and the injection is used in hospital to gain control of severe asthma. Drugs that are not bronchodilators, such as corticosteroids and leukotriene receptor antagonists (see p.60), are not useful for dealing with an acute attack of asthma, but they are effective for long-term protection.

Antihistamines have been tried in the treatment of asthma, but although these drugs are useful for other allergic conditions, they are not very effective in asthma. One antihistamine-like drug, ketotifen, is sometimes given but is not widely used.

HOW THEY WORK

Inhaling a drug directly into the lungs is the best way of getting benefit without excessive side effects. A selection of devices for delivering drugs into the airways is described below.

Inhalers or puffers release a small dose when they are pressed, but require some skill to use effectively. A large, hollow plastic "spacer" can help you to inhale your drug more easily; you release a dose into the spacer, then inhale normally from the spacer's mouthpiece. Insufflation cartridges deliver larger amounts of drug than inhalers and are easier to use because the drug is taken in as you breathe normally.

Nebulizers pump compressed air through a solution of drug to produce a fine mist that is inhaled through a face mask. They deliver large doses of the drug to the lungs, rapidly relieving breathing difficulty.

Bronchodilators act by relaxing the muscles surrounding the bronchioles. Corticosteroids are used for their anti-inflammatory properties. By suppressing airway inflammation they reduce the swelling (oedema) inside the bronchioles, complementing the action of the bronchodilators in opening up the tubes. Reducing the inflammation also has the effect of reducing the amount of mucus produced, and this again helps to clear the airways. Corticosteroids usually start to increase the sufferer's capacity for exercise within a few days, and most people find that the frequency of their attacks of breathlessness is greatly reduced.

Leukotrienes occur naturally in the body. Chemically related to prostaglandins, they are much more potent in producing an inflammatory reaction; they are also much more potent than histamine at causing bronchoconstriction. Leukotrienes seem to play an important part in asthma, and drugs to block their receptors (leukotriene receptor antagonists) have been developed to reduce inflammation and bronchoconstriction in asthma. Sodium cromoglicate and nedocromil act by stabilizing mast cells in the lungs, preventing them from releasing histamine, leukotrienes, and other chemicals that cause inflammation.

RISKS AND SPECIAL PRECAUTIONS

The drugs taken by inhalation act locally and are used in much lower doses than would be needed as tablets. They do not commonly cause serious side effects, although the dry powder inhalations can cause a reflex bronchospasm as the powder hits the lining of the airways; this can be avoided by first using a short-acting sympathomimetic. Inhaled corticosteroids may encourage fungal growth in the mouth and throat (thrush); this can be minimized by using a spacer. High doses of inhaled steroids may suppress adrenal gland function, reduce bone density, and increase the risk of glaucoma. Sympathomimetics and theophylline taken by mouth may affect heart rate, and should be prescribed with caution to people with heart problems, high blood pressure, or an overactive thyroid gland. The effects of theophylline may last longer if you have a viral infection, heart failure, or liver cirrhosis. The drugs also interact with many other drugs. The anticholinergic drugs must be used with caution in patients who have prostate problems or urinary retention. Leukotriene receptor antagonists may produce a syndrome with several potentially serious effects including worsening lung function and heart complications.

COMMON DRUGS

Sympathomimetics Bambuterol, Ephedrine*, Epinephrine (Adrenaline)*, Fenoterol, Formoterol/eformoterol, Orciprenaline, Salbutamol*, Salmeterol*, Terbutaline*
Anticholinergics Ipratropium bromide*, Oxitropium, Tiotropium*
Leukotriene antagonists Montelukast*, Zafirlukast
Corticosteroids Beclometasone*, Budesonide*, Fluticasone*, Prednisolone*
Xanthines Theophylline/aminophylline*
Other drugs Ketotifen, Nedocromil, Sodium cromoglicate*

Decongestants

The usual cause of a blocked nose is swelling of the delicate mucous membrane that lines the nasal passages, and excessive production of mucus as a result of inflammation. This swelling and inflammation may be caused by an infection, such as a common cold, or to an allergy (for example, to pollen) – a condition known as allergic rhinitis or hay fever. Congestion can also occur in the sinuses (the air spaces in the skull), resulting in sinusitis. Decongestants are drugs that reduce the swelling of the mucous membrane and suppress the production of mucus, helping to clear blocked nasal passages and sinuses. Antihistamines (see p.58) counter the allergic response in allergy-related conditions. If the symptoms are persistent, either topical corticosteroids (see p.120) or sodium cromoglicate (see p.386) may be preferred.

WHY THEY ARE USED

Most common colds and blocked noses do not need to be treated with decongestants. Simple home remedies such as steam inhalation, possibly with the addition of an aromatic oil such as menthol or eucalyptus, are often effective. Decongestants are used when such measures are ineffective or when there is a particular risk from untreated congestion – for example, in people who suffer from recurrent middle-ear or sinus infections.

Decongestants are available in the form of drops or sprays applied directly into the nose (topical decongestants), or they can be taken by mouth. Small quantities of decongestant drugs are added to many over-the-counter cold remedies (see Cold cures, p.28).

HOW THEY WORK

When the mucous membrane lining the nose is irritated by infection or allergy, the blood vessels supplying the membrane become enlarged. This leads to fluid accumulation in the surrounding tissue and encourages the production of larger-than-normal amounts of mucus.

Most decongestants belong to the sympathomimetic group of drugs, which stimulate the sympathetic branch of the autonomic nervous system (see p.8). One effect of this action is to constrict the blood vessels, thereby reducing swelling of the lining of the nose and sinuses.

HOW THEY AFFECT YOU

When applied topically in the form of drops or sprays, these drugs start to relieve congestion within a few minutes. Decongestants taken by mouth take a little longer to act, but their effect may also last longer. Used in moderation, topical decongestants have few adverse effects, because they are not absorbed by the body in large amounts.

Used for too long or in excess, topical decongestants can do more harm than good. After giving initial relief, decongestant nose drops and sprays can cause "rebound congestion" when withdrawn or overused. This is a sudden increase in congestion due to widening of the blood vessels in the nasal lining because the blood vessels are no longer constricted by the decongestant. Rebound congestion can be prevented by taking the minimum effective dose and by using decongestant preparations only when absolutely necessary. Decongestants taken by mouth do not cause rebound congestion but are more likely to cause other side effects; they have been linked with strokes.

COMMON DRUGS

Used topically Ephedrine*, Ipratropium bromide*, Oxymetazoline, Phenylephrine, Xylometazoline
Taken by mouth Ephedrine*, Phenylephrine, Phenylpropanolamine*, Pseudoephedrine
* See Part 2

Drugs to treat coughs

Coughing is a natural response to irritation of the lungs and air passages that is designed to expel harmful substances from the respiratory tract. Common causes of coughing include infection of the respiratory tract (such as bronchitis or pneumonia), inflammation of the airways caused by asthma, or exposure to certain irritant substances, such as smoke or chemical fumes. Depending on their cause, coughs may be productive – that is, phlegm-producing – or dry.

In most cases coughing is a helpful reaction that assists the body in ridding itself of excess phlegm and substances that irritate the respiratory system; suppressing a cough may delay recovery. However, repeated bouts of coughing can be distressing and may increase irritation. In such cases, medication to ease the cough may be recommended.

There are two main groups of cough remedies, according to whether the cough is productive or dry.

PRODUCTIVE COUGHS

Mucolytics and expectorants are sometimes recommended for productive coughs when simple home remedies such as steam inhalation have failed to "loosen" the cough and make it easier to cough up phlegm. Mucolytics alter the consistency of the phlegm, making it less sticky and easier to cough up. These drugs are often given by inhalation. However, there is little evidence that they are effective. Dornase alfa may be given to people who suffer from cystic fibrosis; the drug, which is inhaled via a nebulizer, is an enzyme that improves lung function by thinning the mucus. Expectorant drugs, such as ammonium chloride, are taken by mouth to loosen a cough. There is some evidence that guaifenesin is effective. Expectorants are included in many over-the-counter cough remedies.

DRY COUGHS

In dry coughs there is no advantage to be gained from promoting the expulsion of phlegm. Drugs used for dry coughs are given to suppress the coughing mechanism by calming the part of the brain that governs the coughing reflex. Antihistamines are often given for mild coughs, particularly in children. A demulcent (soothing preparation), such as a simple linctus, can be used to soothe a dry, irritating cough. For persistent coughs, mild opioid drugs such as codeine may be prescribed (see also Analgesics, p.9). All cough suppressants have a generally sedating effect on the brain and nervous system and commonly cause drowsiness and other side effects.

SELECTING A COUGH MEDICATION

There is a bewildering variety of over-the-counter medications available for treating coughs. Most consist of a syrupy base to which active ingredients and flavourings are added. Many medications contain a number of different active ingredients, sometimes with contradictory effects: it is not uncommon to find an expectorant (for a productive cough) and a decongestant included in the same preparation.

Cough medicines, although soothing, are not often beneficial and can be harmful. For example, using a cough suppressant for the relief of a productive cough may prevent you from getting rid of excess infected phlegm and may delay your recovery. It is best to choose a preparation with a single active ingredient that is appropriate for your type of cough. Diabetics may need to select a sugar-free product. If you are in any doubt about which medication to select, ask your doctor or pharmacist for advice. Because there is a danger that use of over-the-counter cough remedies to alleviate symptoms may delay the diagnosis of a more serious underlying disorder, it is important that you seek medical advice for any cough that persists for longer than a few days or if a cough is accompanied by additional symptoms such as fever or blood in the phlegm.

COLD CURES

Many preparations are available over the counter to treat different symptoms of the common cold. The main ingredient in most of these preparations is a mild analgesic, such as aspirin or paracetamol, accompanied by a decongestant (see p.26), an antihistamine (see p.58), and sometimes caffeine. In some cases, the dose of each added ingredient is too low to provide any benefit. There is no evidence to suggest that vitamin C (see p.90) speeds recovery. However, zinc supplements (see p.93) may be effective in shortening the duration of a cold.

While some people find these drugs help to relieve symptoms, over-the-counter cold cures do not alter the course of the illness. Most doctors recommend using a product with a single analgesic as the best way of alleviating symptoms. Other decongestants or antihistamines may be taken if needed. These medicines are not harmless, and care should be taken to to avoid overdose if different brands are used.

COMMON DRUGS

Expectorants Ammonium chloride, Guaifenesin
Mucolytics Carbocysteine, Dornase alfa, Mecysteine
Steam inhalation Eucalyptus, Menthol
Opioid cough suppressants Codeine*, Dextromethorphan, Pholcodine
Non-opioid cough suppressants Antihistamines (see p.27)
* See Part 2

HEART AND CIRCULATION

The blood transports oxygen, nutrients, and heat, carries chemical messages in the form of hormones and drugs, and removes waste products from cells for excretion by the kidneys. It is pumped by the heart through the lungs, and then in a separate circuit to the rest of the body, including the brain, digestive organs, muscles, kidneys, and skin.

The heart is a pump with four chambers – two atria and two ventricles. The atrium and ventricle on the left side pump oxygenated blood to the body, while those on the right pump deoxygenated blood to the lungs. Backflow of blood is stopped by one-way valves at the chamber exits. Arteries carry blood away from the heart. Their muscle walls are elastic, contracting and dilating in response to nerve signals. Veins carry blood back to the heart. Their walls are thinner and less elastic than those of arteries.

WHAT CAN GO WRONG

The efficiency of the circulation may be impaired by weakening of the heart's pumping action (heart failure), too fast a heart rate (tachycardia), or irregularity of the heart rate (arrhythmia). In addition, the blood vessels may be narrowed and clogged by fatty deposits (atherosclerosis). This may reduce blood supply to the brain, the extremities (peripheral vascular disease), or the heart muscle (coronary heart disease and angina). These last disorders can be complicated by the formation of clots that may block a blood vessel. A clot in the arteries supplying the heart muscle is known as coronary thrombosis; a clot in an artery inside the brain (cerebral thrombosis) is the most frequent cause of stroke.

One common circulatory disorder is hypertension (abnormally high blood pressure), in which the pressure of circulating blood on the blood vessel walls is increased for reasons not yet fully understood; loss of elasticity of the vessel walls (arteriosclerosis) may be a factor. Several other conditions, such as migraine and Raynaud's disease, are caused by temporary alterations to blood vessel size.

WHY DRUGS ARE USED

Because people with heart disease often have more than one problem, several drugs may be prescribed at once. Many act directly on the heart to alter the heart rate and rhythm. These drugs are known as anti-arrhythmics; they include beta blockers and digoxin.

Other drugs affect the diameter of the blood vessels by either dilating them (vasodilators) to improve the blood flow and reduce blood pressure, or by constricting them (vasoconstrictors).

Drugs may also reduce blood volume and fat levels, and alter its clotting ability. Diuretics (used in the treatment of hypertension and heart failure) increase the body's excretion of water. Lipid-lowering drugs reduce the levels of cholesterol in the blood, thereby minimizing the risk of atherosclerosis. Drugs to reduce blood clotting are administered if there is a risk of abnormal blood clots forming in the heart, veins, or arteries. Drugs that increase clotting are given when the body's natural clotting mechanism is defective.

MAJOR DRUG GROUPS

◆ Digitalis drugs
◆ Beta blockers
◆ Vasodilators
◆ Diuretics
◆ Anti-arrhythmics
◆ Anti-angina drugs
◆ Antihypertensive drugs
◆ Lipid-lowering drugs
◆ Drugs that affect blood clotting

Digitalis drugs

Digitalis is the collective term for the naturally occurring substances (also called cardiac glycosides) found in the leaves of plants of the foxglove family and used to treat certain heart disorders. The principal drugs in this group are digoxin and digitoxin. Digoxin is more commonly used because it is shorter acting and dosage is easier to adjust (see also Risks and special precautions, p.30).

WHY THEY ARE USED

Digitalis drugs do not cure heart disease, but they improve the heart's pumping action and thereby relieve many of the symptoms that result from poor heart function. They are useful for treating conditions in which the heart beats irregularly or too rapidly (notably in atrial fibrillation; see Anti-arrhythmics, p.33), when it pumps too weakly (in congestive heart failure), or when the heart muscle is damaged and weakened following a heart attack.

Digitalis drugs can be used for a short period when the heart is working poorly but have to be taken indefinitely in many cases. Their effect does not diminish with time. In heart failure, these drugs are often given together with a diuretic drug (see p.32).

HOW THEY WORK

The normal heart beat results from electrical impulses generated in nerve tissue within the heart. These impulses cause the heart muscle to contract and pump blood. By reducing the flow of electrical impulses in the heart, digitalis makes the heart beat more slowly.

The force with which the heart muscle contracts depends on chemical changes in the heart muscle. By promoting these chemical changes, digitalis increases the force of muscle contraction each time the heart is stimulated. This compensates for the loss of power that occurs when some of the muscle is damaged following a heart attack. The stronger heart beat increases blood flow to the kidneys. This increases urine production and helps to remove the excess fluid that often accumulates as a result of heart failure.

HOW THEY AFFECT YOU

Digitalis relieves the symptoms of heart failure – fatigue, breathlessness, and swelling of the legs – and increases your capacity for exercise. The frequency with which you need to pass urine is also increased initially.

RISKS AND SPECIAL PRECAUTIONS

Digitalis drugs can be toxic: if blood levels rise too high, symptoms of digitalis poisoning (including nausea, appetite loss, vomiting, diarrhoea, confusion, and visual disturbance) may occur. It is important to report any such symptoms to your doctor promptly.

Digoxin is normally removed from the body by the kidneys; if kidney function is impaired, the drug is more likely to accumulate in the body and cause toxic effects. Digitoxin, which is broken down in the liver, is sometimes preferred in such cases. If liver function is severely impaired, digitoxin can accumulate after repeated dosage.

Both digoxin and digitoxin are more toxic when blood potassium levels are low. Potassium deficiency is commonly due to diuretics; the effects of both drugs and the blood potassium levels of people taking diuretics with digitalis drugs require careful monitoring. Potassium supplements may be required.

COMMON DRUGS

Digitoxin, Digoxin*
* See part 2

Beta blockers

Beta blockers are drugs that interrupt the transmission of stimuli through receptors called beta receptors. The actions that they block originate in the adrenal glands (and elsewhere), so the drugs are also sometimes called beta adrenergic blocking agents. There are two types of beta receptor in the body: beta 1 and beta 2. Beta 1 receptors are located mainly in the heart muscle; beta 2 receptors in the airways and blood vessels. Cardioselective drugs act mainly on beta 1 receptors: non- cardioselective drugs on both types. Used mainly in heart disorders, these drugs are occasionally prescribed for other conditions.

WHY THEY ARE USED

Beta blockers are used for treating angina (see p.35), hypertension (see p.36), and irregular heart rhythms (see p.34). They are usually given after a heart attack to reduce the likelihood of abnormal heart rhythms or further damage to the heart muscle. Beta blockers are also prescribed to improve heart function in heart muscle disorders (which are called cardiomyopathies).

Beta blockers may also be given to prevent migraine headaches (see p.20), and they are sometimes prescribed to reduce the physical symptoms of anxiety (see p.13). These drugs may be given to control symptoms of an overactive thyroid gland. A beta blocker is sometimes given in the form of eye drops to lower the excessive fluid pressure inside the eye that occurs in glaucoma (see p.114).

HOW THEY WORK

By occupying the beta receptors in different parts of the body, beta blockers nullify the stimulating action of norepinephrine (noradrenaline), the main "fight or flight" hormone. Blocking the transmission of signals through beta receptors produces a wide variety of benefits and side effects depending on the disease being treated.

Heart Slowing of the heart rate and reduction of the force of the heart beat reduces the workload of the heart, helping to prevent angina and abnormal heart rhythms. This action may worsen heart failure, however.

Lungs Constriction of the airways may provoke breathlessness in asthmatic people or those with chronic bronchitis.

Brain Dilation of the blood vessels that surround the brain is inhibited, thereby preventing migraine.

Blood vessels Constriction of the blood vessels may cause coldness of the hands and feet.

Blood pressure The pressure is lowered due to reduction in the rate and force at which the heart pumps blood around the body.

Eye Beta blocker eye drops reduce fluid production, lowering pressure inside the eye.

Muscles Muscle tremor caused by anxiety or overactivity of the thyroid gland is reduced.

HOW THEY AFFECT YOU

Beta blockers are taken to treat angina. They reduce the frequency and severity of attacks. As part of the treatment for hypertension, they help to lower the blood pressure and thus reduce the risks that are associated with this condition. Beta blockers help to prevent severe attacks of arrhythmia, in which the heart beat is wild and uncontrolled.

Because beta blockers affect many parts of the body, they often produce minor side effects. By reducing the heart rate and air flow to the lungs, they may reduce the capacity for strenuous exercise. This is unlikely to be noticed by somebody whose physical activity was previously limited by heart problems, however. Many people taking these drugs experience cold hands and feet as a result of a reduction in the blood supply to the limbs. Reduced circulation can, rarely, lead to temporary impotence during treatment.

RISKS AND SPECIAL PRECAUTIONS

The main risk of beta blockers is that they may provoke breathing difficulties due to their blocking effect on beta receptors in the lungs. Cardioselective beta blockers act mainly on the heart and are thought to be less likely than non-cardioselective ones to cause such problems. But all beta blockers are prescribed with caution to people with asthma, bronchitis, or other forms of respiratory disease.

Beta blockers are not commonly prescribed to people with poor circulation in the limbs because they reduce blood flow and may aggravate such conditions. Large doses are not normally given to people subject to heart failure because they may further reduce the force of the heart beat, although small doses are helpful. Diabetics should be aware that they may notice a change in the warning signs of low blood sugar; in particular, they may find that symptoms such as palpitations and tremor are suppressed.

Beta blockers should not be stopped suddenly after prolonged use; this may provoke a sudden and severe recurrence of symptoms of the original disorder, or even a heart attack. The blood pressure may also rise markedly. When treatment with beta blockers needs to be stopped, the drugs should be withdrawn gradually under medical supervision.

COMMON DRUGS

Cardioselective Atenolol*, Betaxolol, Bisoprolol, Celiprolol, Esmolol, Metoprolol*, Nebivolol

Non-cardioselective Acebutolol, Carvedilol, Labetalol, Nadolol, Oxprenolol, Pindolol, Propranolol*, Sotalol*, Timolol*

* **See part 2**

Vasodilators

Vasodilators are drugs that widen blood vessels. Their most obvious use is to reverse narrowing of blood vessels when this leads to reduced blood flow and, consequently, a lower oxygen supply to parts of the body. Vasodilators are often used to treat high blood pressure (hypertension) and angina because the widening of the body's blood vessels reduces the heart's workload.

WHY THEY ARE USED

Vasodilators improve blood flow and thus the oxygen supply to areas of the body where they are most needed. In angina, dilation of blood vessels throughout the body reduces the force with which the heart has to pump and thus eases its workload (see also Anti-angina drugs, p.35). Vasodilators may also be helpful in treating congestive heart failure when other treatments are not effective.

Because blood pressure is partly dependent on the diameter of blood vessels, vasodilators are often helpful for hypertension (see p.36).

In peripheral vascular disease, narrowed blood vessels in the legs cannot supply sufficient blood to the extremities; this often leads to pain in the legs during exercise. Unfortunately, because the vessels are narrowed by atherosclerosis, vasodilators have little effect.

Vasodilators have also been used to treat senile dementia, in the hope of increasing the oxygen supply to the brain, but the benefits of this treatment have not yet been proved.

HOW THEY WORK

Vasodilators widen blood vessels by relaxing the muscles surrounding them. They achieve this either by directly affecting the action of the muscles (nitrates, calcium channel blockers, potassium channel activators, and hydralazine) or by interfering with the nerve signals that govern contraction of the blood vessels (alpha blockers). ACE (angiotensin-converting enzyme) inhibitors are powerful vasodilators that block the action of an enzyme in the bloodstream that is responsible for converting a chemical called angiotensin I into angiotensin II. Angiotensin II encourages constriction of the blood vessels; its absence permits them to dilate.

HOW THEY AFFECT YOU

As well as relieving the symptoms of the disorders for which they are taken, vasodilators can have many minor side effects related to

their action on the circulation. Flushing and headaches are common at the start of treatment; dizziness and fainting may occur due to lowered blood pressure. Dilation of blood vessels can also cause a build-up of fluid, leading to swelling, particularly of the ankles.

RISKS AND SPECIAL PRECAUTIONS

The major risk is that blood pressure may fall too low, and this can lead to dizziness on standing because the blood vessels cannot contract to prevent pooling of the blood in the legs. Therefore, vasodilators are prescribed with caution for people with unstable blood pressure. It is also advisable to sit or lie down after taking the first dose of a vasodilator.

COMMON DRUGS

ACE inhibitors Captopril*, Cilazapril, Enalapril*, Fosinopril, Imidapril, Lisinopril*, Moexipril, Perindopril, Quinapril, Ramipril*, Trandolapril

Potassium channel activators Nicorandil*

Alpha blockers Doxazosin*, Indoramin*, Prazosin, Terazosin*

Calcium channel blockers Amlodipine*, Diltiazem*, Felodipine, Isradipine, Lacidipine, Lercanidipine, Nicardipine, Nifedipine*, Nisoldipine, Verapamil*

Angiotensin II blockers Candesartan, Eprosartan, Irbesartan*, Losartan*, Telmisartan, Valsartan

Nitrates Glyceryl trinitrate*, Isosorbide dinitrate/mononitrate*

Other drugs Hydralazine, Minoxidil*, Naftidrofuryl*
* See part 2

Diuretics

Diuretic drugs help to turn excess body water into urine. As the urine is expelled, two disorders are relieved: oedema is relieved as the tissues become less water-swollen, and the heart's action improves because it has to pump a smaller volume of blood. There are several classes of diuretic, each of which has different uses, modes of action, and effects. But all diuretics act on the kidneys, the organs that govern the body's water content.

WHY THEY ARE USED

Diuretics are most commonly used in the treatment of high blood pressure (hypertension). By removing more water than usual from the bloodstream, the kidneys reduce the total volume of blood circulating. This drop in volume is thought to cause a reduction of the pressure within the blood vessels (see Antihypertensive drugs, p.36).

Diuretics are also widely used to treat heart failure (in which the heart's pumping mechanism has become weak) by removing fluid that has accumulated in the tissues and lungs. The resulting drop in blood volume reduces the work of the heart.

Other conditions for which diuretics are often prescribed include nephrotic syndrome (a kidney disorder that causes oedema), liver cirrhosis (in which fluid may accumulate in the abdominal cavity), and premenstrual syndrome (when hormonal activity can lead to fluid retention and bloating).

Less commonly, diuretics are used to treat glaucoma (see p.114) and Ménière's disease (see also Anti-emetics, p.21).

TYPES OF DIURETIC

Thiazides The most commonly prescribed diuretics, thiazides are often given with potassium supplements, or in conjunction with a potassium-sparing diuretic (see below), because they may lead to potassium deficiency.
Loop diuretics These fast-acting, powerful drugs increase urine output for a few hours and are therefore sometimes used in emergencies. They can cause excessive potassium loss, which may need to be prevented as for thiazides.
Potassium-sparing diuretics These mild diuretics are usually used in conjunction with a thiazide or a loop diuretic to prevent excessive loss of potassium.
Osmotic diuretics Prescribed only rarely, osmotics are used to maintain the flow of urine through the kidneys after surgery or injury, and to reduce pressure rapidly in the brain or the eye.
Acetazolamide This mild diuretic is used mainly to treat glaucoma (see p.114).

HOW THEY WORK

The normal filtration process of the kidneys removes water, salts (mainly potassium and sodium), and waste products from the bloodstream. Most of the salts and water are subsequently returned to the bloodstream, but some

are expelled from the body along with the waste products in the urine. Diuretics interfere with this process by reducing the amount of sodium and water taken back into the bloodstream, thereby increasing the volume of urine produced. Modifying the filtration process in this way means that the water content of the blood is reduced; less water in the blood causes excess water present in the tissues to be drawn out and eliminated in urine.

HOW THEY AFFECT YOU

All diuretics increase the frequency with which you need to pass urine, most noticeably at the start of treatment. People who have had oedema may notice reduction in swelling, particularly of the ankles; and those with heart failure may find that breathlessness is relieved.

RISKS AND SPECIAL PRECAUTIONS

Diuretics can cause blood chemical imbalances, of which hypokalaemia (a fall in potassium levels) is the most common. Hypokalaemia can cause confusion and weakness and can trigger abnormal heart rhythms (especially in people taking digitalis drugs). Potassium supplements or a potassium-sparing diuretic usually corrects the imbalance. A potassium-rich diet (containing plenty of fresh fruits and vegetables) may be helpful.

Some diuretics may raise uric acid levels, increasing the risk of gout; others may raise blood glucose levels, causing problems for diabetics. Thiazides can cause impotence.

COMMON DRUGS

Loop diuretics Bumetanide*, Furosemide*, Torasemide
Potassium-sparing diuretics Amiloride*, Spironolactone, Triamterene*
Thiazides Bendroflumethiazide*, Chlortalidone, Cyclopenthiazide, Hydrochlorothiazide*, Hydroflumethiazide, Indapamide*, Metolazone, Xipamide
* See part 2

Anti-arrhythmics

The heart contains two upper and two lower chambers, which are known as the atria and ventricles (see p.29). The pumping actions of these two sets of chambers are normally co-ordinated by electrical impulses that originate in the heart's pacemaker and then travel along conducting pathways so that the heart beats with a regular rhythm. If this coordination breaks down, the heart will beat abnormally, either irregularly or faster or slower than usual. The general term for abnormal heart rhythm is arrhythmia.

Arrhythmias may occur as a result of a birth defect, coronary heart disease, or other less common heart disorders. A variety of more general conditions, including an overactive thyroid gland, and certain drugs, such as caffeine and anticholinergic drugs, can also disturb heart rhythm.

Arrhythmias can be divided into two groups: tachycardias (such as atrial fibrillation), in which the heart rate is faster than normal; and bradycardias (such as heart block), in which the rate is slower.

Atrial fibrillation In this common type of arrhythmia, the atria contract irregularly at such a high rate that the ventricles cannot keep pace. The condition is treated with digoxin, verapamil, or a beta blocker.

Ventricular tachycardia This condition arises from abnormal electrical activity in the ventricles that causes the ventricles to contract rapidly. Regular treatment with quinidine, disopyramide, or procainamide is usually given. Amiodarone may be used if these drugs are not effective.

Supraventricular tachycardia This condition occurs when extra electrical impulses arise in the pacemaker or atria, stimulating the ventricles into contracting rapidly. Attacks may disappear on their own without treatment, but drugs such as adenosine, digoxin, verapamil, or propranolol may be given.

Heart block When impulses are not conducted from the atria to the ventricles, the ventricles start to beat at a slower rate. Some cases of heart block do not require treatment. For more severe heart block accompanied by dizziness and fainting, the fitting of an artificial pacemaker is usually necessary.

A wide range of drugs, including beta blockers, calcium channel blockers, and digitalis drugs, is used to regulate heart rhythm. Lidocaine, disopyramide, procainamide, and quinidine are also used.

WHY THEY ARE USED

Minor disturbances of heart rhythm are common and do not usually require drug treatment. However, if the heart's pumping action is seriously affected, the circulation of blood throughout the body may become inefficient, and drug treatment may be necessary.

Drugs may be taken to treat individual attacks of arrhythmia, or they may be taken on a regular basis to prevent or control abnormal heart rhythms. The particular drug prescribed depends on the type of arrhythmia to be treated but, because people differ in their response, it may be necessary to try several in order to find the most effective one. When the arrhythmia is sudden and severe, it may be necessary to inject a drug immediately to restore normal heart function.

HOW THEY WORK

The heart's pumping action is governed by electrical impulses under the control of the sympathetic nervous system (see Autonomic nervous system, p.8). These signals pass through the heart muscle, causing the two pairs of chambers – the atria and ventricles – to contract in turn.

All anti-arrhythmic drugs alter the conduction of electrical signals in the heart. However, each drug or drug group has a different effect on the sequence of events controlling the pumping action. Some block the transmission of signals to the heart (beta blockers); some affect the way in which signals are conducted within the heart (digitalis drugs); others affect the response of the heart muscle to the signals received (calcium channel blockers, disopyramide, procainamide, and quinidine).

HOW THEY AFFECT YOU

Anti-arrhythmics usually prevent the symptoms of arrhythmia and may restore a regular heart rhythm. Although they do not prevent all arrhythmias, they usually reduce the frequency and severity of any symptoms.

As well as suppressing arrhythmias, many anti-arrhythmic drugs tend to depress normal heart function, and may produce dizziness on standing or increased breathlessness on exertion. Mild nausea and visual disturbance also occur fairly frequently. Verapamil can cause constipation, especially when prescribed in high doses. Disopyramide may interfere with the parasympathetic nervous system (see Autonomic nervous system, p.8), causing various anticholinergic effects, such as blurred vision, fast heart rate, and urinary retention.

RISKS AND SPECIAL PRECAUTIONS

These drugs, in certain circumstances, may further disrupt heart rhythm and are used only when the likely benefit outweighs the risks.

Quinidine can be toxic if an overdose is taken, causing a syndrome called cinchonism, which includes disturbed hearing, giddiness, and impaired vision (even blindness). Because some people are particularly sensitive to this drug, a test dose is usually given before regular treatment is started.

Amiodarone may, over time, accumulate in the tissues and may lead to light-sensitive rashes, changes in thyroid function, and liver and lung problems.

COMMON DRUGS

Beta blockers (See p.30)
Calcium channel blockers Verapamil*
Digitalis drugs Digitoxin, Digoxin*,
Other drugs Adenosine, Amiodarone*, Bretylium, Disopyramide, Flecainide, Lidocaine, Mexiletine, Moracizine, Procainamide, Propafenone, Quinidine
* See part 2

Anti-angina drugs

Angina is chest pain that is produced when insufficient oxygen reaches the heart muscle. This is usually due to narrowing of the vessels (coronary arteries) that carry blood and oxygen to the heart muscle. In the most common type of angina (classic angina), the pain usually occurs during physical exertion or emotional stress. The pain may also occur at rest (variant angina). In classic angina, the narrowing of the coronary arteries results from fat deposits (atheroma) on the artery walls. In the variant type, however, it is caused by contraction (spasm) of the muscle fibres in the artery walls. Pain that is not relieved by drugs may indicate that a heart attack is imminent (unstable angina) and emergency treatment is needed.

Atheroma deposits build up more rapidly in the arteries of smokers and people who eat a high-fat diet. This is why, as a basic component of angina treatment, doctors recommend that smoking should be given up and the diet changed. Overweight people are also advised to lose weight in order to reduce the demands placed on the heart. While such changes in lifestyle often produce an improvement in symptoms, drug treatment to relieve angina is also frequently necessary.

The drugs used to treat angina include beta blockers, nitrates, calcium channel blockers, and potassium channel activators.

WHY THEY ARE USED

Frequent episodes of angina can be disabling and, if left untreated, can lead to increased risk of a heart attack. Drugs can both relieve angina attacks and reduce their frequency. People who suffer only occasional episodes are usually prescribed a rapid-acting drug to take at the first signs of an attack, or before an activity known to bring on an attack; glyceryl trinitrate is a rapid-acting drug that is usually prescribed for this purpose.

If the attacks become more frequent or more severe, regular preventative treatment may be advised. Beta blockers, calcium channel blockers, and long-acting nitrates are used as regular medication to prevent attacks. The introduction of adhesive patches to administer nitrates through the patient's skin has extended the duration of action of glyceryl trinitrate, making treatment easier.

Drugs can often control angina for many years, but they cannot cure the disorder. When severe angina cannot be controlled by drugs, then surgery to increase the blood flow to the heart may be recommended.

HOW THEY WORK

Nitrates, calcium channel blockers, and potassium channel activators dilate blood vessels by relaxing the muscle layer in the blood vessel walls (see also Vasodilators, p.31). Blood is more easily pumped through the dilated vessels, reducing the strain on the heart.

Beta blockers protect the heart muscle from excessive stimulation by norepinephrine (noradrenaline) during exercise or stress by interrupting signal transmission in the heart. Decreased heart muscle stimulation means that less oxygen is required, reducing the risk of angina attacks. For further information on beta blockers, see p.30.

HOW THEY AFFECT YOU

Treatment with one or more of these medicines usually controls angina effectively. Drugs to prevent attacks allow sufferers to undertake more strenuous activities without provoking pain, and if an attack does occur, nitrates usually provide effective relief.

These drugs do not usually cause serious adverse effects but can produce a variety of minor symptoms. By dilating blood vessels throughout the body, nitrates and calcium channel blockers can cause dizziness (especially on standing up) and may cause fainting. Other possible side effects are throbbing headaches at the start of treatment, flushing (especially on the face), and ankle swelling. Beta blockers often cause cold hands and feet and may sometimes produce tiredness and a feeling of heaviness in the legs.

COMMON DRUGS

Beta blockers (see p.30)
Calcium channel blockers Amlodipine*, Diltiazem*, Felodipine, Nicardipine, Nifedipine*, Nisoldipine, Verapamil*
Nitrates Glyceryl trinitrate*, Isosorbide dinitrate/mononitrate*
Potassium channel activator Nicorandil*
Other drugs Aspirin*, Heparin*
* See part 2

Antihypertensive drugs

Blood pressure is the force exerted by the blood against the walls of the arteries. Two measurements are taken. One indicates force while the heart's ventricles are contracting (systolic pressure). This reading is a higher figure than the other one, which measures the blood pressure during ventricle relaxation (diastolic pressure). Blood pressure varies among individuals, and in each person from moment to moment; it is lower at night, higher with stress or exercise, and normally increases with age. If a person's blood pressure is higher than normal on at least three separate occasions, a doctor may diagnose the condition as hypertension.

Blood pressure may be elevated as a result of an underlying disorder, which the doctor will try to identify. Usually, however, it is not possible to determine a cause. This condition is referred to as essential hypertension.

Hypertension does not usually cause any symptoms, but severely raised blood pressure may produce headaches, palpitations, and a general feeling of ill-health. It is important to reduce high blood pressure because it can have serious consequences, including stroke, heart attack, heart failure, and kidney damage. Diabetics, smokers, people with pre-existing heart damage, and those whose blood contains a high level of fat are at particular risk from high blood pressure. High blood pressure is more common in black people than white and in countries where the diet is high in salt. Processed foods are high in salt, and this contributes to high blood pressure.

A small reduction in blood pressure may be brought about by reducing weight, exercising regularly, and reducing the amount of salt in the diet. For more severely raised blood pressure, one or more antihypertensives may be prescribed. Several classes of drugs have antihypertensive properties, including the centrally acting antihypertensives, diuretics (p.32), beta blockers (p.30), calcium channel blockers (p.35), ACE (angiotensin-converting enzyme) inhibitors (see Vasodilators, p.31), and alpha blockers.

WHY THEY ARE USED

Antihypertensive drugs are prescribed when diet, exercise, and other simple remedies have not reduced blood pressure adequately, and your doctor sees a risk of serious consequences if the condition is not treated. These drugs do not cure hypertension and usually have to be taken indefinitely. However, it is sometimes possible to taper off drug treatment when blood pressure has been reduced to normal for a year or more.

HOW THEY WORK

Blood pressure depends, not only on the force with which the heart pumps blood, but also on the diameter of blood vessels and the volume of blood in circulation. The blood pressure is increased either if the vessels are narrow or the volume of blood is high. Antihypertensives lower blood pressure either by dilating the blood vessels or by reducing blood volume. Each type of antihypertensive acts in a different way to lower blood pressure.

Centrally acting drugs act on the mechanism in the brain that controls the diameter of the blood vessels.

Beta blockers reduce the force of the heart beat.

Diuretics act on the kidneys to reduce blood volume.

ACE inhibitors act on enzymes in the blood to dilate blood vessels.

Vasodilators and calcium channel blockers act on the arterial wall muscles to prevent constriction.

Alpha blockers block nerve signals that trigger constriction of blood vessels.

CHOICE OF DRUG

Drug treatment depends on the severity of hypertension. At the start of treatment for mild or moderately high blood pressure, a single drug is used. A thiazide diuretic or beta blocker is often chosen initially, but it is also increasingly common to use a calcium channel blocker or ACE inhibitor. If a single drug does not reduce the blood pressure sufficiently, a diuretic in combination with one of the other drugs may be used. Some people who have moderate hypertension require a third drug, in which case a vasodilator, centrally acting antihypertensive, or alpha blocker may also be prescribed.

Severe hypertension can usually be controlled using a combination of several drugs, which may need to be given in high doses. Your doctor may need to try a number of drugs before finding a combination that controls your blood pressure without causing unacceptable side effects.

HOW THEY AFFECT YOU

Treatment with antihypertensive drugs relieves symptoms such as headache and palpitations. However, since most people with hypertension have few, if any, symptoms, side effects may be more noticeable than any immediate beneficial effect. Some antihypertensive drugs may cause dizziness and fainting at the start of treatment because they can sometimes cause an excessive fall in blood pressure. It may take a while for your doctor to determine a dosage that avoids such effects. For detailed information on adverse effects of drugs used to treat hypertension, see the individual drug profiles in part 2.

RISKS AND SPECIAL PRECAUTIONS

Since your doctor needs to know exactly how treatment with a particular drug affects your hypertension – the benefits as well as the side effects – it is important for you to keep using the medication as prescribed, even though you may feel the problem is under control. Sudden withdrawal of some antihypertensive drugs may cause a potentially dangerous rebound increase in blood pressure. To stop treatment, the dose needs to be reduced gradually under medical supervision.

COMMON DRUGS

ACE inhibitors (see Vasodilators, p.31)
Beta blockers (see p.30)
Calcium channel blockers Amlodipine*, Diltiazem*, Felodipine, Isradipine, Lacidipine, Lercanidipine, Nicardipine, Nifedipine*, Nisoldipine, Verapamil*
Centrally acting antihypertensives Clonidine, Methyldopa*
Diuretics (see p.32)
Alpha blockers Doxazosin*, Indoramin*, Prazosin, Terazosin
Vasodilators Hydralazine, Minoxidil*
* See part 2

Lipid-lowering drugs

The blood contains several types of fats, or lipids. These are necessary for normal body function but can be damaging if they are present in excess, particularly cholesterol. The main risk is atherosclerosis, in which fatty deposits called atheroma build up in the arteries, restricting and disrupting the flow of blood. This can increase the likelihood of the formation of abnormal blood clots, leading to potentially fatal disorders such as stroke and heart attack.

For most people, reducing their fat intake lowers the risk of atherosclerosis. However, those with an inherited tendency to high levels of fat in the blood (hyperlipidaemia) may also be prescribed lipid-lowering drugs.

WHY THEY ARE USED

Lipid-lowering drugs are usually prescribed only when dietary measures have failed to control hyperlipidaemia. The drugs may be given at an earlier stage to those individuals at increased risk of atherosclerosis (such as diabetics and people who are already suffering from circulatory disorders). Lipid-lowering drugs are also given to people who have had a heart attack to help prevent further attacks. The drugs may remove existing atheroma in the blood vessels and prevent the accumulation of new deposits.

For maximum benefit, these drugs are used in conjunction with a low-fat diet and a reduction in other risk factors such as obesity and smoking. The choice of drug depends on the type of lipid causing problems, so a full medical history, examination, and laboratory analysis of blood samples are needed before drug treatment is prescribed.

HOW THEY WORK

Cholesterol and triglycerides are two of the major fats in the blood. One or both may be raised, influencing the choice of lipid-lowering drug. Bile salts contain a large amount of cholesterol and are normally released into the bowel to aid digestion before being reabsorbed into the blood. Drugs that bind to bile salts reduce cholesterol levels by blocking their reabsorption, allowing them to be lost from the body.

Other drugs act on the liver by altering the way in which the liver converts fatty acids in the blood into different types of lipid. Fibrates and nicotinic acid and its derivatives can reduce the level of both cholesterol and triglycerides in the blood. Statins lower blood cholesterol. Fish oil concentrates, containing omega-3 fatty acids, reduce blood triglycerides, but they may raise cholesterol levels.

Lipid-lowering drugs do not correct the underlying cause of raised levels of fat in the blood, so it is usually necessary to continue with diet and drug treatment indefinitely. Stopping treatment usually leads to a return of high blood lipid levels.

HOW THEY AFFECT YOU

Because hyperlipidaemia and atherosclerosis are usually symptomless, you are unlikely to notice any short-term benefits from these drugs. Rather, the aim of treatment is to reduce long-term complications. There may be minor side effects from some of these drugs.

By increasing the amount of bile in the digestive tract, several lipid-lowering drugs can cause gastrointestinal disturbances such as nausea and constipation or diarrhoea, especially at the start of treatment. The statin drugs appear to be well tolerated and are widely used to lower cholesterol levels when diet alone does not have sufficient effect.

RISKS AND SPECIAL PRECAUTIONS

Drugs that bind to bile salts can limit the absorption of some fat-soluble vitamins, and vitamin supplements may therefore be needed. The fibrates can increase susceptibility to gallstones and can occasionally upset the balance of fats in the blood. Statins are used with caution in people with reduced kidney or liver function, and monitoring of blood samples is often advised.

COMMON DRUGS

Fibrates Bezafibrate*, Ciprofibrate*, Fenofibrate, Gemfibrozil

Statins Atorvastatin*, Fluvastatin, Pravastatin*, Simvastatin*

Drugs that bind to bile salts Colestipol, Colestyramine*, Ispaghula

Nicotinic acid and derivatives Acipimox, Nicotinic acid

Other drugs acting on the liver Omega-3 acid ethyl esters, Omega-3 marine triglycerides

* See part 2

Drugs that affect blood clotting

When bleeding occurs through injury or following surgery, the body normally acts swiftly to stem the flow by sealing the breaks in the blood vessels. This occurs in two stages: first, when cells called platelets accumulate as a plug at the opening in the blood vessel wall, then when these platelets produce chemicals that activate clotting factors in the blood to form a protein known as fibrin. Vitamin K plays an important role in this process. An enzyme in the blood called plasmin ensures that clots are broken down when the injury has been repaired.

Some disorders interfere with this process, either preventing clot formation or creating clots uncontrollably. If the blood does not clot, there is a danger of excessive blood loss. Inappropriate development of clots may block the supply of blood to a vital organ.

DRUGS USED TO PROMOTE BLOOD CLOTTING

Fibrin formation depends on the presence in the blood of several clotting-factor proteins. Lack of these clotting factors can lead to uncontrolled bleeding or excessive bruising following even minor injuries. The inherited disease haemophilia causes absence or low levels of Factor VIII; the symptoms almost always appear only in males. Factor IX deficiency causes the bleeding condition called Christmas disease, named after the person in whom it was first identified.

Regular drug treatment for haemophilia is not normally required. But if severe bleeding or bruising occurs, a concentrated form of the missing factor, extracted from normal blood, may be injected to promote clotting and thereby halt bleeding. Injections may need to be repeated for several days after injury.

It is sometimes useful to promote blood clotting in non-haemophiliacs when bleeding is difficult to stop (for example, after surgery). In such cases, blood clots are sometimes stabilized by reducing the action of plasmin with an antifibrinolytic (or haemostatic) drug such as tranexamic acid; this is also occasionally given to haemophiliacs before minor surgery such as tooth extraction.

A tendency to bleed may also occur with deficiency of vitamin K, which is required for the production of several blood clotting factors. It is absorbed from the intestine in fats, but some diseases of the small intestine or pancreas cause fat to be poorly absorbed. As a result, the level of vitamin K in the circulation is low, causing impaired blood clotting. A similar problem sometimes occurs in newborn babies due to absence

of vitamin K. Injections of phytomenadione, a vitamin K preparation, are used to restore levels to normal.

DRUGS USED TO PREVENT ABNORMAL BLOOD CLOTTING

Blood clots normally form only as a response to injury. In some people, however, there is a tendency for clots to form in the blood vessels without apparent cause. Damage to blood vessels that occurs as a result of the presence of fatty deposits (atheroma) inside them increases the risk of the formation of this type of abnormal clot (a thrombus). In addition, a portion of a blood clot (an embolus) formed in response to injury or surgery may sometimes break off and be removed in the bloodstream. The likelihood of this happening is increased by long periods of little or no activity. When an abnormal clot forms, there is a risk that it may become lodged in a blood vessel and block the blood supply to a vital organ such as the brain or heart.

Three main types of drugs are used to prevent and disperse clots: antiplatelet drugs, anticoagulants, and thrombolytics.

ANTIPLATELET DRUGS

Taken regularly by people with a tendency to form clots in the fast-flowing blood of the heart and arteries, these drugs are also given to prevent clots from forming after heart surgery. They reduce the tendency of platelets to stick together when the blood flow is disrupted.

The most widely used antiplatelet drug is aspirin (see also Analgesics, p.9), which has an antiplatelet action even when given in much lower doses than would be needed to reduce pain. In these low doses, adverse effects that may occur when aspirin is given in pain-relieving doses are unlikely. Other antiplatelet drugs are clopidogrel and dipyridamole.

ANTICOAGULANTS

These drugs help to maintain normal blood flow in people at risk from clot formation. They can either prevent the formation of blood clots in the veins or stabilize an existing clot so that it does not break away and become a circulation-stopping embolism. All anticoagulant drugs reduce the activity of certain blood clotting factors, although the mode of action of each drug differs. These medicines do not dissolve the clots that have already formed, however; these clots are treated with thrombolytic drugs (see right).

Anticoagulants fall into two groups: those that are given by intravenous injection and act immediately, and those that are given by mouth and take effect after a few days.

INJECTED ANTICOAGULANTS

Heparin is the most widely used drug of this type, and it is used mainly in hospital before or after surgery. It is also given during kidney dialysis to prevent clots from forming in the dialysis equipment. Because heparin cannot be taken by mouth, it is less suitable for long-term treatment in the home.

A number of synthetic injected anticoagulants have recently been developed. Some act for a longer time than heparin, and others are alternatives for people who react adversely to heparin.

ORAL ANTICOAGULANTS

Warfarin is the most widely used oral anticoagulant, although newer drugs that require less monitoring are now under study. Anticoagulants are mainly prescribed to prevent the formation of clots in veins and the chambers of the heart; they are less likely to prevent blood clots from forming in arteries. Oral anticoagulants may be given following injury or surgery (in particular, heart valve replacement) when there is a high risk of embolism. They are also given long term as a preventative treatment to people at risk from strokes. A common problem experienced with these drugs is that overdosage may lead to bleeding from the nose or gums or in the urinary tract. For this reason, the dosage needs to be carefully calculated; regular blood tests are performed to ensure that the clotting mechanism is correctly adjusted.

The action of oral anticoagulants may be affected by many other drugs. It may therefore be necessary to alter the dosage of anticoagulant when other drugs also need to be given. People who are taking oral anticoagulants should carry a warning list of the drugs that they should avoid. In particular, none of the anticoagulants should be taken together with aspirin except under the direction of a doctor.

THROMBOLYTICS

Also called fibrinolytics, thrombolytics are used to dissolve clots that have already formed. They are usually administered in hospital to clear a blocked blood vessel (for example, in coronary thrombosis). The sooner they are given after symptoms have started, the more likely they are to reduce the size and severity of a heart attack. Thrombolytics may be given either intravenously or directly into the blocked blood vessel.

The main thrombolytic drugs are streptokinase and alteplase. These drugs act by increasing the blood level of plasmin, the enzyme that breaks up the strands of fibrin that bind the clot together, allowing the clot to disperse and restoring the blood flow to normal. When given promptly, alteplase appears to be tolerated better than streptokinase.

The most common problems with use of these drugs are an increased susceptibility to bleeding and bruising, and allergic reactions to streptokinase, which often take the form of rashes, breathing difficulties, or general discomfort. Once streptokinase has been administered, patients are given a card indicating that they have had it, because further treatment with the same drug is generally not advised for several months.

COMMON DRUGS

Blood clotting factors Factor VIIa, Factor VIII, Factor IX

Antifibrinolytic or haemostatic drugs Aprotinin, Etamsylate, Tranexamic acid

Vitamin K Phytomenadione

Antiplatelet drugs Abciximab, Aspirin*, Clopidogrel*, Dipyridamole*, Eptifibatide, Ticlopidine, Tirofiban

Injected anticoagulants Certoparin, Dalteparin, Danaparoid, Desirudin, Enoxaparin, Epoprostenol, Fondaparinux, Heparin *, Lepirudin, Reviparin, Tinzaparin

Thrombolytic drugs Alteplase, Reteplase, Streptokinase *, Tenecteplase *

Oral anti-coagulants Acenocoumarol/nicoumalone, Warfarin*

  * **See part 2**

GASTROINTESTINAL TRACT

The gastrointestinal tract, also known as the digestive or alimentary tract, is the pathway through which food passes as it is processed to enable the nutrients it contains to be absorbed for use by the body. It consists of the mouth, oesophagus, stomach, duodenum, small intestine, large intestine (including the colon and rectum), and anus. A number of other organs are also involved in the digestion of food: the salivary glands in the mouth, the liver, pancreas, and gallbladder, which, together with the gastrointestinal tract, form the digestive system.

The digestive system breaks down the large, complex chemicals – proteins, fats, and carbohydrates, which are present in the food we eat – into simpler molecules that can be used by the body (see also Nutrition, p.90).

The stomach holds food and passes it into the intestine. The lining of the stomach releases gastric juice that partly digests food. The stomach wall continuously produces thick mucus that forms a protective coating.

The duodenum is the tube that connects the stomach to the intestine. Its lining may be damaged by excess acid from the stomach.

The pancreas produces enzymes that digest proteins, fats, and carbohydrates into simpler substances; pancreatic juices neutralize the acidity of the food passing from the stomach.

The gallbladder stores bile, which is produced by the liver, and releases it into the duodenum. Bile assists the digestion of fats by reducing them to smaller units that are more easily acted upon by digestive enzymes.

The small intestine is a long tube in which food is broken down by digestive juices from the gallbladder and pancreas. The mucous lining of the small intestine consists of tiny, finger-like projections called villi that provide a large surface area through which the products of digestion are absorbed into the bloodstream.

The large intestine receives both undigested food and indigestible material from the small intestine. Water and mineral salts pass through the lining into the bloodstream. When a sufficient mass of undigested or indigestible material, together with some of the body's waste products, has accumulated it is expelled from the body as faeces.

MOVEMENT OF FOOD THROUGH THE GASTROINTESTINAL TRACT

Food is propelled through the gastrointestinal tract by rhythmic waves of muscular contraction called peristalsis.

Muscle contraction in the gastrointestinal tract is controlled by the autonomic nervous system (p.8) and is therefore easily disrupted by drugs that either stimulate or inhibit the activity of the autonomic nervous system. Excessive peristaltic action may cause diarrhoea, and constipation may result from slowed peristalsis.

WHAT CAN GO WRONG

Inflammation of the lining of the stomach or intestine (gastroenteritis) is usually due to infection or parasitic infestation. Damage may also result from inappropriate production of digestive juices, leading to minor complaints such as acidity and more serious disorders such as peptic ulcers. The intestinal lining can be damaged by abnormal functioning of the immune system (inflammatory bowel disease). The rectum and anus can become painful and irritated by damage to the lining, tears in the skin at the opening of the anus (anal fissure), or enlarged veins (haemorrhoids, or piles).

Constipation, diarrhoea, and irritable bowel syndrome are the most frequently experienced gastrointestinal complaints, and they usually occur when something disrupts the normal muscle contractions that propel food residue through the bowel.

WHY DRUGS ARE USED

Many drugs for gastrointestinal disorders are taken by mouth and act directly on the digestive tract without first entering the bloodstream. Such drugs include certain antibiotics and other drugs for treating infestations. Some antacids for peptic ulcers and excess stomach acidity, and the bulk-forming agents for constipation and diarrhoea, also pass through the system unabsorbed.

For certain disorders, drugs with a systemic effect are required, including anti-ulcer drugs, opioid antidiarrhoeal drugs, and some of the drugs for inflammatory bowel disease.

MAJOR DRUG GROUPS

♦ Antacids
♦ Anti-ulcer drugs
♦ Antidiarrhoeal drugs
♦ Drugs for irritable bowel syndrome
♦ Laxatives
♦ Drugs for inflammatory bowel disease
♦ Drugs for rectal and anal disorders
♦ Drug treatment for gallstones
♦ Drug treatment for pancreatic disorders

Antacids

Digestive juices in the stomach contain acid and enzymes that break down food before it passes into the intestine. The wall of the stomach is normally protected from the action of digestive acid by a layer of mucus that is constantly secreted by the stomach lining. Problems arise when the stomach lining is damaged or too much acid is produced and eats away at the mucous layer.

Excess acid that leads to discomfort, commonly referred to as indigestion, may result from anxiety, overeating or eating certain foods, coffee, alcohol, or smoking. Some drugs, most notably aspirin and non-steroidal anti-inflammatory drugs, can irritate the stomach lining and even cause ulcers.

Antacids neutralize acid, thereby relieving pain. They are simple chemical compounds that are mildly alkaline and some also act as chemical buffers. Their chalky taste is often disguised with flavourings.

WHY THEY ARE USED

Antacids may be needed when simple remedies (a change in diet or a glass of milk) fail to relieve indigestion. They are especially useful one to three hours after meals to neutralize the effects of excess acid after meals.

Doctors prescribe antacids to relieve dyspepsia or heartburn (pain in the chest or upper abdomen caused or aggravated by acid) in disorders such as inflammation or ulceration of the oesophagus, stomach lining, and duodenum. Antacids usually relieve the pain of ulcers in the oesophagus, stomach, or duodenum within a few minutes. Regular treatment with antacids reduces the acidity of the stomach, thereby encouraging the healing of any ulcers that may have formed.

TYPES OF ANTACID

Aluminium compounds These drugs have a prolonged action and are widely used, especially for the treatment of indigestion and dyspepsia. They may cause constipation, but this is often countered by combining this type of antacid with one containing magnesium. Aluminium compounds can interfere with the absorption of phosphate from the diet, causing muscle weakness and bone damage if taken in high doses over a long period.

Magnesium compounds Like the aluminium compounds, these have a prolonged action. In large doses magnesium compounds can cause diarrhoea, and in people who have impaired kidney function, a high blood magnesium level may build up, causing weakness, lethargy, and drowsiness.

Sodium bicarbonate This antacid, the only sodium compound used as an antacid, acts quickly, but its effect soon passes. It reacts with stomach acids to produce gas, which may cause bloating and belching. Sodium bicarbonate is not advised for people with heart or kidney disease, because the excess sodium can lead to accumulation of water (oedema) in the legs and lungs and may raise blood pressure.

Combined preparations Antacids may be combined with other substances called alginates and antifoaming agents. Alginates are intended to float on the contents of the stomach and produce a neutralizing layer to subdue acid that can otherwise rise into the oesophagus, causing heartburn.

Antifoaming agents (usually dimeticone) are used to relieve flatulence. In some preparations, a local anaesthetic is combined with the antacid to relieve discomfort in oesophagitis. The value of these additives is dubious.

HOW THEY WORK

By neutralizing stomach acid, antacids prevent inflammation, relieve pain, and allow the mucous layer and lining to mend. When used in the treatment of ulcers, they prevent acid from attacking damaged stomach lining and so allow the ulcer to heal.

HOW THEY AFFECT YOU

If antacids are taken according to the instructions, they are usually effective in relieving abdominal discomfort caused by acid. The speed of action, dependent on the ability to neutralize acid, varies. Their duration of action also varies; the short-acting drugs may have to be taken quite frequently.

Most antacids have few serious side effects when used only occasionally, but some may cause diarrhoea, and others may cause constipation (see Types of antacid, facing page).

RISKS AND SPECIAL PRECAUTIONS

Antacids should not be taken to prevent abdominal pain on a regular basis except under medical supervision, because they may suppress the symptoms of stomach cancer. Your doctor is likely to want to arrange tests such as endoscopy or barium X-rays before prescribing long-term treatment.

All antacids can interfere with the absorption of other drugs. Therefore, if you are taking a prescription medicine, you should check with your doctor or pharmacist before taking an antacid.

COMMON DRUGS

Antacids Aluminium hydroxide*, Calcium carbonate, Hydrotalcite, Magnesium hydroxide*, Magnesium trisilicate, Sodium bicarbonate*
Antifoaming agent Dimeticone
Other drugs Alginates*
* See Part 2

Anti-ulcer drugs

Normally, the linings of the oesophagus, stomach, and duodenum are protected from the irritant action of stomach acids or bile by a thin covering layer of mucus. If this is damaged, or if large amounts of stomach acid are formed, the underlying tissue may become eroded, causing a peptic ulcer (break in the gut lining). If small enough, an ulcer may heal spontaneously. However, an established ulcer can lead to abdominal pain, vomiting,

and changes in appetite. The most common type of ulcer occurs in the duodenum, just beyond the stomach. The exact cause of peptic ulcers is not understood, but a number of risk factors have been identified, including heavy smoking, the regular use of aspirin or similar drugs, and family history. An organism found in almost all patients who have peptic ulcers, *Helicobacter pylori*, is now believed to be the main causative agent (although many people who have the organism show no ulcer symptoms).

Symptoms of ulcers may be relieved by an antacid (see facing page), but healing is slow. The usual treatment is with an anti-ulcer drug, such as an H_2 blocker, a proton pump inhibitor, bismuth, or sucralfate, combined with antibiotics to eradicate *Helicobacter pylori* infection.

WHY THEY ARE USED

Anti-ulcer drugs are used to relieve symptoms and heal the ulcer. Untreated ulcers may erode blood vessel walls or perforate the stomach or duodenum.

Until recently, drugs could heal ulcers but not cure them. However, the eradication of *Helicobacter pylori* by a proton pump inhibitor, or ranitidine bismuth citrate combined with two antibiotics (triple therapy), may provide a cure in one to two weeks. Surgery is reserved for complications such as obstruction, perforation, or haemorrhage, and when there is a possibility of cancer.

HOW THEY WORK

Drugs protect ulcers from the action of stomach acid, allowing the tissue to heal. H_2 blockers, misoprostol, and proton pump inhibitors reduce the amount of acid released; bismuth and sucralfate form a protective coating over the ulcer. Bismuth also has an antibacterial effect. It is combined with an H_2 blocker in ranitidine bismuth citrate.

HOW THEY AFFECT YOU

These drugs begin to reduce pain in a few hours and usually allow the ulcer to heal in four to eight weeks. They produce few side effects, although H_2 blockers can cause confusion in elderly people. Bismuth and sucralfate may cause constipation; misoprostol, diarrhoea; and proton pump inhibitors, either constipation or diarrhoea. Triple therapy is given for one or two weeks. If *Helicobacter pylori* is eradicated, maintenance therapy should not be necessary. Sucralfate is usually prescribed for up to 12 weeks, and bismuth and misoprostol for four to six weeks. As they may mask symptoms of stomach cancer, H_2 blockers and proton pump inhibitors are normally prescribed for older patients only when tests have ruled out this disorder.

COMMON DRUGS

Proton pump inhibitors Esomeprazole, Lansoprazole*, Omeprazole*, Pantoprazole, Rabeprazole

H_2 blockers Cimetidine*, Famotidine, Nizatidine, Ranitidine*

Other drugs Antacids (see p.42), Antibiotics (see p.62), Bismuth, Carbenoxolone, Misoprostol*, Ranitidine bismuth citrate, Sucralfate*, Tripotassium dicitrato-bismuthate (bismuth chelate)

* See Part 2

Antidiarrhoeal drugs

Diarrhoea is an increase in the fluidity and frequency of bowel movements. In some cases, diarrhoea protects the body from harmful substances in the intestine by hastening their removal. The most common causes of diarrhoea are infection with unfamiliar bacteria when abroad ("travellers' diarrhoea"), viral infection, food poisoning, and parasites. Diarrhoea also occurs as a symptom of other illnesses. It can be a side effect of some drugs and may follow radiation therapy for cancer. It may also be caused by anxiety.

Most attacks clear up quickly without medical attention. The best treatment is to abstain from food and to drink plenty of clear fluids. Rehydration solutions containing sugar with sodium and potassium salts are widely recommended to prevent dehydration and chemical imbalances, particularly in children. You should consult your doctor if the condition does not improve within 48 hours; the diarrhoea contains blood; there is severe abdominal pain and vomiting; you have just come back from a foreign country; or if diarrhoea occurs in a small child or an elderly person.

Severe diarrhoea can impair the absorption of drugs; anyone taking prescribed drugs should seek advice from a doctor or pharmacist. Women taking oral contraceptives may require additional contraception (see p.105).

The main types of drug for non-specific diarrhoea are opioids and bulk-forming and adsorbent agents. Antispasmodic drugs may also be used to relieve pain (see Drugs for irritable bowel syndrome, facing page).

WHY THEY ARE USED
An antidiarrhoeal drug may be prescribed to provide relief when simple remedies are not effective, and after ruling out the more severe types of infectious diarrhoea.

Opioids are the most effective antidiarrhoeals. They are used when the diarrhoea is severe and debilitating. Bulking and adsorbent agents have a milder effect and are often used when it is necessary to regulate bowel action over a prolonged period (for example, in people with colostomies or ileostomies).

HOW THEY WORK
Opioids decrease the muscles' propulsive activity so that faecal matter passes more slowly through the bowel. This allows more time for water to be absorbed from the food residue and therefore reduces the fluidity as well as the frequency of bowel movements.

Bulk-forming agents and adsorbents absorb water and irritants in the bowel, resulting in larger, firmer stools at less frequent intervals.

HOW THEY AFFECT YOU
Antidiarrhoeals reduce the urge to move the bowels. Opioids and antispasmodics may relieve abdominal pain. All antidiarrhoeals may cause constipation if used in excess.

RISKS AND SPECIAL PRECAUTIONS
Used in relatively low doses for limited periods, the opioid drugs are unlikely to produce adverse effects. They should be used with caution when diarrhoea is caused by an infection, however, since they may slow the elimination of microorganisms from the intestine. All antidiarrhoeals should be taken with plenty of water, and if the diarrhoea is prolonged or the patient is a child, an oral rehydration solution should be taken. Bulk-forming agents

should not be taken together with opioid or antispasmodic drugs, because a bulky mass could form and obstruct the bowel.

COMMON DRUGS

Antispasmodics Atropine*, Dicycloverine*, Hyoscine*
Opioids Codeine*, Co-phenotrope*, Diphenoxylate, Loperamide*
Bulk-forming agents and adsorbents Guar gum, Ispaghula, Kaolin, Methylcellulose*
Antibacterials Ciprofloxacin*
Oral rehydration solutions
* See Part 2

Drugs for irritable bowel syndrome

Irritable bowel syndrome is a common, often stress-related condition in which the waves of muscular contraction that normally move the bowel contents smoothly through the intestines become strong and irregular. This disruption often causes pain, and may be associated with diarrhoea or constipation.

Symptoms are often relieved by adjusting the amount of fibre in the diet, but medication may also be needed. Bulk-forming agents may be given to regulate the consistency of the bowel contents. If pain is severe, an antispasmodic drug may be given. These drugs are anticholinergics (see Drugs that act on the parasympathetic nervous system, p.9), which reduce the transmission of nerve signals to the bowel wall. Tricyclic antidepressants are sometimes used because their anticholinergic action has a calming effect on the bowel.

COMMON DRUGS

Antispasmodics Atropine* dicycloverine*, hyocine* Mebeverine*
Opioids Loperamide*
Other drugs Peppermint oil

Laxatives

When your bowels do not move as frequently as usual and the faeces are hard and difficult to pass, you are suffering from constipation.

The most common cause of constipation is lack of sufficient fibre in your diet; fibre supplies the bulk that makes the faeces soft and easy to pass. The simplest remedy is more fluid and a diet that contains plenty of high-fibre foods, but laxatives may also be used.

Ignoring the urge to open the bowels can also cause constipation because the faeces become hard and dry, difficult to pass, and too small to stimulate the muscles that propel them through the intestine.

Certain drugs (such as opioid analgesics, tricyclic antidepressants, and antacids containing aluminium) may be constipating. Some disorders, such as hypothyroidism (an underactive thyroid gland; see p.84), and painful conditions of the anus (such as fissures; see p.47) can also lead to constipation.

The onset of constipation in a middle-aged or elderly person may be an early symptom of bowel cancer. Consult your doctor about any persistent change in bowel habit.

TYPES OF LAXATIVE

Bulk-forming agents These are relatively slow-acting but are less likely than other laxatives to interfere with normal bowel action. If the constipation is accompanied by abdominal pain, take them only after consulting your doctor because there is a risk of intestinal obstruction.

Stimulant (contact) laxatives These laxatives are for occasional use when other treatments have failed or when rapid onset of action is needed. They should not normally be used for longer than a week at a time, because they can cause abdominal cramps and diarrhoea.

Softening agents These treatments are often used when hard faeces cause pain as the bowels are opened – especially after surgery, when straining must be avoided, or if you have haemorrhoids (see p.47). Liquid paraffin was once used to relieve faecal impaction (blockage of the bowel by faeces) but, because of its side effects, has largely been replaced by docusate sodium.

Osmotic laxatives Salts such as Epsom salts (magnesium sulphate) may be used to evacuate the bowel before surgery or investigative procedures. They are not normally used for long-term relief of constipation because they can cause chemical imbalances in the blood.

Lactulose is an alternative to bulk-forming laxatives for long-term treatment of chronic constipation. It may cause stomach cramps and flatulence but is usually well tolerated.

WHY THEY ARE USED

Because prolonged use of laxatives is harmful, the drugs should be used only for very short periods. Laxatives may prevent pain and straining in people with haemorrhoids (see facing page) or hernias. Doctors may prescribe them for the same reason after childbirth or abdominal surgery. They are also used to clear the bowel before investigative procedures such as colonoscopy. In addition, they may be prescribed for elderly or bedridden patients because lack of exercise can often lead to constipation.

HOW THEY WORK

Laxatives act on the large intestine. They work by increasing the speed with which faecal matter passes through the bowel or by increasing its bulk and/or water content.

Stimulants cause the bowel muscles to contract, increasing the speed at which faecal matter passes through the intestine. Bulk-forming laxatives absorb water in the bowel, thereby increasing the volume of faeces, making them softer and easier to pass. Lactulose also causes fluid to accumulate in the intestine. Osmotic laxatives act by keeping water in the bowel, and thus make the bowel movements softer. This also increases the bulk of the faeces and enables them to be passed more easily. Lubricant liquid paraffin preparations make bowel movements softer and easier to pass without increasing their bulk.

RISKS AND SPECIAL PRECAUTIONS

Laxatives can cause diarrhoea if taken in overdose, and constipation can occur if they are overused. Prolonged use of liquid paraffin preparations can interfere with the absorption of some vitamins. The most serious risk from prolonged use of most laxatives is developing dependence on them for normal bowel action. Therefore, their use should be discontinued as soon as normal bowel movements have been re-established. Laxatives should not be given to children except in special circumstances on the advice of a doctor.

COMMON DRUGS

Stimulant laxatives Bisacodyl, Co-danthramer, Co-danthrusate, Docusate sodium, Glycerol, Senna, Sodium picosulfate

Bulk-forming agents Bran, Ispaghula, Methylcellulose*, Sterculia

Softening agents Arachis oil, Liquid paraffin

Osmotic laxatives Lactulose*, Macrogols, Magnesium citrate, Magnesium hydroxide*, Magnesium sulphate, Sodium acid phosphate

* See Part 2

Drugs for inflammatory bowel disease

Inflammatory bowel disease is the term used for disorders causing inflammation of the intestinal wall. Such diseases result in symptoms ranging from minor, infrequent attacks of diarrhoea to episodes of life-threatening illness. There may be recurrent attacks of abdominal pain, general feelings of ill-health, and, frequently, diarrhoea containing blood and mucus. Loss of appetite and poor absorption of food may often lead to weight loss.

There are two main types of inflammatory bowel disease: Crohn's disease and ulcerative colitis. In Crohn's disease (also called regional enteritis), any part of the digestive tract may become inflamed, although the small intestine is the most commonly affected site. In ulcerative colitis, it is the large intestine (colon) that becomes inflamed and ulcerated, often producing bloodstained diarrhoea.

The exact cause of these disorders is unknown, but dietary, infectious, genetic, and stress-related factors may all be important.

Establishing a proper diet and less stressful lifestyle may help to alleviate these conditions. Bed rest during attacks is also advisable. However, these simple measures alone do not usually relieve or prevent attacks, and drug treatment is often necessary.

Three types of drug are used to treat inflammatory bowel disease: corticosteroids (p.80), immunosuppressants (p.99), and aminosalicylate anti-inflammatory drugs such as sulfasalazine. Nutritional supplements (used especially for Crohn's disease) and anti-diarrhoeal drugs (p.44) may also be used.

Surgery to remove damaged areas of the intestine may be needed in severe cases. Newer drugs are currently being developed; one new drug, infliximab, offers hope of controlling Crohn's disease.

WHY THEY ARE USED

Drugs cannot cure inflammatory bowel disease, but treatment is needed, not only to control symptoms but also to prevent complications, especially severe anaemia and perforation of the intestinal wall. Aminosalicylates are used to treat acute attacks of ulcerative colitis and Crohn's disease, and they may be continued as maintenance therapy. People who have severe bowel inflammation are usually prescribed a course of corticosteroids, particularly during a sudden flare-up. Once the disease is under control, an immunosuppressant drug may be prescribed to prevent a relapse.

HOW THEY WORK

Corticosteroids and sulfasalazine damp down the inflammatory process, allowing the damaged tissue to recover. They act in different ways to prevent the migration of white blood cells into the bowel wall, which may be partly responsible for the inflammation of the bowel.

HOW THEY AFFECT YOU

Taken to treat attacks, these drugs relieve symptoms within a few days, and general health improves gradually over a period of a few weeks. Aminosalicylates usually provide long-term relief from the symptoms of inflammatory bowel disease.

Treatment with an immunosuppressant drug may take several months before improvement of the condition occurs, and regular blood tests to monitor possible drug side effects are often required.

RISKS AND SPECIAL PRECAUTIONS

Immunosuppressants and corticosteroids can cause serious adverse effects and are only used when potential benefits outweigh the risks.

The side effects of corticosteroids can be reduced by the use of budesonide in a topical preparation which releases the drug at the site of inflammation.

It is important to continue taking these drugs as instructed because stopping them abruptly may cause a sudden flare-up of the disorder. Doctors usually supervise a gradual reduction in dosage when such drugs are stopped, even when they are given as a short course for an attack. Antidiarrhoeal drugs should not be taken on a routine basis because they may mask signs of deterioration or cause sudden bowel dilation or rupture.

HOW THEY ARE ADMINISTERED

Antidiarrhoeals are usually taken in the form of tablets, although mild ulcerative colitis in the last part of the large intestine may be treated with suppositories or an enema containing a corticosteroid or aminosalicylate.

COMMON DRUGS

Corticosteroids Budesonide*, Hydrocortisone*, Prednisolone*
Immunosuppressants Azathioprine*, Mercaptopurine*, Methotrexate*
Aminosalicylates Balsalazide, Mesalazine*, Olsalazine, Sulfasalazine*
Other drugs Infliximab, Metronidazole
* See Part 2

Drugs for rectal and anal disorders

The most common disorder of the rectum (the last part of the large intestine) and anus (the opening from the rectum) is haemorrhoids, or piles. They occur when haemorrhoidal veins are swollen or irritated, often as a result of prolonged local pressure such as that caused by pregnancy or a job requiring long hours of sitting. Haemorrhoids may cause irritation and pain, especially on opening the bowels, and are aggravated by constipation and straining. In some cases haemorrhoids may bleed, and occasionally clots form in the swollen veins, leading to severe pain, a condition called thrombosed haemorrhoids.

Other common disorders include pruritus ani (itching around the anus) and anal fissure (painful cracks in the anus). Anal disorders of all kinds occur less often in people who have soft, bulky stools.

A number of both over-the-counter and prescription-only preparations are available for the relief of such disorders.

WHY THEY ARE USED

Preparations for relief of haemorrhoids and anal discomfort fall into two main groups: creams or suppositories that act locally to relieve inflammation and irritation; and measures that relieve constipation, which contributes to the formation of, and discomfort from, haemorrhoids and anal fissure.

Locally acting treatments often contain a soothing agent with antiseptic, astringent, or vasoconstrictor properties. Such ingredients include zinc oxide, bismuth, hamamelis (witch hazel), and ephedrine. Some products also include a mild local anaesthetic (see p.11) such as lidocaine. In some cases a doctor may prescribe an ointment containing a corticosteroid to relieve inflammation around the anus (see Topical corticosteroids, p.120).

People who suffer from haemorrhoids or anal fissure are generally advised to include in their diets plenty of fluids and fibre-rich foods, such as fresh fruits, vegetables, and whole grain products, both to prevent constipation and to ease bowel movements. A mild bulk-forming or softening laxative (see p.45) may also be prescribed .

Neither of these treatments can shrink large haemorrhoids, although they may provide relief while anal fissures heal naturally. Severe, persistently painful haemorrhoids that continue to be troublesome in spite of these measures may need to be removed surgically or, more commonly, by banding. This is a procedure in which a small rubber band is applied tightly to a haemorrhoid, thereby blocking off its blood supply; the haemorrhoid will eventually wither away.

HOW THEY AFFECT YOU

These treatments usually relieve discomfort, especially during bowel movement. Most people experience no adverse effects, but preparations containing local anaesthetics may cause irritation or even a rash in the anal area. It is rare for ingredients in locally acting preparations to be absorbed into the body in sufficient quantities to cause generalized side effects.

The main risk is that self-treatment of haemorrhoids may delay diagnosis of bowel cancer. It is therefore always wise to consult your doctor if you have symptoms of haemorrhoids, especially if you have noticed bleeding from the rectum or a change in bowel habits.

COMMON DRUGS

Soothing and astringent agents Aluminium acetate, Bismuth, Peru balsam, Zinc oxide
Topical corticosteroids Hydrocortisone*
Local anaesthetics (see p.11)
Laxatives (see p.45)
* **See Part 2**

Drug treatment for gallstones

The formation of gallstones is the most common disorder of the gallbladder. This small sac stores and concentrates bile, which is a digestive juice produced by the liver. During digestion, bile passes from the gallbladder via the bile duct into the small intestine, where it assists in the digestion of fats. Bile is composed of several ingredients, including bile acids, bile salts, and bile pigments. It also contains a significant amount of cholesterol, which is dissolved in the bile acids. If the amount of cholesterol in the bile increases, or if the amount of bile acid is reduced, a proportion of the cholesterol cannot remain dissolved, and under certain circumstances this excess accumulates in the gallbladder to form gallstones.

Gallstones may exist in the gallbladder for years without causing symptoms. Sometimes, however, they may cause the gallbladder to become infected and inflamed. They may also lodge in the bile duct, causing pain and blocking the flow of bile. The bile may then spill over into the blood and result in jaundice.

Drug treatment with ursodeoxycholic acid is only effective against stones that are composed principally of cholesterol (some contain other substances), and even these take many months to dissolve. Therefore, as techniques have improved, surgery and ultrasound treatments have become widely used.

These treatments are always used to remove stones that are blocking the bile duct.

WHY THEY ARE USED

Even if you have not experienced any symptoms, once gallstones have been diagnosed your doctor may advise treatment because of the risk of blockage of the bile duct. Drug treatment is usually preferred to surgery for small cholesterol stones when there is a possibility that surgery may be risky.

HOW THEY WORK

Ursodeoxycholic acid is a substance naturally present in bile. It acts on chemical processes in the liver to regulate the amount of cholesterol in the blood by controlling the amount that passes into the bile. Once the cholesterol level in the bile is reduced, the bile acids can start dissolving the stones in the gallbladder. For maximum effect, ursodeoxycholic acid treatment usually has to be accompanied by adherence to a low-cholesterol, high-fibre diet.

HOW THEY AFFECT YOU

Drug treatment may often take years to dissolve gallstones completely. You will not, therefore, feel any immediate benefit, but you may have some minor side effects, the most usual of which is diarrhoea. If this occurs, your doctor may adjust the dosage. The effect of drug treatment on the gallstones is usually monitored at regular intervals by means of ultrasound or X-ray examinations.

Even after successful drug treatment, gallstones often recur when the drug is stopped. In some cases, to prevent recurrence, drug treatment and dietary restrictions may be continued after the gallstones have dissolved.

Although the drug reduces cholesterol in the gallbladder, it increases the cholesterol level in the blood because it reduces excretion in the bile. Doctors therefore prescribe it with caution to people with atherosclerosis (fatty deposits in the blood vessels). The drug is not usually given to people who have liver disorders because it can interfere with normal liver function; instead, surgical or ultrasound treatment is used.

COMMON DRUGS

Drugs for gallstones Ursodeoxycholic acid

Drug treatment for pancreatic disorders

The pancreas releases certain enzymes into the small intestine that are necessary for digestion of a range of foods. If the release of pancreatic enzymes is impaired (by chronic pancreatitis or cystic fibrosis, for example), enzyme replacement therapy may be necessary. Replacement of enzymes does not cure the underlying disorder, but it restores normal digestion. Pancreatic enzymes should be taken just before or with meals, and usually take effect immediately. Your doctor will probably advise you to eat a diet that is high in protein and carbohydrates and low in fat. Pancreatin, the generic name for those preparations containing pancreatic enzymes, is extracted from pig pancreas. Treatment must be continued indefinitely as long as the pancreatic disorder persists.

COMMON DRUGS

Pancreatic enzymes Amylase, Lipase, Pancreatin, Protease

MUSCLES, BONES, AND JOINTS

The basic architecture of the human body comprises 206 bones, over 600 muscles, and a complex variety of other tissues that enable the body to move efficiently.

Bones support the body, provide protection for organs, and enable movement.

Tendons attach the muscles that control body movement to the bones.

Muscles work bones that act as levers: when the muscle contracts, movement occurs at the joint.

Ligaments are bands of tough fibrous tissue that hold joints together.

Cartilage covers each bone end, reducing friction between the ends of two bones.

WHAT CAN GO WRONG

Although tough, these structures often suffer damage. Muscles, tendons, and ligaments can be strained or torn by violent movement, which may cause inflammation, making the affected tissue swollen and painful. Joints, especially those that bear the body's weight – the hips, knees, ankles, and vertebrae – are prone to wear and tear. The cartilage covering the bone ends may tear, causing pain and inflammation. Joint damage also occurs in rheumatoid arthritis, which is thought to be a form of autoimmune disorder. Gout, in which uric acid crystals form in some joints, may also cause inflammation, a condition known as gouty arthritis.

Another type of problem affecting the muscles and joints is nerve injury or degeneration, which alters nerve control over muscle contraction. Myasthenia gravis, in which transmission of signals between nerves and muscles is reduced, affects muscle strength as a result. Bones may also be weakened by vitamin, mineral, or hormone deficiencies.

WHY DRUGS ARE USED

A simple analgesic drug or one that has an anti-inflammatory effect will provide pain relief in most of the conditions described above. For severe inflammation, a doctor may inject a drug with a more powerful anti-inflammatory effect, such as a corticosteroid, into the affected site. In cases of severe progressive rheumatoid arthritis, antirheumatic drugs may halt the disease's progression and relieve symptoms.

Drugs that help to eliminate excess uric acid from the body are often prescribed to treat gout. Muscle relaxants that inhibit transmission of nerve signals to the muscles are used to treat muscle spasm. Drugs that increase nervous stimulation of the muscle are prescribed for myasthenia gravis. Bone disorders in which the mineral content of the bone is reduced are treated with supplements of minerals, vitamins, and hormones.

MAJOR DRUG GROUPS

◆ Non-steroidal anti-inflammatory drugs
◆ Antirheumatic drugs
◆ Corticosteroids for rheumatic disorders
◆ Drugs for gout
◆ Muscle relaxants
◆ Drugs used for myasthenia gravis
◆ Drugs for bone disorders

Non-steroidal anti-inflammatory drugs

Drugs in this group, often referred to as NSAIDs, are used to relieve the pain, stiffness, and inflammation of painful conditions affecting the muscles, bones, and joints. For this reason, they are effective in rheumatoid arthritis. They are less effective in osteoarthritis, however, because there is usually pain, due to worn joints, without inflammation. NSAIDs are called "non-steroidal" to distinguish them from corticosteroid drugs (see p.80), which also relieve inflammation.

There are many NSAIDs currently available, and others are being investigated in the hope of finding new compounds with fewer side effects.

WHY THEY ARE USED

NSAIDs are widely prescribed for the treatment of osteoarthritis, rheumatoid arthritis, and other rheumatic conditions. They do not alter the progress of these diseases but reduce inflammation and thus relieve pain and swelling of joints.

The response to the various drugs in this group varies between individuals and the first drug chosen may not be effective. The doctor may sometimes need to prescribe a number of different NSAIDs before he or she finds one best suited to a particular person.

Because NSAIDs do not change the progress of the disease, additional treatment may be required, particularly for rheumatoid arthritis (see p.52).

NSAIDs are also commonly prescribed for back pain, headaches, gout (see p.53), menstrual pain (see p.104), mild pain following surgery, and pain from soft tissue injuries such as sprains and strains (see also Analgesics, p.9).

HOW THEY WORK

Prostaglandins are chemicals released by the body at the site of injury. They are responsible for producing inflammation and pain following tissue damage and in immune reactions. NSAIDs block prostaglandin production, reducing pain and inflammation.

HOW THEY AFFECT YOU

NSAIDs are usually effective in reducing joint pain and swelling. They are rapidly absorbed from the digestive system, and most start to relieve pain within an hour. When used regularly, NSAIDs reduce pain, inflammation, and stiffness and may restore or improve the function of a joint if this has been impaired.

Most NSAIDs are short-acting and need to be taken a few times a day to provide optimal relief from pain. Some need to be taken only twice daily. Others, such as piroxicam, are very slowly eliminated from the body and are effective when taken once a day.

RISKS AND SPECIAL PRECAUTIONS

Most NSAIDs carry a low risk of serious adverse effects although nausea, indigestion, and altered bowel action are common. The main risk from NSAIDs, however, is that they can occasionally cause bleeding in the stomach or duodenum. They should therefore be avoided by people who have suffered from peptic ulcers.

Most NSAIDs are not recommended during pregnancy or for breast-feeding mothers.

Caution is also advised for those people with kidney or liver abnormalities or with a history of hypersensitivity to other drugs.

NSAIDs may impair blood clotting and are, therefore, prescribed with caution to people with bleeding disorders or who are taking drugs that reduce blood clotting.

MISOPROSTOL

An NSAID causes bleeding when its antiprostaglandin action occurs where it is not wanted, such as in the digestive tract. To protect against this side effect, a prostaglandin-like drug called misoprostol is sometimes prescribed with the NSAID. Preparations are available that incorporate both misoprostol and an NSAID. Misoprostol is also used to help heal peptic ulcers (see p.43). As an alternative to giving drugs such as misoprostol, NSAIDs are being developed that work selectively by preventing prostaglandin production in the joints but not in the digestive tract.

COX-2 INHIBITORS

NSAIDs block the action of the enzyme cyclo-oxygenase (COX), which is involved in the manufacture of prostaglandins at different sites in the body. Research has shown that they block two types of COX (COX-1 and COX-2) and that blocking COX-1 leads to the stomach irritation of NSAIDs, while blocking COX-2 leads to the anti-inflammatory effect. As a result, a new class of NSAID, COX-2 inhibitors, has been developed, to block COX-2 but not COX-1. In this way, the benefits of NSAIDs can be obtained with less risk of stomach pain, peptic ulcers, or intestinal bleeding. COX-2 inhibitors include celecoxib and etodolac, and are useful in people at high risk of stomach problems.

COMMON DRUGS

Aceclofenac, Acemetacin, Aspirin*, Azapropazone, Benorylate, Benzydamine, Diclofenac*, Diflunisal, Etodolac, Felbinac, Fenbufen, Fenoprofen, Flurbiprofen, Ibuprofen*, Indometacin, Ketoprofen*, Mefenamic acid*, Nabumetone, Naproxen*, Phenylbutazone, Piroxicam*, Sulindac, Tenoxicam, Tiaprofenic acid

Cox-2 inhibitors Celecoxib*, Etodolac, Meloxicam*

* See Part 2

Antirheumatic drugs

These drugs are used in the treatment of various rheumatic disorders, the most crippling and deforming of which is rheumatoid arthritis: an autoimmune disease in which the body's mechanism for fighting infection contributes to the damage of its own joint tissue. The disease causes pain, stiffness, and swelling of the joints that can, over many months, lead to deformity. Flare-ups of rheumatoid arthritis also cause a general feeling of being unwell, fatigue, and loss of appetite.

Treatments for rheumatoid arthritis include drugs, rest, physiotherapy, changes in diet, and immobilization of joints. The disorder cannot yet be cured, but in many cases it does not progress far enough to cause permanent disability. It sometimes subsides spontaneously for prolonged periods.

WHY THEY ARE USED

The aim of drug treatment is to relieve the symptoms of pain and stiffness, maintain mobility, and prevent deformity. There are two main forms of drug treatment for rheumatoid arthritis: the first alleviates symptoms, and the second modifies, halts, or slows the underlying disease process. Drugs in the first category include aspirin (see p.146) and the NSAIDs (see Nonsteroidal anti-inflammatory drugs, p.50). These drugs are usually prescribed as a first treatment.

However, if the rheumatoid arthritis is severe, or the initial drug treatment has proved ineffective, the second category of drugs may be given. These drugs may prevent any further joint damage and disability. They are not prescribed routinely because they have potentially severe adverse effects and because the disease may stop spontaneously.

Corticosteroids (see p.80) are sometimes used in the long-term treatment of rheumatoid arthritis, but high doses are only used for limited periods of time because the risks from adverse effects outweigh the benefits.

TYPES OF ANTIRHEUMATIC DRUG

Chloroquine Originally developed to treat malaria (see p.75), chloroquine and related drugs are less effective than penicillamine or gold. Prolonged use may cause eye damage, but only if too high a dose is used.

Immunosuppressants These are prescribed if other drugs do not provide relief and if the rheumatoid arthritis is severe and disabling. Regular observation and blood tests must be carried out because immunosuppressants can cause severe complications.

Sulfasalazine Used mainly for ulcerative colitis (p.46), sulfasalazine was originally introduced to treat rheumatoid arthritis and is effective in some cases.

Gold-based drugs These are effective and may be given orally or by injection for many years. Side effects can include a rash and digestive disturbances. Gold may sometimes damage the kidneys, which recover once treatment is stopped; regular urine tests are usually carried out, however. Gold can also suppress blood cell production in bone marrow. Therefore, periodic blood tests are also carried out.

Penicillamine This drug may be used when rheumatoid arthritis is worsening, or when gold cannot be given. Improvement in symptoms may take 3 to 6 months. It has similar side effects to gold, and periodic blood and urine tests are usually performed.

HOW THEY WORK

It is not known precisely how most antirheumatic drugs stop or slow the disease process. Some may reduce the body's immune response, which is thought to be partly responsible for the disease (see also Immunosuppressant drugs, p.99). When they are effective, antirheumatic drugs prevent damage to the cartilage and bone, thereby reducing progressive deformity and disability. The effectiveness of each drug varies depending on the individual response.

HOW THEY AFFECT YOU

These drugs are generally slow-acting; it may be weeks or even months before benefit is felt. Therefore, aspirin or other NSAID treatment is usually continued until remission occurs. Prolonged treatment with antirheumatic drugs can cause a marked improvement in symptoms. Arthritic pain is relieved, joint mobility increased, and general symptoms of ill health fade. Side effects (which vary between individual drugs) may be noticed before any beneficial effect, so patience is required. Severe adverse effects may necessitate abandoning the treatment.

COMMON DRUGS

Immunosuppressants Azathioprine*, Cyclophosphamide*, Ciclosporin*, Leflunomide, Methotrexate*
NSAIDs (see p.50)
Gold-based drugs Auranofin, Sodium aurothiomalate
Other drugs Chloroquine*, Hydroxychloroquine, Penicillamine, Sulfasalazine*
* See Part 2

Corticosteroids for rheumatic disorders

The adrenal glands, which lie on the top of the kidneys, produce a number of important hormones. Among these are the corticosteroids, so named because they are made in the outer part (cortex) of the glands. The corticosteroids play an important role, influencing the immune system and regulating the carbohydrate and mineral metabolism of the body. A number of drugs that mimic the natural corticosteroids have been developed.

These drugs have many uses and are discussed in detail under Corticosteroids (see p.80). This section concentrates on those corticosteroids injected into an affected site to treat joint disorders.

WHY THEY ARE USED

Corticosteroids given by injection are particularly useful for treating joint disorders (notably rheumatoid arthritis and osteoarthritis) when only one or a few joints are involved, and when pain and inflammation have not been relieved by other drugs. In such cases, it is possible to relieve symptoms by injecting each affected joint individually. Corticosteroids may also be injected to relieve pain and inflammation caused by strained or contracted muscles, ligaments, and/or tendons (in frozen shoulder or tennis elbow, for example). They may also be used to treat bursitis, tendinitis, or swelling that is compressing a nerve. Corticosteroid injections are sometimes used to relieve pain and stiffness sufficiently for physiotherapy to be carried out.

HOW THEY WORK

Corticosteroids have two important actions that are believed to account for their effectiveness: they block the production of prostaglandins – chemicals responsible for triggering inflammation and pain – and they depress the accumulation and activity of the white blood cells that cause the inflammation. Injection concentrates the corticosteroids, and their effects, at the site of the problem, thereby giving the maximum benefit where it is most needed.

HOW THEY AFFECT YOU

Corticosteroids usually produce dramatic relief of symptoms when the drug is injected into a joint. Often a single injection is sufficient to relieve pain and swelling, and to improve mobility. When used to treat muscle or tendon pain, they may not always be effective because it is difficult to position the needle so that the drug reaches the right spot. In some cases, repeated injections are necessary.

Because these drugs are concentrated in the affected area, rather than being dispersed in significant amounts in the body, the generalized adverse effects that sometimes occur when corticosteroids are taken by mouth are unlikely. Minor effects, such as loss of skin pigment at the injection site, are uncommon. Occasionally, a temporary increase in pain (steroid flare) may occur. In such cases, rest, local application of ice, and analgesic medication may relieve the condition. Sterile injection technique is critically important.

COMMON DRUGS

Dexamethasone*, Hydrocortisone*, Methylprednisolone, Prednisolone*, Triamcinolone
* See Part 2

Drugs for gout

Gout is a disorder that arises when the blood contains increased levels of uric acid, which is a by-product of normal body metabolism.

When its concentration in the blood is excessive, uric acid crystals may form in various parts of the body, especially in the joints of the foot (most often the big toe), the knee, and the hand, causing intense pain and inflammation known as gouty arthritis. Crystals may form as white masses, known as tophi, in soft tissue, and in the kidneys as stones. Attacks of gouty arthritis can recur, and may lead to damaged joints and deformity. Kidney stones can cause kidney damage.

Excess uric acid can be due either to increased production or decreased elimination by the kidneys (which remove it from the body). Gout tends to run in families and is far more common in men than women. The risk of attack is increased by high alcohol intake, the consumption of certain foods (red meat, sardines, anchovies, and offal), and obesity. An attack may be triggered by drugs such as thiazide diuretics (see p.32) or anti-cancer drugs (see p.96), or excessive drinking. Changes in diet and reduced alcohol intake may be an important part of treatment.

Drugs to treat acute attacks of gouty arthritis include NSAIDs (see Non-steroidal anti-inflammatory drugs, p.50), and colchicine. Other drugs, which lower blood levels of uric acid, are for the long-term prevention of gout. These include the uricosuric drugs probenecid and sulfinpyrazone (both of which are now rarely used) and allopurinol. Aspirin is not prescribed for pain relief because it slows the excretion of uric acid.

WHY THEY ARE USED

Drugs may be prescribed either to treat an attack of gout or to prevent recurrent attacks that could lead to deformity of the affected joints and to kidney damage. The NSAIDs and colchicine are both used to treat an attack of gout and should be taken as soon as it begins. Because colchicine is relatively specific in relieving the pain and inflammation arising from gout, doctors sometimes administer it in order to confirm their diagnosis of the condition before prescribing an NSAID.

If symptoms recur, your doctor may advise long-term treatment with either allopurinol or a uricosuric drug. One of these drugs usually has to be taken indefinitely. Because these drugs can trigger acute attacks of gout

at the beginning of treatment, they are only given once the attack has settled. NSAIDs are widely used to treat acute attacks.

HOW THEY WORK

Allopurinol lowers uric acid levels in the blood by reducing the activity of xanthine oxidase, an enzyme involved in the production of uric acid in the body. Both sulfinpyrazone and probenecid increase the rate at which the kidneys excrete uric acid. The process by which colchicine reduces inflammation and relieves pain is not understood. The actions of NSAIDs are described on p.51.

HOW THEY AFFECT YOU

Drugs for long-term gout treatment are usually successful in preventing attacks and joint deformity, but response may be slow. Colchicine can disturb the digestive system, causing abdominal pain and diarrhoea, which your doctor can control by prescribing other drugs.

RISKS AND SPECIAL PRECAUTIONS

Because they increase the output of uric acid through the kidneys, uricosuric drugs can cause uric acid crystals to form in the kidneys. They are not, therefore, usually prescribed for those people who already have kidney problems. In such cases, allopurinol is preferred. It is always important to drink plenty of fluids while taking drugs for gout in order to prevent kidney crystals from forming. Blood tests to monitor levels of uric acid may be required until its concentration in the blood has been successfully reduced.

COMMON DRUGS

Drugs to treat attacks Colchicine*, NSAIDs (but not aspirin; see p.48)
Drugs to prevent attacks Allopurinol*, Probenecid, Sulfinpyrazone
Drugs to treat high uric acid caused by cytotoxic drugs Rasburicase
* See Part 2

Muscle relaxants

Several drugs are available to treat muscle spasm – involuntary, painful contraction of a muscle or a group of muscles that can stiffen an arm or leg, or make it nearly impossible to straighten your back. Muscle spasm has various causes. It can follow an injury, or come on without warning. It may also be brought on by a disorder such as osteoarthritis, the pain in the affected joint triggering abnormal tension in a nearby muscle.

Spasticity is another form of muscle tightness seen in some neurological disorders, such as multiple sclerosis, stroke, or cerebral palsy. Spasticity can sometimes be helped by physiotherapy, but in severe cases drugs may be used to relieve symptoms.

WHY THEY ARE USED

Muscle spasm resulting from direct injury is usually treated with an NSAID (see Nonsteroidal anti-inflammatory drugs, p.50) or an analgesic. However, if the spasm is severe, a muscle relaxant drug may also be tried for a short period.

In spasticity, the legs may become so stiff and uncontrollable that walking unaided is impossible. In such cases, a drug may be used to relax the muscles. Relaxation of the muscles often permits physiotherapy to be given for longer-term relief from spasms.

The muscle relaxant botulinum toxin may be injected locally to relieve muscle spasm in small groups of accessible muscles, such as those around the eye or in the neck.

HOW THEY WORK

Muscle-relaxant drugs work in one of several ways. The centrally acting drugs damp down the passage of the nerve signals from the brain and spinal cord that cause muscles to contract, thus reducing excessive stimulation of muscles as well as unwanted muscular contraction. Tizanidine stimulates the alpha receptors in the blood vessels. Dantrolene reduces the sensitivity of the muscles to nerve signals. When injected locally, botulinum toxin prevents the transmission of impulses between nerves and muscles.

HOW THEY AFFECT YOU

Drugs taken regularly for a spastic disorder of the central nervous system usually reduce stiffness and improve mobility. They may restore the use of the arms and legs when this has been impaired by muscle spasm.

Unfortunately, most centrally acting drugs can have a generally depressant effect on nervous activity and produce drowsiness, particularly at the beginning of treatment. Too high a dosage can excessively reduce the muscles' ability to contract and can therefore cause weakness. For this reason, the dosage needs to be carefully adjusted to find a level that controls symptoms while maintaining sufficient muscle strength.

RISKS AND SPECIAL PRECAUTIONS

The main long-term risk associated with centrally acting muscle relaxants is that the body becomes dependent. If the drugs are withdrawn suddenly, the stiffness may become worse than before drug treatment.

Rarely, dantrolene can cause serious liver damage, especially when it is given in high doses. Anyone taking this drug should have his or her blood tested regularly to assess liver function.

Unless used very cautiously, botulinum toxin can paralyse unaffected muscles, and might interfere with functions such as speech and swallowing.

COMMON DRUGS

Centrally acting drugs Baclofen*, Carisoprodol, Cyclobenzaprine, Diazepam*, Methocarbamol, Orphenadrine*
Other drugs Botulinum toxin*, Dantrolene, Quinine*, Tizanidine
* See Part 2

Drugs used for myasthenia gravis

Myasthenia gravis occurs when the immune system (see p.95) becomes defective and produces antibodies that disrupt the signals being transmitted between the nervous system and muscles that are under voluntary control. As a result, the body's muscular response is progressively weakened. The first muscles to be affected are those controlling the eyes, eyelids, face, pharynx, and larynx, with muscles in the arms and legs becoming involved as the disease progresses. Typical symptoms that result include drooping eyelids, double vision, and a weak voice, which worsens during the day. The disease is often linked to a disorder of the thymus gland. Located in the upper part of the chest, this gland is thought to be partly responsible for the disease because it is the source of the destructive antibodies concerned.

Various methods can be used in the treatment of myasthenia gravis, including removal of the thymus gland (thymectomy) or temporarily clearing the blood of antibodies using a procedure known as plasmapheresis. Drugs that improve muscle function, principally neostigmine and pyridostigmine, may be prescribed. They may be used either alone or together with other drugs that depress the immune system – usually azathioprine (see Immunosuppressant drugs, p.99) or corticosteroids (see p.80).

WHY THEY ARE USED

Drugs that improve the muscle response to nerve impulses have several uses. One such drug, edrophonium, acts very quickly and, once administered, brings about a dramatic improvement in the symptoms. This effect is used to confirm the diagnosis of myasthenia gravis. However, because of its short duration of action, edrophonium is not used for long-term treatment. Pyridostigmine and neostigmine are preferred for long-term treatment, especially when surgery to remove the thymus gland is not feasible or does not provide adequate relief.

These drugs may also be given following surgery in order to counteract the effects of a muscle-relaxant drug given prior to certain surgical procedures.

HOW THEY WORK

Normal muscle action occurs when a nerve impulse triggers a nerve ending to release a neurotransmitter, which combines with a specialized receptor on the muscle cells and causes contraction of the muscles. In myasthenia gravis, the body's immune system destroys many of these receptors, so that the muscles are less responsive to nervous stimulation. Drugs used to treat the disorder increase the amount of neurotransmitter at the nerve ending by blocking the action of an enzyme that normally breaks it down.

Increased levels of the neurotransmitter permit the remaining receptors to function more efficiently.

HOW THEY AFFECT YOU

These drugs usually restore the muscle function to a normal or near-normal level, particularly when the myasthenia gravis takes a mild form. Unfortunately, the drugs can produce unwanted muscular activity by enhancing the transmission of nerve impulses elsewhere in the body.

Common side effects include vomiting, nausea, diarrhoea, and muscle cramps in the arms, legs, and abdomen.

RISKS AND SPECIAL PRECAUTIONS

Muscle weakness can suddenly worsen even when it is being treated with drugs. Should this occur, it is important not to take larger doses of the drug in an attempt to relieve the symptoms, since excessive levels can interfere with the transmission of nerve impulses to muscles, causing further weakness. The administration of other drugs, including some antibiotics, can also markedly increase the symptoms of myasthenia gravis. If your symptoms suddenly become worse, you should consult your doctor.

COMMON DRUGS

Azathioprine*, Distigmine, Edrophonium, Neostigmine, Pyridostigmine*, Corticosteroids (see p.80)
* See Part 2

Drugs for bone disorders

Bone is a living structure. Its hard, mineral quality is created by the action of the bone cells. These cells continuously deposit and remove phosphorus and calcium, which are stored in a honeycombed protein framework called the matrix. Because the rates of deposit and removal (the bone metabolism) are about equal in adults, the bone mass remains fairly constant.

Removal and renewal is regulated by hormones and influenced by a number of factors, notably the level of calcium in the blood; this, in turn, depends on the intake of calcium and vitamin D from the diet, the actions of various hormones, plus everyday movement and weight-bearing stress. When normal bone metabolism is altered, various bone disorders result.

OSTEOPOROSIS

In osteoporosis, the strength and density of bone are reduced. Such wasting occurs when the rate of removal of mineralized bone exceeds the rate of deposit. In most people, bone density decreases very gradually from the age of 30. But bone loss can dramatically increase when a person is immobilized for a period, and this is an important cause of osteoporosis in elderly people. Hormone deficiency is another important cause, commonly occurring in women with lowered oestrogen levels after the menopause or removal of the ovaries. Osteoporosis is therefore much more common with increasing age in women than in men. It also occurs in disorders in which there is excess production of adrenal or thyroid hormones, and it is a major adverse effect of long-term treatment with corticosteroid drugs.

People with osteoporosis often have no symptoms, but, if the vertebrae become so weakened that they are unable to bear the body's weight, they may collapse spontaneously or after a minor accident. Subsequently, the individual suffers from back pain, reduced height, and a round-shouldered appearance. Osteoporosis also makes a fracture of a wrist, thigh, or hip bone more likely.

Most doctors stress the need to prevent osteoporosis by ensuring an adequate intake of protein and calcium, giving up smoking, and taking regular exercise throughout adult life. Oestrogen supplements, however, are no longer usually recommended to prevent osteoporosis.

The condition of bones damaged by osteoporosis cannot usually be improved, but drug treatment can help prevent further deterioration and help fractures to heal. For people whose diet is deficient in calcium or vitamin D, supplements may be prescribed. However, these are of limited value and are often less useful than drugs that inhibit the removal of calcium from the bones. In the past, the hormone calcitonin was used, but it has now been largely superseded by drugs such as etidronate and alendronate. These drugs, known as bisphosphonates, bind very tightly to bone matrix, preventing its removal by bone cells. They reduce the incidence of vertebral fractures, but there is less evidence of their effectiveness in reducing hip fractures.

OSTEOMALACIA AND RICKETS

In osteomalacia (called rickets when it affects children), lack of vitamin D leads to loss of calcium, resulting in softening of the bones. Sufferers experience pain, tenderness, and reduced muscle strength, and there is a risk of fracture and bone deformity. In children, growth is retarded.

Osteomalacia is most commonly caused by a lack of vitamin D. This can result from an inadequate diet, inability to absorb the vitamin, or insufficient exposure of the skin to sunlight (the action of the sun on the skin produces vitamin D inside the body). People at special risk include those whose absorption of vitamin D is impaired by an intestinal disorder such as Crohn's disease or coeliac disease. Dark-skinned people living in Northern Europe are also susceptible. Chronic kidney disease is an important cause of rickets in children and of osteomalacia in adults, since healthy kidneys play an essential role in the body's metabolism of vitamin D.

Long-term relief depends on treating the underlying disorder where possible. In rare cases, treatment may be lifelong.

VITAMIN D

A number of substances that are related to vitamin D may be used in the treatment of bone disorders. These include alfacalcidol, calcitriol, and ergocalciferol. The drug prescribed depends on the underlying problem.

COMMON DRUGS

Alendronate*, Alfacalcidol, Calcitonin, Calcitriol, Calcium carbonate, Ergocalciferol, Etidronate*, Fluoride, Risendronate, Salcatonin (calcitonin (salmon)), Vitamin D

* **See Part 2**

ALLERGY

Allergy, a hypersensitivity to certain substances, is a reaction of the body's immune system. Through a variety of mechanisms (see Malignant and immune disease, p.95), the immune system protects the body by eliminating unrecognized foreign substances such as microorganisms (bacteria or viruses).

One such mechanism is the production of antibodies. When the body encounters a particular allergen (foreign substance) for the first time, one type of white blood cell (a lymphocyte) produces antibodies that attach themselves to another type of white blood cell (a mast cell). If that substance is encountered again, the allergen binds to the antibodies on the mast cells, causing the release of chemicals called mediators.

The most important mediator is histamine. Released in response to injury or allergens, it acts on H_1 receptors in the skin, blood vessels, nasal passages, and airways, and on H_2 receptors in the stomach lining. This can produce a rash, swelling, narrowed airways, and a drop in blood pressure. Although important in protecting the body against infection, these effects may be triggered inappropriately in an allergic reaction. (See also Antihistamines, right, and Anti-ulcer drugs, p.43.)

WHAT CAN GO WRONG

Hay fever, one of the most common allergic disorders, is caused by an allergic reaction to inhaled grass pollen, leading to allergic rhinitis (swollen and irritated nasal passages and watering nose and eyes). Other substances, such as house-dust mites and fur, may cause a similar reaction in susceptible people.

Asthma (see p.24) may be due to the action of leukotrienes rather than histamine. Other allergic conditions include urticaria (hives) or other rashes (sometimes in response to a drug), and some forms of eczema and dermatitis. Anaphylaxis is a serious, systemic reaction that occurs when an allergen reaches the tissues. (See also Epinephrine, p.233.)

WHY DRUGS ARE USED

Antihistamines and drugs that inhibit mast cell activity are used to prevent and treat allergic reactions. Other drugs minimize symptoms, such as decongestants (see p.26) to clear the nose in allergic rhinitis, bronchodilators (see p.23) to widen the airways in asthma, and corticosteroids applied to skin affected by eczema (see p.125).

MAJOR DRUG GROUPS
◆ Antihistamines
◆ Leukotriene antagonists
◆ Corticosteroids (see p.80)

Antihistamines

Antihistamines are the most widely used drugs for treating allergic reactions of all kinds. They can be subdivided according to their chemical structure; each subgroup has slightly different actions and characteristics (see table, p.60). Their main action is to counter the effects of histamine, one of the chemicals released in the body when there is an allergic reaction (see left).

Histamine is also involved in other body functions, including blood-vessel dilation and constriction, contraction of muscles in the respiratory and gastrointestinal tracts, and the release of digestive juices. The antihistamines described here are also known as H_1 blockers because they only block the action of histamine on certain receptors, called H_1 receptors. Another group of antihistamines, called H_2 blockers, is used in the treatment of peptic ulcers (see Anti-ulcer drugs, p.43).

Some antihistamines have a marked anticholinergic action (see Drugs that act on the parasympathetic nervous system, p.9). This is used to advantage in various conditions but also accounts for certain undesired effects.

WHY THEY ARE USED

Antihistamines relieve allergy-related symptoms when it is not possible to prevent exposure to the substance that has provoked the reaction. They are most commonly used in preventing allergic rhinitis (hay fever). In this condition, histamine released in response to an allergen, such as pollen, dust, animal fur, or feathers, acts on histamine receptors and produces dilation of the blood vessels supplying the lining of the nose, leading to swelling and increased mucus production. There is also irritation that causes sneezing and, often, redness and watering of the eyes. The drugs are more effective when taken before an attack starts; if taken after the start of an attack, beneficial effects may be delayed.

Antihistamines are not usually effective in asthma caused by similar allergens because the symptoms of this allergic disorder are not solely caused by the action of histamine, but are likely to be the result of more complex mechanisms. Antihistamines are usually the first drugs to be tried in the treatment of allergic disorders but alternatives can be prescribed (see Other allergy treatments, p.60).

Antihistamines are also prescribed for the itching, swelling, and redness of allergic reactions involving the skin (such as urticaria (hives) and dermatitis) and the irritation of chickenpox. The drugs may also reduce allergic reactions to insect stings. In such cases they may be taken by mouth or applied topically. Applied as drops, antihistamines can reduce inflammation and irritation of the eyes and eyelids in allergic conjunctivitis.

Antihistamines are often included in cold and cough preparations (see p.28), when the anticholinergic effect and sedative effect on the coughing mechanism may be helpful.

Because most antihistamines have a depressant effect on the brain, they are sometimes used to promote sleep, especially when it is disturbed by itching (see also Sleeping drugs, p.11). Antihistamines' depressant effect on the brain also extends to the centres that control nausea and vomiting. The drugs are therefore often effective in preventing and controlling these symptoms (see Anti-emetics, p.21).

Occasionally, antihistamines are used to treat fever, rash, and breathing difficulties that may occur in adverse reactions to blood transfusions and allergic reactions to drugs. Promethazine and trimeprazine are also used as premedication and to dry secretions during surgery, particularly in children.

HOW THEY WORK

Antihistamines block the action of histamine on H_1 receptors, which are found in various body tissues, particularly the small blood vessels in the skin, nose, and eyes. This helps prevent the dilation of the vessels, caused by the release of histamine in allergic reactions, thus reducing the redness, watering, and swelling typical of many types of allergy. Also, the drugs' anticholinergic action contributes to this effect by reducing secretions from tear glands and nasal passages. Antihistamines pass from the blood into the brain, where they produce general sedation and depression of various brain functions, including the vomiting and coughing mechanisms.

HOW THEY AFFECT YOU

Some antihistamines can cause a degree of drowsiness and may adversely affect coordination, leading to clumsiness. However, there are a number of newer drugs which have little or no sedative effect (see table, p.60).

Anticholinergic side effects, including dry mouth, blurred vision, and difficulty passing urine, are common. Most diminish with continued use and can often be helped by adjusting the dose or changing to a different drug.

RISKS AND SPECIAL PRECAUTIONS

It is advisable not to drive or operate machinery while taking antihistamines, particularly those more likely to cause drowsiness (see table, p.60). The sedative effects of alcohol, sleeping drugs, opioid analgesics, and anti-anxiety drugs add to those of antihistamines.

In high doses, or in children, some antihistamines can cause excitement, agitation, and, in extreme cases, hallucinations and convulsions. Abnormal heart rhythms have occurred after high doses or when drugs that interact with them (such as antifungals and antibiotics) have been taken at the same time. Heart-rhythm problems may also affect people with liver disease, electrolyte disturbances, or abnormal heart activity. People with these conditions, or glaucoma or prostate trouble, should seek medical advice before taking antihistamines because the various actions of these drugs may make such conditions worse.

COMMON DRUGS

Non-sedating Acrivastine, Cetirizine*, Fexofenadine, Levocetirizine, Loratadine/Desloratadine *, Mizolastine

Sedating Alimemazine, Azatadine, Brompheniramine, Chlorphenamine*, Cinnarizine*, Clemastine, Cyclizine, Dimenhydrinate, Diphenhydramine, Diphenylpyraline, Doxylamine, Hydroxyzine, Promethazine*, Triprolidine

* See Part 2

OTHER ALLERGY TREATMENTS

Sodium cromoglicate This drug (see p.386) prevents the release of histamine from mast cells (see p.58) in response to exposure to an allergen, thereby preventing the physical symptoms of allergies. Sodium cromoglicate is commonly given by inhaler for the prevention of allergy-induced rhinitis (hay fever) or asthma attacks and by drops for the treatment of allergic eye disorders.

Leukotriene antagonists Like histamine, leukotrienes are substances that occur naturally in the body and seem to play an important part in asthma. Drugs such as montelukast (see p.323) and zafirlukast (leukotriene antagonists) have been developed to prevent asthma attack from occurring. They are not bronchodilators, however, and will not relieve an existing attack (see Drugs for asthma, p.24).

Corticosteroids These drugs for allergic rhinitis and asthma are usually given by inhaler, providing a high dose to the affected area. The dose of the drug to the rest of the body is very low, reducing the risk of long-term adverse effects.

Desensitization This may be tried in conditions such as allergic rhinitis due to pollen sensitivity and insect venom hypersensitivity, when avoidance, antihistamines, and other treatments have not been effective and tests have shown one or two specific allergens to be responsible. Desensitization often provides incomplete relief and can be time-consuming.

Treatment involves a series of injections containing increasing doses of an extract of the allergen. It is not understood how this prevents allergic reactions, but controlled exposure may trigger the immune system into producing increasing levels of antibodies so that the body no longer responds dramatically when the allergen is encountered naturally.

Desensitization must be carried out under medical supervision because it can provoke a severe allergic response. It is important to remain near emergency medical facilities for at least one hour after each injection.

COMPARISON OF ANTIHISTAMINES

The table below indicates the main uses of some common antihistamines and lists their relative strength of anticholinergic action, sedative effects, and duration of action.

KEY

● Drug used ■ Strong ◪ Medium □ Minimal
▲ Long (over 12 hours) ▲ Medium (6–12 hours)
△ Short (4–6 hours)

DRUGS	COMMON USES Allergic rhinitis	Skin allergy	Sedation	Premedication	Nausea/vomiting	Cough/cold remedies	ACTIONS AND EFFECTS Sedation/ drowsiness	Anticholinergic action	DURATION OF ACTION
Alimemazine	●	●	●				■	□	▲
Azatadine	●	●					◪	◪	▲
Brompheniramine	●	●				●	◪	□	△
Cetirizine	●	●					□	□	▲
Chlorphenamine	●	●	●				◪	◪	△
Cyclizine					●		◪	◪	△
Diphenhydramine			●		●	●	◪	◪	△
Diphenylpyraline	●	●					■	◪	▲
Hydroxyzine		●	●				◪	◪	▲
Loratadine	●	●					□	□	▲
Promethazine	●	●	●	●		●	■	◪	▲
Triprolidine	●	●				●	□	□	▲

INFECTIONS AND INFESTATIONS

The human body provides a suitable environment for the growth of many types of microorganism, including bacteria, viruses, fungi, yeasts, and protozoa. It may also become the host for animal parasites such as insects, worms, and flukes.

Microorganisms (microbes) exist all around us and can be transmitted from person to person in many ways: direct contact, inhalation of infected air, and consumption of contaminated food or water. Not all microorganisms cause disease; many types of bacteria exist on the skin surface or in the bowel without causing ill effects, while others cannot live either in or on the body.

Normally the immune system protects the body from infection. Invading microbes are killed before they can multiply in sufficient numbers to cause serious disease. (See also Malignant and immune disease, p.95.)

TYPES OF INFECTING ORGANISM

A typical bacterium consists of a single cell with a protective wall. Some bacteria are aerobic (requiring oxygen) and are therefore more likely to infect surface areas such as the skin or respiratory tract. Others are anaerobic and multiply in oxygen-free surroundings such as the bowel or deep wounds. Bacteria can cause symptoms of disease in two principal ways: by releasing toxins that harm body cells and by provoking an inflammatory response in the infected tissues.

Viruses are smaller than bacteria and consist simply of a core of genetic material surrounded by a protein coat. A virus can multiply only in a living cell, by using the host tissue's replicating material.

Protozoa are single-celled parasites and are slightly bigger than bacteria. Many protozoa live in the human intestine and are harmless. However, other types cause malaria, sleeping sickness, and dysentery.

INFESTATIONS

Invasion by parasites that live on the body (such as lice) or in the body (such as tapeworms) is known as infestation. Since the body lacks strong natural defences against infestation, antiparasitic treatment is necessary. Infestation is often associated with tropical climates and poor standards of hygiene.

WHAT CAN GO WRONG

Infectious diseases occur when the body is invaded by microbes. This may be caused by the body having little or no natural immunity to the invading organism, or the number of invading microbes being too great for the body's immune system to overcome. Serious infections can occur when the immune system does not function properly, as in malnourished or elderly people, or when a disease weakens or destroys the immune system, as occurs in AIDS (acquired immune deficiency syndrome).

Infections can cause generalized illness (as in childhood infectious diseases or those with flu-like symptoms), or they may affect a specific part of the body (as in wound infections). Some parts are more susceptible to infection than others – respiratory tract infections are relatively common, whereas bone and muscle infections are rare.

Some symptoms are the result of damage to body tissues by the infection, or by toxins released by the microbes. In other cases, they result from the body's defence mechanisms.

Most bacterial and viral infections cause fever; bacterial infections may also result in pus and inflammation in the affected area.

WHY DRUGS ARE USED

Treatment of an infection is necessary only when the type or severity of symptoms shows that the immune system has not overcome the infection.

Bacterial infection can be treated with antibiotic or antibacterial drugs. Some of these drugs kill the infecting bacteria; others simply prevent them from multiplying. Unnecessary use of antibiotics, however, may result in the development of resistant bacteria.

Some antibiotics can be used to treat a broad range of infections, while others are effective against particular types of bacteria or in a certain part of the body. Antibiotics are most commonly given by mouth, or by injection in severe infections, but they may be applied topically for a local action.

Antiviral drugs are used for severe viral infections that threaten body organs or survival. Antivirals may be used in topical preparations, given by mouth, or administered in hospital by injection.

Other drugs used to fight infection include antiprotozoal drugs for protozoal infections such as malaria; antifungal drugs for infection by fungi and yeasts, including *Candida* (thrush); and anthelmintics to eradicate worm and fluke infestations. Infestation by skin parasites is usually treated with the topical application of insecticides (see p.118).

MAJOR DRUG GROUPS
- Antibiotics
- Drugs for meningitis
- Antibacterial drugs
- Drug treatment for Hansen's disease
- Antituberculous drugs
- Antiviral drugs
- Vaccines and immunization
- Antiprotozoal drugs
- Antimalarial drugs
- Antifungal drugs
- Anthelmintic drugs

Antibiotics

One in six prescriptions that British doctors write every year is for antibiotics. These drugs are usually safe and effective in the treatment of bacterial disorders ranging from minor infections, such as conjunctivitis, to life-threatening diseases such as pneumonia, meningitis, and septicaemia. They are similar in function to the antibacterial drugs (see p.66), but the early antibiotics all had a natural origin in moulds and fungi, although most are now synthesized.

Since 1941, when the first antibiotic, penicillin, was introduced, many different classes have been developed. Each one has a different chemical composition and is effective against a particular range of bacteria. None is effective against viral infections (see Antiviral drugs, p.69).

Some of the antibiotics have a broad spectrum of activity against a wide variety of bacteria. Others are used in the treatment of infection by only a few specific organisms. For a description of each common class of antibiotic, see Classes of antibiotic, p.64.

WHY THEY ARE USED
We are surrounded by bacteria – in the air we breathe, on the mucous membranes of our mouth and nose, on our skin, and in our intestines – but we are protected, most of the time, by our immunological defences. When these break down, or when bacteria already present migrate to a vulnerable new site, or when harmful bacteria not usually present invade the body, infectious disease sets in.

The bacteria multiply uncontrollably, destroying tissue, releasing toxins, and, in some cases, threatening to spread via the bloodstream to such vital organs as the heart, brain, lungs, and kidneys. The symptoms of infectious disease vary widely, depending on the site of the infection and type of bacteria.

Confronted with a sick person and suspecting a bacterial infection, the doctor identifies the organism causing the disease before prescribing any drug. However, tests to analyse blood, sputum, urine, stool, or pus usually take 24 hours or more. In the meantime, especially if the person is in discomfort or pain, the doctor usually makes a preliminary drug choice, based on an educated guess as to the causative organism. In starting this "empirical" treatment, as it is called, the doctor is guided by the site of the infection, the nature and severity of the symptoms, the likely source of infection, and the prevalence of any similar illnesses in the community at that time.

In such circumstances, pending laboratory identification of the trouble-making bacteria, the doctor may initially prescribe a broad-spectrum antibiotic, which is effective against a wide variety of bacteria. As soon as tests provide more exact information, the doctor may switch the person to the recommended antibiotic treatment for the identified bacteria. In some cases, more than one antibiotic is prescribed, to be sure of eliminating all strains of bacteria.

In most cases, antibiotics can be given by mouth. However, in serious infections when

USES OF ANTIBIOTICS

The table below shows common drugs in each class of antibiotic used to treat infections in different parts of the body. (It is not intended as a guide to prescribing.) For comparison, some antibacterial drugs (p.66) are included under "Sulphonamides" and "Other drugs".

ANTIBIOTIC / SITE OF INFECTION	Ear, nose, throat, and mouth	Respiratory tract	Skin and soft tissue	Gastrointestinal tract	Eye	Kidney and urinary tract	Brain and nervous system	Heart and blood	Bones and joints	Genital tract
Penicillins										
Amoxicillin	●	●	●			●		●	●	●
Ampicillin	●	●	●			●	●		●	●
Benzylpenicillin	●	●	●			●	●	●	●	
Co-amoxiclav	●	●	●			●			●	
Flucloxacillin	●		●					●	●	
Phenoxymethylpenicillin	●	●	●							
Cephalosporins										
Cefaclor	●	●				●				
Cefalexin		●	●			●				
Cefotaxime		●		●			●	●		
Cefoxitin		●	●			●				●
Macrolides										
Azithromycin	●	●	●							●
Clarithromycin	●	●	●	●						
Erythromycin	●	●	●	●					●	●
Tetracyclines										
Doxycycline	●	●				●				●
Oxytetracycline	●	●								
Tetracycline	●	●			●	●				●
Aminoglycosides										
Amikacin		●	●	●		●	●		●	
Gentamicin		●	●	●	●	●	●	●	●	
Neomycin		●	●							
Netilmicin		●	●	●		●	●		●	
Streptomycin		●						●		
Tobramycin		●	●	●		●	●		●	
Sulphonamides										
Co-trimoxazole		●				●				
Other drugs										
Chloramphenicol	●	●		●	●	●				
Ciprofloxacin		●		●		●				●
Clindamycin		●	●	●					●	
Colistin		●				●				
Dapsone			●							
Fusidic acid			●					●	●	
Metronidazole	●		●	●			●	●	●	●
Nalidixic acid						●				
Nitrofurantoin						●				
Teicoplanin				●				●	●	
Trimethoprim		●		●		●				
Tinidazole	●									●
Vancomycin				●				●		

high blood levels of the drug are needed rapidly, or when a type of antibiotic is needed that cannot be given by mouth, the drug may be given by injection. Antibiotics are also included in topical preparations for localized skin, eye, and ear infections (see also Anti-infective skin preparations, p.120, and Drugs for ear disorders, p.117).

HOW THEY WORK

Depending on the type of drug and the dosage, antibiotics are either bactericidal, killing organisms directly, or bacteriostatic, halting the multiplication of bacteria and enabling the body's natural defences to overcome the remaining infection.

Penicillins and cephalosporins are bactericidal, destroying bacteria by preventing them from making normal cell walls. Most other antibiotics act inside the bacteria by interfering with the chemical activities essential to their life cycle.

CLASSES OF ANTIBIOTIC

Penicillins The first antibiotic drugs to be developed, penicillins are still widely used to treat many common infections. Some are not effective when they are taken by mouth and therefore have to be given by injection in hospital. Unfortunately, certain strains of bacteria are resistant to penicillin treatment, and other drugs may have to be substituted. Penicillins often cause allergic reactions.

Cephalosporins These broad-spectrum antibiotics, similar to the penicillins, are often used when penicillin treatment has proved ineffective. Some can be given by mouth, but others are only given by injection. About 10 per cent of people who are allergic to penicillins are also allergic to cephalosporins. Some cephalosporins can occasionally damage the kidneys, particularly if used with aminoglycosides. Another serious, although rare, adverse effect of a few cephalosporins is that they may interfere with normal blood clotting, leading to abnormally heavy bleeding, especially in elderly people.

Macrolides Erythromycin is the most common drug in this group. It is a broad-spectrum antibiotic that is often prescribed as an alternative to penicillins or cephalosporins. Erythromycin is also effective against certain diseases, such as Legionnaires' disease (a rare type of pneumonia), that cannot be treated with other antibiotics. The main risk with erythromycin is that it can occasionally impair liver function.

Tetracyclines These have a broader spectrum of activity than other classes of antibiotic. However, increasing bacterial resistance (see Antibiotic resistance, facing page) has limited their use, but they are still widely prescribed. As well as being used for the treatment of infections, tetracyclines are also used in the long-term treatment of acne, although this application is probably not related to their antibacterial action. A major drawback to the use of tetracycline antibiotics in pregnant women and young children is that they are deposited in developing bones and teeth.

With the exception of doxycycline, drugs from this group are poorly absorbed through the intestines, and when given by mouth they have to be administered in high doses in order to reach effective levels in the blood. Such high doses increase the likelihood of diarrhoea as a side effect. The absorption of tetracyclines can be further reduced by interaction with calcium and other minerals. Drugs from this group should not therefore be taken with iron tablets or milk products. Tetracyclines deteriorate and may become poisonous with time, so leftover tablets or capsules should always be discarded.

Aminoglycosides These potent drugs are effective against a wide range of bacteria. They are not as widely used as some other antibiotics, however, since they have to be given by injection and have potentially serious side effects. Their use is therefore limited to hospital treatment of serious infections. They are often given with other antibiotics. Possible adverse effects include a severe skin rash and damage to the kidneys and nerves in the ear.

Lincosamides The lincosamide clindamycin is not commonly used because it is more likely than other antibiotics to cause serious disruption of bacterial activity in the bowel. It is reserved mainly for treating bone, joint, abdominal, and pelvic infections that do not respond well to the safer antibiotics. It is also used topically for acne and vaginal infections.

Quinolones These drugs, often called antibacterials, are derived from chemicals rather than living organisms. Quinolones have a wide spectrum of activity. They are used in the treatment of urinary infections and are widely effective in acute diarrhoeal diseases, including that caused by salmonella, as well as in the treatment of enteric fever.

The absorption of quinolones is reduced by antacids containing magnesium and aluminium. Quinolones are well tolerated but should be avoided by people with epilepsy because they may, rarely, cause convulsions. Their use should also be avoided in children because studies have shown that they may cause arthritis.

HOW THEY AFFECT YOU

Antibiotics stop most common types of infection within days. Because they do not relieve symptoms directly, your doctor may advise additional medication, such as analgesics (see p.9), to relieve pain and fever until the antibiotics take effect.

It is important to complete the course of medication as prescribed by your doctor, even if all your symptoms have disappeared. Failure to do this can lead to a resurgence of the infection in an antibiotic-resistant form (see Antibiotic resistance, below).

Most antibiotics used in the home do not cause adverse effects if taken in the recommended dosage. In people who do experience adverse effects, nausea and diarrhoea are common. (See also individual drug profiles in Part 2.) Some people may be sensitive to certain types of antibiotic, which can result in a variety of serious adverse effects.

ANTIBIOTIC RESISTANCE

The increasing use of antibiotics in the treatment of infection has led certain types of bacteria to become resistant to the effects of particular antibiotics. This resistance to the drug usually occurs when bacteria develop mechanisms of growth and reproduction that are not disrupted by the effects of the antibiotics. In other cases, bacteria produce enzymes that neutralize the antibiotics.

Antibiotic resistance may develop in a person during prolonged treatment when a drug has failed to eliminate the infection quickly. The resistant strain of bacteria is able to multiply, thereby prolonging the illness. It may also infect other people and result in the spread of resistant infection.

One particularly important example is methicillin-resistant staphylococcus aureus (MRSA), which resists most antibiotics but can be treated with other drugs such as teicoplanin and vancomycin.

Doctors try to prevent the development of antibiotic resistance by selecting the drug most likely to eliminate the bacteria present in each individual case as quickly and as thoroughly as possible. Failure to complete a course of antibiotics that has been prescribed by your doctor increases the likelihood that the infection will recur in a resistant form.

RISKS AND SPECIAL PRECAUTIONS

Most antibiotics that are used for short periods outside of a hospital setting are safe for most people. The most common risk, especially with cephalosporins and penicillins, is a severe allergic reaction to the drug that can cause a rash and sometimes swelling of the face and throat. If this happens, you should stop taking the drug and seek immediate medical advice. If you have had a previous allergic reaction to an antibiotic, all other drugs in that class and related classes should be avoided. It is therefore important to inform your doctor if you have previously suffered an adverse reaction to treatment with an antibiotic (with the exception of minor bowel disturbances).

Another risk of antibiotic treatment, especially if it is prolonged, is that the balance among microorganisms normally inhabiting the body may be disturbed. In particular, antibiotics may destroy the bacteria that normally limit the growth of *Candida*, a yeast that is often present in small amounts in the body. This can lead to overgrowth of *Candida* (thrush) in the mouth, vagina, or bowel, and an antifungal drug (p.76) may be needed.

A rarer, but more serious, result of the disruption of normal bacterial activity in the body is a disorder known as pseudomembranous colitis, in which bacteria that are resistant to the antibiotic multiply in the bowel, causing violent, bloody diarrhoea. This potentially fatal disorder can occur with any antibiotic but is most common with the lincosamides.

COMMON DRUGS

Aminoglycosides Amikacin, Gentamicin*, Neomycin, Netilmicin, Streptomycin, Tobramycin

Cephalosporins Cefaclor, Cefadroxil, Cefalexin*, Cefamandole, Cefixime, Cefoxitin, Cefpodoxime, Ceftazidime

Lincosamides Clindamycin

Macrolides Azithromycin, Clarithromycin*, Erythromycin*

Penicillins Amoxicillin*, Ampicillin, Azlocillin, Benzylpenicillin, Co-amoxiclav, Co-fluampicil, Flucloxacillin*, Phenoxymethylpenicillin*, Piperacillin

Tetracyclines Doxycycline*, Oxytetracycline, Tetracycline*

Other drugs Aztreonam, Chloramphenicol*, Colistin, Fusidic acid, Imipenem, Linezolid, Metronidazole*, Rifampicin*, Teicoplanin, Trimethoprim*, Vancomycin

* **See Part 2**

Drugs for meningitis

Meningitis is inflammation of the meninges (the membranes surrounding the brain and spinal cord), and it can be caused by both bacteria and viruses. Bacterial meningitis can kill previously well individuals within hours.

If bacterial meningitis is suspected, intramuscular or intravenous antibiotics will be needed immediately, and admission to hospital is arranged.

In cases of bacterial meningitis caused by *Haemophilus influenzae* or *Neisseria meningitidis*, people who have been in contact with an infected person are advised to have a preventative course of antibiotics, usually rifampicin (see p.373).

Antibacterial drugs

This broad class of drugs comprises agents similar to the antibiotics (p.62) in function but dissimilar in origin. The original antibiotics were derived from living organisms such as moulds and fungi. Antibacterials were developed from chemicals. The sulphonamides were the first drugs to be used for bacterial infections and were the mainstay of infection treatment before penicillin (the first antibiotic) became generally available. Increasing bacterial resistance and the development of more effective and less toxic antibiotics have reduced the use of sulphonamides.

WHY THEY ARE USED

Sulphonamides are especially useful for treating urinary tract infections because high concentrations of the drug reach the urine. They are also often used for chlamydial pneumonia and some middle ear infections.

Trimethoprim is used for chest and urinary tract infections. The drug used to be combined with sulfamethoxazole as co-trimoxazole, but because of the side effects of sulfamethoxazole, trimethoprim on its own is usually preferred now.

Antibacterials used in the treatment of tuberculosis are discussed on p.67. Others, sometimes classified as antimicrobials, include metronidazole, which is prescribed to treat a variety of genital infections and for some serious infections of the abdomen, pelvic region, heart, and central nervous system. Certain antibacterials are used to treat urinary infections. These include nitrofurantoin and drugs in the quinolone group, such as nalidixic acid (see Classes of antibiotic, p.64), which is used as a urinary tract antiseptic and to cure or prevent recurrent infections. The quinolones are effective against a broad spectrum of bacteria. More potent relatives of nalidixic acid include norfloxacin, used to treat urinary tract infections, and ciprofloxacin, levofloxacin, and ofloxacin. These are all used to treat many serious bacterial infections.

HOW THEY WORK

Most antibacterials function by preventing the growth and multiplication of bacteria. As an example, folic acid, a chemical necessary for the growth of bacteria, is produced within bacterial cells by an enzyme that acts on a chemical called para-aminobenzoic acid. Sulphonamides interfere with the release of the enzyme. This prevents folic acid from being formed. The bacterium is therefore unable to function properly and dies.

HOW THEY AFFECT YOU

Antibacterials usually take several days to eliminate bacteria. During this time your doctor may recommend additional medication to alleviate pain and fever. Possible side effects of sulphonamides include loss of appetite, nausea, a rash, and drowsiness.

RISKS AND SPECIAL PRECAUTIONS

Like antibiotics, most antibacterials can cause allergic reactions in susceptible people. Possible symptoms that should always be brought to your doctor's attention include rashes and fever. If such symptoms occur, a change to another drug is likely to be necessary. Treatment with sulphonamides carries a number of serious but rare risks. Some drugs in this group can cause crystals to form in the kidneys, a risk that can be reduced by drinking adequate amounts of fluid during prolonged treatment. Sulphonamides may also occasionally damage the liver, so they are not usually prescribed for people with impaired liver function. There is also a slight risk of damage to bone marrow, lowering the production of white blood cells and increasing the chances of infection. Doctors therefore try to avoid prescribing sulphonamides for prolonged periods. If long-term treatment is unavoidable, liver function and blood composition are often regularly monitored.

COMMON DRUGS

Quinolones Ciprofloxacin*, Levofloxacin*, Nalidixic acid, Norfloxacin, Ofloxacin
Sulphonamides Co-trimoxazole*, Sulfadiazine
Urinary antiseptic Nitrofurantoin
Other drugs Clofazimine, Dapsone, Metronidazole*, Tinidazole, Trimethoprim*
* See Part 2

Drug treatment for Hansen's disease

Hansen's disease, more commonly known as leprosy, is a bacterial infection caused by *Mycobacterium leprae*. It is rare in the United Kingdom but relatively common in parts of Africa, Asia, and Latin America.

Hansen's disease progresses slowly, first affecting the peripheral nerves and causing loss of sensation in the hands and feet. This leads to frequent unnoticed injuries and consequent scarring. Later, the nerves of the face may also be affected.

Treatment involves the use of three drugs together to prevent the development of resistance. Usually, dapsone, rifampicin, and clofazimine will be given for at least 2 years. If one of these drugs cannot be used, then a second-line drug (ofloxacin, minocycline, or clarithromycin) might be substituted. Complications during treatment may require use of prednisolone, aspirin, chloroquine, or even thalidomide.

Antituberculous drugs

Tuberculosis is an infectious bacterial disease that is acquired, often in childhood, by inhaling tuberculosis bacilli from spray sneezed or coughed by someone who is actively infected. It may also be acquired from infected cow's milk. The disease usually starts in a lung and takes one of two forms: either primary infection or reactivated infection.

In 90 to 95 per cent of those people with a primary infection, the body's immune system suppresses the infection, but it does not kill the bacilli. They remain alive but dormant and may cause the reactivated form of tuberculosis. After the tuberculosis bacilli are reactivated, they may spread throughout the body via the lymphatic system and the bloodstream.

The first symptoms of the primary infection may include a cough, fever, tiredness, night sweats, and loss of weight. Tuberculosis is confirmed through clinical investigations, which may include a chest X-ray, isolation of the bacilli from the person's sputum, and a positive reaction (localized inflammation) to the Mantoux test, an injection of tuberculin (a protein extracted from tuberculosis bacilli) into the skin.

The gradual emergence in adults of the destructive and progressive form of tuberculosis is caused by the reactivated infection. It occurs in 5 to 10 per cent of those who have had a previous primary infection. Another form, reinfection tuberculosis, occurs when someone with the dormant, primary form is reinfected. This type of tuberculosis is clinically identical to the reactivated form.

Reactivation is more likely in those people whose immune system is suppressed, such as the elderly, those on corticosteroids or other immunosuppressant drugs, and those who have AIDS. Reactivation tuberculosis may be difficult to identify because the symptoms may start in any part of the body seeded with the bacilli. It is most often first seen in the upper lobes of the lung, and is frequently diagnosed after a chest X-ray. The early symptoms may be identical to those of primary infection: a cough, tiredness, night sweats, fever, and loss of weight.

If left untreated, tuberculosis continues to destroy tissue, spreading throughout the body and eventually causing death. It was one of the most common causes of death in the United Kingdom until the 1940s and the disease is on the increase again. Vulnerable groups are people with suppressed immune systems and the homeless.

WHY THEY ARE USED

A person diagnosed as having tuberculosis is likely to be treated with three or four antituberculous drugs. This helps to overcome the risk of drug-resistant strains of the bacilli emerging (see Antibiotic resistance, p.65).

The standard drug combination for the treatment of tuberculosis consists of four drugs, usually including rifampicin, isoniazid, pyrazinamide, and ethambutol. Other drugs may be substituted if the initial treatment fails or if drug sensitivity tests indicate that the bacilli are resistant to these drugs.

The standard duration of treatment for a newly diagnosed tuberculosis infection is a six-month regimen as follows: isoniazid, rifampicin, pyrazinamide, and ethambutol daily for two months, followed by isoniazid and rifampicin for four months. The duration of treatment can be extended from nine months to up to two years in people at particular risk, such as those whose immune system has been suppressed. Ethambutol can sometimes be omitted if resistance is unlikely. Corticosteroids may be added to the treatment, if the immune system is not suppressed, to reduce the amount of tissue damage; and pyridoxine (see Vitamins, p.90) is also often prescribed to protect the nerves from damage by isoniazid.

Both the number of drugs required and the long duration of treatment may make treatment difficult, particularly for those who are homeless. To help with this problem, supervised administration of treatment is available when required, both in the community and in hospital.

Tuberculosis infection in patients with HIV infection or AIDS is treated with the standard antituberculous drug regimen, but lifelong preventative treatment with isoniazid may be necessary.

HOW THEY WORK

Antituberculous drugs act in the same way as antibiotics, either by killing bacilli or preventing them from multiplying. (See also antibiotics, p.62.)

HOW THEY AFFECT YOU

Although the drugs start to combat the disease within days, the benefits of drug treatment are not usually noticeable for a few weeks. As the infection is eradicated, the body repairs the damage caused by the disease. Symptoms such as fever and coughing gradually subside, and the appetite and general health improve.

RISKS AND SPECIAL PRECAUTIONS

Antituberculous drugs may cause adverse effects (nausea, vomiting, and abdominal pain), and they occasionally lead to serious allergic reactions. When this happens, another drug is substituted.

Rifampicin and isoniazid may affect liver function; isoniazid may adversely affect the nerves as well. Ethambutol can cause changes in colour vision. Dosage is carefully monitored, especially in children, the elderly, and those with reduced kidney function.

TUBERCULOSIS PREVENTION

A vaccine prepared from an artificially weakened strain of cattle tuberculosis bacteria can provide immunity from tuberculosis by provoking the development of natural resistance to the disease (see Vaccines and immunization, p.70). The BCG (Bacille Calmette-Guérin) vaccine is a form of tuberculosis bacillus that provokes the body's immune response but does not cause the illness because it does not invade tissues. The vaccine is usually given to children between the ages of 10 and 14 years who are shown to have no natural immunity when given a skin test. BCG vaccination may be given to newborn babies if, for example, someone in the family has tuberculosis.

The vaccine is usually injected into the upper arm. A small pustule usually appears 6–12 weeks later, by which time the person can be considered immune.

COMMON DRUGS

Capreomycin, Cycloserine, Ethambutol*, Isoniazid*, Pyrazinamide, Rifabutin, Rifampicin*, Streptomycin
* See Part 2

Antiviral drugs

Viruses are simpler and smaller organisms than bacteria and are less able to sustain themselves. These organisms can survive and multiply only by penetrating body cells. In order to reproduce, a virus requires a living cell. The invaded cell eventually dies and the new viruses are released, spreading and infecting other cells. Because viruses perform few functions independently, medicines that disrupt or halt their life cycle without harming human cells have been difficult to develop.

There are many different types of virus, and viral infections cause illnesses with various symptoms and degrees of severity. Common viral illnesses include colds, influenza and flu-like illnesses, cold sores, and childhood diseases such as chickenpox and mumps. Throat infections, pneumonia, acute bronchitis, gastroenteritis, and meningitis are often, but not always, caused by a virus.

Fortunately, the body's natural defences are usually strong enough to overcome infections such as these, with drugs given to ease pain and lower fever. However, the more serious viral diseases, such as pneumonia and meningitis, need close medical supervision.

Another difficulty with viral infections is the speed at which the virus multiplies. By the time symptoms appear, the viruses are so numerous that antiviral drugs have little effect. Antivirals must be given early in the course of the infection; they may also be used as a prophylactic (preventative). Some viral infections can be prevented by vaccination (see p.70).

WHY THEY ARE USED

Antiviral drugs are helpful in the treatment of the various herpes virus infections: cold sores, encephalitis, genital herpes, chickenpox, and shingles.

Aciclovir and penciclovir are applied topically to treat cold sores, herpes eye infections, and genital herpes. They can reduce the severity and duration of an outbreak, but they do not eliminate the infection permanently. The drugs aciclovir, famciclovir, and valaciclovir are given by mouth or, under exceptional circumstances, by injection to prevent chickenpox or severe, recurrent attacks of the herpes virus infections in those already weakened by other conditions.

Influenza may sometimes be prevented by oseltamivir or treated with zanamivir. Oseltamivir may also be used to treat at-risk people (such as those aged over 65 or those who have respiratory diseases such as COPD (chronic obstructive pulmonary disease) or asthma, cardiovascular disease, kidney disease, immunosuppression, or diabetes mellitus).

Interferons are proteins produced by the body and involved in the immune response and cell function. Interferon alpha and beta are effective in reducing the activity of hepatitis B and hepatitis C. Lamivudine is also used to treat hepatitis B, and ribavirin is used for hepatitis C.

Ganciclovir is sometimes used for cytomegalovirus (CMV). Respiratory syncytial virus (RSV) has been treated with ribavirin, and prevented by palivizumab. Drug treatment for AIDS is discussed on p.100.

HOW THEY WORK

Some antiviral drugs, such as idoxuridine, act by altering the cell's genetic material (DNA) so that the virus cannot use it to multiply. Other drugs stop the multiplication of viruses by blocking enzyme activity within the host cell. Halting multiplication prevents the virus from spreading to uninfected cells and improves symptoms rapidly. However, in herpes infections, it does not eradicate the virus from the body. Infection may therefore flare up on another occasion.

HOW THEY AFFECT YOU

Topical antiviral drugs usually start to act at once. Providing that the treatment is applied early enough, an outbreak of herpes can be cut short. Symptoms usually clear up within two to four days. Antiviral ointments may cause irritation and redness. Antiviral drugs given by mouth or injection can occasionally cause nausea and dizziness.

RISKS AND SPECIAL PRECAUTIONS

Because some of these drugs may adversely affect the kidneys, they are prescribed with caution to people with reduced kidney function. Some antivirals can adversely affect the activity of normal body cells, particularly those in the bone marrow. For this reason, idoxuridine is available only in topical form.

COMMON DRUGS

Aciclovir*, Amantadine, Cidofovir, Famciclovir, Fomivirsen, Foscarnet, Ganciclovir, Idoxuridine, Inosine pranobex, Interferon*, Lamivudine, Oseltamivir, Palivizumab, Penciclovir, Ribavirin, Valaciclovir, Valganciclovir, Zanamivir*

* See Part 2

Vaccines and immunization

Many infectious diseases, including most of the common viral infections, occur only once during a person's life. The reason is that the antibodies produced in response to the disease remain afterwards, prepared to repel any future invasion as soon as the first infectious germs appear. The duration of such immunity varies, but it can last a lifetime.

Protection against many infections can now be provided artificially by use of vaccines derived from altered forms of the infecting organism. These vaccines stimulate the immune system in the same way as a genuine infection, and provide lasting, active immunity. Since each type of microbe stimulates production of a specific antibody, a different vaccine must be given for each disease.

Another type of immunization, called passive immunization, relies on giving antibodies (see Immune globulins, p.72).

WHY THEY ARE USED

Some infectious diseases cannot be treated effectively or are potentially so serious that prevention is the best treatment. Routine immunization not only protects the individual but may gradually eradicate the disease completely, as has been achieved with smallpox.

Newborn babies receive antibodies for many diseases from their mothers, but this protection lasts only for about three months. Most children between the ages of 2 months and 15 years are routinely vaccinated against common childhood infectious diseases. In addition, travellers to many underdeveloped countries, especially those in the tropics, are often advised to be vaccinated against the diseases common in those regions. Rabies, yellow fever, and hepatitis B vaccines may be required for remote areas.

Effective lifelong immunization can sometimes be achieved by a single dose of the vaccine. However, in many cases, reinforcing doses, commonly called booster shots, are needed later to maintain reliable immunity.

Vaccines do not provide immediate protection against infection and it may be up to four weeks before full immunity is able to develop. When immediate protection from infectious disease is needed – for example, following exposure to infection – it may be necessary to establish passive immunity with immune globulins (see p.72).

HOW THEY WORK

Vaccines provoke the immune system into creating antibodies that help the body to resist specific infectious diseases. Many vaccines (known as live vaccines) are made from artificially weakened forms of the disease-causing germ; even these weakened germs are effective in stimulating sufficient growth of antibodies. Other vaccines rely either on inactive (or killed) disease-causing germs, or inactive derivatives of these germs, but their effect on the immune system remains the same. Effective antibodies are created, thereby establishing active immunity.

HOW THEY AFFECT YOU

The degree of protection offered by different vaccines varies. Some of them provide reliable lifelong immunity, whereas others may

COMMON VACCINATIONS

Most vaccinations are given during infancy and childhood as part of a routine immunization schedule, and most are given by injection. Those people at particular risk through their work or travel can have additional immunization in adulthood.

DISEASE	AGE AT WHICH VACCINATION IS GIVEN
Diphtheria	2 months, 3 months, 4 months, 3–5 years. Booster 13–18 years.
Tetanus	2 months, 3 months, 4 months, 3–5 years. Booster 13–18 years. 5 doses usually gives adults lifelong immunity.
Acellular pertussis (whooping cough)	2 months, 3 months, 4 months, 3–5 years
Inactivated polio	2 months, 3 months, 4 months, 3–5 years. Booster 13–18 years.
Haemophilus influenzae type b (Hib)	2 months, 3 months, 4 months.
Rubella (German measles)	12–15 months and 3–5 years.
Measles	12–15 months and 3–5 years.
Mumps	12–15 months and 3–5 years.
Tuberculosis (BCG) (Bacille Calmette-Guérin)	6 weeks or 10–14 years.
Influenza	People of any age who are at risk of serious illness or death if they develop influenza.
Hepatitis A	Single dose for people of any age who are at risk. Booster 6–12 months after initial shot. Boosters every 10 years if needed.
Hepatitis B	3 inoculations at any age, with the second and third shots 1 and 6 months after the first. Booster after 5 years if needed.
Pneumococcal pneumonia	Single dose for people of any age who are at risk.
Meningococcal meningitis A+C	Single dose for people of any age who are at risk.
Meningococcal meningitis C	2 months, 3 months, 4 months
Typhoid	Single dose for people of any age who are at risk.

not give full protection against a disease, or the effects may last for as little as six months. Influenza vaccines usually protect only against the variety of virus that is causing the latest outbreak of flu. New varieties appear during most years.

Any vaccine may cause side effects but they are usually mild and soon disappear. The most common reactions are a red, slightly raised, tender area at the site of injection and a slight fever or a flu-like illness lasting for one or two days.

RISKS AND SPECIAL PRECAUTIONS

Serious reactions are rare and, for most children, the risk is far outweighed by the protection given. Children who have had fits may be advised against vaccinations for pertussis (whooping cough) or measles. Children who have any infection more severe than a common cold will not be given any routine vaccination until they have recovered.

Live vaccines should not be given during pregnancy because they can affect the developing baby, nor should they be given to people whose immune systems are weakened by disease or drug treatment, although HIV-positive people can have MMR unless they are severely immunosuppressed. It is also advisable for people taking high doses of corticosteroids (p.80) to delay their vaccinations until they have completed their drug treatment.

The risk of the development of a high fever following vaccination with DTaP/IPV/Hib (combined diphtheria, tetanus, acellular pertussis, inactivated polio vaccine, and *Haemophilus influenzae* type b) can be reduced by giving paracetamol at the time of the vaccination. The pertussis vaccine may rarely cause a mild fit, which is brief, usually associated with fever, and stops without treatment. Children who have experienced such fits recover completely without neurological or developmental problems.

IMMUNE GLOBULINS

Antibodies, which can result from exposure to snake and insect venom as well as infectious disease, are found in the serum of the blood (the part remaining after the red cells and clotting agents are removed). The concentrated serum of people who have survived diseases or poisonous bites is called immune globulin. Given by injection, it creates passive immunity. Immune globulin from blood donated by a wide cross-section of donors is likely to contain antibodies to most common diseases. Specific immune globulins against rare diseases or toxins are derived from the blood of selected donors who are likely to have high levels of antibodies to that disease. These are called hyperimmune globulins. Some immune globulins are extracted from horse blood following repeated doses of the toxin.

Because immune globulins do not stimulate the body to produce its own antibodies, their effect is not long-lasting and diminishes progressively over three or four weeks. Continued protection requires repeated injections of immune globulins.

Adverse effects from immune globulins are uncommon. Some people are sensitive to horse globulins, and approximately a week after the injection they may experience a reaction known as serum sickness, in which they have fever, a rash, joint swelling, and pain. Serum sickness usually ends in a few days but should be reported to your doctor before any further immunization.

TRAVEL VACCINATIONS

These are not normally needed for travel to Western Europe, North America, Australia, or New Zealand (but you should make sure that your tetanus and polio boosters are up to date). Consult your doctor if you are visiting other destinations. Check that children travelling with you have had all the routine childhood vaccinations as well as any that are necessary for the areas in which you will be travelling.

If you are visiting an area where there is yellow fever, an International Certificate of Vaccination will be needed. You may also need this certificate in the future. Many countries that you might want to visit require an International Certificate of Vaccination if you have already been to a country where yellow fever is present.

You are at risk of other infectious diseases in many parts of the world, and appropriate vaccinations are a wise precaution. For example, a zone called the "Meningitis Belt" runs in a wide band across Africa from the Sahara down to Kenya. Anyone intending to visit this zone should have meningococcal vaccine A, C, W135, and Y. Visitors to Saudi Arabia at certain times of the year may also be required to have had the meningitis group A, C, W135, and Y vaccine.

You may need extra vaccinations if you are backpacking or planning a lengthy stay. For example, hepatitis A vaccine would be sensible for anyone travelling to a developing country, but a long-stay traveller should consider having the hepatitis B vaccine and BCG (tuberculosis) as well. Rabies vaccination is recommended to anyone travelling into remote areas.

All immunization should be completed well before departure as the vaccinations do not give instant protection (BCG needs 3 months), and some (for example, typhoid) need more than one dose to be effective.

The Department of Health publishes a booklet called "Health Advice for Travellers Anywhere in the World". This booklet gives information on the requirements for vaccination and is available from some travel agents and post offices.

TRAVEL IMMUNIZATION

The immunizations needed before travelling depend on the part of the world you intend to visit, but some diseases can be contracted almost anywhere. Make sure that you have been immunized against tetanus and polio and have had boosters if necessary. Ask your doctor or pharmacist for the most up-to-date information on vaccination for specific areas.

DISEASE	NUMBER OF DOSES	WHEN EFFECTIVE	PERIOD OF PROTECTION	WHO SHOULD BE IMMUNIZED
Diphtheria	1 injection	Immediately	10 years	People travelling to the countries of the former USSR and expatriates living in developing countries
Hepatitis A	2 injections 6–12 months apart	2–4 weeks after 1st dose	10 years	Frequent travellers to the Mediterranean or developing countries
Hepatitis B	3 injections, 1 month between 1st and 2nd doses, 5 months between 2nd and 3rd doses	Immediately after 2nd dose	3–5 years	People travelling to countries in which hepatitis B is prevalent; those who might need medical or dental treatment while travelling in a developing country; and people likely to have unprotected sex
Japanese B encephalitis	2–3 injections 1–2 weeks apart	10–14 days after last dose	About 2 years	People staying for an extended period in rural areas of the Indian subcontinent, China, Southeast Asia, and the Far East
Meningitis A, C, W135, and Y	1 injection	After 15 days	3–5 years	People travelling to sub-Saharan Africa. Immunization certificate needed if travelling to Saudi Arabia for the Hajj and Umrah pilgrimages
Rabies	3 injections. 1 week between 1st and 2nd doses, 3 weeks between 2nd and 3rd doses	Immediately after 3rd dose	2–3 years	People travelling to areas where rabies is endemic and who are at high risk (such as veterinary surgeons, people working with animals, and those travelling into remote country)
Typhoid	1 injection or 3 oral doses	10 days after last dose or injection	3 years	People travelling to areas with poor sanitation
Yellow fever	1 injection	After 10 days	10 years	People travelling to parts of South America and Africa
Cholera	No satisfactory vaccine exists. Travellers to countries where cholera exists must pay scrupulous attention to food, water, and personal hygiene.			

Antiprotozoal drugs

Protozoa are single-celled organisms that are present in soil and water. They may be transmitted to or between humans through contaminated food or water, sexual contact, or insect bites. There are many different types of protozoal infection, each causing a different disease, depending on the organism involved.

Many types of protozoa infect the bowel, causing diarrhoea and generalized symptoms of ill-health. Others may infect the genital tract or skin. Some protozoa may penetrate vital organs such as the lungs, brain, and liver. Prompt diagnosis and treatment are important in order to limit the spread of the infection within the body and, in some cases, prevent it from spreading to other people. Increased attention to hygiene is an important factor in controlling the spread of the disease.

A variety of medicines is used in the treatment of these diseases. Some, such as metronidazole and tetracycline, are also commonly used for their antibacterial action. Others, such as pentamidine, are rarely used except in treating specific protozoal infections.

HOW THEY AFFECT YOU

Protozoa are often difficult to eradicate from the body. Drug treatment may therefore need to be continued for several months in order to eliminate the infecting organisms completely and thus prevent recurrence of the disease. In addition, unpleasant side effects such as nausea, diarrhoea, and abdominal cramps are often unavoidable because of the limited choice of drugs and the need to maintain dosage levels that will effectively cure the disease. For detailed information on the risks and adverse effects of individual antiprotozoal drugs, consult the appropriate drug profile in Part 2.

TYPES OF PROTOZOAL DISEASE

Amoebiasis (*Entamoeba histolytica*), or amoebic dysentery, is an infection of the bowel (and sometimes the liver and other organs) usually transmitted in contaminated food or water. Its major symptom is violent, sometimes bloody, diarrhoea. Treatment is with diloxanide, metronidazole, or tinidazole.

Balantidiasis (*Balantidium coli*) is an infection of the bowel, specifically the colon, that is usually transmitted through contact with infected pigs. Possible symptoms include diarrhoea and abdominal pain. Treatment of the infection is with tetracycline, metronidazole, or diodohydroxyquinoline.

Cryptosporidiosis (*Cryptosporidium*) affects the bowel (and occasionally the respiratory tract and bile ducts). Cryptosporidiosis is spread through contaminated food or water or by contact with animals or other humans. Symptoms include diarrhoea and abdominal pain. There are no specific drugs to treat it, but paromomycin, azithromycin, or eflornithine may be effective.

Giardiasis (*Giardia lamblia*), or lambliasis, affects the bowel and is usually transmitted in con-

taminated food or water; but it may also be spread by some types of sexual contact. Its major symptoms are generalized ill-health, diarrhoea, flatulence, and abdominal pain. Treatment is with mepacrine, metronidazole, or tinidazole.

Leishmaniasis (*Leishmania*) is a mainly tropical and subtropical disease caused by organisms spread through sandfly bites. It affects the mucous membranes of the mouth, nose, and throat and may, in its severe form, invade organs such as the liver. Treatment is with paromomycin, sodium stibogluconate, pentamidine, or amphotericin.

Pneumocystis pneumonia (*Pneumocystis carinii*) is a potentially fatal lung infection usually affecting only those people with reduced resistance to infection, such as AIDS sufferers. Symptoms include cough, breathlessness, fever, and chest pain. Treatment is with drugs such as atovaquone, co-trimoxazole, pentamidine, and dapsone with trimethoprim.

Toxoplasmosis (*Toxoplasma gondii*) is usually spread via cat faeces or by eating undercooked meat. Although usually symptomless, toxoplasmosis may cause generalized ill-health, mild fever, and eye inflammation. Treatment is necessary only if the eyes are involved or the patient is immunosuppressed (such as in AIDS). It may also pass from mother to baby during pregnancy, leading to severe disease in the fetus. Treatment usually consists of pyrimethamine with sulfadiazine, azithromycin, clarithromycin, or clindamycin, or, during pregnancy, spiramycin.

Trichomoniasis (*Trichomonas vaginalis*) most often affects the vagina, causing irritation and an offensive discharge. In men, it may occur in the urethra. It is usually sexually transmitted. Treatment is with metronidazole or tinidazole.

Trypanosomiasis (*Trypanosoma*), or African trypanosomiasis (sleeping sickness), is spread by the tsetse fly and causes fever, swollen glands, and drowsiness. South American trypanosomiasis (Chagas' disease) is spread by assassin bugs and causes inflammation, enlargement of internal organs, and infection of the brain. Sleeping sickness is treated with pentamidine, suramin, eflornithine, or melarsoprol. Chagas' disease is treated with primaquine or nifurtimox.

Trichomoniasis, toxoplasmosis, crypto-sporidium, giardiasis, and pneumocystis pneumonia are probably the most common protozoal infections seen in the United Kingdom. The rarer infections are usually contracted as a result of exposure to infection in another part of the world.

Antimalarial drugs

Malaria is one of the main killing diseases in the tropics and is most likely to affect people who live in or travel to such places.

The disease is caused by protozoa (see p.73) whose life cycle is far from simple. The malaria parasite, which is called *Plasmodium*, lives in and depends on the female *Anopheles* mosquito during one part of its life cycle. It lives in and depends on human beings during other parts of its life cycle.

Transferred to humans in the saliva of the female mosquito as she penetrates ("bites") the skin, the malaria parasite enters the bloodstream and settles in the liver, where it multiplies asexually.

Following its stay in the liver, the parasite (or plasmodium) enters another phase of its life cycle, circulating in the bloodstream, penetrating and destroying red blood cells, and reproducing again. If the plasmodia then transfer back to a female *Anopheles* mosquito via another "bite", they breed sexually, and are again ready to start a human infection.

Following the emergence of plasmodia from the liver, the symptoms of malaria occur: episodes of high fever and profuse sweating alternate with equally agonizing episodes of shivering and chills. One of the four strains of malaria (*Plasmodium falciparum*) can produce a single severe attack that can be fatal unless treated. The others cause recurrent attacks, sometimes extending over many years.

A number of drugs are available for preventing malaria, the choice depending on the region in which the disease can be contracted and the resistance to the commonly used drugs. In most malarial areas, *Plasmodium falciparum* is resistant to chloroquine. (See Choice of drug, above right.) In all regions, four drugs are commonly used for treating malaria: quinine, mefloquine, Malarone, and Riamet.

CHOICE OF DRUG

The parts of the world in which malaria is prevalent, and travel to which may make antimalarial drug treatment advisable, can be divided into six zones. Due to drug resistance, specific antimalarials are recommended for each zone.

Zone 1 North Africa and the Middle East Chloroquine, plus proguanil in areas of chloroquine resistance

Zone 2 Sub-Saharan Africa Mefloquine, or chloroquine with proguanil, or doxycycline, or Malarone

Zone 3 South Asia Mefloquine, or chloroquine with proguanil, or doxycycline, or Malarone

Zone 4 Southeast Asia Mefloquine in high-risk areas, or chloroquine with proguanil; doxycycline or Malarone in mefloquine-resistant areas

Zone 5 Oceania Mefloquine, or doxycycline, or Malarone

Zone 6 Latin America Central America: chloroquine or proguanil. South America: mefloquine, or doxycycline, or Malarone in high-risk areas, or chloroquine with proguanil

Because prevalent strains of malaria change very rapidly, you must always seek specific medical advice before travelling to any of these areas.

WHY THEY ARE USED

The medical response to malaria takes three forms: prevention, treatment of attacks, and the complete eradication of the plasmodia (radical cure).

For an individual planning a trip to an area where malaria is prevalent, drugs are given that destroy the parasites as they enter the liver. This preventive treatment needs to start up to 3 weeks before departure and continue for 1–4 weeks after returning (the exact timings depend on the drugs taken).

Drugs such as mefloquine, Riamet, and Fansidar can produce a radical cure, but chloroquine does not. Therefore, following chloroquine treatment of non-falciparum malaria, a 14- to 21-day course of primaquine is administered. Although it is highly effective in destroying the plasmodia in the liver, primaquine is weak against the plasmodia circulating in the bloodstream. The drug is recommended only after a person leaves the malarial area because of the high risk of reinfection.

HOW THEY WORK

Taken to prevent the disease, the drugs kill plasmodia in the liver, preventing them from multiplying. Once the plasmodia have multiplied in the liver, the same drugs may be used in higher doses to kill those that re-enter the bloodstream. If these drugs are not effective, primaquine may be used to destroy any plasmodia still present in the liver.

HOW THEY AFFECT YOU

The low doses of antimalarial drugs taken to prevent the disease rarely produce noticeable effects. Drugs taken for an attack usually begin to relieve symptoms within a few hours. Most of them can cause nausea, vomiting, and diarrhoea. Quinine can cause disturbances in vision and hearing. Mefloquine can cause sleep disturbance, dizziness, and difficulties in coordination.

RISKS AND SPECIAL PRECAUTIONS

When drugs are given to prevent or cure malaria, the full course of treatment must be taken. No drugs give long-term protection; a new course of treatment is needed for each journey.

Most of these drugs do not produce severe adverse effects, but primaquine can cause the blood disorder haemolytic anaemia, particularly in people with glucose-6-phosphate dehydrogenase (G6PD) deficiency. Blood tests are taken before treatment to identify susceptible individuals. Mefloquine is not prescribed for those who have had psychological disorders or convulsions.

OTHER PROTECTIVE MEASURES

Because *Plasmodium* strains continually develop resistance to the available drugs, prevention of malaria with the use of drugs is not absolutely reliable. Therefore, protection from mosquito bites is of the highest priority. Such protection includes the use of insect repellents, such as DEET, and mosquito nets impregnated with permethrin insecticide, as well as covering any areas of exposed skin after dark, when mosquitoes are active.

COMMON DRUGS

Drugs for prevention Chloroquine*, Doxycycline*, Mefloquine*, Proguanil*, Proguanil with atovaquone (Malarone)*

Drugs for treatment Artemether with lumefantrine (Riamet), Chloroquine*, Mefloquine*, Primaquine, Proguanil with atovaquone (Malarone)*, Pyrimethamine with sulfadoxine (Fansidar)*, Quinine*

* See Part 2

Antifungal drugs

We are continually exposed to fungi – in the air we breathe, the food we eat, and the water we drink. Fortunately, most fungi cannot live in the body, and few are harmful. But some can grow in the mouth, skin, hair, or nails, causing irritating or unsightly changes, and a few can cause serious and possibly fatal disease. The most common fungal infections are caused by the tinea group. These include tinea pedis (athlete's foot), tinea corporis (ringworm), tinea cruris (groin ringworm), and tinea capitis (scalp ringworm). Caused by a variety of organisms, they are spread by direct or indirect contact with infected humans or animals. Infection is encouraged by warm, moist conditions.

Problems may also result from the proliferation of a fungus that is normally present in the body; the most common example is excessive growth of *Candida*, a yeast that causes thrush infection of the mouth, vagina, and bowel. It can also infect other organs if it spreads through the body via the bloodstream. Overgrowth of *Candida* may occur in people taking antibiotics (p.62) or oral contraceptives (p.105), pregnant women, or those with diabetes or immune system disorders such as AIDS.

Superficial fungal infections – those that attack only the outer layer of the skin and mucous membranes – are relatively common and, although irritating, do not usually present a threat to general health. Internal fungal infections – for example, of the lungs, heart, or other organs – are rare but may be serious and prolonged.

Because antibiotics and other antibacterial drugs have no effect on fungi and yeasts, it is necessary to use a different type of drug.

CHOICE OF ANTIFUNGAL DRUG

The table below shows the range of uses for some of the more common antifungal drugs. The particular drug chosen in each case depends on the precise nature and site of the infection. The usual route of administration for each drug is also indicated.

DRUG	Oesophageal thrush	Cryptococcal meningitis	Skin ringworm	Scalp ringworm	Nail infection	Mouth thrush	Vaginal thrush	Candida of the skin	Systemic candida	Topical	Injection	Oral
Amphotericin	●	●				●		●	●	▲	▲	
Clotrimazole			●	●		●	●	●		▲		
Fluconazole	●	●					●		●		▲	▲
Flucytosine	●	●							●		▲	▲
Griseofulvin			●	●	●							▲
Ketoconazole			●	●			●	●	●	▲		▲
Miconazole						●	●	●		▲		▲
Nystatin						●	●	●		▲		▲
Terbinafine			●	●	●							▲

Drugs for fungal infections are either applied topically to treat minor infections of the skin, nails, and mucous membranes, or they are given by mouth or injection to eliminate serious fungal infections of the internal organs and nails.

WHY THEY ARE USED

Drug treatment is necessary for most fungal infections since they rarely improve alone. Measures such as careful washing and drying of affected areas may help, but they are not a substitute for antifungal drugs. The use of over-the-counter preparations to increase the acidity of the vagina is not usually effective except when it is accompanied by drug treatment.

Fungal infections of the skin and scalp are usually treated with a cream or shampoo. Drugs for vaginal thrush are most commonly applied in the form of vaginal pessaries or cream applied with a special applicator. For very severe or persistent vaginal infections, fluconazole or itraconazole may be given as a short course by mouth. Mouth infections are usually eliminated by lozenges dissolved in the mouth or an antifungal solution or gel applied to the affected areas. When Candida infects the bowel, an antifungal drug that is not absorbed into the bloodstream, such as nystatin, is given in the form of tablets. For severe or persistent infections of the nails, either griseofulvin or terbinafine are given by mouth and are continued until the infected nails have grown out.

In the rare cases of fungal infections affecting internal organs, such as the blood, the heart, or the brain, potent drugs such as fluconazole and itraconazole are given by mouth, or amphotericin and flucytosine are given by injection. These drugs pass into the bloodstream to fight the fungi.

HOW THEY WORK

Most antifungals alter the permeability of the fungal cell's walls. Chemicals needed for cell life leak out and the fungal cell dies.

HOW THEY AFFECT YOU

The speed with which antifungal drugs provide benefit varies with the type of infection. Most fungal or yeast infections of the skin, mouth, and vagina improve within a week. The condition of nails affected by fungal infections improves only when new nail growth occurs, which takes months. Systemic infections of the internal organs can take weeks to cure.

Antifungal drugs applied topically rarely cause side effects, although they may irritate the skin. However, treatment by mouth or injection for systemic and nail infections may produce more serious side effects.

Amphotericin, injected in cases of life-threatening, systemic infections, can cause potentially dangerous effects, including kidney damage.

COMMON DRUGS

Amorolfine, Amphotericin*, Benzoyl peroxide*, Clotrimazole*, Econazole, Fenticonazole, Fluconazole*, Griseofulvin, Isoconazole, Itraconazole, Ketoconazole*, Lucytosine, Miconazole*, Nystatin*, Sulconazole, Terbinafine*, Tioconazole

* See Part 2

Anthelmintic drugs

Anthelmintics are drugs used to eliminate the many types of worm (helminth) that can enter the body and live there as parasites. The worms may produce a general weakness in some cases and serious harm in others. The body may be host to many different worms (see Types of infestation, right). Most species spend part of their life cycle in another animal, and the infestation is often passed on to humans in food contaminated with the eggs or larvae. In some cases, such as hookworm, larvae enter the body through the skin. Larvae or adults may attach themselves to the intestinal wall and feed on the bowel contents; others feed off the intestinal blood supply, causing anaemia. Worms can also infest the bloodstream or lodge in the muscles or internal organs.

Many people have worms at some time during their life, especially during childhood. Most infestations can be effectively eliminated with anthelmintic drugs.

WHY THEY ARE USED

Most worms common in the United Kingdom cause only mild symptoms and usually do not pose a serious threat to general health. Anthelmintic drugs are usually necessary, however, because the body's natural defences against infection are not effective against most worm infestations. Certain types of infestation must always be treated because they can cause serious complications. In some cases, such as threadworm infestation, doctors may recommend anthelmintic drug treatment for the whole family to prevent reinfection. If worms have invaded the tissues and formed cysts, they may have to be removed surgically. Laxatives are given with some anthelmintics to hasten the expulsion of worms from the bowel. Other drugs may be prescribed to ease symptoms or to compensate for any blood loss or nutritional deficiency.

TYPES OF INFESTATION

Threadworm (*enterobiasis*) The most common worm infection in the UK, especially among young children. The worm lives in the intestine but travels to the anus at night to lay eggs, causing itching; scratching leaves eggs on the fingers, usually under the fingernails. Sucking the fingers or eating food with unwashed hands often transfers these eggs to the mouth. Keeping the nails short; good hygiene, including washing the hands after using the toilet and before each meal; and an early morning bath to remove the eggs are important in eradicating the infection.
Drugs Mebendazole, piperazine
All members of the household should be treated simultaneously.

Common roundworm (*ascariasis*) The most common worm infection worldwide. It is transmitted to humans in contaminated raw food or in soil. The worms are large, and they infect the intestine, which can be blocked by dense clusters of them.
Drugs Levamisole, mebendazole, piperazine

Tropical threadworm (*strongyloidiasis*) Occurs in the tropics and southern Europe. The larvae from contaminated soil penetrate the skin, pass into the lungs, are swallowed, and pass into the gut.
Drugs Albendazole, tiabendazole, ivermectin

Whipworm (*trichuriasis*) Mainly occurs in tropical areas of the world as a result of eating contaminated raw vegetables. The worms infest the intestines.
Drug Mebendazole

Hookworm (*uncinariasis*) Mainly found in tropical areas. The worm larvae penetrate the skin and pass via the lymphatic system and bloodstream to the lungs. They then travel up the airways, are swallowed, and attach themselves to the intestinal wall, where they feed off the intestinal blood supply.
Drug Mebendazole

Pork roundworm (*trichinosis*) Transmitted in infected undercooked pork. Initially, the worms lodge in the intestines, but larvae may invade muscle to form cysts that are often resistant to drug treatment and may require surgery.

Drugs Mebendazole, tiabendazole

Toxocariasis (*visceral larva migrans*) Usually occurs as a result of eating soil or eating with fingers contaminated with dog or cat faeces. The eggs hatch in the intestine and may travel to the lungs, liver, kidney, brain, and eyes. Treatment is not always effective.

Drugs Mebendazole, tiabendazole, diethylcarbamazine

Creeping eruption (*cutaneous larva migrans*) Mainly occurs in tropical areas and coastal areas of the southeastern US as a result of skin contact with larvae from cat and dog faeces. Infestation is usually confined to the skin.

Drugs Tiabendazole, ivermectin, albendazole

Filariasis (including *onchocerciasis* and *loiasis*) Occurs in tropical areas only. It may affect the lymphatic system, blood, eyes, and skin. Infection by this group of worms is spread by the bites of insects that are carriers of worm larvae or eggs.

Drugs Diethylcarbamazine, ivermectin

Flukes Sheep liver fluke (*fascioliasis*) is indigenous to the UK. Infestation usually results from eating watercress grown in contaminated water. It mainly affects the liver and biliary tract. Other flukes only found abroad may infect the lungs, intestines, or blood.

Drug Praziquantel

Tapeworms (including beef, pork, fish, and dwarf tapeworms) Depending on the type, it may be carried by cattle, pigs, or fish and transmitted to humans in undercooked meat. Most types affect the intestines. Larvae of the pork tapeworm may form cysts in muscle and other tissues.

Drugs Niclosamide, praziquantel

Hydatid disease (*echinococciasis*) The eggs are transmitted in dog faeces, and the larvae may form cysts over many years, commonly in the liver. Surgery is the usual treatment for cysts.

Drug Albendazole

Bilharzia (*schistosomiasis*) Occurs in polluted water in tropical areas. The larvae may be swallowed or penetrate the skin. Once inside the body, they migrate to the liver; adult worms live in the bladder.

Drug Praziquantel

HOW THEY WORK

The anthelmintic drugs act in several ways. Many of them kill or paralyse the worms, which pass out of the body in the faeces. Others, which act systemically, are used to treat infection in the tissues.

Many anthelmintics are specific for particular worms, and the doctor must identify the worm before selecting the most appropriate treatment (see Types of infestation, facing page). Most of the common intestinal infestations are easily treated, often with only one or two doses of the drug. However, tissue infections may require more prolonged treatment.

HOW THEY AFFECT YOU

Once the drug has eliminated the worms, symptoms caused by infestation rapidly disappear. Taken as a single dose or a short course, anthelmintics do not usually produce side effects. However, treatment can disturb the digestive system, causing abdominal pain, nausea, and vomiting.

COMMON DRUGS

Albendazole, Diethylcarbamazine, Ivermectin, Levamisole, Mebendazole, Niclosamide, Piperazine, Praziquantel, Tiabendazole

* See Part 2

HORMONES AND ENDOCRINE SYSTEM

The endocrine system is a collection of endocrine glands located throughout the body. These glands produce hormones and release them into the bloodstream. Each endocrine gland produces one or more hormones, each of which governs a particular body function, including growth and repair of tissues, sexual development and reproductive function, and the body's response to stress.

The pituitary gland produces hormones that regulate growth and sexual and reproductive development, and also stimulate other endocrine glands (see p.85).

The thyroid gland regulates metabolism. Hyperthyroidism or hypothyroidism may occur if the thyroid does not function well (see p.84).

The adrenal glands produce hormones that regulate the body's mineral and water content and reduce inflammation (see Corticosteroids, below right).

The pancreas produces insulin to regulate blood glucose levels, and glucagon, which helps the liver and muscles to store glucose (see p.82).

The kidneys produce a hormone, erythropoietin, needed for red blood cell production. Patients with kidney failure lack this hormone and become anaemic; they may be given epoetin (p.237), a version of the hormone.

The ovaries (in women) secrete oestrogen and progesterone, responsible for female sexual and physical development (see p.88).

The testes (in men) produce testosterone, which controls the development of male sexual and physical characteristics (see p.87).

Most hormones are released continuously from birth, but the amount produced fluctuates with the body's needs. Others are produced mainly at certain times; for example, growth hormone is released mainly during childhood and adolescence, and sex hormones are produced by the testes and ovaries from puberty onwards (see p.103).

Many endocrine glands release their hormones in response to triggering hormones produced by the pituitary gland. This gland releases a variety of pituitary hormones, each of which, in turn, stimulates the appropriate endocrine gland to produce its hormone.

A "feedback" system usually regulates blood hormone levels; if the blood level rises too high, the pituitary responds by reducing the amount of stimulating hormone produced, thereby allowing the blood hormone level to return to normal.

WHAT CAN GO WRONG

Endocrine disorders, usually resulting in too much or too little of a particular hormone, have a variety of causes. Some are congenital in origin. Others may be caused by autoimmune disease (including some forms of diabetes mellitus), malignant or benign tumours, injury, or certain drugs.

WHY DRUGS ARE USED

Natural hormone preparations or their synthetic versions are often prescribed to treat deficiency. Sometimes, drugs are given to stimulate increased hormone production in the endocrine gland, such as oral antidiabetic drugs, which act on the insulin-producing cells of the pancreas. When too much hormone is produced, drug treatment may be used to reduce the activity of the gland.

Hormones or related drugs are also used to treat certain other conditions. Corticosteroids related to adrenal hormones are prescribed to relieve inflammation and to suppress immune system activity (see p.99). Several types of cancer (see p.96) are treated with sex hormones. Female sex hormones are used as contraceptives (see p.105) and to treat menstrual disorders (see p.104).

MAJOR DRUG GROUPS

◆ Corticosteroids
◆ Drugs used in diabetes
◆ Drugs for thyroid disorders
◆ Drugs for pituitary disorders
◆ Male sex hormones
◆ Female sex hormones

Corticosteroids

Corticosteroid drugs, often referred to simply as steroids, are derived from, or are synthetic variants of, the natural corticosteroid hormones formed in the outer part (cortex) of the adrenal glands, situated on top of each kidney. Release of these hormones is governed by the pituitary gland (see p.85).

Corticosteroids mainly have either glucocorticoid or mineralocorticoid effects. Glucocorticoid effects include the maintenance of normal levels of sugar in the blood and the promotion of recovery from injury and stress. The main mineralocorticoid effects are the regulation of the balance of mineral salts and the water content of the body. When present in large amounts, corticosteroids reduce inflammation and suppress allergic reactions and immune system activity. They are distinct from another group of steroid hormones, the anabolic steroids (see p.88).

Although corticosteroids have broadly similar actions, they vary in their relative strength and duration of action. Their mineralocorticoid effects also vary in strength.

WHY THEY ARE USED

Corticosteroids are used primarily for their effect in controlling inflammation, whatever its cause. Topical corticosteroid preparations are often used for the treatment of many inflammatory skin disorders (see p.120). These drugs may also be injected directly into a joint or around a tendon to relieve inflammation due to injury or disease (see p.53). However, when local administration of the drug is either not possible or not effective, corticosteroids may be given systemically, either by mouth or by intravenous injection.

Corticosteroids are commonly part of the treatment of many disorders in which inflammation is thought to be due to excessive or inappropriate activity of the immune system. These disorders include inflammatory bowel disease (p.46), rheumatoid arthritis (p.52), glomerulonephritis (a kidney disease), and some rare connective tissue disorders, such as systemic lupus erythematosus. In these conditions corticosteroids relieve symptoms and may also temporarily halt the disease.

Corticosteroids may be given regularly, by mouth or inhaler, to treat asthma but are not effective for the relief of asthma attacks that are in progress (see Bronchodilators, p.23, and Drugs for asthma, p.24).

An important use of oral corticosteroids is to replace deficiencies in the levels of natural hormones resulting from reduced adrenal gland function, as in Addison's disease. In these cases, the drugs most closely resembling the actions of the natural hormones are selected and a combination may be used.

Some cancers of the lymphatic system (lymphomas) and blood (leukaemias) may also respond to corticosteroid treatment. These drugs are also widely used to prevent or treat rejection of organ transplants, usually in conjunction with other drugs, such as azathioprine (see Immunosuppressants, p.99).

HOW THEY WORK

Given in high doses, corticosteroids reduce inflammation by blocking the action of chemicals called prostaglandins that are responsible for triggering the inflammatory response. These drugs also temporarily depress the immune system by reducing the activity of certain types of white blood cell.

HOW THEY AFFECT YOU

Corticosteroids often dramatically improve symptoms. Given systemically, they may also act on the brain to produce a heightened sense of well-being and, in some people, a sense of euphoria.

Troublesome day-to-day side effects are rare. Long-term corticosteroid treatment, however, carries a number of serious risks for the patient.

RISKS AND SPECIAL PRECAUTIONS

In the treatment of Addison's disease, corticosteroids can be considered as "hormone replacement therapy", with the drugs replacing the natural hormone hydrocortisone. Because replacement doses are given, the adverse effects of high-dose corticosteroids do not occur.

Drugs with strong mineralocorticoid effects, such as fludrocortisone, may cause water retention, swelling (especially of the ankles), and an increase in blood pressure. Because corticosteroids reduce the effect of insulin, they may create problems in people with diabetes, and may even give rise to diabetes in susceptible individuals. They can also cause peptic ulcers.

Corticosteroids suppress the immune system, so they increase susceptibility to infection. In addition, they suppress symptoms of infectious disease. People taking corticosteroids should avoid exposure to chickenpox or shingles, but if they catch either disease, aciclovir tablets may be prescribed.

With long-term use, corticosteroids may cause various adverse effects, such as mood changes, acne, a moon-shaped face, increased blood pressure and fluid retention, peptic ulcers, reduction in the effect of insulin, a fat pad on the top of the back, muscle weakness and wasting, osteoporosis, cataracts, thin skin, and easy bruising. Doctors try to avoid prescribing corticosteroids to children in the long term because it may retard growth.

Long-term use of corticosteroids also suppresses production of the body's own corticosteroid hormones. Therefore, treatment lasting longer than a few weeks should be withdrawn gradually to give the body time to adjust. Stopping abruptly may lead to sudden collapse due to lack of the hormones.

People taking corticosteroids by mouth for longer than one month are advised to carry a warning card. If someone taking steroids long term has an accident or serious illness, his or her defences against shock may need to be quickly strengthened with extra hydrocortisone, administered intravenously.

COMMON DRUGS

Alclometasone, Beclometasone*, Betamethasone*, Budesonide*, Clobetasol*, Clobetasone, Deflazacort, Desoximetasone, Dexamethasone*, Diflucortolone, Fludrocortisone, Fludroxycortide, Flunisolide, Flumetasone, Fluocinolone, Fluocinonide, Fluocortolone, Fluticasone*, Halcinonide, Hydrocortisone*, Methylprednisolone, Mometasone*, Prednisolone*, Triamcinolone

* See Part 2

Drugs used in diabetes

The body obtains most of its energy from glucose, a simple form of sugar made in the intestine from the breakdown of starch and other sugars. Insulin, one of the hormones produced in the pancreas, enables body tissues to take up glucose from the blood either to use for energy or to store. In diabetes mellitus (or sugar diabetes), insulin production is defective. As a result, the tissues take up less glucose than usual, and therefore the glucose level in the blood rises abnormally. This is known medically as hyperglycaemia.

There are two main types of diabetes mellitus. Insulin-dependent (Type 1) diabetes usually affects young people; 50 per cent of cases occur at puberty. The insulin-secreting cells in the pancreas are gradually destroyed. An autoimmune condition in which the body identifies its own pancreas as "foreign" and tries to eliminate it, or a childhood viral infection, is the most likely cause. Despite slow insulin production, the condition often appears suddenly, brought on by periods of stress (such as infection or puberty), when insulin requirements are high. Symptoms of Type 1 diabetes include extreme thirst, increased urination, lethargy, and weight loss. Left untreated, this type of diabetes is fatal.

In Type 1 diabetes, insulin treatment is the only treatment option. It has to be continued for the rest of the patient's life. Several types of insulin are available, which are broadly classified by their duration of action (short-, medium-, and long-acting).

Non-insulin-dependent diabetes mellitus (NIDDM), also called Type 2 or maturity-onset diabetes, appears at an older age (usually over 40) and tends to come on much more gradually – there may be a delay in its diagnosis for several years because of the gradual onset of symptoms. In this type of diabetes, insulin is present but the cells of the body are often resistant to its effects and have a reduced glucose uptake despite the presence of insulin. This results in hyperglycaemia. Obesity is the most common cause of Type 2 diabetes.

In both types of diabetes, an alteration in diet is vital. A healthy diet that is low in fat, high in fibre, low in simple sugar (cakes, sweets), and high in complex sugar (pasta, rice, potatoes) is advised.

In Type 2 diabetes, a reduction in weight alone may be sufficient to lower the body's energy requirements and restore blood glucose to normal levels. If an alteration in diet fails, oral antidiabetic drugs, such as metformin, acarbose, or sulphonylureas, are prescribed. Insulin may need to be given to people with Type 2 diabetes if the above treatments fail, or in pregnancy, during severe illness, and before the patient undergoes any surgery requiring a general anaesthetic.

IMPORTANCE OF TREATING DIABETES

If diabetes is left untreated, the continuous high blood glucose levels damage various parts of the body. The major problems are caused by the build-up of atherosclerosis in arteries, which narrows the vessels, reducing blood flow. This can result in heart attacks, blindness, kidney failure, reduced circulation in the legs, and even gangrene. With treatment, the risk of these conditions is greatly reduced. Careful control of diabetes in young people, during puberty and afterwards, is of great importance in reducing possible long-term complications. Good diabetic control before conception reduces the chance of miscarriage or abnormalities in the baby.

HOW ANTIDIABETIC DRUGS WORK

Insulin treatment directly replaces the natural hormone that is deficient in diabetes mellitus. Human and pork insulins are the most widely available. When transferring between animal and human insulin, alteration of the dose may be required.

Unfortunately, insulin cannot be given by mouth because it is broken down in the digestive tract before it reaches the bloodstream. Regular injections are therefore necessary (see Administration of insulin, below).

Sulphonylurea oral antidiabetics encourage the pancreas to produce insulin; they are, therefore, effective only when some insulin-secreting cells remain active. This is why they are ineffective in the treatment of Type 1 diabetes. Metformin alters the way in which the body metabolizes sugar, and acarbose slows the digestion of starch and sugar. Both slow the increase in blood sugar that occurs after a meal. Nateglinide and repaglinide stimulate insulin release. Pioglitazone and rosiglitazone reduce the body's resistance to insulin.

ADMINISTRATION OF INSULIN

The body normally produces a background level of insulin, with additional insulin being produced as required in response to meals.

The insulin delivery systems currently available cannot mimic this process precisely. In people with Type 1 diabetes, short-acting insulin is usually given before meals, and medium-acting either before the evening meal or at bedtime. Insulin pen injectors are especially useful for daytime administration because they are discreet and easy to carry and use. In patients with Type 2 diabetes who require insulin, a mixture of short- and medium-acting insulin may be given twice a day. Special pumps that deliver continuous subcutaneous insulin seem to have no advantage over multiple subcutaneous injections. Some new insulin types called "insulin analogues" (such as Insulin lispro) act very rapidly and may be better at mimicking the insulin-producing behaviour of the normal pancreas.

INSULIN TREATMENT AND YOU

The insulin requirements in diabetes vary greatly between individuals and also depend on physical activity and calorie intake. Hence, insulin regimens are tailored to each person's particular needs, and if you have diabetes you will be encouraged to take an active role in your own health management.

You should keep a regular record of home blood glucose monitoring. This is the basis on which insulin doses are adjusted, preferably by yourself. You need to check either your blood or urine glucose level, although blood tests give the most accurate results. Home blood-testing kits are available; these consist of a special card testing strip to which blood samples are applied, and a programmable meter that reads the glucose levels.

You should learn to recognize the warning signs of hypoglycaemia (low blood glucose). A hypoglycaemic event may be induced by giving insulin under medical supervision. The symptoms of sweating, faintness, or palpitations are produced but disappear with the administration of glucose, so you should always carry glucose tablets or sweets. Recurrent "hypos" at specific times of the day or night may require a reduction of insulin dose. Rarely, undetected low glucose levels may lead to coma. The injection of glucagon (a substance that raises blood glucose) rapidly reverses the coma. A relative may be instructed how to perform this procedure.

Repeated injections at the same site may disturb the fat layer beneath the skin, producing either swelling or dimpling. This alters the rate at which insulin is absorbed. It can, however, be avoided by regularly rotating the injection sites.

Insulin requirements are increased during illness and pregnancy. During an illness, the urine should be checked for ketones, which are produced when there is insufficient insulin to permit the normal uptake of glucose by the tissues. If high ketone levels occur in your urine during an illness, you should seek urgent medical advice. The combination of high blood glucose, high urinary ketones, and vomiting is a diabetic emergency; in this situation, you should attend an Accident and Emergency department immediately.

Exercise increases the body's need for glucose, so you should take extra calories prior to exertion. The effects of vigorous exercise on blood glucose levels may last for up to 18 hours, and the subsequent (post-exercise) doses of insulin may need to be reduced by 10–25 per cent to avoid hypoglycaemia (low blood glucose).

It is advisable for diabetic people to carry a card or bracelet detailing their treatment. This may be useful in an emergency.

ANTIDIABETIC DRUGS AND YOU

The sulphonylureas may lower the blood glucose too much, producing hypoglycaemia. This condition can be avoided by starting treatment with low doses and ensuring a regular intake of food. Rarely, sulphonylureas cause a decrease in the blood cell count, a rash, or intestinal or liver disturbances. Interactions may occur with other drugs; therefore, your doctor should be informed of your treatment before any medicines are prescribed for you.

Unlike the sulphonylureas, metformin does not cause hypoglycaemia. Its most common side effects are nausea, weight loss, abdominal distension, and diarrhoea. It should not be used in people with liver, kidney, or heart problems. Acarbose does not cause hypoglycaemia if used on its own. The tablets must either be chewed with the first mouthful of food at mealtimes or swallowed whole with a little liquid immediately before food.

COMMON DRUGS

Sulphonylurea drugs Chlorpropamide, Glibenclamide*, Gliclazide*, Glimepiride, Gliquidone, Glipizide, Tolbutamide*
Other drugs Acarbose, Glucagon, Insulin*, Insulin lispro, Metformin*, Nateglinide, Pioglitazone, Repaglinide*, Rosiglitazone*
* See Part 2

Drugs for thyroid disorders

The thyroid gland produces the hormone thyroxine, which regulates the body's metabolism. During childhood, thyroxine is essential for normal physical and mental development. Calcitonin, also produced by the thyroid, regulates calcium metabolism and is used as a drug for certain bone disorders (see p.56).

HYPERTHYROIDISM

In this condition (often called thyrotoxicosis), the thyroid is overactive and produces too much thyroxine. Women are more commonly affected than men. Symptoms include anxiety, palpitations, weight loss, increased appetite, heat intolerance, diarrhoea, and menstrual disturbances. Graves' disease, the most common form of hyperthyroidism, is an autoimmune disease in which the body produces antibodies that stimulate the thyroid to produce excess thyroxine. Patients with Graves' disease may develop exophthalmos (protuberant eyes) or pretibial myxoedema (a swelling involving the skin over the shins).

Hyperthyroidism can be caused by a benign single tumour of the thyroid. It can also be the result of a pre-existing multinodular goitre (see below). Rarely, an overactive thyroid may follow a viral infection, a condition known as thyroiditis. Inflammation of the thyroid gland leads to the release of stored thyroxine.

Goitre is a swelling of the thyroid gland. It may occur only temporarily, during puberty or pregnancy, or may be due to abnormal growth of thyroid tissue that requires surgical removal. Goitre may also, rarely, be brought about by iodine deficiency, which can be prevented or treated with iodine supplements.

MANAGEMENT OF HYPERTHYROIDISM

There are three possible treatments: antithyroid drugs, radio-iodine, and surgery. The most commonly used antithyroid drug is carbimazole, which inhibits the formation of thyroid hormones and reduces their levels to normal over a period of 4–8 weeks. In the early stage of treatment, a beta blocker (see p.30) may be prescribed to control symptoms. This should be stopped once thyroid function returns to normal. Long-term carbimazole is usually given for 18 months to prevent relapse. A "block and replace" regimen may also be used. This treatment involves blocking the thyroid gland by high doses of carbimazole and adding thyroxine when the thyroid hormone level in the blood falls below normal.

Carbimazole may produce minor side effects such as nausea, vomiting, rashes, or headaches. Rarely, the drug may reduce the white blood cell count. Propylthiouracil may be used as an alternative antithyroid drug.

Radio-iodine (radioactive iodine) is often chosen as first-line therapy, especially in the elderly, usually after giving a course of carbimazole until up to a week before treatment. It is the second choice if hyperthyroidism recurs following use of carbimazole. It acts by destroying thyroid tissue. Hypothyroidism occurs in up to 80 per cent of people within 20 years after treatment. Long-term studies show radio-iodine to be safe, but its use should be avoided during pregnancy.

Surgery is a third-line therapy. Its use may be favoured for patients with a large goitre, particularly if it causes difficulty in swallowing or breathing. Exophthalmos may require corticosteroids (see p.80) as it does not respond to other treatments.

HYPOTHYROIDISM

This condition results from too little thyroxine. Sometimes it may be due to an autoimmune disorder in which the body's immune system attacks the thyroid gland. Other cases may follow treatment for hyperthyroidism. In newborn babies, hypothyroidism may be due to an inborn enzyme disorder. Rarely, it arises from deficiency of iodine in the diet.

The symptoms of adult hypothyroidism develop slowly. They include weight gain, constipation, mental slowness, dry skin, hair loss, increased sensitivity to cold, and heavy menstrual periods. In babies, low thyroxine levels cause permanent mental and physical retardation. For this reason, babies are tested for hypothyroidism within a week of birth.

MANAGEMENT OF HYPOTHYROIDISM

Lifelong oral treatment with the synthetic thyroid hormones levothyroxine or liothyronine is the only option. Blood tests are performed regularly to monitor treatment and permit dosage adjustments. In elderly people and those with heart disease, levothyroxine is introduced gradually to prevent heart strain.

In severely ill patients, thyroid hormone may be given by injection. This method of administration may also be used to treat newborn babies with low levels of thyroxine.

Symptoms of thyrotoxicosis may appear if excess thyroxine replacement is given. Otherwise, no adverse events occur since treatment is adjusted to replace the natural hormone that the body should produce itself.

COMMON DRUGS

Drugs for hyperthyroidism Carbimazole*, Iodine, Nadolol, Propranolol*, Propylthiouracil,* Radio-iodine
Drugs for hypothyroidism Levothyroxine*, Liothyronine
* See Part 2

Drugs for pituitary disorders

The pituitary gland, which lies at the base of the brain, produces a number of hormones that regulate physical growth, metabolism, sexual development, and reproductive function. Many of these hormones act indirectly by stimulating other glands, such as the thyroid, adrenal glands, ovaries, and testes, to release their own hormones.

Thyroid-stimulating hormone stimulates production and release of thyroid hormones.
Prolactin stimulates glands in the breast to produce milk in women and helps sperm production in men.
Corticotrophin (ACTH) controls production and release of adrenal corticosteroid hormones.

Gonadotrophins called follicle-stimulating hormone (FSH) and luteinizing hormone (LH) act on the sex glands to stimulate egg production and release in females and sperm production in males. They also control the output of the sex hormones oestrogen, progesterone, and testosterone.

Growth hormone promotes normal growth and development.

Melanocyte-stimulating hormone controls skin pigmentation.

Antidiuretic hormone (ADH or vasopressin) regulates the output of water in the urine.

An excess or a lack of one of the pituitary hormones may produce serious effects, the nature of which depends on the hormone involved. Abnormal levels of a particular hormone may be caused by a pituitary tumour, which may be treated with surgery, radiotherapy, or drugs. In other cases, drugs may be used to correct the hormonal imbalance.

The more common pituitary disorders that can be treated with drugs are those involving growth hormone, antidiuretic hormone, prolactin, adrenal hormones, and the gonadotrophins. The first three are discussed below. For information on the use of drugs to treat infertility arising from inadequate levels of gonadotrophins, see p.109. Lack of corticotrophin, leading to inadequate production of adrenal hormones, is usually treated with corticosteroids (see p.80).

DRUGS FOR GROWTH HORMONE DISORDERS

Growth hormone (somatotropin) is the principal hormone required for normal growth in childhood and adolescence. Lack of growth hormone impairs normal physical growth. Doctors administer hormone treatment only after tests have proven that a lack of this hormone is the cause of the disorder. If treatment is started at an early age, regular injections of somatropin, a synthetic form of natural growth hormone administered until the end of adolescence, usually allow normal growth and development to take place.

Less often, the pituitary produces excess growth hormone. In children this can result in pituitary gigantism; in adults, it can produce a disorder known as acromegaly. This disorder, which is usually the result of a pituitary tumour, is characterized by thickening of the skull, face, hands, and feet, and enlargement of some internal organs.

A pituitary tumour may be either surgically removed or destroyed by radiotherapy. In frail or elderly people, drugs such as bromocriptine and octreotide are used to reduce growth hormone levels. Octreotide is also used as an adjunctive treatment before surgery and in those with increased growth hormone levels occurring after surgery. People who have undergone surgery and/or radiotherapy may require long-term replacement with other hormones (such as sex hormones, thyroid hormone, or corticosteroids).

DRUGS FOR DIABETES INSIPIDUS

Antidiuretic hormone (also known as ADH or vasopressin) acts on the kidneys, controlling the amount of water retained in the body and returned to the blood. Lack of ADH is usually caused by damage to the pituitary; this, in turn, causes diabetes insipidus. In this rare condition, the kidneys cannot retain water, and large quantities pass into the urine. The chief symptoms are constant thirst and the production of large volumes of urine.

Diabetes insipidus is treated with ADH or a related synthetic drug, desmopressin. These replace naturally produced ADH. They may be given by injection or in the form of a nasal spray. Chlorpropamide may be used to treat mild cases; it works by increasing ADH release from the pituitary and by sensitizing the kidneys to the effect of ADH.

Alternatively, a thiazide diuretic (such as chlortalidone) may be prescribed for mild cases (see Diuretics, p.32). The usual effect of such drugs is to increase urine production, but in diabetes insipidus they have the opposite effect, reducing water loss from the body.

DRUGS TO REDUCE PROLACTIN LEVELS

Prolactin, also called lactogenic hormone, is produced in both men and women. In women, prolactin controls the secretion of breast milk following childbirth. The function of this hormone in men is not understood, although it appears to be necessary for normal sperm production.

The disorders associated with prolactin are all to do with overproduction. High levels in women can cause galactorrhoea (lactation that is not associated with pregnancy and birth), amenorrhoea (lack of menstruation), and infertility. If excessive prolactin is produced in men, the result may be galactorrhoea, impotence, or infertility.

Some drugs, notably methyldopa, oestrogen, and the phenothiazine antipsychotics, can raise the prolactin level in the blood. More often, however, the increased prolactin results from a pituitary tumour; it is usually treated with bromocriptine or cabergoline, which inhibit prolactin production.

COMMON DRUGS

Drugs for growth hormone disorders
Bromocriptine*, Lanreotide, Octreotide, Somatropin
Drugs for diabetes insipidus Carbamazepine*,
Chlorpropamide, Chlortalidone, Desmopressin*,
Vasopressin (ADH)
Drugs to reduce prolactin levels Bromocriptine*,
Cabergoline, Quinagolide
* See Part 2

Male sex hormones

Male sex hormones, or androgens, are responsible for the development of male sexual characteristics. The principal androgen is testosterone, which in men is produced by the testes from puberty onwards. Women produce testosterone in small amounts in the adrenal glands, but its exact function in the female body is not known.

Testosterone has two major effects: an androgenic effect and an anabolic effect. Its androgenic effect is to stimulate the appearance of the secondary sexual characteristics at puberty, such as the growth of body hair, deepening of the voice, and an increase in genital size. Its anabolic effects are to increase muscle bulk and accelerate growth rate.

There are a number of synthetic derivatives of testosterone that produce varying degrees of the androgenic and anabolic effects mentioned above. Derivatives that have a mainly anabolic effect are known as anabolic steroids (see p.88).

Testosterone and its derivatives have been used under medical supervision in both men and women to treat a number of conditions.

WHY THEY ARE USED

Male sex hormones are mainly given to men to promote the development of male sexual characteristics when hormone production is deficient. This problem may result from an abnormality of the testes or from inadequate production of the pituitary hormones that stimulate the testes to release testosterone.

A course of treatment with male sex hormones is sometimes prescribed for adolescent boys in whom the onset of puberty is delayed by pituitary problems. The treatment may also help to stimulate development of secondary male sexual characteristics and to increase sex drive (libido) in adult men who are producing inadequate testosterone levels. However, this type of hormone treatment has been found to reduce the production of sperm. (For information on the drug treatment of male infertility, see p.109.)

Androgens may also be prescribed for women to treat certain types of cancer of the breast and uterus (see Anticancer drugs, p.96). Testosterone can be given by injection, capsules, patches, or pellets that are surgically inserted.

HOW THEY WORK

Taken in low doses as part of replacement therapy when natural production is low, male sex hormones act in the same way as the natural hormones. In adolescents suffering from delayed puberty, hormone treatment produces both androgenic and anabolic effects, initiating the development of secondary sexual characteristics over a few months; full sexual development usually takes place over three to four years. When sex hormones are given to adult men, the effects on physical appearance and libido may begin to be felt within a few weeks.

RISKS AND SPECIAL PRECAUTIONS

The main risks with these drugs occur when they are given to boys with delayed puberty and to women with breast cancer. Given to initiate the onset of puberty, they may stunt growth by prematurely sealing the growing ends of the long bones. Doctors normally try to avoid prescribing hormones in these circumstances until growth is complete. High doses given to women have various masculinizing effects, including increased facial and body hair, and a deeper voice. The drugs may also produce enlargement of the clitoris, changes in libido, and acne.

ANABOLIC STEROIDS

Anabolic steroids are synthetically produced variants that mimic the anabolic effects of the natural hormones. They increase muscle bulk and body growth.

Doctors occasionally prescribe anabolic steroids and a high-protein diet to promote recovery after serious illness or major surgery. The steroids may also help to increase the production of blood cells in some forms of anaemia and to reduce itching in chronic obstructive jaundice.

Anabolic steroids have been widely abused by athletes because these drugs speed up the recovery of muscles after a session of intense exercise. This enables the athlete to go through a more demanding daily exercise programme, which results in a significant improvement in muscle power. The use of anabolic steroids by athletes to improve their performance is condemned by doctors and athletic organizations because of the risks to health, particularly for women. The side effects range from acne and baldness to psychological changes, fluid retention, testicular atrophy and impotence (men), reduced fertility (women), hardening of the arteries, a long-term risk of liver disease, and certain forms of cancer.

COMMON DRUGS

Primarily androgenic Mesterolone, Testosterone*
Primarily anabolic Nandrolone
Anti-androgens Cyproterone, Finasteride*
* See Part 2

Female sex hormones

There are two natural female sex hormones: oestrogen and progesterone. In women, they are secreted by the ovaries from puberty until the menopause. Each month, oestrogen and progesterone levels fluctuate, producing the menstrual cycle (see p.104). At the start of pregnancy, progesterone is made by the corpus luteum (empty egg follicle); both

hormones are made by the placenta thereafter. The adrenal gland also makes small amounts of oestrogen. Production of oestrogen and progesterone is regulated by the two gonadotrophin hormones (FSH and LH) produced by the pituitary gland (see p.85).

Oestrogen is responsible for the development of female sexual characteristics, including breast development, growth of pubic hair, and widening of the pelvis. Progesterone prepares the lining of the uterus for implantation of a fertilized egg; it is also important for the maintenance of pregnancy.

Synthetic forms of these hormones, known as oestrogens and progestogens, are used medically to treat a number of conditions.

WHY THEY ARE USED

The best known use of oestrogens and progestogens is in oral contraceptives. These drugs are discussed on p.105. Other uses include the treatment of menstrual disorders (p.104) and certain hormone-sensitive cancers (p.96). This page discusses the drug treatments that are used for natural hormone deficiency.

HORMONE DEFICIENCY

Deficiency of female sex hormones may result from a deficiency of gonadotrophins, which may be caused by a pituitary disorder or by abnormal development of the ovaries (ovarian failure). This may lead to the absence of menstruation and lack of sexual development. If tests show a deficiency of gonadotrophins, preparations of these hormones may be prescribed (see p.109). These preparations trigger the release of oestrogen and progesterone from the ovaries. If pituitary function is normal and ovarian failure is diagnosed as the cause of hormone deficiency, oestrogens and progestogens may be given as supplements. In this situation, these supplements ensure development of normal female sexual characteristics but cannot stimulate ovulation.

MENOPAUSE

A decline in the levels of oestrogen and progesterone occurs naturally after the menopause, when the menstrual cycle ceases. The sudden reduction in levels of oestrogen often causes distressing symptoms, and many doctors suggest that hormone supplements be used around the time of the menopause (see Effects of hormone replacement therapy (HRT), right). HRT may also be prescribed for women who have undergone premature menopause following surgical removal of the ovaries.

HRT helps to reduce the symptoms of the menopause, including hot flushes and vaginal dryness. It is no longer normally recommended for long-term use or for the treatment of osteoporosis (see p.57), however, because of the increased risk of disorders such as breast cancer, stroke, and thromboembolism. If dryness of the vagina is a particular problem, a cream containing an oestrogen drug may be prescribed for short-term use.

HOW THEY AFFECT YOU

Hormones given to treat ovarian failure or delayed puberty take three to six months to produce a noticeable effect on sexual development. Taken for menopausal symptoms, they can dramatically reduce the number of hot flushes within a week.

Both oestrogens and progestogens can cause fluid retention; and oestrogens may cause nausea, vomiting, breast tenderness, headache, dizziness, and depression. Progestogens may cause "breakthrough" bleeding between menstrual periods. In the comparatively low doses used to treat these disorders, side effects are unlikely.

RISKS AND SPECIAL PRECAUTIONS

Because oestrogens increase the risk of hypertension (high blood pressure), thrombosis (abnormal blood clotting), and breast cancer, there are risks associated with long-term HRT. Therefore, a balance between the benefits and risks for each individual woman must be considered.

HRT may not be recommended for women with heart or circulatory disorders, or those who are overweight or who smoke. Oestrogens may also trigger the onset of diabetes mellitus in susceptible people or may aggravate blood glucose control in diabetic women. Tibolone has both oestrogen and progestogen properties and can be used on its own.

EFFECTS OF HORMONE REPLACEMENT THERAPY (HRT)

Besides alleviating the symptoms of the menopause, such as hot flushes and vaginal dryness, HRT may have a beneficial effect on certain parts of the body. Such benefits must, however, be weighed against an increased risk of disorders such as breast cancer, stroke and thromboembolism.

Breasts There is an increased risk of breast cancer with long-term use of HRT. The increase in risk is related to the length of time for which HRT is used. If HRT is stopped, however, the risk reduces to its pre-treatment level within about five years.

Bones For women who go through premature menopause, HRT reduces the thinning of bone that occurs in osteoporosis and thus protects against fractures.

Reproductive organs Thinning of the vaginal tissues leading to painful intercourse can be prevented by HRT.

COMMON DRUGS

Oestrogens Conjugated oestrogens*, Estradiol*, Estriol, Estrone, Estropipate, Tibolone*

Progestogens Dydrogesterone*, Hydroxyprogesterone, Levonorgestrel*, Medroxyprogesterone*, Norethisterone*, Norgestrel, Progesterone, Raloxifene*

* See Part 2

NUTRITION

Food provides energy in the form of calories. It also provides materials called nutrients, which are needed for growth and renewal of tissues. Protein, carbohydrate, and fat are the major nutrient components of food.

Proteins are vital for tissue growth and repair. The moderate amounts required can be found in meat and dairy products, cereals, and pulses.

Carbohydrates are a major energy source, and are stored as fat when taken in excess. They can be found in cereals, sugar, and vegetables. Starchy foods are preferable to sugar.

Fats are a concentrated energy form needed only in small quantities. They are contained in animal products such as butter and in the oils of plants such as corn and nuts.

Vitamins and minerals are found only in small amounts in food but are very important for the normal functioning of the body.

Fibre (non-starch polysaccharides) is the indigestible part of any fruit, vegetable, or food or product derived from plants. It is needed for a healthy digestive system. Fibre contains no nutrients but adds bulk to faeces.

During digestion, large molecules of food are broken down into smaller molecules, releasing nutrients that are absorbed into the bloodstream. Carbohydrates and fats are then metabolized by body cells to produce energy. They may also be incorporated, with protein, into the cell structure. Each metabolic process is promoted by a specific enzyme and often requires the presence of a particular vitamin or mineral.

WHY DRUGS ARE USED

Dietary deficiency of essential nutrients can lead to illness. In poorer countries where there is a shortage of food, marasmus (resulting from lack of food energy) and kwashiorkor (from lack of protein) are common. In the developed world, however, excessive food intake leading to obesity is more common. Nutritional deficiencies in developed countries result from poor food choices and usually stem from a lack of a specific vitamin or mineral, as in iron-deficiency anaemia.

Some nutritional deficiencies may be caused by an inability of the body to absorb nutrients from food (malabsorption) or to utilize them once they have been absorbed. Malabsorption may be caused by the lack of an enzyme or an abnormality of the digestive tract. Errors of metabolism are often inborn and are not yet fully understood. They may be caused by failure of the body to produce the chemicals needed to process nutrients for use.

WHY SUPPLEMENTS ARE USED

Deficiencies such as kwashiorkor or marasmus are usually treated by dietary improvement and, in some cases, food supplements, rather than drugs. Vitamin and mineral deficiencies are usually treated with appropriate supplements. Malabsorption disorders may require changes in diet or long-term use of supplements. Metabolic errors are not easily treated with supplements or drugs, and a special diet may be the main treatment.

The preferred treatment of obesity is reduction of food intake, altered eating patterns, and increased exercise. When these methods are not effective, and the body mass index, or BMI (a figure indicating healthy or unhealthy body weight) is 30 or more, an anti-obesity drug may be used.

MAJOR DRUG GROUPS
◆ Vitamins
◆ Minerals

Vitamins

Vitamins are complex chemicals that are essential for a variety of body functions. With the exception of vitamin D, the body cannot manufacture these substances itself, so we need to include them in our diet.

There are 13 major vitamins: A, C, D, E, K, and the B complex vitamins – thiamine (B_1), riboflavin (B_2), niacin (B_3), pantothenic acid (B_5), pyridoxine (B_6), cobalamin (B_{12}), folic acid, and biotin. Most vitamins are required in very small amounts and each vitamin is present in one or more foods (see Main food sources of vitamins, p.92). Vitamin D is also produced in the body when the skin is exposed to sunlight. Vitamins fall into two groups, depending on whether they dissolve in fat or water.

Water-soluble vitamins Vitamin C and the B vitamins dissolve in water. Most are stored in the body for only a short period and are rapidly excreted by the kidneys if taken in higher amounts than the body needs. Vitamin B_{12} is the exception; it is stored in the liver, which may hold up to six years' supply. For these reasons, foods containing water-soluble vitamins need to be eaten daily. These vitamins are easily lost in cooking, so uncooked foods containing them should be eaten regularly. An overdose does not usually cause toxic effects, but adverse reactions to large dosages of vitamin C and pyridoxine (vitamin B_6) have been reported.

Fat-soluble vitamins Vitamins A, D, E, and K are absorbed from the intestine into the bloodstream together with fat. Deficiency of these vitamins may occur as a result of any disorder that affects the absorption of fat (for example, coeliac disease). These vitamins are stored in the liver and reserves of some of them may last for several years. Taking an excess of a fat-soluble vitamin for a long period may cause it to build up to a harmful level in the body. Ensuring that foods rich in these vitamins are regularly included in the diet usually provides a sufficient supply without the risk of overdosage.

A number of vitamins, such as vitamins A, C, and E, have now been recognized as having strong antioxidant properties (neutralizing the effect of free radicals, which are believed to play a role in aging and disease).

A balanced diet that includes a variety of different types of food is likely to contain adequate amounts of all the vitamins. Inadequate intake of any vitamin over an extended period, however, can lead to symptoms of deficiency. The nature of these symptoms depends on the vitamin concerned.

A doctor may recommend supplements of one or more vitamins in a variety of circumstances: to prevent deficiency occurring in people who are considered at special risk, to treat symptoms of deficiency, and in the treatment of certain medical conditions.

WHY VITAMINS ARE USED

Preventing deficiency Most people in the UK obtain enough vitamins from their diet, and supplements are not usually necessary. If you are unsure whether your diet is adequate, you are advised to look at the table on p.92 to check that you are regularly eating vitamin-rich foods. Vitamin intake can often be boosted simply by increasing the quantities of fresh food and raw fruit and vegetables in the diet.

Certain groups of people are at increased risk of vitamin deficiency. They include people with an increased need of certain vitamins that may not be met from dietary sources – in particular, pregnant or breast-feeding women, and infants and young children. Elderly people who may not be eating a varied diet may also be at risk. Strict vegetarians, vegans, and other people on restricted diets may not receive adequate amounts of all vitamins.

People who have disorders in which absorption of nutrients from the bowel is impaired, or who take drugs that reduce vitamin absorption (such as some types of lipid-lowering drugs), are usually given additional vitamins.

In these cases, the doctor is likely to advise supplements of one or more vitamins; most are available without prescription, but it is important to seek specialist advice before starting a course, so that a proper assessment of your individual requirements can be made.

Vitamin supplements should not be used as a tonic to improve your general well-being – they are ineffective for this purpose – nor as a substitute for a balanced diet.

Treating deficiency It is rare for a diet to lack a particular vitamin completely. If, however, intake of a vitamin is regularly lower than the body needs (see Vitamin requirements, p.92), the stores of vitamins may, over time, become depleted and symptoms of deficiency may begin to appear. In the UK, vitamin deficiency disorders are most common among vagrants and alcoholics, and in those on low incomes who fail to eat an adequate diet. Deficiencies of water-soluble vitamins are more likely since most of these are not stored in large quantities in the body.

Dosages of vitamins prescribed to treat deficiency are likely to be larger than those used to prevent it. Medical supervision is required when correcting vitamin deficiency.

MAIN FOOD SOURCES OF VITAMINS

The table below lists especially good sources of particular vitamins. A balanced diet helps to maintain adequate intake without the need for supplements. Processed and overcooked foods are likely to contain fewer vitamins than fresh, raw, or lightly cooked foods.

VITAMINS	Red meat	Poultry	Liver	Milk	Cheese	Butter/margarine	Eggs	Fish	Cereals and bread	Green vegetables	Root vegetables	Pulses/legumes	Nuts	Fruit
Biotin			•				•					•	•	
Folic acid			•				•			•				•
Niacin as nicotinic acid	•	•	•					•	•			•	•	
Pantothenic acid			•					•	•					
Pyridoxine	•	•	•				•	•	•					
Riboflavin			•	•	•		•		•			•	•	•
Thiamine	•		•						•			•	•	
Vitamin A			•	•	•	•	•			•	•			•
Vitamin B12	•		•	•	•		•	•						
Vitamin C										•	•			•
Vitamin D				•		•	•	•						
Vitamin E						•	•		•	•			•	•
Vitamin K										•	•			

Other medical uses of vitamins Various claims have been made for the value of vitamins in the treatment of other medical disorders. High doses of vitamin C have been said to be effective in preventing and treating the common cold. Such claims are not proved (although the mineral zinc may be helpful for this purpose). Supplements do not improve IQ in well-nourished children, but quite small dietary deficiencies can cause poor academic performance. This problem may be reversed once the deficiency has been remedied.

Certain vitamins also have recognized medical uses. Vitamin D has long been used to treat bone-wasting disorders (see p.56). Niacin is sometimes used (in the form of nicotinic acid) as a lipid-lowering drug (see p.37). Vitamin A derivatives (retinoids) are an established part of the treatment for severe acne (see p.123). Many women with pre-menstrual syndrome take pyridoxine (vitamin B_6) supplements to relieve their symptoms. See also Drugs used to treat menstrual disorders, p.104.

VITAMIN REQUIREMENTS

Normal daily vitamin requirements are usually based on the Reference Nutrient Intake (RNI). Deficiency needs much higher doses, which should be determined by your doctor.

Biotin No RNI established; 10–200 micrograms is safe.

Folic acid (as folate) 50 micrograms (birth–1 year); 70 micrograms (1–3 years); 100 micrograms (4–6 years); 150 micrograms (7–10 years); 200 micrograms (11 years and over). For women planning pregnancy, 400 micrograms per day, before conception and during first 12 weeks of pregnancy (to prevent first occurrence of neural tube defects). To prevent recurrence of a neural tube defect, 5mg per day before conception and during first 12 weeks of pregnancy.

Niacin 3mg (birth–3 months); 4mg (7–9 months); 5mg (10–12 months); 8mg (1–3 years); 11mg (4–6 years); 12mg (males 7–10 years and females 7–14 years); 15mg (males 11–14 years); 18mg (males 15–18 years); 14mg (females 15–18 years); 17mg (males 19–50 years); 13mg (females 19–50 years); 16mg (males 51 years and over); 12mg (females 51 years and over). No extra requirement in pregnancy; 2mg extra during breast-feeding.

Pantothenic acid No RNI established; adults require 3–7mg daily.

Pyridoxine 0.2mg (birth–6 months); 0.3mg (7–9 months); 0.4mg (10 months–1 year); 0.7mg (1–3 years); 0.9mg (4–6 years); 1mg (males 7–10 years and females 7–14 years);

1.2mg (males 11–14 years); 1.5mg (males 15–18 years); 1.2mg (females 15 and over); 1.4mg (males 19 and over).

Riboflavin 0.4mg (birth–1 year); 0.6mg (1–3 years); 0.8mg (4–6 years); 1mg (7–10 years); 1.2mg (males 11–14 years); 1.1mg (females 11 and over); 1.3mg (males 15 and over). Requirements rise by 0.3mg in pregnancy and 0.5mg during breast-feeding.

Thiamine 0.2mg (birth–9 months); 0.3mg (10–12 months); 0.5mg (1–3 years); 0.7mg (males 4–10 years and females 4–14 years); 0.9mg (males 11–14 years); 1.1mg (males 15–18 years); 0.8mg (females 15 and over); 1mg (males 19–50 years); 0.9mg (males 51 and over). Extra 0.1mg in last three months of pregnancy; 0.2mg during breast-feeding.

Vitamin A 350 micrograms (up to 1 year); 400 micrograms (1–3 years); 500 micrograms (4–10 years); 600 micrograms (males 11–14 years, females 11 years and over); 700 micrograms (males 15 and over, and pregnant women); 950 micrograms (breast-feeding).

Vitamin B$_{12}$ Only minute quantities required. 0.3 micrograms (birth–6 months); 0.4 micrograms (7–12 months); 0.5 micrograms (1–3 years); 0.8 micrograms (4–6 years); 1 microgram (7–10 years); 1.2 micrograms (11–14 years); 1.5 micrograms (15 years and over). No extra requirements in pregnancy; 2 micrograms during breast-feeding.

Vitamin C 25mg (birth–1 year); 30mg (1–10 years); 35mg (11–14 years); 40mg (15 years and over). Extra 50mg in pregnancy; 70mg during breast-feeding.

Vitamin D 8.5 micrograms (birth–6 months); 7 micrograms (7 months–3 years); 10 micrograms (over 65 years, pregnancy, and breast-feeding). Most people outside these groups do not require supplements.

Vitamin E No UK recommendations. Requirement depends on intake of polyunsaturated fatty acid, which varies widely; 3–15mg (approx.) recommended.

Vitamin K 10 micrograms (newborn); no RNI established (other age groups). No extra requirements for pregnancy and breast-feeding.

RISKS AND SPECIAL PRECAUTIONS

Vitamins are essential for health, and supplements can be taken without risk by most people. It is important not to exceed the recommended dosage, however, particularly in the case of fat-soluble vitamins, which may accumulate in the body. Dosage needs to be carefully calculated, taking into account the degree of deficiency, dietary intake, and duration of treatment. Overdosage has no therapeutic value, and may even have serious harmful effects. Multivitamin preparations containing a large number of different vitamins are widely available, but the amounts of each vitamin in each tablet are not usually large and are not likely to be harmful unless the dose is greatly exceeded. Single vitamin supplements can be harmful; excess of one vitamin may increase requirements for others. They should be used only on medical advice

Minerals

Minerals are chemical elements (the simplest form of substance) many of which are essential in trace amounts for normal metabolic processes. A balanced diet usually contains all of the minerals that the body needs; mineral deficiency diseases, except iron-deficiency anaemia, are uncommon.

Dietary supplements are necessary only when a doctor has diagnosed a specific deficiency, or as part of the prevention or treatment of a medical disorder. Doctors often prescribe minerals for people with intestinal diseases that reduce the absorption of minerals from the diet. Iron supplements are often advised for pregnant or breast-feeding women, and iron-rich foods are recommended for infants over six months.

Taking mineral supplements unless under medical direction is not advisable. Exceeding the body's daily requirements is not beneficial, and large doses may be harmful.

MINERAL REQUIREMENTS

As with vitamins, normal daily mineral requirements are usually based on the Reference Nutrient Intake (RNI).

Calcium 525mg (birth–1 year); 350mg (1–3 years); 450mg (4–6 years); 550mg (7–10 years); 1,000mg (males 11–18 years); 800mg (females 11–18 years); 700mg (19 years and older). No extra requirement in pregnancy; 550mg extra during breast-feeding.

MAIN FOOD SOURCES OF MINERALS

The table below indicates foods that are especially good sources of particular minerals. A balanced diet usually contains all the minerals required by the body, without the need for supplements. Some, known as trace elements, are required in only minute amounts.

MINERALS	Red meat	Poultry	Liver	Milk	Cheese	Butter/margarine	Eggs	Fish	Cereals and bread	Green vegetables	Root vegetables	Pulses/legumes	Nuts	Fruit
Calcium				•	•				•	•		•	•	
Chromium	•				•				•	•				
Copper	•	•	•					•	•	•		•	•	
Fluoride								•						
Iodine				•	•			•	•					
Iron	•	•	•				•	•	•	•				
Magnesium				•				•	•	•		•	•	
Phosphorus	•	•	•	•	•		•	•	•	•	•	•	•	•
Potassium								•	•	•	•	•	•	•
Selenium	•		•	•				•	•					
Sodium	•	•	•	•	•	•	•	•	•					
Zinc	•				•					•		•		

Chromium Only minute quantities needed. RNI not established; about 25 micrograms is safe.

Copper 0.2mg (birth–3 months); 0.3mg (4 months–1 year); 0.4mg (1–3 years); 0.6mg (4–6 years); 0.7mg (7–10 years); 0.8mg (11–14 years); 1.0mg (15–18 years); 1.2mg (19 years and over). No extra requirement in pregnancy; 0.3mg extra during breast-feeding.

Fluoride No RNI established; about 0.15mg (infants under 3 months) and 0.5mg (up to 2 years) is safe.

Iodine 50 micrograms (birth–3 months); 60 micrograms (4–12 months); 70 micrograms (1–3 years); 100 micrograms (4–6 years); 110 micrograms (7–10 years); 130 micrograms (11–14 years); 140 micrograms (15 years and over). Slightly increased requirement during breast-feeding; one vitamin tablet with calcium and iodine is recommended.

Iron 1.7mg (birth–3 months); 4.3mg (4–6 months); 7.8mg (7–12 months); 6.9mg (1–3 years); 6.1mg (4–6 years); 8.7mg (7–10 years); 11.3mg (males 11–18 years); 14.8mg (females 11–50 years); 8.7mg (males 19 and over, and females 51 and over). Requirements may be increased in pregnancy and for 2 to 3 months after childbirth.

Magnesium 55mg (birth–3 months); 60mg (4–6 months); 75mg (7–9 months); 80mg (10–12 months); 85mg (1–3 years); 120mg (4–6 years); 200mg (7–10 years); 280mg (11–14 years); 300mg (males 15 and over, and females 15–18 years); 270mg (females 19 and over). No extra requirement in pregnancy; 50mg extra during breast-feeding.

Potassium 0.8g (birth–3 months); 0.85g (4–6 months); 0.7g (7–12 months); 0.8g (1–3 years); 1.1g (4–6 years); 2g (7–10 years); 3.1g (11–14 years); 3.5g (15 years and over).

Selenium 10 micrograms (birth–3 months); 13 micrograms (4–6 months); 10 micrograms (7–12 months); 15 micrograms (1–3 years); 20 micrograms (4–6 years); 30 micrograms (7–10 years); 45 micrograms (11–14 years); 70 micrograms (males 15–18 years); 60 micrograms (females 15 and over); 75 micrograms (males 19 and over). No extra requirement in pregnancy; 15 micrograms extra during breast-feeding.

Sodium 0.21g (birth–3 months); 0.28g (4–6 months); 0.32g (7–9 months); 0.35g (10–12 months); 0.5g (1–3 years); 0.7g (4–6 years); 1.2g (7–10 years); 1.6g (11 years and over).

Zinc 4mg (birth–6 months); 5mg (7 months–3 years); 6.5mg (4–6 years); 7mg (7–10 years); 9mg (11–14 years); 9.5mg (males 15 years and over); 7mg (females 15 years and over). No extra requirement in pregnancy; 13mg during first 4 months of breast-feeding and 9.5mg thereafter.

MALIGNANT AND IMMUNE DISEASE

New cells are continuously needed by the body to replace those that wear out and die naturally and to repair injured tissue. In normal circumstances, the rate at which cells are created is carefully regulated. Sometimes, however, abnormal cells are formed that multiply uncontrollably. The cells may form lumps of abnormal tissue called tumours. Most tumours, such as warts, are confined to one place and cause few problems; these are known as benign growths. In other types of tumour, the cells may invade or destroy the structures around the tumour, and abnormal cells may spread to other parts of the body, forming satellite or metastatic tumours. These are malignant growths, also called cancers.

Opposing the development of tumours is the body's immune system. This identifies and deals with foreign material – not only invading bacteria and viruses, but also transplanted tissue and cells that have become cancerous. Interferons are natural proteins that limit viral infection by inhibiting viral replication within body cells. Some of these substances also assist in the destruction of cancer cells. The immune system relies on different types of white blood cells, produced in the lymph glands and bone marrow.

TYPES OF CANCER

Uncontrolled multiplication of cells leads to the formation of tumours that may be benign or malignant. Benign tumours do not spread to other tissues; malignant (cancerous) tumours do, however.

Carcinomas affect the skin and cells in the tissue lining internal organs.

Sarcomas affect muscles, bones, and fibrous tissues and lining cells of blood vessels.

Leukaemia affects white blood cells.

Lymphomas affect the lymph glands.

WHAT CAN GO WRONG

A single cause for cancer has not been identified; an individual's risk of developing cancer may depend both upon genetic predisposition (some types of cancer run in families) and upon exposure to external risk factors, known as carcinogens. These include tobacco smoke, which increases the risk of lung cancer, and ultraviolet light, which makes skin cancer more likely to occur in those people who spend long periods in the sun. Long-term suppression of the immune system through disease (as occurs in AIDS) or by the use of drugs (such as those given to prevent rejection of transplanted organs) also increases the risk of developing not only infections but also certain cancers. This demonstrates the importance of the immune system in removing abnormal cells with the potential to cause a tumour.

Overactivity of the immune system may also cause problems. It may respond excessively to an innocuous stimulus, as in hay fever (see Allergy, p.58), or may mount a reaction against normal tissues, leading to a variety of disorders known as autoimmune diseases. These include rheumatoid arthritis, certain inflammatory skin disorders (for example, systemic lupus erythematosus), pernicious anaemia, and some forms of hypothyroidism. Increased immune system activity can also occur following an organ or tissue transplant, when it may lead to rejection of the foreign tissue. This shows the need for medication that can dampen the immune system and enable the body to accept the foreign tissue.

WHY DRUGS ARE USED

In cancer treatment, cytotoxic (cell-killing) drugs are used to eliminate abnormally dividing cells. This has the effect of slowing the growth rate of tumours and sometimes leading to their complete disappearance. However, because these drugs act against all rapidly dividing cells, they also reduce the number of normal cells, including blood cells, being produced from the bone marrow. This can cause serious adverse effects, such as anaemia and neutropenia (decreased numbers of certain white blood cells), but it can be useful in limiting white cell activity in autoimmune disorders. Some newer anticancer drugs are more selective in the cells they target.

Other drugs that have immunosuppressant effects include corticosteroids and ciclosporin, which are used following transplant surgery. No drugs are yet available that directly stimulate the entire immune system. However, growth factors may be used to increase the number and activity of some white blood cells, and antibody infusions may help those individuals with deficient white blood cell production, or may be used against specific targets in organ transplantation and cancer.

MAJOR DRUG GROUPS
◆ Anticancer drugs
◆ Immunosuppressant drugs
◆ Drugs for HIV and AIDS

Anticancer drugs

Cancer is a general term that covers a wide range of disorders, ranging from the leukaemias (blood cancers) to solid tumours of the lung, breast, and other organs. In all cancers, a group of cells escape from the normal controls on cell growth and multiplication. As a result, the malignant (cancerous) cells begin to crowd out the normal cells and a tumour develops. Cancerous cells are frequently unable to perform their usual functions, and this may lead to progressively impaired function of the organ or area concerned. Cancers may develop from cells of the blood, skin, muscle, or any other tissue.

Malignant tumours spread into nearby structures, blocking blood vessels and compressing nerves and other structures. Fragments of the tumour may become detached and carried in the bloodstream to other parts of the body, where they form secondary growths (metastases).

Many different factors, or a combination of them, can provoke cancerous changes in cells. These include an individual's genetic background, immune system failure, and exposure to cancer-causing agents (carcinogens). Known carcinogens include strong sunlight, tobacco smoke, radiation, certain chemicals, viruses, and dietary factors.

Treating cancer is a complicated process that depends on the type of cancer, its stage of development, and the patient's condition and wishes. Any of the following treatments may be used, either alone or in combination with the others: surgery, radiation treatment, and drug therapy.

Until recently, drug treatment of cancer relied heavily on hormonal drugs and cytotoxic agents (usually referred to collectively as chemotherapy). Hormone treatments are suitable for only a few types of cancer and cytotoxic drugs, although valuable, can have severe side effects because of the damage that they do to normal tissues. In recent years, as understanding of cancer biology has increased, new drugs have been developed. These include cytokines, such as interferon and interleukin-2, that stimulate the immune system to attack certain cancers, and monoclonal antibodies and growth-factor inhibitors that attack the cancer cells much more selectively.

WHY THEY ARE USED
Cytotoxic drugs can cure rapidly growing cancers and are the treatment of choice for leukaemias, lymphomas, and certain cancers of the testis. They are less effective against slow-growing solid tumours, however, such as those of the breast and bowel, but they can relieve symptoms and prolong life when they are given as palliative chemotherapy (treatment that relieves symptoms but does not cure the disease). Adjuvant (effect-enhancing) chemotherapy is increasingly being used following surgery, especially for breast and bowel tumours, to prevent regrowth of the cancer from cells left behind after surgery. Neoadjuvant, or primary, chemotherapy is sometimes used before surgery to reduce the size of the tumour.

Hormone therapy is offered to patients whose cancer is hormone-sensitive. Such cancers include many cancers of the breast, uterus, and prostate. In hormone therapies, the hormones can be used to relieve symptoms of the disease or, in advanced disease, provide palliative treatment.

Cytokines, monoclonal antibodies, and growth-factor inhibitors are used, either alone or alongside chemotherapy, sometimes with the aim of cure but more often with the aim of producing disease remission.

Most anticancer drug treatments, especially cytotoxic treatments, have side effects, sometimes severe, so treatment decisions have to balance possible benefits against the risk of side effects. More aggressive treatments may be appropriate for patients who have curable cancers.

Often a combination of several drugs is used, either simultaneously or successively. Special regimes of different drugs are used together and in succession have been devised to maximize their activity and minimize the side effects.

Certain anticancer drugs are also used for their effect in suppressing immune system activity (see p.99).

HOW THEY WORK

Anticancer drugs work in many different ways. The main groups of drugs and how they work are described below.

Cytotoxic drugs There are several classes of cytotoxic drug, including alkylating agents, antimetabolites, taxanes, and cytotoxic antibiotics. Each class has a different mechanism of action, but all act by interfering with basic processes of cell replication and division. They are particularly potent against rapidly dividing cells; these include cancer cells but also certain normal cells, especially those in the hair follicles, gut lining, and bone marrow. This action explains the drugs' side effects and the need to schedule treatment carefully.

Hormone therapies Hormone treatments act by counteracting the effects of the hormone that is encouraging growth of the cancer. For example, some breast cancers are stimulated by the female sex hormone oestrogen, whose action is opposed by the drug tamoxifen. Other cancers are damaged by high doses of a particular sex hormone. For example, medroxyprogesterone, a progestogen, is often used to halt the spread of endometrial cancer.

Cytokines The cytokines, interferon alfa and interleukin-2, stimulate the immune system to attack certain cancers. The mechanisms responsible for this action are not entirely understood.

Monoclonal antibodies Antibodies are special proteins that form a fundamental element of the immune system. They recognize, and bind very specifically to, "foreign" proteins on the surface of bacteria, viruses, and parasites, marking them out for destruction. Monoclonal antibodies are produced in tissue culture using cells that have been genetically engineered to make antibodies against a particular target protein.

If the target protein is carefully selected, the antibodies can be used to identify cancer cells for destruction by the immune system. If the target protein is found only on cancer cells, or on the cancer cells and the normal tissue from which it arose, the damage to healthy tissues during treatment is very limited. Once they have bound to a cell, antibodies interact with the immune system to kill cells in a variety of ways; for example, by attracting white blood cells called killer leukocytes and provoking a series of chemical reactions that dissolve the cell walls; this process is known as "complement fixation".

To date, there are three monoclonal antibodies in routine use as cancer treatment: trastuzumab, which binds to a protein produced in particularly large quantities in about one-fifth of breast cancer cells; rituximab, which recognizes a protein found on most lymphatic cancer cells as well as some normal white blood cells; and alemtuzumab, which recognizes and kills certain leukaemic cells in addition to some normal white blood cells. Because these antibodies are so specific, they are useful only against particular cancers, in which they cause little of the toxicity of conventional chemotherapy. They do, however, often cause allergy-type reactions, especially at the beginning of treatment.

Growth-factor inhibitors It has recently been discovered that the growth of cells, including cancer cells, is controlled by a complex network of growth factors that bind very specifically to receptor sites on the cell surface. This triggers a complex series of chemical reactions that transmit the "grow" message to the nucleus, triggering cell growth and replication. In many cancers, this system is faulty and there are either too many receptors on the cell surface or other abnormalities that result in the nucleus receiving inappropriate "grow" messages. The extra or abnormal cell surface receptors can be selected as targets for monoclonal antibodies (see above).

Other defects in this system are being used as the basis for other new drugs. For example, imatinib very selectively interferes with an abnormal version of an enzyme that is found in certain leukaemic cells. This abnormal enzyme causes the cell nucleus to receive a "grow" signal continuously, resulting in the uncontrolled growth of cancer. By stopping the enzyme working, it is possible to selectively "turn off" the growth of the abnormal cells. Imatinib is proving very successful in treating certain types of leukaemia, with few serious side effects.

HOW THEY AFFECT YOU

Cytotoxic drugs are generally associated with more side effects than other anti-cancer drugs. At the start of treatment, adverse effects of the drugs may be more noticeable than benefits. The most common side effect is nausea and vomiting, for which an anti-emetic (see p.21) will usually be prescribed. Effects on the blood are also common. Many cytotoxic drugs cause hair loss because of the effect of their activity on hair follicle cells, but the hair usually starts to grow back after chemotherapy has been completed. Individual drugs may produce other side effects.

Cytotoxic drugs are, in most cases, administered in the highest doses that can be tolerated in order to kill as many cancer cells as quickly as possible.

The unpleasant side effects of intensive chemotherapy, combined with a delay of several weeks before any beneficial effects are seen and the seriousness of the underlying disease, often lead to depression in those who are receiving anticancer drugs. Specialist counselling, support from family and friends, and, in some cases, treatment with anti-depressant drugs may be helpful.

SUCCESSFUL CHEMOTHERAPY

Not all cancers respond to treatment with anticancer drugs. Some cancers can be cured by drug treatment. In others, drug treatment can slow or temporarily halt the disease's progress. In certain cases, drug treatment has no beneficial effect, but other treatments, such as surgery, often produce significant benefits. The main cancers that fall into each of the first two groups are described here:

Cancers that can often be cured by drugs
◆ Some cancers of the lymphatic system (including Hodgkin's disease)
◆ Acute leukaemias (forms of blood cancer)
◆ Choriocarcinoma (cancer of the placenta)
◆ Germ cell tumours (cancers affecting sperm and egg cells)
◆ Wilms' tumour (a rare form of kidney cancer that affects children)
◆ Cancer of the testis

Cancers in which drugs may produce worthwhile benefits
◆ Breast cancer
◆ Ovarian cancer
◆ Some leukaemias
◆ Multiple myeloma (a bone marrow cancer)
◆ Many types of lung cancer
◆ Head and neck cancers
◆ Cancer of the stomach
◆ Cancer of the prostate
◆ Some cancers of the lymphatic system
◆ Bladder cancer
◆ Endometrial cancer (cancer affecting the lining of the uterus)
◆ Cancer of the large intestine
◆ Cancer of the oesophagus
◆ Cancer of the pancreas
◆ Cancer of the cervix

Successful drug treatment of cancer usually requires repeated courses of anticancer drugs because the treatment needs to be halted periodically to allow the blood-producing cells in the bone marrow to recover.

RISKS AND SPECIAL PRECAUTIONS

All cytotoxic anticancer drugs interfere with the activity of noncancerous cells and, for this reason, they often produce serious adverse effects during long-term treatment. In particular, these drugs often adversely affect rapidly dividing cells such as the blood-producing cells in the bone marrow. The numbers of red and white blood cells and the number of platelets (particles in the blood responsible for clotting) may all be reduced.

In some cases, symptoms of anaemia (which include weakness and fatigue) and an increased risk of abnormal or excessive bleeding may develop as a result of treatment with anticancer drugs. Reduction in the number of white blood cells may result in an increased susceptibility to infection. A simple infection such as a sore throat may be a sign of depressed white-cell production in a patient taking anticancer drugs, and it must be reported to the doctor without delay. In addition, wounds may take longer to heal, and susceptible people can develop gout as a result of increased uric acid production due to cells being broken down.

Because of these problems, anticancer chemotherapy is often undertaken in hospital, where the adverse effects can be closely monitored. Several short courses of drug treatment are usually given, thereby allowing the bone marrow time to recover in the period between courses of treatment (see Successful chemotherapy, facing page). Blood tests are performed regularly. When necessary, blood transfusions, antibiotics, or other forms of treatment are used in order to overcome the adverse effects. When relevant, contraceptive advice is given early in the treatment because most anticancer drugs can damage a developing baby.

In addition to these general effects, individual drugs may have adverse effects on particular organs.

By contrast, other anticancer drugs, such as hormonal drugs, antibodies, and growth-factor inhibitors are much more selective in their actions, and they generally have less serious side effects.

COMMON DRUGS

Alkylating agents Chlorambucil, Cyclophosphamide*, Melphalan

Antimetabolites Azathioprine*, Cytarabine, Fluorouracil, Mercaptopurine*, Methotrexate*

Taxanes Docetaxel, Paclitaxel

Cytotoxic antibiotics Doxorubicin*, Epirubicin

Hormone treatments Anastrozole*, Bicalutamide, Cyproterone acetate, Flutamide*, Formestane, Goserelin*, Letrozole, Leuprorelin, Medroxyprogesterone*, Megestrol*, Tamoxifen*

Cytokines Interferon alfa*, Interleukin-2

Monoclonal antibodies Alemtuzumab, Rituximab, Trastuzumab

Growth-factor inhibitors Imatinib

Other drugs Carboplatin, Cisplatin*, Etoposide, Irinotecan

* See Part 2

Immunosuppressant drugs

The body is protected against attack from bacteria, fungi, and viruses by the specialized cells and proteins in the blood and tissues that make up the immune system. They respond to foreign cells in a variety of ways. White blood cells known as lymphocytes respond to infection and foreign tissue, either by killing invading organisms directly or by producing special proteins (antibodies) to destroy them; B-lymphocytes produce antibodies to attack invading organisms, whereas T-lymphocytes attack invading cells directly. Other blood cells help the action of the B- and T-cells. These mechanisms are also responsible for eliminating abnormal or unhealthy cells that could otherwise multiply and develop into a cancer.

In certain conditions it is medically necessary to dampen the immune system's activity. They include a number of autoimmune disorders (in which the immune system attacks normal body tissue), which may affect a single organ (such as the adrenal glands in Addison's disease or the thyroid gland in Hashimoto's disease), or they may result in widespread damage (as in rheumatoid arthritis or systemic lupus erythematosus).

Immune system activity may also need to be reduced following an organ transplant, when the body's defences would otherwise attack and reject the transplanted tissue.

Several types of drug are used as immunosuppressants.

Anticancer drugs (see p.96) slow the production of all cells in the bone marrow.

Corticosteroids (see p.80) reduce the activity of both B- and T-lymphocytes.

Ciclosporin (see p.182) inhibits the activity of T-lymphocytes only and not B-lymphocyte activity.

WHY THEY ARE USED

Immunosuppressants are given for autoimmune disorders such as rheumatoid arthritis when symptoms are severe and other treatments have not given adequate relief. Corticosteroids are usually prescribed initially; their anti-inflammatory effect and immunosuppressant action help to promote the healing of tissue damaged by abnormal immune system activity. A drug such as methotrexate may be used in addition to corticosteroids, to reduce the activity of lymphocytes, if these drugs do not produce sufficient improvement or if their effect wanes (see also Antirheumatic drugs, p.52).

Immunosuppressant drugs are given before and after organ and other tissue transplants. Treatment may have to be continued indefinitely to prevent rejection. Several drugs and drug combinations are used, depending on the organ being transplanted and the underlying condition. However, ciclosporin, along with the related drug tacrolimus, is now the most widely used drug for preventing organ rejection. It is also increasingly used to treat autoimmune disorders. It is often used in combination with a corticosteroid or the more specific drug mycophenolate mofetil.

Monoclonal antibodies that attack the parts of the immune system responsible for organ rejection are also used after transplantation.

HOW THEY WORK

Immunosuppressant drugs reduce the effectiveness of the immune system, either by depressing the production of lymphocytes or by altering their activity.

HOW THEY AFFECT YOU

When immunosuppressants are given to treat an autoimmune disorder, they reduce the severity of symptoms and may temporarily halt the progress of the disease. They cannot repair major tissue damage, however.

Immunosuppressants can produce a range of unwanted side effects. The side effects of corticosteroids are described on p.80. Anticancer drugs prescribed as immunosuppressants are given in low doses that produce only mild side effects. They may cause nausea and vomiting, for which an anti-emetic drug (see p.21) may be prescribed. Hair loss is rare and regrowth usually occurs when treatment is stopped. Ciclosporin may cause increased facial hair growth, swelling of the gums, and tingling in the hands.

RISKS AND SPECIAL PRECAUTIONS

All of these drugs may produce potentially serious adverse effects. By reducing the activity of the patient's immune system, immuno-suppressant drugs can affect the body's ability to fight invading microorganisms, thereby increasing the risk of serious infections. Because lymphocyte activity is also important for preventing the multiplication of abnormal cells, there is an increased risk of certain types of cancer. A major drawback of anticancer drugs is that, in addition to their effect on the production of lymphocytes, they interfere with the growth and division of other blood cells in the bone marrow. Reduced production of red blood cells can cause anaemia; when the production of blood platelets is suppressed, blood clotting may be less efficient.

Although ciclosporin is more specific than either corticosteroids or anticancer drugs in its action, it can cause kidney damage. In addition, in too high a dose it may affect the brain, causing hallucinations or seizures. Ciclosporin also has a tendency to raise the blood pressure, and another drug may be required to counteract this effect (see Antihypertensive drugs, p.36).

COMMON DRUGS

Anticancer drugs Azathioprine*, Chlorambucil, Cyclophosphamide*, Methotrexate*, Mycophenolate mofetil

Corticosteroids (see p.80)

Antibodies Anti-lymphocyte globulin, Basiliximab, Daclizumab

Other drugs Ciclosporin*, Tacrolimus

* See Part 2

Drugs for HIV and AIDS

The disease AIDS (acquired immune deficiency syndrome) is caused by infection with HIV (human immunodeficiency virus). HIV invades certain cells of the immune system, particularly white blood cells called T-helper lymphocytes (or CD_4 cells), which normally activate other cells in the immune system to fight infection. Since HIV kills T-helper lymphocytes, the body cannot fight the virus or subsequent infections. Over the past few years the number of drugs available to treat HIV has increased considerably, as well as the knowledge about how best to use the drugs in combination.

ANTIRETROVIRAL DRUGS

DRUG NAME	FORMULATION	STANDARD ADULT DOSE
Reverse transcriptase inhibitors		
Abacavir *Ziagen*	Tablets (300mg) Oral solution (20mg/ml)	300mg twice daily
Didanosine (ddI, DDI) *Videx*	Enteric-coated capsules (400mg, 250mg, 200mg, 125mg) Tablets (200mg, 150mg, 100mg, 25mg)	Adults over 60kg: 400mg daily in 1 or 2 divided doses. Adults under 60kg:250mg in 1 or 2 divided doses
Efavirenz *Sustiva*	Capsules (200mg, 100mg, 50mg) Tablets (600mg)	600mg once daily
Lamivudine (3TC) *Epivir*	Tablets (300m, 150mg) Oral solution (50mg/5ml)	300mg in 1 or 2 divided doses
Lamivudine, zidovudine (AZT) Combivir	Combivir is the brand name of a tablet containing lamivudine (150mg) and zidovudine (300mg).	1 tablet twice daily
Lamivudine, zidovudine (AZT), abacavir *Trizivir*	Trizivir is the brand name of a tablet containing lamivudine (150mg), zidovudine (300mg), and abacavir (300mg).	1 tablet twice daily
Nevirapine *Viramune*	Tablets (200mg) Suspension (50mg/5ml)	200mg daily for 2 weeks then 200mg twice daily
Stavudine (d4T) *Zerit*	Capsules (40mg, 30mg, 20mg, 15mg) Oral solution (1mg/ml)	Adults over 60kg: 40mg twice daily. Adults under 60kg: 30mg twice daily
Tenofovir disoproxil *Viread*	Tablets (245mg as disoproxil fumarate = 300mg tenofovir)	1 tablet once daily
Zalcitabine (ddC, DDC) *Hivid*	Tablets (750mcg, 375mcg)	750mcg every 8 hours
Zidovudine (AZT) *Retrovir*	Capsules (250mg, 100mg) Injection (10mg/5ml) Syrup (50mg/5ml)	500–600mg in 2–3 divided doses
Protease inhibitors		
Amprenavir *Agenerase*	Capsules (150mg) Oral solution (15mg/ml)	Over 50kg in weight: tablets 1.2g twice daily
Indinavir *Crixivan*	Capsules (400mg, 100mg)	800mg every 8 hours
Lopinavir with ritonavir *Kaletra*	Each capsule contains 133.3mg of lopinavir and 33.3mg of ritonavir	Three capsules twice daily
Nelfinavir *Vircept*	Tablet (250mg) Oral powder	1.25g twice daily or 750mg three times daily
Ritonavir *Norvir*	Capsules (100mg) Oral solution (400mg/5ml)	600mg twice daily
Saquinavir *Fortovase* *Invirase*	Capsule (200mg)	Invirase: 1g every 12 hours; Fortovase: 1.2g every 8 hours

WHY THEY ARE USED

Drug treatments for HIV infection can be divided into treatment of the initial infection with HIV, and the treatment of diseases and complications that are associated with AIDS.

Drugs that act directly against HIV are known as antiretrovirals and they can be divided into two groups. Both work by interfering with enzymes that are vital for virus replication. The first group, which inhibit an enzyme known as reverse transcriptase, are divided, according to their chemical structure, into nucleoside and non-nucleoside inhibitors. The second group interfere with an enzyme called protease. The drugs in each group, with standard adult doses, are listed in the table on p.101.

Antiretrovirals are much more effective when used in combination. Treatment is now usually started with a combination of two nucleoside transcriptase inhibitors plus a non-nucleoside drug or a protease inhibitor. If combination antiretroviral therapy, also called highly active antiretroviral therapy (HAART), is started before damage to the immune system is too great, it can dramatically reduce the level of HIV in the body and improve the outlook for HIV-infected individuals. However, it is not a cure for the disease and people remain infectious.

The mainstay of drug treatment for AIDS-related diseases are the antimicrobial drugs for the bacterial, viral, fungal, and protozoal infections to which people with AIDS are susceptible. These drugs include the antituberculous drugs (see p.67), co-trimoxazole for the treatment of pneumocystis carinii pneumonia (PCP), and ganciclovir for the treatment of cytomegalovirus (CMV) infection.

COMMON DRUGS

Reverse transcriptase inhibitors Abacavir, Didanosine, Efavirenz*, Lamivudine, Nevirapine, Stavudine, Tenofovir disoproxil, Zalcitabine, Zidovudine (AZT)/lamivudine*

Protease inhibitors Amprenavir, Indinavir, Lopinavir/Ritonavir*, Nelfinavir, Saquinavir

* See Part 2

REPRODUCTIVE & URINARY TRACTS

The reproductive systems of men and women consist of the organs that produce and release sperm (male), or store and release eggs, and then nurture a fertilized egg until it develops into a baby (female). The urinary system filters wastes and water from the blood, producing urine, which is then expelled from the body. The reproductive and urinary systems of men are partially linked, but those of women form two physically close but functionally separate systems.

The female reproductive organs comprise the ovaries, fallopian tubes, and uterus (womb). The uterus opens via the cervix (neck of the uterus) into the vagina (birth canal). The principal male reproductive organs are the two sperm-producing glands, the testes (testicles), which lie within the scrotum, and the penis. Other structures of the male reproductive tract include the prostate gland and several tubular structures – the tightly coiled epididymides (singular: epididymis), the vas deferens, the seminal vesicles, and the urethra.

The urinary organs in both sexes comprise the kidneys, which filter the blood and excrete urine (see also Diuretics, p.32), the ureters, down which urine passes, and the bladder, where urine is stored until it is released from the body via the urethra.

WHAT CAN GO WRONG

The reproductive and urinary tracts are both subject to infection. The short female urethra allows urinary tract infections, especially cystitis (infection of the bladder) and urethritis (infection of the urethra), to occur commonly. The female reproductive tract is also vulnerable to infection, which, in some cases, is sexually transmitted. Such infections (apart from those that are transmitted by sexual activity) are relatively uncommon in men because the long male urethra prevents bacteria and other organisms from passing easily to the bladder and upper urinary tract and to the male sex organs.

Reproductive function may also be disrupted by hormonal disturbances that lead to reduced fertility. Women may be troubled by symptoms arising from normal activity of the reproductive organs, including menstrual disorders as well as problems associated with childbirth.

The most common urinary problems, apart from infection, are those that are related to bladder function. Urine may be released involuntarily (incontinence), or it may be retained in the bladder. Such disorders are usually the result of damage occurring during childbirth. The filtering action of the kidneys may be affected by alteration in the composition of the blood or of the hormones that regulate urine production, or by damage (from infection or inflammation) to the filtering units of the kidneys themselves.

WHY DRUGS ARE USED

Antibiotic drugs (see p.62) are used to eliminate infections of both the urinary and the reproductive tracts (including sexually transmitted infections). Certain infections of the vagina are caused by fungi or yeasts and require antifungal drugs (see p.76).

Hormone drugs are used both to reduce fertility deliberately (oral contraceptives) and to increase fertility in certain conditions in which it has not been possible for a couple to conceive. Hormones may also be used to regulate menstruation when it is irregular or excessively painful or heavy. Analgesic drugs (p.9) are used to treat menstrual period pain and are also widely used for pain relief in labour. Other drugs used in labour include those that increase contraction of the muscles of the uterus and those that limit blood loss after the birth. Drugs may also be used to halt premature labour.

Drugs that alter the transmission of nerve signals to the bladder muscles have an important role in the treatment of urinary incontinence and retention. Drugs that increase the kidneys' filtering action are commonly used to reduce blood pressure and fluid retention (see Diuretics, p.32). Other drugs may alter the composition of the urine – for example, the uricosuric drugs used in the treatment of gout (see p.53) increase the amount of uric acid.

THE MENSTRUAL CYCLE

A monthly cycle of hormone interactions allows an egg to be released and, if it is fertilized, creates the correct environment for it to implant in the uterus. Major changes occur in the body, the most obvious of which is monthly vaginal bleeding (menstruation). The menstrual cycle usually starts between the ages of 11 and 14 years and continues until the menopause, which occurs at around the age of 50. After the menopause, childbearing is no longer possible. The cycle is usually 28 days, but this varies from one individual to another.

Menstruation If no egg is fertilized, the endometrium is shed (days 1–5).

Fertile period Conception may take place in the two days after ovulation (days 14–16).

MAJOR DRUG GROUPS

◆ Drugs used to treat menstrual disorders
◆ Oral contraceptives
◆ Drugs for infertility
◆ Drugs used in labour
◆ Drugs used for urinary disorders

Drugs used to treat menstrual disorders

The menstrual cycle results from the actions of female sex hormones that cause ovulation (the release of an egg) and thickening of the endometrium (the lining of the uterus) each month in preparation for pregnancy. Unless the egg is fertilized, the endometrium will be shed about two weeks later during menstruation (see also The menstrual cycle, above).

The main problems associated with menstruation that may require medical treatment are menorrhagia (excessive blood loss), dysmenorrhoea (pain during menstruation), and premenstrual syndrome (distressing physical and psychological symptoms occurring prior to menstruation). Another possible problem is amenorrhoea (absent periods); the most common cause, in women of childbearing age, is pregnancy.

The drugs most commonly used to treat the main menstrual disorders described above include oestrogens and progestogens (synthetic hormones), danazol, and analgesics.

WHY THEY ARE USED

Drug treatment for menstrual disorders is undertaken only when the doctor has ruled out the possibility of an underlying gynaecological disorder, such as a pelvic infection or fibroids. In some cases, especially in women over the age of 35, a D and C (dilatation and curettage) may be recommended. When no underlying reason for the problem is found, drug treatment aimed primarily at the relief of symptoms is usually prescribed.

Dysmenorrhoea is pain associated with menstrual periods. The condition is usually treated initially with a simple analgesic drug. NSAIDs (see Non-steroidal anti-inflammatory drugs, p.50) are often the most effective because they counter the effects of prostaglandins, chemicals that are partly responsible for the painful cramps of the uterus that occur. Diclofenac and mefenamic acid are also used to reduce the excessive blood loss of menorrhagia (see below).

When these drugs are not sufficient to provide adequate pain relief, hormonal drug treatment may be recommended. If contraception is also required, treatment may involve an oral contraceptive pill containing both an oestrogen and a progestogen, or a progestogen alone. Non-contraceptive progestogen preparations may also be prescribed. These are usually taken for only a few days during each month.

Menorrhagia is excessive blood loss during menstruation. This problem can sometimes be reduced by some NSAIDs. Tranexamic acid, an antifibrinolytic drug, is also an effective treatment for menorrhagia. Alternatively, danazol, a drug that reduces production of the female sex hormone oestrogen, may be prescribed to reduce blood loss.

Premenstrual syndrome is a collection of psychological and physical symptoms that affect many women to some degree in the days before menstruation. Psychological symptoms include mood changes such as increased irritability, depression, and anxiety. Principal physical symptoms are bloating, headache, and breast tenderness. Because some doctors believe that premenstrual syndrome is the result of a drop in progesterone levels in the last half of the menstrual cycle, non-contraceptive supplements of this hormone may be given in the week or so before menstruation. Oral contraceptives may be considered as an alternative. Other drugs sometimes used include pyridoxine (vitamin B_6), diuretics (see p.32) if bloating due to fluid retention is a problem, and bromocriptine when breast tenderness is the major symptom. Antidepressants (see p.14) may be prescribed in cases where severe premenstrual psychological disturbance is experienced.

Endometriosis is a condition in which fragments of endometrial tissue (uterine lining) occur outside the uterus in the pelvic cavity. It causes severe pain during menstruation, often causes pain during intercourse, and may sometimes lead to infertility. Drugs used for this disorder are similar to those prescribed for heavy periods (menorrhagia). In this case, however, the intention is to suppress endometrial development for an extended period so that the abnormal tissue eventually withers away. Progesterone supplements that suppress endometrial thickening may be prescribed throughout the menstrual cycle. Alternatively, danazol, which suppresses endometrial development by reducing oestrogen production, may be prescribed. Any drug treatment usually needs to be continued for a minimum of six months. When drug treatment is unsuccessful, surgical removal of the abnormal tissue is usually necessary.

HOW THEY WORK

Drugs used to treat menstrual disorders act in a variety of ways: hormonal treatments are aimed at suppressing the pattern of hormonal changes that is causing troublesome symptoms; contraceptive preparations override the woman's normal menstrual cycle. Ovulation does not occur, and the endometrium does not thicken normally. Bleeding that occurs at the end of a cycle is less likely to be abnormally heavy, to be accompanied by severe discomfort, or to be preceded by distressing symptoms. For further information on oral contraceptives, see right.

Non-contraceptive progestogen preparations taken in the days before menstruation do not suppress ovulation. Increased progesterone during this time reduces premenstrual symptoms and prevents excessive thickening of the endometrium.

Danazol is a potent drug that prevents the thickening of the endometrium, thereby correcting excessively heavy periods. Blood loss is reduced, and in some cases menstruation ceases altogether during treatment.

COMMON DRUGS

Oestrogens and progestogens (see p.88)
NSAID analgesics Aspirin*, Diclofenac*, Diflunisal, Etoricoxib, Flurbiprofen, Ibuprofen*, Ketoprofen*, Mefenamic acid*, Naproxen*
Diuretics (see p.32)
Other drugs Bromocriptine*, Buserelin, Danazol*, Gestrinone, Goserelin*, Leuprorelin, Nafarelin, Pyridoxine, Tranexamic Acid, Triptorelin
* **See Part 2**

Oral contraceptives

There are many different methods of ensuring that conception and pregnancy do not follow sexual intercourse, but for most women the oral contraceptive is the most effective method.

The following list indicates the number of pregnancies occurring with each method of contraception per 100 users each year. The wide variation that occurs with some of these methods takes into account those pregnancies that occur through incorrect use of the method.

- ◆ Combined and phased pills 2–3
- ◆ Progestogen-only pill 2.5–10
- ◆ IUD (Intrauterine device) 4–9
- ◆ Condom 3–4
- ◆ Diaphragm 10–20
- ◆ Rhythm method 25–30
- ◆ Contraceptive sponge 9–27
- ◆ Vaginal spermicide alone 2–30
- ◆ Norethisterone implant Less than 1
- ◆ No contraception 80–85
- ◆ "Morning after" pill 20–25.

Oral contraceptives have the added advantage of being convenient and unobtrusive during lovemaking. Approximately 25 per cent of those women in Britain who seek contraceptive protection choose a form of oral contraceptive.

There are three main types: the combined pill, the progestogen-only pill, and the phased pill. All three types contain a progestogen (a synthetic form of the female sex hormone, progesterone). Both the combined and phased pills also contain a natural or synthetic oestrogen.

WHY THEY ARE USED

The combined pill contains a fixed dose of an oestrogen and a progestogen drug. It is the most widely prescribed form of oral contraceptive and has the lowest failure rate in terms of unwanted pregnancies. It is the type thought most suitable for young women who want to use hormonal contraception. The combined pill is particularly suitable for those women who regularly experience exceptionally painful, heavy, or prolonged periods (see Drugs used to treat menstrual disorders, p.104).

There are many different products available. They are generally divided into three groups, according to their oestrogen content (see Hormone content of common oral contraceptives, below). Low-dose products are chosen when possible to minimize the risk of adverse effects.

The progestogen-only pill is often recommended for women who react adversely to the oestrogen in the combined pill or for whom this pill is not considered suitable due to their age or medical history (see Risks and special precautions, facing page). It is also prescribed during breast-feeding since it does not reduce milk production. The progestogen-only pill has a higher failure rate than the combined pill and must be taken at precisely the same time each day for maximum contraceptive effect.

Phased pills are a pack of pills divided into two or three groups or phases. Each phase contains a different proportion of an oestrogen and a progestogen. The aim is to provide a hormonal balance that closely resembles the fluctuations of a normal menstrual cycle. Phased pills provide effective protection for many women who suffer side effects from other available forms of oral contraceptive.

HOW THEY WORK

In a normal menstrual cycle, the ripening and release of an egg and the preparation of the uterus for implantation of the fertilized

HORMONE CONTENT OF COMMON ORAL CONTRACEPTIVES

The oestrogen-containing forms are classified according to oestrogen content as follows: low: 20 micrograms; standard: 30–35 micrograms; high: 50 micrograms; phased pills: 30–40 micrograms; morning after pills: 100 micrograms dose.

TYPE OF PILL (oestrogen content)	BRAND NAMES
Combined (20 micrograms)	Loestrin 20, Femodette, Mercilon
(30–35 micrograms)	Brevinor, Cilest, Eugynon 30, Femodene, Femodene ED, Loestrin 30, Norimin, Marvelon, Microgynon 30, Microgynon 30 ED, Minulet, Ovran 30, Ovranette, Ovysmen, Yasmin
(50 micrograms)	Norinyl-1
Phased (30–40 micrograms)	Binovum, Logynon, Logynon ED, Synphase, Triadene, Tri-Minulet, Trinordiol, TriNovum
Progestogen-only (no oestrogen)	Cerazette, Femulen, Micronor, Microval, Neogest, Norgeston, Noriday
Post-coital (morning after) (no oestrogen)	Levonelle, Levonelle-2

egg are the result of a complex interplay between four naturally occurring hormones. These are the female sex hormones oestrogen and progesterone, and the pituitary hormones FSH (follicle-stimulating hormone) and LH (luteinizing hormone). (See also p.88.) The oestrogens and progestogens that are contained in oral contraceptives disrupt the normal menstrual cycle in such a way that conception is less likely to occur.

With combined and phased pills, the increased levels of oestrogen and progesterone produce similar effects to the hormonal changes of pregnancy. The actions of the hormones inhibit the production of FSH and LH, preventing the egg from ripening in the ovary and from being released.

The progestogen-only pill has a slightly different effect. It does not always prevent the release of an egg; its main contraceptive action may be on the mucus that lines the cervix, which thickens so that sperm cannot cross it. This effect occurs to some extent with combined pills and phased pills.

HOW THEY AFFECT YOU

Each course of combined and phased pills lasts for 21 days, followed by a pill-free seven days, during which time menstruation occurs. Some brands contain seven additional inactive pills. With these, the new course directly follows the last so that the habit of taking the pill daily is not broken. Progestogen-only pills are taken for 28 days each month. Menstruation usually occurs during the last few days of the menstrual cycle.

Women who are taking the oral contraceptive pill, especially types that contain oestrogen, usually find that their menstrual periods are lighter and relatively pain-free. Some women cease to menstruate altogether. This is not a cause for concern in itself, provided no pills have been missed, but it may make it difficult to determine if pregnancy has occurred. An apparently missed period probably indicates a light one, rather than pregnancy. However, if you have missed two consecutive periods and you feel that you may be pregnant, it is advisable to have a pregnancy test.

All forms of oral contraceptive may cause "breakthrough bleeding" (spotting of blood in mid-cycle), especially at first, but this can be a particular problem with the progestogen-only pill.

Oral contraceptives that contain oestrogen may produce any of a large number of mild side effects, depending on the dose. Symptoms similar to those experienced early in pregnancy may occur, particularly in the first few months of pill use: some women complain of nausea and vomiting, weight gain, depression, altered libido, increased appetite, and abdominal and leg cramps. The pill may also affect the circulation, producing minor headaches and dizziness. All of these effects usually disappear within a few months, but if they persist, changing to a brand containing a lower dose of oestrogen or to some other contraceptive method may be advisable.

RISKS AND SPECIAL PRECAUTIONS

All oral contraceptives need to be taken regularly for maximum protection against pregnancy. Contraceptive protection can be reduced by missing a pill (see What to do if you miss a pill, p.109). It may also be reduced by vomiting or diarrhoea. If you have either of these symptoms, it is advisable to act as if you had missed your last pill. Many drugs may also affect the action of oral contraceptives; it is essential to tell your doctor that you are taking oral contraceptives before you take additional prescribed medications.

Oral contraceptives, particularly those containing an oestrogen, have been found to carry a number of risks (see Balancing the risks and benefits of oral contraceptives, p.108). One of the most serious potential adverse effects of oestrogen-containing pills is development of a thrombus (blood clot) in a vein or artery that may travel to the lungs or cause a stroke or heart attack. The risk of thrombus formation increases with age and other factors, notably obesity, high blood pressure, and smoking. Doctors assess these risk factors for each person when prescribing oral contraceptives. A woman aged over 35 may be advised against taking a combined pill, especially if she smokes or has an underlying medical condition such as diabetes mellitus. Concerns have been expressed about contraceptive pills containing the progestogens gestodene or desogestrel because several studies have found these preparations to carry a higher risk of thrombus formation than those containing other progestogens. The Committee on the Safety of Medicines has advised that these preparations should be used only by those women who are intolerant of other contraceptive pills and are aware of the higher risk. The drugs that contain desogestrel include Cerazette, Marvelon, and Mercilon, while those that contain gestodene include Femodene, Femodene ED, Minulet, Triadene, and Tri-Minulet.

For some women, high blood pressure is a possible complication of oral contraceptives. All women prescribed oral contraceptives are advised to have their blood pressure measured before they start taking them, and every six months thereafter.

Some very rare liver cancers have occurred in pill-users, and breast cancer may be slightly more common, but cancers of the ovaries and uterus are less common.

There is no evidence that oral contraceptives reduce a woman's fertility or damage the babies conceived after they are discontinued; but doctors recommend that you wait for at least one normal menstrual period before attempting to become pregnant.

BALANCING THE RISKS AND BENEFITS OF ORAL CONTRACEPTIVES

Oral contraceptives are safe for the vast majority of young women. However, every woman who is considering oral contraception should discuss with her doctor the risks and possible adverse effects of the drugs before deciding whether or not a hormonal contraception is the most suitable method in her case. A variety of factors must be taken into account, including the woman's age, her own medical history and that of her close relatives, and factors such as whether she is a smoker. The importance of such factors varies depending on the type of contraceptive. The main advantages and disadvantages of oestrogen-containing and progestogen-only pills are listed below.

Advantages of oestrogen-containing combined and phased pills Very reliable; convenient and unobtrusive; regularize menstruation; reduce menstrual pain and blood loss; reduce risk of benign breast disease, endometriosis, ectopic pregnancy, ovarian cysts, pelvic infection, ovarian and endometrial cancer.

Advantages of progestogen-only pill Reasonably reliable; convenient and unobtrusive; suitable during breast-feeding; avoids any oestrogen-related side effects and risks; allows rapid return to fertility.

Side effects of oestrogen-containing combined and phased pills Weight gain; depression; breast swelling; reduced sex drive; headaches; increased vaginal discharge; nausea.

Side effects of progestogen-only pill Irregular menstruation.

Risks of oestrogen-containing combined and phased pills Thrombosis/embolism; heart disease; high blood pressure; jaundice; cancer of the liver (rare); gallstones.

Risks of progestogen-only pill Ectopic pregnancy; ovarian cysts.

Factors that may prohibit use of oestrogen-containing combined and phased pills Previous thrombosis*; heart disease; high levels of lipid in blood; liver disease; blood disorders; high blood pressure; unexplained vaginal bleeding; migraine; otosclerosis; presence of several risk factors (see below).

Factors that may prohibit use of progestogen-only pill Previous ectopic pregnancy; heart or circulatory disease; unexplained vaginal bleeding.

Factors that increase risks of oestrogen-containing combined and phased pills Smoking*; obesity*; increasing age; diabetes mellitus; family history of heart or circulatory disease*; current treatment with other drugs.

Factors that increase risks of progestogen-only pill As for oestrogen-containing pills, but to a lesser degree.

* Products containing desogestrel or gestodene have a higher excess risk with these factors than other progestogens.

HOW TO MINIMIZE YOUR HEALTH RISKS WHILE TAKING THE PILL

◆ Give up smoking.
◆ Maintain a healthy weight and diet.
◆ Have regular blood pressure and blood lipid checks.
◆ Have regular cervical smear tests.
◆ Remind your doctor that you are taking oral contraceptives before taking other prescription drugs.

◆ Stop taking oestrogen-containing oral contraceptives four weeks before planned major surgery (use alternative contraception).

WHAT TO DO IF YOU MISS A PILL

Contraceptive protection may be reduced if blood levels of the hormones in the body fall as a result of missing a pill. It is particularly important to ensure that the progestogen-only pills are taken punctually. If you miss a pill, the action you should take depends on the degree of lateness and the type of pill being used (see below).

Combined and phased pills If you are 3–12 hours late, take the missed pill now; no additional precautions are necessary. If you are over 12 hours late, take the missed pill now and take the next pill on time (even if it is on the same day). If more than one pill has been missed, take the latest missed pill now and the next on time; take additional precautions for the next 7 days. If the 7 days extends into the pill-free (or inactive pill) period, start the next packet without a break (or without taking inactive pills).

Progestogen-only pills If you are 3–12 hours late, take the missed pill now; take additional precautions for the next 7 days. If you are over 12 hours late, take the missed pill now, and take the next on time; take additional precautions for the next 7 days.

POSTCOITAL CONTRACEPTION

Pregnancy following intercourse without contraception may be avoided by taking a postcoital ("morning after") pill. The preparation used for this purpose contains a progestogen and is taken, as soon as possible after intercourse, as a single dose within 12 hours but no later than after 72 hours. It postpones ovulation and acts on the lining of the uterus to prevent implantation of the egg. The high dose needed makes it unsuitable for regular frequent use, however. This method has a higher failure rate than the usual oral contraceptives.

COMMON DRUGS

Progestogens Desogestrel, Drospirenone, Etynodiol, Gestodene, Levonorgestrel*, Norethisterone*, Norgestimate

Oestrogens Ethinylestradiol*, Mestranol

* **See Part 2**

Drugs for infertility

Conception and the establishment of pregnancy require a healthy reproductive system in both partners. The man must be able to produce sufficient numbers of healthy sperm; the woman must be able to produce a healthy egg that is able to pass freely down the fallopian tube to the uterus. The lining of the uterus must be in a condition that allows the implantation of the fertilized egg.

The cause of infertility may sometimes remain undiscovered, but in the majority of cases it is due to one of the following factors: intercourse taking place at the wrong time during the menstrual cycle; the man producing too few or unhealthy sperm; the woman either failing to ovulate (release an egg) or having blocked fallopian tubes perhaps as a result of previous pelvic infection. Alternatively, production of gonadotrophin hormones – follicle-stimulating hormone (FSH) and luteinizing hormone (LH) – needed for ovulation and implantation of the egg may be affected by illness or psychological stress.

If no simple explanation can be found, the man's semen will be analysed. If these tests show abnormally low sperm production, or if a large proportion of the sperm produced are unhealthy, drug treatment may be tried.

If no abnormality of sperm production is found, the woman will be given a thorough medical examination. Ovulation is monitored and blood tests may be performed to assess hormone levels. If ovulation does not occur, the woman may be offered drug treatment.

WHY THEY ARE USED

In men, low sperm production may be treated with gonadotrophins (FSH or HCG) or a pituitary-stimulating drug (for example, clomifene) and some problems may be controlled with corticosteroids.

In women, drugs are useful in helping to achieve pregnancy only when a hormone defect inhibiting ovulation has been diagnosed. Treatment may continue for months and does not always produce a pregnancy. Women in whom the pituitary gland produces some FSH and LH may be given courses of clomifene for several days during each month. Usually, up to three courses may be tried. An effective dose produces ovulation five to ten days after the last tablet is taken.

Clomifene may thicken cervical mucus, impeding the passage of sperm, but the advantage of achieving ovulation outweighs the risk of this side effect. If treatment with clomifene fails to produce ovulation, or if a disorder of the pituitary gland prevents production of FSH and LH, treatment with FSH and human chorionic gonadotrophin (HCG) may be given. FSH is given during the second week of the menstrual cycle, followed by an injection of HCG.

HOW THEY WORK

Ovulation (release of an egg) and implantation are governed by hormones produced by the pituitary gland. FSH stimulates ripening of the egg follicle. LH triggers ovulation and ensures that progesterone is produced to prepare the uterus for the implantation of the egg. Drugs for female infertility boost the actions of these hormones.

Fertility drugs raise the chance of ovulation by boosting levels of LH and FSH. Clomifene stimulates the pituitary gland to increase its output of these hormones. Artificially produced FSH and HCG mimic the action of naturally produced FSH and LH respectively. Both treatments, when successful, stimulate ovulation and implantation of the fertilized egg.

HOW THEY AFFECT YOU

Clomifene may produce hot flushes, nausea, headaches, and, rarely, ovarian cysts and visual disturbance, while HCG can cause tiredness, headaches, and mood changes. FSH can cause the ovaries to enlarge, producing abdominal discomfort. These drugs increase the likelihood of multiple births, usually twins.

DRUGS FOR IMPOTENCE

Impotence is a common male disorder defined as inability to achieve or maintain an erection. The penis contains three cylinders of erectile tissue: the two corpora cavernosa and the corpus spongiosum. Normally, when a man is sexually aroused, the arteries in the penis relax and widen, allowing more blood than usual to flow into the organ, filling the corpora cavernosa and corpus spongiosum. As these tissues expand and harden, the veins that carry blood out of the penis are compressed, reducing outflow and resulting in an erection. In some forms of impotence, this does not happen. Drugs can be used to increase blood flow into the penis to produce an erection.

Sildenafil (see p.383), taken by mouth, not only increases the blood flow into the penis but also prevents the muscle wall from relaxing, so the blood does not drain out of the blood vessels and the penis remains erect.

Alprostadil (see p.135) is a prostaglandin drug that helps men achieve an erection by widening the blood vessels, but it must be injected directly into the penis, or applied into the urethra using a special pipette.

COMMON DRUGS

Buserelin, Cetrorelix, Chorionic gonadotrophin (HCG)*, Clomifene*, Follicle-stimulating hormone (FSH), Follitropin, Ganirelix, Goserelin*, Luteinizing hormone (LH), Menotrophin, Menopausal gonadotrophins, Nafarelin, Tamoxifen*, Urofollitropin

Drugs for impotence Alprostadil*, Apomophine*, Sildenafil*

* **See Part 2**

Drugs used in labour

Normal labour has three stages. In the first stage, the uterus begins to contract, initially irregularly and then gradually more regularly and powerfully, while the cervix dilates until it is fully stretched. During the second stage, powerful contractions of the uterus push the baby down the mother's birth canal and out of her body. The third stage involves the delivery of the placenta.

Drugs may be needed during one or more stages of labour for any of the following reasons: to induce or augment labour, delay premature labour (see Uterine muscle relaxants, facing page), and relieve pain. The administration of some drugs may be viewed as part of normal obstetric care; for example, ergometrine, a uterine stimulant, may be injected routinely before the third stage of labour. Other drugs are given only when the condition of the mother or baby requires intervention. The possible adverse effects of the drug on both mother and baby are always carefully balanced against the benefits.

DRUGS TO INDUCE OR AUGMENT LABOUR

Induction of labour may be advised when a doctor considers it risky for the health of the mother or baby for the pregnancy to continue (for example, if natural labour does not occur within two weeks of the due date or when a woman has pre-eclampsia). Other common reasons for inducing labour include premature rupture of the membrane surrounding the baby (breaking of the waters), slow growth of the baby due to poor nourishment by the placenta, or death of the fetus (unborn baby) in the uterus.

If it is necessary to induce labour, oxytocin, a uterine stimulant, may be administered intravenously. Alternatively, a prostaglandin pessary may be given to soften and dilate the cervix. If these methods are ineffective or cannot be used because they may have potential adverse effects (see Risks and special precautions, below), a caesarean delivery may have to be performed.

Oxytocin may also be used to strengthen the force of uterine contractions in labour that has started spontaneously but has not continued normally.

A combination of oxytocin and another uterine stimulant, ergometrine, is given to most women as the baby is being born or immediately following birth to prevent excessive bleeding after the delivery of the placenta. This combination encourages the uterus to contract after delivery, which restricts the flow of blood.

RISKS AND SPECIAL PRECAUTIONS

When oxytocin is used to induce labour, the dosage is carefully monitored throughout to prevent the possibility of excessively violent contractions. It is administered to women who have had surgery of the uterus only with careful monitoring. The drug is not known to affect the baby adversely. Ergometrine is not given to women who have had high blood pressure during the course of pregnancy.

DRUGS USED FOR PAIN RELIEF

Opioid analgesics Pethidine, morphine, or other opioids may be given once active labour has been established (see Analgesics, p.9). Possible side effects for the mother include drowsiness, nausea, and vomiting.

Opioid drugs may cause breathing difficulties for the newborn baby, but these problems can be reversed by the antidote naloxone, if necessary.

Epidural anaesthesia This provides pain relief during labour and birth by numbing the nerves leading to the uterus and pelvic area. It is often used during a planned caesarean delivery, thus enabling the mother to be fully conscious for the birth.

An epidural involves the injection of a local anaesthetic drug (see p.11) into the epidural space, between the spinal cord and the vertebrae. An epidural may block the mother's urge to push during the second stage, and a forceps delivery may be necessary. Headaches may occasionally occur following epidural anaesthesia.

Oxygen and nitrous oxide These gases are combined to produce a mixture that reduces the pain caused by contractions. During the first and second stages of labour, gas is self-administered by inhalation through a mouthpiece or mask. If it is used over too long a period, it may produce nausea, confusion, and dehydration in the mother.

Local anaesthetics These drugs are injected inside the vagina or near the vaginal opening and are used to numb sensation during forceps delivery, before an episiotomy (an incision made to enlarge the vaginal opening), and when stitches are necessary. Side effects of these drugs are rare.

UTERINE MUSCLE RELAXANTS

When contractions of the uterus start before the 34th week of pregnancy, doctors usually advise bed rest and may also administer a drug that relaxes the muscles of the uterus and thus halts labour. Initially, the drug is given in hospital by injection, but it may be continued orally at home. These drugs work by stimulating the sympathetic nervous system (see Autonomic nervous system, p.8) and may cause palpitations and anxiety in the mother. They have not been shown to have adverse effects on the baby.

DRUGS USED TO TERMINATE PREGNANCY

Drugs may be used in a hospital or clinic to terminate pregnancy up to 20 weeks, or to empty the uterus after the death of the baby.

Mifepristone may be given first to sensitize the tissues before a prostaglandin is given to dilate the cervix. Before 14 weeks, the fetus is then removed under anaesthetic. After 14 weeks, labour is induced with a prostaglandin. These methods may be supplemented by oxytocin given by intravenous drip (see Drugs to induce or augment labour, p.110).

COMMON DRUGS

Prostaglandins Carboprost, Dinoprostone, Gemeprost

Pain relief Entonox® (oxygen and nitrous oxide), Fentanyl, Morphine*, Pethidine

Antiprogestogen Mifepristone

Uterine muscle relaxants Atosiban, Ritodrine, Salbutamol*, Terbutaline*

Uterine stimulants Ergometrine, Oxytocin

Local anaesthetics Bupivacaine, Lidocaine (lignocaine)

* See Part 2

Drugs used for urinary disorders

Urine is produced by the kidneys and stored in the bladder. As the urine accumulates, the bladder's walls stretch and pressure inside it increases. Eventually, the stretching stimulates nerve endings that produce the urge to urinate. The ring of muscle (sphincter) around the bladder neck normally keeps the bladder closed until it is consciously relaxed, allowing urine to pass out of the body via the urethra.

A number of disorders can affect the urinary tract. The most common of these disorders are infection in the bladder (cystitis) or the urethra (urethritis), and loss of reliable control over urination (urinary incontinence). A less common problem is inability to expel urine (urinary retention). Drugs used to treat these problems include antibiotics and antibacterial drugs, analgesics, drugs to increase the acidity of the urine, and drugs that act on nerve control over the muscles of the bladder and sphincter.

DRUGS FOR URINARY INFECTION

Almost all infections of the bladder are caused by bacteria. Symptoms include a continual urge to urinate, although often nothing is passed; pain on urinating; and lower abdominal pain.

Many antibiotic and antibacterial drugs are used to treat urinary tract infections. Among the most widely used – because of their effectiveness – are trimethoprim and amoxicillin (see Antibiotics, p.62, and Antibacterial drugs, p.66).

Measures are also sometimes taken to increase the acidity of the urine, thereby making it hostile to bacteria. Ascorbic acid (vitamin C) and acid fruit juices have this effect, although making the urine less acidic with potassium or sodium citrate during an attack of cystitis helps to relieve the discomfort. Symptoms are commonly relieved within a few hours of the start of treatment.

For maximum effect, all drug treatments prescribed for urinary tract infections need to be accompanied by increased fluid intake.

DRUGS FOR URINARY INCONTINENCE

Urinary incontinence can occur for a several reasons. A weak sphincter muscle allows the involuntary passage of urine when abdominal pressure is raised by coughing or physical exertion. This is known as stress incontinence and commonly affects women who have had children. Urgency – a sudden need to urinate – stems from oversensitivity of the bladder muscle; small quantities of urine stimulate the urge to urinate frequently.

Incontinence can also occur due to loss of nerve control in neurological disorders such as multiple sclerosis. In children, inability to control urination at night (nocturnal enuresis) is also a form of urinary incontinence.

Drug treatment is not necessary or appropriate for all forms of incontinence. In stress incontinence, exercises to strengthen the pelvic floor muscles or surgery to tighten stretched ligaments may be effective. In urgency, regular emptying of the bladder often avoids the need for medical intervention. Incontinence caused by loss of nerve control is unlikely to be helped by drug treatment. Frequency of urination in urgency may be reduced by anticholinergic drugs (see Autonomic nervous system, p.8) and antispasmodic drugs. These reduce nerve signals from the muscles in the bladder, allowing greater volumes of urine to accumulate without stimulating the urge to pass urine. Tricyclic antidepressants, such as imipramine, have a strong anticholinergic action and have been prescribed to treat nocturnal enuresis (bed-wetting) in children. However, many doctors believe the risk of overdosage is unacceptable. Desmopressin, a synthetic derivative of antidiuretic hormone (see p.85), is also used to treat nocturnal enuresis.

DRUGS FOR URINARY RETENTION

Urinary retention is the inability to empty the bladder. This usually results from failure of the bladder muscle to contract sufficiently to expel accumulated urine. Possible causes include an enlarged prostate gland, a prostate tumour, or a longstanding neurological disorder. In addition, some drugs can cause urinary retention.

Most cases of urinary retention need to be relieved by inserting a tube (catheter) into the urethra. Surgery may be needed to prevent a recurrence of the problem. Drugs that relax the sphincter or stimulate bladder contraction are now rarely used in the treatment of urinary retention, but two types of drug are used in the long-term management of prostatic enlargement. Finasteride prevents the production of male hormones that stimulate prostatic growth, and alpha blockers, such as prazosin, indoramin, and terazosin, relax prostatic and urethral smooth muscle, thereby improving urine outflow. Long-term drug treatment can relieve symptoms and delay the need for surgery.

COMMON DRUGS

Antibiotics and antibacterials (see pp.62–66)
Anticholinergics Flavoxate, Imipramine*, Oxybutynin*, Propiverine, Tolterodine*, Trospium
Parasympathomimetic Distigmine
Alpha blockers Alfuzosin, Doxazosin*, Indoramin*, Prazosin, Tamsulosin*, Terazosin*
Other drugs Desmopressin*, Finasteride*, Potassium citrate, Vitamin C
* See Part 2

EYES AND EARS

The eyes and ears are the two sense organs that provide us with the most information about the world around us. The eye is the organ of vision; it converts light images into nerve signals, which are transmitted to the brain for interpretation. The ear not only provides the means by which sound is detected and communicated to the brain, but it also contains the organ of balance that tells the brain about the position and movement of the body. It is divided into three parts – outer, middle, and inner ear.

WHAT CAN GO WRONG

The most common eye and ear disorders are infection and inflammation (sometimes caused by allergy). Many parts of the eye may be affected, notably the conjunctiva (the membrane that covers the front of the eye and lines the eyelids) and the iris. The middle and outer ear are more commonly affected by infection than the inner ear.

The eye may also be damaged by glaucoma, a disorder in which pressure of fluid within the eye builds up and may eventually threaten vision. Eye problems such as retinopathy (disease of the retina) or cataracts (clouding of the lens) may occur as a result of diabetes or for other reasons, but both are now treatable. Disorders for which no drug treatment is appropriate are beyond the scope of this book.

Other disorders affecting the ear include build-up of wax (cerumen) in the outer ear canal and disturbances to the balance mechanism within the ear (vertigo and Ménière's disease; see Anti-emetics, p.21).

WHY DRUGS ARE USED

Doctors usually prescribe antibiotics (see p.62) to clear eye and ear infections. These may be given by mouth or topically. Topical eye and ear preparations may contain a corticosteroid (see p.80) to reduce inflammation. When inflammation has been caused by allergy, antihistamines (see p.58) may also be taken. Decongestant drugs (see p.26) are often prescribed to help clear the eustachian tube in middle ear infections.

Various drugs are used to reduce fluid pressure in glaucoma. These include diuretics (see p.32), beta blockers (see p.30), and miotics (to narrow the pupil). In other cases, the pupil may need to be widened by mydriatic drugs. (See also Drugs affecting the pupil, p.116.)

MAJOR DRUG GROUPS
◆ Drugs for glaucoma
◆ Drugs affecting the pupil
◆ Drugs for ear disorders

Drugs for Glaucoma

Glaucoma is the name given to a group of conditions in which the pressure in the eye builds up to an abnormally high level. This compresses the blood vessels that supply the nerve connecting the eye to the brain (optic nerve) and may result in irreversible nerve damage and permanent loss of vision.

In the most common form, chronic (open-angle) glaucoma, reduced fluid drainage from the eye causes pressure inside the eye to build up slowly. Progressive reduction in the peripheral field of vision may take months or years to be noticed.

Acute (closed-angle) glaucoma arises when fluid drainage is suddenly blocked by the iris. Fluid pressure usually builds up rapidly, blurring vision in that eye. The eye becomes red and painful, and a headache and sometimes vomiting also occur. The main attack is often preceded by milder warning attacks, such as seeing haloes around lights, in the previous weeks or months. Elderly, far-sighted people are particularly at risk of acute glaucoma. The angle may also narrow suddenly after injury or taking certain drugs, such as anticholinergics (see Drugs that act on the parasympathetic nervous system, p.9). Some cases of closed-angle glaucoma may develop more slowly (chronic closed-angle glaucoma).

Drugs are used in the treatment of both types of glaucoma. They include miotics (see Drugs affecting the pupil, p.116), beta blockers (see p.30), and the diuretics (see p.32) carbonic anhydrase inhibitors and osmotics.

WHY THEY ARE USED

Chronic glaucoma In this form of glaucoma, drugs are used to reduce pressure inside the eye. These drugs will prevent further deterioration of vision but cannot restore damage that has already been sustained, and therefore they may be required for life.

In most patients, treatment is begun with eye drops containing a beta blocker to reduce the production of fluid inside the eye. Miotic eye drops to constrict the pupil and improve fluid drainage may be given. The prostaglandin analogue latanoprost is also used to increase fluid outflow. If none of these drugs are effective, epinephrine, dipivefrine, or brimonidine may be tried to reduce secretion and help outflow. Sometimes a carbonic anhydrase inhibitor such as acetazolamide may be given by mouth to reduce fluid production. Laser treatment and surgery may also be used to improve fluid drainage from the eye.

Acute glaucoma In acute glaucoma, immediate medical treatment is required in order to prevent total loss of vision. Drugs are used initially to bring down the pressure within the eye. Laser treatment or surgery is then carried out to prevent a recurrence of the problem so that long-term drug treatment is seldom required.

Acetazolamide is often the first drug to be administered when the condition is diagnosed. This drug may be injected for rapid effect and thereafter administered by mouth. Frequent applications of eye drops containing pilocarpine or carbachol are given. An osmotic diuretic such as mannitol may be administered. This drug draws fluid out of all body tissues, including the eye, and reduces pressure within the eye.

HOW THEY WORK

Drugs for glaucoma act in various ways to reduce the pressure of fluid in the eye. Miotics improve drainage of fluid out of the eye. In chronic glaucoma, this is achieved by increasing the outflow of aqueous humour via the drainage channel called the trabecular meshwork. In acute glaucoma, the pupil-constricting effect of miotics pulls the iris away from the drainage channel, allowing the aqueous humour to flow out in the normal way. Prostaglandin analogues act by increasing fluid outflow from the eye. Beta blockers and carbonic anhydrase inhibitors act on the fluid-producing cells inside the eye to reduce the output of aqueous humour. Sympathomimetic drugs such as epinephrine (adrenaline), brimonidine, and apraclonidine are also thought to act partly in this way and partly by improving fluid drainage.

HOW THEY AFFECT YOU

Drugs for acute glaucoma relieve pain and other symptoms within a few hours of their being used. The benefits of treatment in chronic glaucoma, however, may not be immediately apparent since treatment is only able to halt a further deterioration of vision.

People receiving miotic eye drops are likely to notice darkening of vision and difficulty seeing in the dark. Increased shortsightedness may be noticeable. Some miotics also cause irritation and redness of the eyes.

Beta blocker eye drops have few day-to-day side effects but carry risks for a few people (see below). Acetazolamide usually causes an increase in frequency of urination and thirst; nausea and general malaise are also common.

RISKS AND SPECIAL PRECAUTIONS

Miotics can cause alteration in vision. Beta blockers are absorbed into the body and can affect the lungs, heart, and circulation. As a result, a cardioselective beta blocker such as betaxolol may be prescribed with caution to people with asthma or certain circulatory disorders; in some cases, such drugs are withheld altogether. The amount of the drug absorbed into the blood can be reduced by pressing on the lacrimal (tear) duct in the corner of the eye while applying the number of eye drops prescribed by your doctor. Acetazolamide may cause troublesome adverse effects such as painful tingling of the hands and feet, the formation of kidney stones, and, rarely, kidney damage. People with existing kidney problems are not usually given this drug.

COMMON DRUGS

Miotics Carbachol, Pilocarpine*
Carbonic anhydrase inhibitors Acetazolamide, Brinzolamide, Dorzolamide*
Prostaglandin analogues Bimatoprost, Latanoprost*, Travoprost

Beta blockers Betaxolol, Carteolol, Levobunolol, Metipranolol, Timolol*
Sympathomimetics Apraclonidine, Brimonidine, Dipivefrine, Epinephrine*, Guanethidine
* See Part 2

Drugs affecting the pupil

The pupil of the eye is the circular opening in the centre of the iris (the coloured part of the eye) through which light enters. It continually changes in size to adjust to variations in the intensity of light; in bright light it becomes quite small (constricts), but in dim light the pupil enlarges (dilates).

Eye drops containing drugs that act on the pupil are widely used by specialists. There are two categories: mydriatics, which dilate the pupil, and miotics, which constrict it.

WHY THEY ARE USED

Mydriatics are most often used to allow the doctor to view the inside of the eye – particularly the retina, the optic nerve head, and the blood vessels that supply the retina. Many of these drugs cause temporary paralysis of the eye's focusing mechanism. This state, called cycloplegia, is sometimes induced to help determine the presence of any focusing errors, especially in babies and young children. By producing cycloplegia, it is possible to determine the precise optical prescription required for a small child, especially in the case of a squint.

Dilation of the pupil is part of the treatment for uveitis, an inflammatory disease of the iris and focusing muscle. In uveitis, the inflamed iris may stick to the lens, severely damaging the eye. This complication can be prevented by early dilation of the pupil so that the iris is no longer in contact with the lens.

Constriction of the pupil with miotic drugs is often required in the treatment of glaucoma (see p.114). Miotics can also be used to restore the pupil to a normal size after dilation is induced by mydriatics.

HOW THEY WORK

The size of the pupil is controlled by two separate sets of muscles in the iris: the circular muscle and the radial muscle. The two sets of muscles are governed by separate branches of the autonomic nervous system (see p.8): the radial muscle is controlled by the sympathetic nervous system, and the circular muscle is controlled by the parasympathetic nervous system.

Individual mydriatic and miotic drugs affect different parts of the autonomic nervous system, and cause the pupil to dilate or contract, depending on the type of drug used.

HOW THEY AFFECT YOU

Mydriatic drugs – especially the long-acting types – impair the ability to focus the eye(s) for several hours after use. This interferes particularly with close activities such as reading. Bright light may cause discomfort. Miotics often interfere with night vision and may cause temporary short sight.

Normally, these eye drops produce few serious adverse effects. Sympathomimetic mydriatics may raise the blood pressure, and they are used with caution in people who have hypertension or heart disease. Miotics may irritate the eyes, but they rarely cause generalized effects.

ARTIFICIAL TEAR PREPARATIONS

Tears are continually produced to keep the front of the eye covered with a thin, moist film. This is essential for clear vision and for keeping the front of the eye free from dirt and other irritants. In some conditions, known collectively as dry eye syndromes (for example, Sjögren's syndrome), inadequate tear production may make the eyes feel dry and sore. Sore eyes can also occur in disorders where the eyelids do not close properly, causing the eye to become dry.

Why they are used Since prolonged deficiency of natural tears can damage the cornea, regular application of artificial tears in the form of eye drops is recommended for all of the conditions described above. Artificial tears may also be used to provide temporary relief from any feeling of discomfort and dryness in the eye caused by irritants or exposure to wind or sun, or following the initial wearing of contact lenses.

Although artificial tears are non-irritating, they often contain a preservative (such as thimerosal or benzalkonium chloride) that may cause irritation. This risk of irritation is increased for wearers of soft contact lenses, who should ask their optician for advice before using any type of eye drops.

COMMON DRUGS

Sympathomimetic mydriatics Epinephrine*, Phenylephrine

Miotics Carbachol, Pilocarpine*

Anticholinergic mydriatics Atropine*, Cyclopentolate, Homatropine, Tropicamide

*** See Part 2**

Drugs for ear disorders

Inflammation and infection of the outer and middle ear are the most common ear disorders treated with drugs. Drug treatment for Ménière's disease, which affects the inner ear, is described under Anti-emetics, p.21.

The type of drug treatment given for ear inflammation depends on the cause of the trouble and the site affected.

INFLAMMATION OF THE OUTER EAR

Inflammation of the external ear canal (otitis externa) can be caused by eczema or a bacterial or fungal infection. The risk of inflammation is increased by swimming in dirty water, accumulation of wax in the ear, or scratching or poking too frequently at the ear.

Symptoms vary, but in many cases there is itching, pain (which may be severe if there is a boil in the ear canal), tenderness, and possibly some loss of hearing. If the ear is infected there will probably be a discharge.

Drug treatment A corticosteroid (see p.80) in the form of ear drops may be used to treat inflammation of the outer ear when there is no infection. Aluminium acetate solution, as drops or applied on a piece of gauze, may also be used. Relief is usually obtained within a day or two. Prolonged use of corticosteroids is not advisable because they may reduce the ear's resistance to infection.

If there is both inflammation and infection, your doctor may prescribe ear drops containing an antibiotic (see p.62) combined with a corticosteroid to relieve the inflammation. Usually, a combination of antibiotics is prescribed to make the treatment effective against a wide range of bacteria. Commonly used antibiotics include framycetin, neomycin, and polymyxin B. These are not used if the eardrum is perforated and are not usually applied for long periods because they can irritate the skin lining the ear canal.

Sometimes an antibiotic given as drops is not effective, and another type of antibiotic may have to be taken by mouth as well.

INFECTION OF THE MIDDLE EAR

Infection of the middle ear (otitis media) often causes severe pain and hearing loss. It is particularly common in young children, in whom infecting organisms are able to spread easily into the middle ear from the nose or throat via the eustachian tube.

Viral infections of the middle ear usually cure themselves and are less serious than those caused by bacteria. Bacterial infections often cause the eustachian tube to swell and become blocked. When a blockage occurs, pus builds up in the middle ear and puts pressure on the eardrum, which may perforate as a result.

Drug treatment Doctors usually prescribe a decongestant (see p.26) or an antihistamine (see p.58) to reduce swelling in the eustachian tube, thus allowing the pus to drain out of the middle ear. Usually, an antibiotic is also given by mouth or administered by injection to clear the infection.

Although antibiotics are not effective against viral infections, it is often difficult to distinguish between a viral and a bacterial infection of the middle ear, so your doctor may prescribe an antibiotic as a precautionary measure. Paracetamol, an analgesic (see p.9), may be given to relieve pain.

COMMON DRUGS

Antibiotic and antibacterial ear drops
Chloramphenicol*, Clioquinol, Framycetin, Gentamicin*, Neomycin

Decongestants Ephedrine*, Oxymetazoline, Xylometazoline

Corticosteroids Betamethasone*, Dexamethasone*, Flumethasone, Hydrocortisone*, Prednisolone*, Triamcinolone

Other drugs Aluminium acetate, Antihistamines (see p.58), Choline salicylate, Clotrimazole*

*** See Part 2**

SKIN

The skin waterproofs, cushions, and protects the body and is its largest organ. It provides a barrier against innumerable infections and infestations, helps the body to retain its vital fluids, plays a major role in temperature control, and houses the sensory nerves of touch.

The skin consists of two main layers: a thin, tough top layer, the epidermis; and a thicker layer, the dermis, beneath. The epidermis also has two layers: the skin surface, or stratum corneum (horny layer), consisting of dead cells, and below, a layer of active cells. The cells in the active layer divide and finally die, maintaining the horny layer. Living cells produce the protein keratin, which toughens the epidermis and is the basic substance of hair and nails. Some living cells in the epidermis produce melanin, a pigment released in increased amounts following exposure to sunlight.

The dermis contains different types of nerve ending for sensing pain, pressure, and temperature; sweat glands to cool the body; sebaceous glands to lubricate and waterproof the skin; and white blood cells to help keep the skin free of infection.

WHAT CAN GO WRONG

Most skin complaints are not serious but may be distressing if visible. They include infection, inflammation and irritation, infestation by skin parasites, and changes in skin structure and texture (such as psoriasis, eczema, and acne). Serious skin conditions include cancers such as malignant melanoma.

WHY DRUGS ARE USED

Skin problems often clear up without drug treatment. Preparations containing drugs are available over the counter, but their use is generally discouraged without medical supervision because they can aggravate some skin conditions if used inappropriately. Prescribed drugs, including antibiotics (see p.62) for bacterial infections, antifungals (see p.76) for fungal infections, agents for skin parasites (see p.122), and topical corticosteroids (see p.120) for inflammatory conditions are often highly effective, however. Specialized drugs are available for conditions such as psoriasis and acne.

Although many drugs are topical, they must be used carefully because, like drugs taken orally, they can also cause adverse effects; and some can lead to allergy when they are used on the skin.

MAJOR DRUG GROUPS
◆ Antipruritics
◆ Topical corticosteroids
◆ Anti-infective skin preparations
◆ Drugs to treat skin parasites
◆ Drugs used to treat acne
◆ Drugs for psoriasis
◆ Treatments for eczema
◆ Drugs for dandruff
◆ Drugs for hair loss
◆ Sunscreens

Antipruritics

Itching (irritation of the skin that creates the urge to scratch), also called pruritus, most often occurs as a result of minor physical irritation or chemical changes in the skin due to disease, allergy, inflammation, or exposure to irritant substances. People have differing tolerance thresholds, which can be altered by stress and other psychological factors.

Itching is a common symptom of many skin disorders, such as eczema and psoriasis, and allergic conditions, such as urticaria (hives). It is also sometimes caused by a localized fungal infection, parasitic infestation, or diseases such as chickenpox. Less commonly, itching may also occur as a symptom of diabetes mellitus, jaundice, and kidney failure.

Generalized itching is caused, in many cases, by dry skin. Itching in particular parts of the body is often due to a specific problem. For example, itching around the anus (pruritus ani) may result from haemorrhoids or worm infestation, while genital itching in women (pruritus vulvae) may be due to vaginal infection or diabetes or, in older women, may be the result of a hormone deficiency.

Although scratching frequently provides temporary relief, it can often increase inflammation and make the condition worse.

Continued scratching of irritated skin may occasionally lead to a vicious cycle of scratching and itching that continues long after the original cause has been removed.

Many types of medication, including soothing topical preparations and drugs taken by mouth, relieve skin irritation. The main drugs in antipruritic products include local anaesthetics (see p.11), topical corticosteroids (see p.120), and antihistamines (see p.58). Simple emollient or cooling creams or ointments, such as emulsifying ointment, contain no active ingredients and are often recommended.

WHY THEY ARE USED

For mild itching arising from sunburn, urticaria, or insect bites, a cooling lotion such as calamine, perhaps containing menthol, phenol, or camphor, may be the most appropriate treatment. Local anaesthetic creams can be helpful for small areas of irritation such as insect bites, but are unsuitable for widespread itching. The itching caused by dry skin is often soothed by a simple emollient. Avoiding excessive use of soap and water and using moisturizing bath oils may also help.

Severe itching in eczema or other inflammatory skin conditions may be treated with a topical corticosteroid preparation. When the irritation prevents sleep, a doctor may prescribe an oral antihistamine for use at night to promote sleep as well as to relieve the itching (see also Sleeping drugs, p.11). Antihistamines are also often included in topical preparations for the relief of skin irritation, but their effectiveness when administered in this way is doubtful. For the treatment of pruritus ani, see Drugs for rectal and anal disorders (p.47). Post-menopausal pruritus vulvae may be helped by vaginal creams containing oestrogen (see Female sex hormones, p.88). Itching caused by an underlying illness cannot be helped by skin creams and requires treatment for the principal disorder.

HOW THEY WORK

Irritation of the skin causes the release of substances such as histamine, which cause blood vessels to dilate and fluid to accumulate under the skin; this results in itching and inflammation. Antipruritic drugs act either by reducing inflammation and thus irritation, or by numbing the nerve impulses that transmit sensation to the brain.

Corticosteroids applied to the skin reduce itching caused by allergy within a few days, but the cream's soothing effect may produce an immediate improvement. The drugs pass into the underlying tissues and blood vessels and reduce the release of histamine, the chemical that causes itching and inflammation.

Antihistamines act within a few hours to reduce allergy-related skin inflammation. Applied to the skin, they pass into the underlying tissue and block the effects of histamine on the blood vessels beneath the skin. Taken by mouth, they also act on the brain to reduce the perception of irritation.

Local anaesthetics absorbed through the skin numb the transmission of signals from the nerves in the skin to the brain.

Soothing and emollient creams such as calamine lotion, applied to the skin surface, reduce inflammation and itching by cooling the skin. Emollient creams lubricate the skin surface and prevent dryness.

RISKS AND SPECIAL PRECAUTIONS

The main risk of any antipruritic (except simple emollient and soothing preparations) is skin irritation, and therefore aggravated itching, caused by prolonged or heavy use. Antihistamine and local anaesthetic creams are especially likely to cause a reaction and must be stopped if they do so. Antihistamines taken by mouth to relieve itching are likely to cause drowsiness. The special risks of topical corticosteroids are discussed on p.120.

Because itching can be a symptom of many underlying conditions, self-treatment should be continued for no longer than a week before medical advice is sought.

COMMON DRUGS

Antihistamines (see also p.58) Alimemazine, Antazoline, Diphenhydramine, Mepyramine, Trimeprazine
Corticosteroids (see also p.80) Hydrocortisone*
Local anaesthetics Benzocaine, Lidocaine, Tetracaine
Emollient and cooling preparations Aqueous cream, Calamine lotion, Cold cream, Emulsifying ointment
Other drugs Colestyramine*, Crotamiton, Doxepin
* See Part 2

Topical corticosteroids

Corticosteroid drugs (which are often simply known as steroids) are related to the hormones that are produced naturally by the adrenal glands. For a full description of these drugs, see p.80. Topical preparations containing a corticosteroid are often used to treat skin conditions in which inflammation is a prominent symptom.

WHY THEY ARE USED

Corticosteroid creams and ointments are most commonly given to relieve the itching and inflammation that is associated with skin diseases such as eczema and dermatitis. These preparations may also be prescribed for the treatment of psoriasis (see p.124). Corticosteroids do not affect the underlying cause of the skin irritation; therefore, the condition is likely to recur unless the substance (allergen or irritant) that has provoked the irritation is removed or the underlying condition is treated.

A doctor might not prescribe a corticosteroid as the initial treatment, preferring to try a topical medicine that has fewer adverse effects (see Antipruritics, p.118).

In most cases, treatment is started with a preparation containing a low concentration of a mild corticosteroid drug. A stronger preparation may be prescribed subsequently if the first product is ineffective.

HOW THEY WORK

Irritation of the skin, caused by exposure to allergens or irritant factors, provokes white blood cells to release substances that dilate the blood vessels, making the skin hot, red, and swollen.

Applied to the skin surface, corticosteroids are absorbed into the underlying tissue. There, they inhibit the action of the substances that cause inflammation, allowing the blood vessels to return to normal and reducing the swelling.

HOW THEY AFFECT YOU

Because corticosteroids prevent the release of chemicals that trigger inflammation, conditions that are treated with these drugs improve within a few days of starting the drug. Applied topically, corticosteroids rarely cause side effects. There are, however, certain risks associated with the stronger drugs used in high concentrations.

RISKS AND SPECIAL PRECAUTIONS

Prolonged use of potent corticosteroids in high concentrations usually leads to permanent skin changes – most commonly, thinning of the skin, sometimes resulting in permanent stretch marks. Fine blood vessels under the skin may become prominent (a condition known as telangiectasia). Because the skin on the face and genital area is especially vulnerable to such damage, only weak corticosteroids should be prescribed for use on these parts of the body. Dark-skinned people sometimes suffer temporary reduction in pigmentation at the site of application.

When topical corticosteroids are used for a prolonged period, abrupt discontinuation can cause rebound erythroderma (a reddening of the skin). This may be avoided by a gradual reduction in dosage. Corticosteroids suppress the body's immune system (see p.80), increasing the risk of infection. For this reason, they are never used alone to treat skin inflammation caused by bacterial or fungal infection. However, they are sometimes included in a topical preparation also containing an antibiotic or antifungal agent (see Anti-infective skin preparations, below).

COMMON DRUGS

Very potent Clobetasol*, Halcinonide
Potent Beclometasone*, Betamethasone*, Desoxymetasone, Diflucortolone, Fluocinolone, Fluocinonide, Fluticasone*, Mometasone*, Triamcinolone
Moderate Alclometasone, Clobetasone, Fludroxycortide, Fluocortolone
Mild Hydrocortisone*
* See Part 2

Anti-infective skin preparations

The skin is the body's first line of defence against infection. Yet the skin itself can also become infected, especially if the outer layer (epidermis) is damaged by a burn, scrape, cut, insect bite, or an inflammatory skin condition such as eczema or dermatitis.

Several different types of organism may infect the skin, including bacteria, viruses, fungi, and yeasts. This section concentrates on topical drugs for bacterial skin infections and includes antiseptics, antibiotics, and other antibacterial agents. Infection by other organisms is covered elsewhere (see Antiviral drugs, p.69; Antifungal drugs, p.76; and Drugs used to treat skin parasites, p.122).

WHY THEY ARE USED

Bacterial infection of a skin wound can usually be prevented by thorough cleansing of the damaged area and the application of antiseptic creams or lotions. If infection does occur, the wound usually becomes inflamed and swollen, and pus may form. If you develop these signs, you should see your doctor. The usual treatment for a wound infection is an antibiotic taken orally, although often an antibiotic cream is also prescribed.

An antibiotic or antibacterial skin cream may also be used to prevent infection when your doctor considers this to be a particular risk (for example, in the case of severe burns).

Other skin disorders in which topical antibiotic treatment may be prescribed include impetigo and infected eczema, skin ulcers, bedsores, and nappy rash.

Often, a preparation containing two or more antibiotics is used to ensure that all bacteria are eradicated. The antibiotics selected for inclusion in topical preparations are usually drugs that are poorly absorbed through the skin (such as aminoglycosides); thus the drug remains concentrated on the surface and in the skin's upper layers, where it is intended to have its effect. However, if the infection is deep under the skin, or is causing fever and malaise, antibiotics may need to be given by mouth or injection.

RISKS AND SPECIAL PRECAUTIONS

Any topical antibiotic product can irritate the skin or cause an allergic reaction. Irritation is sometimes provoked by another ingredient of the preparation rather than the active drug (such as a preservative contained in the product). An allergic reaction causing

swelling and reddening of the skin is more likely to be caused by the antibiotic itself. Any adverse reaction of this kind should be reported to your doctor, who may substitute another drug or a different preparation.

Always follow your doctor's instructions on how long the treatment with antibiotics should be continued. Stopping too soon may cause the infection to flare up again.

Never use a skin preparation that has been prescribed for someone else, because it may aggravate your condition. Always throw away any unused medication.

BASES FOR SKIN PREPARATIONS

Drugs applied to the skin are usually contained in a preparation known as a base (or vehicle), such as a cream, lotion, ointment, or paste. Many bases are beneficial on their own.

Creams These have an emollient effect. They are usually composed of an oil-in-water emulsion and are used in the treatment of dry skin disorders, such as psoriasis and dry eczema. They may contain other ingredients, such as camphor or menthol.

Barrier preparations These may be creams or ointments. They protect the skin against water and irritating substances. They may be used in the treatment of nappy rash and to protect the skin around an open sore. Barrier preparations may contain powders and water-repellent substances, such as silicones.

Lotions These thin, semi-liquid preparations are often used to cool and soothe inflamed skin. They are most suitable for use on large, hairy areas. Preparations called shake lotions contain fine powder that remains on the skin surface when the liquid has evaporated. They are used to encourage scabs to form.

Ointments These are usually greasy and are suitable for treating wet (weeping) eczema.

Pastes These are ointments containing large amounts of finely powdered solids such as starch or zinc oxide. Pastes protect the skin and absorb unwanted moisture. They are used for skin conditions that affect clearly defined areas, such as psoriasis.

Collodions These are preparations that, when applied to damaged areas of the skin such as ulcers and minor wounds, dry to form a protective film. They are sometimes used to keep a dissolved drug in contact with the skin.

COMMON DRUGS

Antibiotics Bacitracin, Colistin, Framycetin, Fusidic acid, Gramicidin, Mupirocin, Neomycin, Polymyxin B

Antiseptics and other antibacterials Cetrimide, Chlorhexidine, Hexachlorophene, Metronidazole*, Povidone iodine, Silver sulfadiazine, Triclosan

* See Part 2

Drugs to treat skin parasites

Mites and lice are the most common parasites that live on the skin. One common mite causes the skin disease scabies. The mite burrows into the skin and lays eggs, causing intense itching. Scratching the affected area results in bleeding and scab formation, as well as increasing the risk of infection.

There are three types of lice, each of which infests a different part of the human body: the head louse, the body (or clothes) louse, and the crab louse, which often infests the pubic areas but is also sometimes found on other hairy areas such as the eyebrows. All of these lice cause itching and lay eggs (nits) that look like white grains attached to hairs.

Both mites and lice are passed on by direct contact with an infected person (during sexual intercourse in the case of pubic lice) or, particularly in the case of body lice, by contact with infected bedding or clothing.

The drugs most often used to eliminate skin parasites are insecticides that kill both the adult insects and their eggs. The most effective drugs for scabies are malathion and permethrin; benzyl benzoate is occasionally used. Very severe scabies may require oral ivermectin as well. For lice infestations, carbaryl, malathion, permethrin, and phenothrin are used.

WHY THEY ARE USED

Skin parasites do not represent a serious threat to health, but their prompt eradication is necessary because they can cause severe irritation and can spread rapidly if left untreated. Drugs are used to eradicate them from the body, but bedding and clothing should be disinfected to avoid the possibility of reinfestation.

ELIMINATING PARASITES FROM BEDDING AND CLOTHING

Most skin parasites may also infest bedding and clothing that has been next to an infected person's skin. To avoid reinfestation following treatment of the body, any insects and eggs lodged in the bedding or clothing must also be eradicated.

Washing Since all skin parasites are killed by heat, washing affected items of clothing and bedding in hot water and drying them in a hot dryer is an effective and convenient method of dealing with the problem.

Non-washable items Items that cannot be washed should be isolated in plastic bags. The insects and their eggs cannot survive for long without their human hosts and die within days. The length of time they can survive, and therefore the period of isolation, varies depending on the type of parasite.

HOW THEY ARE USED

Lotions for the treatment of scabies are applied to the whole body following a bath or shower. Many people find that the preparations are messy to use; however, they should not be washed off for 12 hours (malathion) or 48 hours (benzyl benzoate), otherwise they will not be effective. It is probably most convenient to apply malathion before going to bed. The lotion may then be washed off the following morning.

One or two treatments are normally sufficient to remove the scabies mites. However, the itch that is associated with scabies may persist after the mite has been removed. Therefore, a soothing cream or medication containing an antipruritic drug (see p.118) may be necessary to ease it. People who have direct skin-to-skin contact with a sufferer from scabies, such as family members, classmates, and sexual partners, should also be treated with antiparasitic preparations at the same time.

Head and pubic lice infestations are usually treated by applying a preparation of one of the products and washing it off with water as and when instructed by the leaflet given with the preparation. If the skin has become infected as a result of scratching, a topical antibiotic (see Anti-infective skin preparations, p.120) may also be prescribed.

RISKS AND SPECIAL PRECAUTIONS

Lotions prescribed to control parasites can cause intense irritation and stinging if they are allowed to come into contact with the eyes, mouth, or other moist membranes. Therefore, lotions and shampoos should be applied carefully, following the instructions of your doctor or the manufacturer.

Because antiparasitic drugs are topical, they do not usually have generalized effects. Nevertheless, it is important not to apply these preparations more often than directed.

COMMON DRUGS

Benzyl benzoate, Carbaryl*, Crotamiton, Ivermectin, Malathion*, Permethrin*, Phenothrin
* See Part 2

Drugs used to treat acne

Acne, known medically as acne vulgaris, is a common condition caused by excess production of the skin's natural oil (sebum), leading to blockage of hair follicles. It chiefly affects adolescents but may occur at any age, due to certain drugs, exposure to industrial chemicals, oily cosmetics, or hot, humid conditions.

Acne primarily affects the face, neck, back, and chest. The main symptoms are blackheads, papules (inflamed spots), and pustules (raised, pus-filled spots with a white centre). Mild acne may produce only blackheads and an occasional papule or pustule. Moderate cases are characterized by larger numbers of pustules and papules. In severe cases, painful, inflamed cysts also develop, causing permanent pitting and scarring.

Medication for acne can be divided into two groups: topical preparations applied directly to the skin and systemic treatments taken by mouth.

WHY THEY ARE USED

Mild acne usually does not need medical treatment. It can be controlled by regular washing and by moderate exposure to sunlight or ultraviolet light. Over-the-counter antibacterial soaps and lotions are limited in use and may cause irritation.

Acne that is severe enough to need medication is usually treated with a topical preparation containing benzoyl peroxide or salicylic acid. If this does not produce an improvement, an ointment containing tretinoin (a drug related to vitamin A), azelaic acid, or tetracycline (an antibiotic), may be prescribed.

If acne is very severe or does not respond to topical treatments, a doctor may prescribe a course of antibiotics by mouth (usually tetracycline or minocycline). If these measures are unsuccessful, isotretinoin (a more powerful vitamin A-like drug, taken by mouth, may be prescribed.

Oestrogen drugs may have a beneficial effect on acne. A woman with acne who also needs contraception may be given an oral contraceptive (see p.105) containing oestrogen. Alternatively, a preparation containing an oestrogen and cyproterone (a drug that opposes male sex hormones) may be prescribed.

HOW THEY WORK

Drugs used to treat acne act in different ways. Some have a keratolytic effect – that is, they loosen the dead cells on the skin surface. Others work by countering bacterial activity in the skin or reducing sebum production.

Topical preparations, such as benzoyl peroxide, salicylic acid, and tretinoin, have a keratolytic effect. Benzoyl peroxide also has an antibacterial effect. Topical or systemic tetracyclines reduce bacteria but may also have a direct anti-inflammatory effect on the skin. Isotretinoin reduces sebum production, soothes inflammation, and helps to unblock hair follicles.

HOW THEY AFFECT YOU

Keratolytic preparations often cause soreness of the skin, especially at the start of treatment. If this persists, a change to a milder preparation may be recommended. Day-to-day side effects are rare with antibiotics.

Treatment with isotretinoin often causes dry and scaly skin, particularly on the lips. The skin may become itchy and some hair loss may occur.

RISKS AND SPECIAL PRECAUTIONS

Antibiotics in skin ointments may, rarely, provoke an allergic reaction requiring discontinuation of treatment. The tetracyclines, which are some of the most commonly used antibiotics for acne, have the advantage of being effective both topically and systemically. They are not suitable for use by mouth in pregnancy, however, since they can affect the bones and teeth of the developing baby.

Isotretinoin sometimes increases blood lipid levels. More seriously, it is known to damage the developing baby if taken during pregnancy. Women need to ensure that they avoid conception during treatment.

COMMON DRUGS

Topical treatments Adapalene, Azelaic acid, Benzoyl peroxide*, Isotretinoin*, Nicotinamide (Niacin), Salicylic acid, Tretinoin

Oral and topical antibiotics Clindamycin, Doxycycline*, Erythromycin*, Minocycline*, Tetracycline*, Trimethoprim*

Other oral drugs Co-cyprindiol (women only), Isotretinoin*

* **See Part 2**

Drugs for psoriasis

The skin is constantly being renewed; as fast as dead cells in the outer layer (epidermis) are shed, they are replaced by cells from the base of the epidermis. Psoriasis occurs when production of new cells increases while shedding of old cells remains normal. As a result, the live skin cells accumulate and produce patches of inflamed, thickened skin covered by silvery scales. In some cases, the affected area is extensive and causes severe embarrassment and physical discomfort. Psoriasis may occasionally be accompanied by arthritis, in which the joints become swollen and painful.

The underlying cause of psoriasis is not known. The disorder usually first occurs between the ages of 10 and 30 and recurs throughout life. Outbreaks may be triggered by stress, skin damage, drugs, and physical illness. Psoriasis can also occur as a consequence of the withdrawal of corticosteroid drugs.

There is no complete cure for psoriasis; simple measures, including careful sunbathing or using an ultraviolet lamp, may help to clear mild cases. An emollient cream (see Antipruritics, p.118) often soothes the irritation. When such measures fail to provide adequate relief, additional drug therapy is needed.

WHY THEY ARE USED

Drugs are used to decrease the size of affected areas and reduce inflammation and scaling. Mild and moderate psoriasis are usually treated topically. Calcipotriol, applied as an ointment, is very effective for treating small areas of skin. Coal tar creams, pastes, or bath additives are also often helpful, but some people dislike the smell. Dithranol is also widely used. Applied to the affected areas, it is left for a few minutes or overnight (depending on the product), before being washed off. Dithranol and coal tar can stain clothes and bed linen.

If these agents alone do not produce adequate benefit, ultraviolet light therapy in the form of regulated exposure to natural sunlight or ultraviolet lamps (UVB) may be advised. Salicylic acid may be applied to help remove thick scale and crusts, especially from the scalp.

Topical corticosteroids (see p.120) may be used in difficult cases that do not respond to those treatments. They are particularly useful for the skin-fold areas and may be given to counter irritation caused by dithranol.

If psoriasis is very severe, and other treatments have not been effective, specialist treatment may include the use of more powerful drugs. These drugs include vitamin A derivatives (acitretin), taken by mouth in courses lasting approximately six months, and methotrexate, which is an anticancer drug.

PUVA

PUVA is the combined use of a psoralen drug (methoxsalen) and ultraviolet A light (UVA). The psoralen is applied topically or taken by mouth; then, some hours later, the skin is exposed to UVA, which enhances the effect of the drug on skin cells. The drug is activated by exposure of the skin to the ultraviolet light; it acts on the cell's genetic material (DNA) to regulate its rate of division.

This therapy is given two to three times a week and produces an improvement within about four to six weeks. Possible adverse effects include nausea, itching, and painful reddening of the normal areas of skin. More seriously, there is a risk of the skin ageing prematurely and a long-term risk of skin cancer, particularly in fair-skinned people.

For these reasons, PUVA therapy is generally recommended only for severe psoriasis, when other treatments have failed.

HOW THEY WORK

Dithranol and methotrexate slow down the rapid rate of cell division that causes skin thickening. Acitretin also reduces production of keratin, the hard protein that forms in the outer skin layer. Salicylic acid and coal tar remove layers of dead skin cells. Corticosteroids reduce inflammation of the underlying skin.

HOW THEY AFFECT YOU

Appropriate treatment of psoriasis usually improves the appearance of the skin. However, since drugs cannot cure the underlying cause, psoriasis tends to recur, even following successful treatment of an outbreak.

Individual drugs may cause side effects. Topical preparations can cause stinging and inflammation, especially if they are applied to normal skin. Coal tar increases the skin's sensitivity to sunlight; excessive sunbathing or overexposure to artificial ultraviolet light may damage skin and worsen the condition.

Acitretin and methotrexate can have several serious side effects, including gastrointestinal upset, liver damage, and bone marrow damage (methotrexate). Both are unsuitable in pregnancy, and women are advised to avoid pregnancy for two years after completing treatment with acitretin. Topical corticosteroids may cause rebound worsening of psoriasis when they are stopped.

COMMON DRUGS

Acitretin, Calcipotriol*, Calcitriol, Ciclosporin*, Coal tar, Dithranol, Hydroxycarbamide, Methotrexate*, Methoxsalen, Salicylic acid, Tacalcitol, Tazarotene, Topical corticosteroids (see p.120)

* See Part 2

Treatments for eczema

Eczema, often called dermatitis, is a skin condition causing a dry, itchy rash that may be inflamed and blistered. It can be triggered by allergy but often occurs for no known reason. In the long term, eczema can thicken the skin as a result of persistent scratching.

The most common type, atopic eczema, may appear in infancy, but many children grow out of it. There is often a family history of eczema, asthma, or allergic rhinitis. Atopic eczema commonly appears over joints such as the fronts of the wrists and behind the knees. Contact dermatitis, another common form of eczema, is caused by chemicals, detergents, or soap. It may only appear after repeated exposure to the substance, but strong acids or alkalis can cause a reaction within minutes. It can also result from irritation of the skin by traces of detergent on clothes and bedding.

Allergic contact dermatitis can appear days or even years after initial contact has been made with triggers such as nickel, rubber, elastic, or drugs (such as antibiotics, antihistamines, antiseptics, or local anaesthetics). Sunlight can also trigger contact dermatitis following use of aftershave or perfume.

In nummular eczema, circular dry, scaly, itchy patches develop anywhere on the body, and bacteria are often found in these areas. The cause of nummular eczema is unknown.

Seborrhoeic dermatitis is a skin condition that mainly affects the scalp and face (see Drugs for dandruff, p.126).

WHY THEY ARE USED

Emollients are used to soften and moisten the skin. Oral antihistamines (see p.58) may be prescribed for a particularly itchy rash (topical antihistamines make the skin more sensitive and should not be used). Coal tar or ichthammol may be used for chronic atopic eczema, but topical corticosteroids (see p.120) may be needed to help control a flare-up.

Rarely, severe cases that are resistant to other treatments may need treatment with the immunosuppressant drug ciclosporin (see p.182). Oral corticosteroids (see p.80) may be used for contact dermatitis. Nummular eczema usually needs corticosteroid treatment. If it persists despite treatment there is a likelihood of infection, and antibiotics (see p.62) may be prescribed.

HOW THEY WORK

Emollients make the skin less dry and itchy. They are available as ointments, creams, lotions, soap substitutes, or bath oils. Because their effect is not long-lasting, they need to be applied frequently. Emollients do not usually contain an active drug.

Antihistamines block the action of histamine, a chemical found in all cells. Histamine dilates the blood vessels in the skin, causing redness and swelling of the surrounding tissue due to fluid leaking from the circulation. Antihistamines also prevent histamine from irritating nerve fibres, and thus relieve itching.

Topical corticosteroids are absorbed into the tissues to relieve itching and inflammation. The least potent one that is effective is given. Hydrocortisone 1 per cent is often used in 1 to 2-week courses.

Oral or topical antibiotics destroy the bacteria sometimes present in broken, oozing, or blistered skin.

Ciclosporin blocks the action of white blood cells, which are involved in the immune response. The drug is given in short courses when the immune system responds inappropriately to an allergen.

RISKS AND SPECIAL PRECAUTIONS

All types of eczema can become infected, and antibiotics may be needed. Herpes virus may infect atopic eczema, so direct contact with people who have a herpes infection, such as a cold sore, should be avoided. Emollients are generally well tolerated, as are mild topical corticosteroids used in the short term. Ciclosporin, however, may produce some adverse effects.

PREVENTING ECZEMA

Trigger substances can be identified using patch testing (see below), and then avoided. PVC gloves should be worn to protect the hands from detergents; and cotton, rather than wool or synthetic, garments should be worn next to the skin. Cosmetic moisturizers should be avoided because they usually contain perfumes and other sensitizers.

PATCH TESTING

Low concentrations of suspected substances are applied to the skin of the back and are held in place with non-absorbent adhesive tape. This method allows a number of potential allergens (substances that can cause an allergic reaction) to be tested at the same time. After 48 hours, the adhesive tape is removed and the skin inspected for any redness, swelling, or blistering, which would indicate a positive reaction. The skin is checked after a further 24 and 48 hours, in case the reaction has taken longer to develop.

COMMON DRUGS

Emollient and cooling preparations Aqueous cream, Cold cream, Calamine lotion, Emulsifying ointment

Corticosteroids (see also p.80) Hydrocortisone*

Antihistamines (see also p.58) Alimemazine, Chlorphenamine*, Clemastine, Diphenhydramine, Mepyramine, Trimeprazine

Other drugs Azathioprine*, Ciclosporin*, Coal tar, Ichthammol, Mycophenolate mofetil, Tacrolimus

* **See Part 2**

Drugs for dandruff

Dandruff is an irritating but harmless condition that involves an acceleration in the normal shedding of skin cells from the scalp. Extensive dandruff is considered to be a mild form of a type of dermatitis known as seborrhoeic dermatitis, which is caused by an overgrowth of a yeast organism that lives in the scalp. In severe cases, a rash and reddish-yellow, scaly pimples appear along the hairline and on the face.

WHY THEY ARE USED

Frequent washing with a detergent shampoo usually keeps the scalp free of dandruff, but more persistent dandruff can be treated with a shampoo containing the antifungal drug ketoconazole (see p.280), or medicated shampoos containing zinc pyrithione or selenium sulphide, or with shampoos containing coal tar or salicylic acid. Ointments containing coal tar and salicylic acid are also available. Corticosteroid gels and lotions may be needed to treat an itchy rash, especially in cases of severe seborrhoeic dermatitis or psoriasis on the scalp (see p.124).

HOW THEY WORK

Coal tar and salicylic acid preparations reduce the overproduction of new skin cells and break down scales, which are then washed off during shampooing. Antifungals (see p.76) reduce the overgrowth of yeast on the scalp by altering the permeability of the fungal cell walls. Corticosteroids (see p.80) help to relieve an itchy rash by reducing inflammation of the underlying skin.

COMMON DRUGS

Antifungals Ketoconazole*, Zinc pyrithione
Other drugs Coal tar, Salicylic acid, Selenium sulphide, Topical corticosteroids (see p.120)
* **See Part 2**

Drugs for hair loss

Hair loss (alopecia) is the result of greater-than-normal shedding of hairs or reduced hair production. Some forms of hair loss can be caused by a skin condition such as scalp ringworm or scalp psoriasis. Other forms are due to a disorder of the follicles themselves in response to illness or malnutrition, or as a reaction to some drugs, such as anticancer drugs or anticoagulants. The hair loss may be diffuse, or it may occur in a pattern – as in male-pattern baldness, which is caused by oversensitivity to testosterone.

WHY THEY ARE USED

If the hair loss is caused by a skin disorder such as scalp ringworm, an antifungal will be used to kill the fungal growth. If male-pattern baldness is a response to the male hormone testosterone, finasteride may be used to reduce the hormone's effect. The antihypertensive drug minoxidil (see p.320) can be applied to the scalp to promote hair growth.

HOW THEY WORK

Hair loss can be reversed when the underlying illness is treated, or when drug treatment stops. Oral finasteride inhibits the conversion of testosterone to its more active form and reduces sensitivity to androgens. The role of minoxidil in hair growth is not fully understood, but it is thought to stimulate follicles.

RISKS AND SPECIAL PRECAUTIONS

Finasteride can lead to loss of libido or impotence. Anyone with a history of heart disease or hypertension should consult their doctor before using minoxidil, because the drug can be absorbed through the skin.

COMMON DRUGS

Antifungals Griseofulvin, Ketoconazole*, Terbinafine*
Other drugs Finasteride*, Minoxidil*
* **See Part 2**

Sunscreens

Sunscreens and sunblocks are chemicals, usually formulated as creams or oils, that protect the skin from the damaging effects of ultraviolet radiation from the sun.

People vary in their sensitivity to sunlight. Fair-skinned people generally have the least tolerance and tend to burn easily when exposed to the sun, while those with darker, especially brown or black, skin can withstand exposure for longer periods. Fair skin unprotected by a sunscreen suffers damage as ultraviolet rays pass through to the layers beneath, causing pain and inflammation. Sunscreens act by blocking out some of these ultraviolet rays, while allowing a proportion of them to pass through the skin surface to the epidermis to stimulate the production of melanin, the pigment that gives the skin a tan and helps to protect it during further exposure to the sun.

In a few cases, the skin's sensitivity to sunlight is increased by a disease such as pellagra or herpes simplex infection. Some drugs, such as thiazide diuretics, phenothiazine antipsychotics, psoralens, sulphonamide antibacterials, tetracycline antibiotics, and nalidixic acid, can also increase the skin's sensitivity.

Apart from sunburn and premature skin aging, the most serious effect from sunlight is skin cancer. Reducing the skin's exposure to sunlight can help to prevent skin cancers.

HOW THEY WORK

Sunlight consists of different wavelengths of radiation. Of these, ultraviolet (UV) radiation is particularly harmful to the skin. UV radiation is mainly composed of UVA and UVB rays, both of which prematurely age the skin. In addition, UVA rays cause tanning and UVB rays cause burning. Excessive exposure to UV radiation also increases a person's risk of developing skin cancer. Fair-skinned people, and those being treated with immunosuppressant drugs, are especially vulnerable to skin damage.

Sunscreens absorb some of the UVB radiation, ensuring that less of it reaches the skin. They are graded using the Sun Protection Factor (SPF), which refers to the degree of protection given by a sunscreen against sunburn. SPF is a measure of the amount of UVB radiation a sunscreen absorbs; the higher the number, the greater the protection. This number only describes the protection against UVB radiation. Some sunscreens, which contain chemicals such as zinc oxide and titanium dioxide, protect against UVA radiation as well; these are often called sunblocks. Certain preparations carry a "star" classification for the UVA protection they give; the stars do not describe an absolute measure but indicate a ratio of UVA to UVB protection. Four stars means that the product gives balanced protection against both UVA and UVB. Ratings of 1, 2, or 3 stars mean that the sunscreen has more protection against UVB than UVA.

Sunscreens are particularly advisable for visitors to tropical, subtropical, and mountainous areas, and for those who wish to sunbathe, because they can prevent burning while allowing the skin to tan. Sunscreens must be applied before exposure to the sun. People with fair skin should use a sunscreen with a higher SPF than people with darker skin.

RISKS AND SPECIAL PRECAUTIONS

Sunscreens only form a physical barrier to the passage of UV radiation – they do not alter the skin to make it more resistant to sunlight. Sunscreen lotions must be applied frequently during exposure to the sun in order to maintain protection. People who are very fair-skinned or who are known to be particularly sensitive to sunlight should never expose their skin to direct sunlight, even if they are using a sunscreen, since not even sunscreens with high SPF values will give them complete protection.

Sunscreens can irritate the skin and some preparations may cause an allergic rash. People who are sensitive to some drugs, such as procaine and benzocaine, and some hair dyes, may develop a rash after applying a sunscreen containing aminobenzoic acid or a benzophenone derivative such as oxybenzone.

COMMON DRUGS

Ingredients in sunscreens and sunblocks

Aminobenzoic acid, Benzones, Dibenzoylmethanes, Drometizole trisiloxane, Ethylhexyl methoxycinnamate, Methylbenzylidene camphor, Mexenone, Octocrylene, Oxybenzone, Padimate-O, Titanium dioxide, Zinc oxide

PART 2

A–Z OF DRUGS

This part of the book contains 259 generic drugs, individually profiled, and written to a standard format to help you find specific information quickly and easily; cross-references to the relevant major drug groups are provided.

Acamprosate

Brand name Campral EC
Used in the following combined preparations
None

QUICK REFERENCE
Drug group Alcohol abuse treatment
Overdose danger rating Low
Dependence rating Low
Prescription needed Yes
Available as generic No

GENERAL INFORMATION

Acamprosate has a chemical structure that is similar to some neurotransmitters, and it can cross the blood–brain barrier. Studies show that acamprosate affects alcohol dependence, decreasing the voluntary intake of alcohol without affecting the intake of other fluids or food. Acamprosate is used, together with counselling, in the treatment of alcohol dependence. Treatment with this drug is started after withdrawal of alcohol has been achieved. The drug should be continued if the patient relapses, but there is no point in continuing the treatment if regular alcohol abuse is resumed.

Mental problems are frequently reported in alcoholic patients. Any psychiatric disorders (predominantly depression) that occur while the patient is under treatment with acamprosate could be caused either by the drug or by the patient's underlying condition.

INFORMATION FOR USERS

Your drug prescription is tailored for you. Do not alter dosage without checking with your doctor.
How taken Tablets.
Frequency and timing of doses 3 x daily: at breakfast, midday, and at night.
Adult dosage range For body weight of 60kg or more: 1,998mg daily. For body weight of less than 60kg: 1,332mg daily.
Onset of effect The drug is slowly absorbed. Steady levels are only reached after 7 days.
Duration of action 8 hours.
Diet advice None, but taking the drug with food reduces its absorption.
Storage Keep in a closed container in a cool, dry place out of reach of children.

Missed dose Take as soon as you remember. If your next dose is due within 2 hours, take a single dose now and skip the next.
Stopping the drug If you wish to stop taking the drug, discuss it with your doctor first.
Exceeding the dose An occasional unintentional extra dose is unlikely to be a cause for concern. However, if a large overdose has been taken, diarrhoea will probably result; notify your doctor.

POSSIBLE ADVERSE EFFECTS

Adverse effects associated with acamprosate tend to be mild and transient in nature. They predominantly involve the skin and gastrointestinal tract, commonly causing diarrhoea, nausea and vomiting, abdominal pain, and itching. Contact your doctor if any of these symptoms are severe. If you suffer from depression or loss of libido, or if you develop a rash, seek medical advice; all of these are rare adverse effects of acamprosate.

INTERACTIONS

None.

SPECIAL PRECAUTIONS

Be sure to consult your doctor or pharmacist before taking this drug if:
◆ You have kidney problems.
◆ You have severe liver impairment.
◆ You know that you are allergic to the drug.
Pregnancy Safety not established. Discuss with your doctor.
Breast-feeding Safety not established. Acamprosate passes into the breast milk and may affect the baby adversely. Discuss with your doctor.
Infants and children Not recommended.
Over 60 Not recommended.
Driving and hazardous work No special problems.
Alcohol Alcohol is not permitted while this drug is being taken.

PROLONGED USE

Acamprosate is not taken in the long term. The recommended treatment period for the drug is 1 year.
Monitoring Counselling and regular monitoring for psychiatric problems will be performed .

Aciclovir

Brand names Boots Avert, Herpetad, Soothelip, Virasorb, Virovir, Zovirax
Used in the following combined preparations None

QUICK REFERENCE

Drug group Antiviral drug (p.69)
Overdose danger rating Low
Dependence rating Low
Prescription needed No (cold sore cream); Yes (other preparations)
Available as generic Yes

GENERAL INFORMATION

Aciclovir is an antiviral drug used in the treatment of herpes infections, which can cause cold sores and genital herpes. It is available as a cream, tablets, eye ointment, and injection. The cream is commonly used to treat cold sores, and can speed up the healing of the lesions, provided it is started as soon as symptoms occur and before the lesions appear. The tablets and injection are used to treat severe herpes infections, shingles, chickenpox, and genital herpes. The tablets can also be used to prevent herpes infection from developing in people with reduced immunity. Herpes infection affecting the eye can be treated with an eye ointment.

INFORMATION FOR USERS

Follow instructions on the label. Call your doctor if symptoms worsen.
How taken Tablets, liquid, injection, cream, eye ointment.
Frequency and timing of doses 2–5 x daily. Start as soon as possible.
Adult dosage range *Treatment* 1–4g daily (tablets, liquid). *Prevention* 800mg–1.6g daily (tablets, liquid); 5 x daily (cream, eye ointment).
Onset of effect Within 24 hours.
Duration of action Up to 8 hours.
Diet advice It is necessary to drink plenty of water when taking high doses by mouth or injection.
Storage Keep in a closed container in a cool, dry place out of reach of children. Protect from light.
Missed dose Take as soon as you remember (tablets, liquid, cream, eye ointment).

Stopping the drug Complete the full course as directed, unless rash, confusion, or hallucinations occur.
Exceeding the dose An occasional unintentional extra dose is unlikely to be a cause for concern. But if you notice any unusual symptoms, or if a large overdose has been taken, notify your doctor.

POSSIBLE ADVERSE EFFECTS

Serious adverse effects are rare. The cream may cause stinging or itching at the site of application. Taken by mouth, aciclovir can occasionally cause nausea, vomiting, headache, or dizziness. Confusion or hallucinations may occur rarely with injections; if these or a rash occur, stop taking the drug and consult your doctor without delay.

INTERACTIONS (by mouth or injection only)

General note Any drug that affects the kidneys increases the risk of side effects with aciclovir.
Probenecid and cimetidine This drug may increase the level of aciclovir in the blood.
Mycophenolate mofetil Aciclovir may increase blood levels of this drug and vice versa.

SPECIAL PRECAUTIONS

Be sure to consult your doctor or pharmacist before taking this drug if:
◆ You have a long-term kidney problem.
◆ You have reduced immunity.
◆ You are taking other medications.
Pregnancy No known risk with topical preparations; oral and injectable forms are not usually prescribed, as effects on the developing baby are unknown. Discuss with your doctor.
Breast-feeding No evidence of risk with topical forms. The drug passes into the breast milk following injection or oral administration. Discuss with your doctor.
Infants and children Reduced dose necessary in young children.
Over 60 Reduced dose may be necessary.
Driving and hazardous work No known problems.
Alcohol No known problems.

PROLONGED USE

Aciclovir is usually given as single courses of treatment and is not given long term, except to people with reduced immunity.

Alendronate

Brand names Fosamax, Fosamax Once Weekly
Used in the following combined preparations
None

QUICK REFERENCE

Drug group Drug for bone disorders (p.56)
Overdose danger rating Medium
Dependence rating Low
Prescription needed Yes
Available as generic Yes

GENERAL INFORMATION

Alendronate is used to treat osteoporosis in men and postmenopausal osteoporosis in women. A calcium supplement and vitamin D may be prescribed with the drug if dietary amounts are not adequate, but calcium should not be taken at the same time as alendronate because calcium is one of many substances that reduce its absorption. Combined use of alendronate with HRT (see p.89) in postmenopausal women is more effective than either treatment alone.

Alendronate tablets should be taken on getting up in the morning, swallowed whole with a full glass of tap water (not even mineral water is acceptable because of the minerals' possible effect on absorption). After taking the tablet(s), remain upright for at least 30 minutes; do not go back to bed. This is to prevent the drug from sticking in the oesophagus, where it could cause ulcers or irritation. Breakfast may be eaten and any other medicines taken not less than 30 minutes (preferably longer) after taking alendronate.

INFORMATION FOR USERS

Your drug prescription is tailored for you. Do not alter dosage without checking with your doctor.
How taken Tablets.
Frequency and timing of doses Once daily, first thing. Once weekly, first thing (postmenopausal women).
Adult dosage range *Treatment* men, 10mg; postmenopausal women, 70mg (weekly). *Prevention* 5mg (postmenopausal women). *Prevention and treatment of corticosteroid-induced osteoporosis* 5mg; postmenopausal women not taking HRT, 10mg.

Onset of effect It may take months for any improvement to appear.
Duration of action Some effects may persist for months or years.
Diet advice None.
Storage Keep in a closed container in a cool, dry place out of the reach of children.
Missed dose Take the next dose at the usual time next morning.
Stopping the drug Do not stop the drug without consulting your doctor. Stopping the drug may lead to worsening of the underlying condition.
Exceeding the dose An occasional unintentional extra dose is unlikely to cause problems. Large overdoses, however, may cause stomach problems including heartburn, irritation, and ulcers; if this happens, notify your doctor at once, and try to remain upright.

POSSIBLE ADVERSE EFFECTS

The most frequent adverse effect of alendronate is abdominal pain as a result of irritation to the oesophagus, stomach, or small intestine. Alendronate also commonly causes diarrhoea, constipation, muscle and bone pain, headache, and rarely, nausea and vomiting. If the drug causes a rash and photosensitivity or eye inflammation, however, consult your doctor.

INTERACTIONS

Antacids, calcium, and iron salts These substances reduce the absorption of alendronate.

SPECIAL PRECAUTIONS

Be sure to tell your doctor if:
◆ You have an abnormality of the oesophagus.
◆ You have stomach problems or a history of ulcers.
◆ You are unable to stand or sit upright for at least 30 minutes.
◆ You have hypocalcaemia.
◆ You have kidney impairment.
◆ You are taking any other medications.
Pregnancy Not recommended.
Breast-feeding Not recommended.
Infants and children Not recommended.
Over 60 No special problems.
Driving and hazardous work No special problems.
Alcohol May cause further stomach irritation.

PROLONGED USE

The drug is usually prescribed indefinitely for osteoporosis without causing problems.
Monitoring Blood and urine tests may be carried out at intervals.

Alginates

Brand names Gaviscon Infant (oral); Algisite M, Algosteril, Kaltostat, Melgisorb, Seasorb, Sorbalgon, Sorbsan (dressings)
Used in the following combined preparations
Algicon, Gastrocote, Gaviscon, Peptac, Rennie Duo, Topal

QUICK REFERENCE
Drug group Antacid (p.42)
Overdose danger rating Low
Dependence rating Low
Prescription needed No
Available as generic Yes

GENERAL INFORMATION

"Alginates" is a group term that refers to a mixture of acidic compounds extracted from brown algae (seaweeds). When the powder extract is mixed with water, alginates become a thick, viscous fluid or gel depending on the chemicals used.

Alginates are used to treat mild gastro-oesophageal reflux disease. Combined with antacids, they form a "raft" that floats on the surface of the stomach contents, which reduces reflux and protects the lining of the oesophagus. A number of indigestion remedies on sale to the public also contain alginates.

In addition, the properties of alginates are used in wound dressings where, in the form of a woven pad, they absorb fluids from the surface of the wound, keeping it moist and allowing it to heal.

INFORMATION FOR USERS

Follow instructions on the label. Call your doctor if symptoms worsen.
How taken Tablets, liquid, powder.
Frequency and timing of doses 4 x daily after meals and at bedtime.
Adult dosage range 800–2,000mg daily.
Onset of effect 10–20 minutes.
Duration of action 3–4 hours.
Diet advice None.

Storage Keep in a closed container in a cool, dry place out of reach of children.
Missed dose Take as soon as you remember, if you need it.
Stopping the drug Alginates can be safely stopped as soon as you no longer need them.
Exceeding the dose Overdose of alginates is likely to produce abdominal distension, without any other symptoms. Notify your doctor if symptoms are severe.

POSSIBLE ADVERSE EFFECTS

The antacid salts in combined oral preparations may cause abdominal discomfort and distension, and rarely, nausea. Consult your doctor if the symptoms are severe.

INTERACTIONS
None.

SPECIAL PRECAUTIONS

Be sure to consult your doctor or pharmacist before taking this drug if:
◆ You are on a salt-restricted diet.
◆ You are taking any other medications.
Pregnancy No evidence of risk to the developing baby. Some products can be used for heartburn in pregnancy.
Breast-feeding No evidence of risk.
Infants and children Reduced dose necessary.
Over 60 No special problems.
Driving and hazardous work No known problems.
Alcohol No known problems.

PROLONGED USE
No problems expected.

Allopurinol

Brand names Caplenal, Cosuric, Rimapurinol, Xanthomax, Zyloric
Used in the following combined preparations
None

QUICK REFERENCE
Drug group Drug for gout (p.53)
Overdose danger rating Medium
Dependence rating Low
Prescription needed Yes
Available as generic Yes

GENERAL INFORMATION

Allopurinol is used to prevent gout, which is caused by deposits of uric acid crystals in joints. The drug blocks an enzyme called xanthine oxidase, which is involved in forming uric acid. It is also used to lower high uric acid levels (hyperuricaemia) caused by other drugs, such as anticancer drugs. A course of allopurinol should never be started until an acute attack of gout is over because it may cause a further episode. Treatment with the drug should be continued indefinitely to prevent further attacks.

At the start of treatment, an acute attack may occur, and colchicine (see p.199) or an anti-inflammatory drug may also be given until uric acid levels are reduced. If an acute attack occurs while you are taking allopurinol, treatment should continue along with an anti-inflammatory drug.

INFORMATION FOR USERS

Your drug prescription is tailored for you. Do not alter dosage without checking with your doctor.

How taken Tablets.

Frequency and timing of doses Once daily after food.

Adult dosage range 100–300mg daily.

Onset of effect Within 24–48 hours. Full effect may not be felt for several weeks.

Duration of action Up to 30 hours. Some effect may last for 1–2 weeks after the drug has been stopped.

Diet advice A high fluid intake (2 litres daily) is recommended.

Storage Keep in a closed container in a cool, dry place out of reach of children.

Missed dose If your next dose is not due for another 12 hours or more, take a dose as soon as you remember and take the next one as usual. Otherwise, skip the missed dose and take your next dose on schedule.

Stopping the drug Unless rash, sore throat, fever, or shivering occur, do not stop taking the drug without consulting your doctor; symptoms may recur.

Exceeding the dose An occasional unintentional extra dose is unlikely to cause problems. Large overdoses, however, may cause nausea, vomiting, abdominal pain, diarrhoea, and dizziness; notify your doctor.

POSSIBLE ADVERSE EFFECTS

Adverse effects of allopurinol are not very common. The most serious are allergic rash, sore throat, fever, or shivering, which may require the drug to be substituted. Nausea can be avoided by taking allopurinol after food. Very rarely, the drug causes visual disturbance; always discuss this with your doctor.

INTERACTIONS

Mercaptopurine and azathioprine Allopurinol blocks the breakdown of these drugs, requiring a reduction in their dosage.

Aspirin Large doses of this drug may reduce the effects of allopurinol.

Anticoagulant drugs Allopurinol may increase the effects of these drugs.

Theophylline Allopurinol may increase levels of this drug.

Chlorpropamide The hypoglycaemic effects of this drug may be increased with allopurinol.

Ciclosporin Allopurinol may increase the effects of this drug.

ACE inhibitors Allopurinol may increase the effects of these drugs.

SPECIAL PRECAUTIONS

Be sure to tell your doctor if:
◆ You have long-term liver or kidney problems.
◆ You have had a previous sensitivity reaction to allopurinol.
◆ You have a current attack of gout.
◆ You are taking other medications.

Pregnancy Safety in pregnancy not established. Discuss with your doctor.

Breast-feeding The drug passes into the breast milk and may affect the baby. Discuss with your doctor.

Infants and children Reduced dose necessary.

Over 60 Reduced dose may be necessary.

Driving and hazardous work No problems expected.

Alcohol Keep consumption low. Large amounts of alcohol may worsen gout.

PROLONGED USE

Apart from an increased risk of gout in the first weeks or months, no problems expected.

Monitoring Periodic checks on uric acid levels in the blood are usually performed and the dose of allopurinol adjusted if necessary.

Alprostadil

Brand names Caverject, MUSE, Prostin VR, Viridal
Used in the following combined preparations
None

QUICK REFERENCE

Drug group Prostaglandin and drug for impotence (p.109)
Overdose danger rating Medium
Dependence rating Low
Prescription needed Yes
Available as generic No

GENERAL INFORMATION

Alprostadil is a member of the prostaglandin group of drugs and is used to help impotent men to achieve an erection. The drug is either injected directly into the penis or applied as a gel into the urethra (using a pipette). The most common side effect of alprostadil is pain in the penis.

The first dose must be given by medically trained personnel, and self-administration may only be undertaken after proper training.

Alprostadil is also used to treat patent ductus arteriosus, a congenital heart disorder that occurs in newborn babies. The drug is usually only administered in hospital and works by keeping the ductus blood vessel (normally shut off at birth) open until it can be closed permanently by surgery. Side effects such as heart, circulatory, and respiratory problems are common, and there is a risk of unusual bone growth, particularly after long use.

INFORMATION FOR USERS

Your drug prescription is tailored for you. Do not alter dosage without checking with your doctor.
How taken Injection, gel.
Frequency and timing of doses Up to 3 x per week. Not more than one dose in any 24-hour period.
Dosage range 2.5mcg (starting dose), individually adjusted by your doctor to produce an erection that lasts for no longer than 1 hour.
Onset of effect Within a few minutes.
Duration of action Erection should not last more than 1 hour.

Diet advice None.
Storage Store in a refrigerator, out of reach of children. Do not freeze.
Missed dose Take the next dose when needed. Use no more than one dose in any 24-hour period and no more than 3 doses per week.
Stopping the drug The drug can be safely stopped as soon as you no longer need it.
Exceeding the dose An occasional unintentional extra dose is unlikely to be a cause for concern. But if you notice any unusual symptoms, or if a large overdose has been taken, notify your doctor.

POSSIBLE ADVERSE EFFECTS

In men, pain or bruising may occur at the injection site, and there is a risk of prolonged erection. Any erection that lasts for more than 4 hours should be reported to your doctor, and the drug stopped, immediately.

Breathing difficulties are a side effect of the drug in newborn babies. Less often, it may cause convulsions.

INTERACTIONS

Antihypertensive and vasodilator drugs The effects of these drugs may be increased by alprostadil.

SPECIAL PRECAUTIONS

Be sure to tell your doctor if:
◆ You are taking other medications for impotence.
Pregnancy Not prescribed.
Breast-feeding Not prescribed.
Infants and children Other than for newborn babies, not prescribed.
Over 60 Doses are adjusted individually.
Driving and hazardous work No special problems.
Alcohol Excessive use of alcohol with alprostadil can contribute to erectile problems.

PROLONGED USE

Prolonged use of alprostadil injections for impotence may cause scarring of the penis to develop. Prolonged use of alprostadil in newborn babies may cause abnormal bone development and weakening of some blood vessel walls.
Monitoring Regular examinations are required to check for penile scarring.

Aluminium Hydroxide

Brand names Alu-Cap, Aludrox
Used in the following combined preparations
Algicon, Asilone, Co-magaldrox, Gaviscon, Maalox, Mucaine, Mucogel, Topal, and others

QUICK REFERENCE

Drug group Antacid (p.42)
Overdose danger rating Low
Dependence rating Low
Prescription needed No
Available as generic Yes

GENERAL INFORMATION

Aluminium hydroxide is a common ingredient of many over-the-counter indigestion and heartburn remedies. The drug neutralizes stomach acid. This action makes it useful in preventing pain in stomach and duodenal ulcers or heartburn. It can also promote the healing of ulcers.

Because aluminium hydroxide is constipating (it is sometimes used to treat diarrhoea), it is usually combined with a magnesium-containing antacid that has a balancing laxative effect (a combination sometimes known by the generic name co-magaldrox).

Aluminium hydroxide may be more effective as an antacid in liquid form rather than as tablets. Some antacid preparations include large amounts of sodium, and should be used with caution by people on a low-sodium diet.

In the intestine, aluminium hydroxide binds with, and thereby reduces absorption of, phosphate. This makes it helpful in treating high blood phosphate (hyperphosphataemia), which occurs in some people with impaired kidney function. Prolonged heavy use, however, can lead to phosphate deficiency and consequent weakening of the bones.

INFORMATION FOR USERS

Follow instructions on the label. Call your doctor if symptoms worsen.

How taken Tablets, capsules, liquid (gel suspension). The tablets should be well chewed.

Frequency and timing of doses *As antacid* 4–6 x daily as needed, or 1 hour before and after meals. *Peptic ulcer* 6–7 x daily. *Hyperphosphataemia* 3–4 x daily with meals. *Diarrhoea* 2–6 x daily.

Dosage range *Adults* Up to 70ml daily (liquid), 2–10g daily (tablets or capsules). *Children over 6 years* Reduced dose according to age and weight.

Onset of effect Within 15 minutes.

Duration of action 2–4 hours.

Diet advice For hyperphosphataemia, a low-phosphate diet may be advised in addition to treatment with aluminium hydroxide.

Storage Keep in a closed container in a cool, dry place out of reach of children.

Missed dose Do not take the missed dose. Take your next dose as usual.

Stopping the drug Treatment for indigestion can be safely stopped as soon as you no longer need it. If you are taking the drug as ulcer treatment, or for hyperphosphataemia resulting from kidney failure, do not stop without consulting your doctor.

Exceeding the dose An occasional unintentional extra dose is unlikely to be a cause for concern. But if you notice any unusual symptoms, or if a large overdose has been taken, notify your doctor.

POSSIBLE ADVERSE EFFECTS

Constipation is a common adverse effect. More rarely, nausea and vomiting may occur due to the granular, powdery nature of the drug. If vomiting is severe, see your doctor. Bone pain may occur, but only if large doses have been taken regularly for months or years.

INTERACTIONS

General note Aluminium hydroxide may interfere with the absorption or excretion of many drugs, including oral anticoagulants, digoxin, many antibiotics, penicillamine, corticosteroids, antipsychotics, and phenytoin. It should only be taken at least 2 hours before or after other drugs.

Enteric-coated tablets Aluminium hydroxide may cause enteric-coated tablets (such as bisacodyl or prednisolone) to start breaking up before they leave the stomach, producing stomach irritation.

SPECIAL PRECAUTIONS

Be sure to consult your doctor or pharmacist before taking this drug if:

◆ You have a long-term kidney problem.
◆ You have heart problems.

- ◆ You have high blood pressure.
- ◆ You suffer from constipation.
- ◆ You have a bone disease.
- ◆ You have porphyria.
- ◆ You are taking other medications.

Pregnancy Safety in pregnancy not established. Discuss with your doctor.

Breast-feeding No evidence of risk.

Infants and children Not recommended under 6 years except on the advice of a doctor.

Over 60 Increased likelihood of adverse effects. Reduced dose may therefore be necessary.

Driving and hazardous work No known problems.

Alcohol No known problems.

PROLONGED USE

Aluminium hydroxide should not be used for longer than 4 weeks without consulting your doctor. Prolonged high doses may deplete blood phosphate and calcium levels, leading to weakening of the bones and fractures.

Amiloride

Brand names Amilamont, Amilospare
Used in the following combined preparations
Burinex A, Co-amilofruse, Co-amilozide, Moduretic, Navispare, and others

QUICK REFERENCE

Drug group Potassium-sparing diuretic (p.32)
Overdose danger rating Low
Dependence rating Low
Prescription needed Yes
Available as generic Yes

GENERAL INFORMATION

Amiloride is a diuretic drug that acts on the kidneys to increase the amount of urine that is passed. It is used in the treatment of oedema (fluid retention), which can result from heart failure or liver disease, and for hypertension (high blood pressure).

The effect on urine flow may last for several hours. The drug should, preferably, be taken in the morning and no later than about 4 pm, otherwise you may need to pass urine during the night.

Because amiloride is a "potassium-sparing" diuretic (which causes the kidneys to conserve potassium), it should not be used when blood levels of potassium are high. The drug is prescribed with caution in people with kidney disease or those who are taking potassium supplements and is usually combined with other diuretics.

INFORMATION FOR USERS

Your drug prescription is tailored for you. Do not alter dosage without checking with your doctor.

How taken Tablets, liquid.

Frequency and timing of doses Once daily, usually in the morning.

Adult dosage range 5–20mg daily.

Onset of effect Within 2–4 hours.

Duration of action 12–24 hours.

Diet advice Avoid foods that are high in potassium (such as dried fruit, bananas, tomatoes, and salt substitutes).

Storage Keep in a closed container in a cool, dry place out of reach of children.

Missed dose Take as soon as you remember. However, if it is late in the day, do not take the missed dose, or you may need to get up at night to pass urine. Take the next scheduled dose as usual.

Stopping the drug Unless a rash occurs, do not stop taking the drug without consulting your doctor; symptoms may recur.

Exceeding the dose An occasional unintentional extra dose is unlikely to cause problems. If you notice any symptoms, or if a large overdose has been taken, notify your doctor.

POSSIBLE ADVERSE EFFECTS

Amiloride has few adverse effects, which should all be reported to your doctor. It may cause digestive disturbance, a dry mouth and thirst, confusion, and dizziness, The main problem is the possibility of potassium being retained by the body, causing muscle weakness and numbness. If you develop a rash, stop taking the drug and consult your doctor.

INTERACTIONS

Lithium Amiloride may increase the blood levels of lithium, leading to an increased risk of lithium poisoning.

ACE inhibitors, ciclosporin, and NSAIDs These drugs may increase the risk of potassium retention if they are taken with amiloride.

SPECIAL PRECAUTIONS

Be sure to tell your doctor if:
◆ You have long-term liver or kidney problems.
◆ You have diabetes.
◆ You are taking other medications.

Pregnancy Not usually prescribed during pregnancy. Amiloride may cause a reduction in the blood supply to the developing baby. Discuss with your doctor.

Breast-feeding Not usually prescribed during breast-feeding. Discuss with your doctor.

Infants and children Not recommended.

Over 60 Increased likelihood of adverse effects. Reduced dose necessary.

Driving and hazardous work No known problems.

Alcohol No special problems.

PROLONGED USE

Monitoring Blood tests may be carried out to monitor levels of body salts.

Amiodarone

Brand name Cordarone X
Used in the following combined preparations
None

QUICK REFERENCE

Drug group Anti-arrhythmic drug (p.33)
Overdose danger rating Medium
Dependence rating Low
Prescription needed Yes
Available as generic Yes (tablets)

GENERAL INFORMATION

Introduced in the 1950s, amiodarone is used to treat a variety of abnormal heart rhythms (arrhythmias). It works by slowing nerve impulses in the heart muscle.

Amiodarone is given to prevent recurrent atrial and ventricular fibrillation and to treat ventricular and supraventricular tachycardias and Wolff-Parkinson-White Syndrome. Due to its potentially serious adverse effects, it is often used only when other treatments have failed, especially in the long term. Treatment should be started only under specialist supervision or in hospital, and the dosage is carefully controlled to achieve the desired effect using the lowest possible dose.

INFORMATION FOR USERS

Your drug prescription is tailored for you. Do not alter dosage without checking with your doctor.

How taken Tablets, injection.

Frequency and timing of doses 3 x daily or by injection initially, then reduced to twice daily, then once daily or every other day (maintenance dose).

Adult dosage range 600mg daily, reduced to 400mg, then 100–200mg daily.

Onset of effect Some effects may be noticed within 72 hours (tablets), but full benefits may not be felt for some weeks; effects may be noticed within 30 minutes (injection).

Duration of action Up to 1 month.

Diet advice None.

Storage Keep in a closed container in a cool, dry place out of reach of children. Protect from light.

Missed dose Take as soon as you remember. If your next dose is due within 12 hours, do not take the missed dose, but take your next scheduled dose as usual.

Stopping the drug Do not stop taking the drug without consulting your doctor; symptoms may recur.

Exceeding the dose An occasional unintentional extra dose is unlikely to cause problems. But if you notice any unusual symptoms, or if a large overdose has been taken, notify your doctor at once.

POSSIBLE ADVERSE EFFECTS

Amiodarone produces a number of unusual adverse effects, including a metallic taste in the mouth, photosensitivity (increased skin sensitivity to sunlight), and a greyish skin colour. High-factor sun block should be used, and exposed skin covered. The drug can also cause nausea, headache, disturbed vision or eye damage, and liver, lung, and thyroid problems. If nervousness, tremor, weight loss, or shortness of breath occur, or jaundice develops, consult your doctor.

INTERACTIONS

General note Amiodarone can interact with many drugs. Consult your doctor or pharmacist before taking any other medications.

Diuretics The potassium loss caused by these drugs may increase amiodarone's toxic effects.

Other anti-arrhythmic drugs Amiodarone may increase the effects of drugs such as beta blockers, digoxin, diltiazem, or verapamil.

Warfarin Amiodarone may increase the anti-coagulant effect of warfarin.

SPECIAL PRECAUTIONS

Be sure to tell your doctor if:
◆ You have long-term liver or kidney problems.
◆ You have a lung disorder such as asthma or bronchitis.
◆ You have eye disease.
◆ You have a thyroid disorder.
◆ You are sensitive to iodine.
◆ You are taking other medications.

Pregnancy Not prescribed.

Breast-feeding The drug passes into the breast milk and may affect the baby. Discuss with your doctor.

Infants and children Not recommended.

Over 60 Increased likelihood of adverse effects. Reduced dose necessary.

Driving and hazardous work Avoid such activities until you have learned how amiodarone affects you because the drug can cause dazzling of the eyes by bright light.

Alcohol No known problems.

PROLONGED USE

Prolonged use of this drug may cause a number of adverse effects on the eyes, lungs, thyroid gland, and liver.

Monitoring A chest X-ray may be taken before with treatment with amiodarone starts. Blood tests are carried out before treatment starts and then every 6 months to check thyroid and liver function. Regular eye examinations are required.

Amisulpride/sulpiride

Brand names Solian [amisulpride], Dolmatil, Sulpitil [sulpiride]

Used in the following combined preparations None

QUICK REFERENCE

Drug group Antipsychotic drug (p.15)
Overdose danger rating Medium
Dependence rating Low
Prescription needed Yes
Available as generic No

GENERAL INFORMATION

Amisulpride and sulpiride are antipsychotic drugs that are used to treat acute and chronic schizophrenia. In this condition, a person may have "positive" symptoms such as delusions, hallucinations, and thought disorders, and/or "negative" symptoms such as emotional and social withdrawal. Patients with mainly positive symptoms are treated with higher doses; patients with mainly negative symptoms are treated with lower doses. Sulpiride has also been used to treat Tourette's syndrome (a rare inherited neurological disorder that causes people to make uncontrolled movements and noises), anxiety disorders, and vertigo.

An advantage of amisulpride, a so-called atypical antipsychotic drug, is that it is less likely than the older drugs to cause parkinsonism (tremor and rigidity) or tardive dyskinesia (involuntary movements of the tongue and face).

INFORMATION FOR USERS

Your drug prescription is tailored for you. Do not alter dosage without checking with your doctor.

How taken Tablets, liquid.

Frequency and timing of doses 1–2 x daily (doses of up to 300mg may be once daily).

Dosage range *Amisulpride* 50–300mg daily (mainly negative symptoms); 400–1,200mg daily (mainly positive symptoms). *Sulpiride* 400–800mg daily (mainly negative symptoms); 400–2,400mg daily (mainly positive symptoms).

Onset of effect 1 hour.

Duration of action 12–24 hours.

Diet advice None.

Storage Keep in a closed container in a cool, dry place out of reach of children.

Missed dose Take as soon as you remember. If your next dose is due within 2 hours, take a single dose now and skip the next dose.

Stopping the drug Unless palpitations or dizziness occur, do not stop taking the drug without consulting your doctor; symptoms may recur.

Exceeding the dose An occasional unintentional extra dose is unlikely to cause problems. Large overdoses, however, may produce drowsiness and low blood pressure. If a large overdose has been taken, notify your doctor immediately.

POSSIBLE ADVERSE EFFECTS

Most of the side effects of antipsychotic drugs such as amisulpride and sulpiride are mild. Insomnia is the most common problem, but agitation, drowsiness, nausea, breast swelling, weight gain, parkinsonism (tremor and rigidity), palpitations, and dizziness may also occur. If you develop palpitations, or if dizziness occurs, stop taking the drug and call your doctor immediately.

INTERACTIONS

Antihypertensive drugs Both amisulpride and sulpiride may reduce the blood-pressure-lowering effect of certain antihypertensive drugs.

Central nervous system depressants These drugs may all increase the sedative effects of amisulpride and sulpiride.

SPECIAL PRECAUTIONS

Be sure to tell your doctor if:
◆ You have liver or kidney problems.
◆ You have heart problems or hypertension.
◆ You have epilepsy.
◆ You have Parkinson's disease.
◆ You have phaeochromocytoma.
◆ You have a pituitary tumour or breast cancer.
◆ You have porphyria.
◆ You have had blood problems.
◆ You are taking other medications.

Pregnancy Safety in pregnancy not established. Discuss with your doctor.

Breast-feeding Safety in breast-feeding not established. Discuss with your doctor.

Infants and children Not recommended.

Over 60 Reduced dose may be necessary.

Driving and hazardous work Avoid these activities. Amisulpride and sulpiride can slow your reaction times, and they may also occasionally cause drowsiness or loss of concentration.

Alcohol Avoid. Alcohol increases the sedative effects of these drugs.

PROLONGED USE

Tardive dyskinesia may, rarely, occur during long-term use of these drugs.

Amitriptyline

Brand names None
Used in the following combined preparation
Triptafen

QUICK REFERENCE

Drug group Tricyclic antidepressant drug (p.14)
Overdose danger rating High
Dependence rating Low
Prescription needed Yes
Available as generic Yes

GENERAL INFORMATION

Amitriptyline belongs to a class of antidepressant drugs known as the tricyclics. Used mainly in the long-term treatment of depression, it elevates mood, increases physical activity, improves appetite, and restores interest in everyday activities.

More sedating than similar drugs, amitriptyline is useful when the depression is accompanied by anxiety or insomnia. Taken at night, amitriptyline encourages sleep and helps to eliminate the need to take additional sleeping drugs. It is sometimes used to treat nocturnal enuresis (bedwetting) in children.

In overdose, amitriptyline may cause coma, fits, and abnormal heart rhythms.

INFORMATION FOR USERS

Your drug prescription is tailored for you. Do not alter dosage without checking with your doctor.

How taken Tablets, SR-capsules, liquid, injection.

Frequency and timing of doses 1–4 x daily, usually as a single dose at night.

Adult dosage range 50–200mg daily.

Onset of effect Sedation can occur within hours; full antidepressant effect may not be felt for 2–4 weeks.

Duration of action Antidepressant effect may last for 6 weeks; common adverse effects may last for a few days.

Diet advice None.

Storage Keep in a closed container in a cool, dry place out of reach of children. Protect from light.

Missed dose Take as soon as you remember. If your next dose is due within 3 hours, take a single dose now and skip the next.

Stopping the drug Unless severe adverse effects occur (see below), do not stop taking the drug without consulting your doctor; he or she may supervise a gradual reduction in dosage. Stopping the drug abruptly can cause withdrawal symptoms and a recurrence of the original trouble.

OVERDOSE ACTION

Seek immediate medical advice in all cases. Take emergency action if palpitations are noted or consciousness is lost.

POSSIBLE ADVERSE EFFECTS

The possible adverse effects of amitriptyline are mainly due to its anticholinergic (see Autonomic nervous system, p.8) action and blocking action on the transmission of signals through the heart. Drowsiness, blurred vision, dry mouth, constipation, and sweating may occur. If you have difficulty in passing urine, a sore throat, or palpitations, stop taking the drug and call your doctor immediately.

INTERACTIONS

MAOIs When, rarely, these drugs are given with amitriptyline, serious interactions are possible.

Sedatives All drugs that have sedative effects intensify those of amitriptyline.

Anti-arrhythmic drugs There is an increased risk of abnormal heart rhythms when these drugs are taken with amitriptyline.

Anticonvulsant drugs The effects of these drugs are reduced by amitriptyline as it lowers the seizure threshold.

SPECIAL PRECAUTIONS

Be sure to tell your doctor if:
◆ You have heart problems.
◆ You have had epileptic fits.
◆ You have long-term liver or kidney problems.
◆ You have glaucoma.
◆ You have prostate trouble.
◆ You have had mania or a psychotic illness.
◆ You have thyroid disease.
◆ You are taking other medications.

Pregnancy Safety in pregnancy not established. Discuss with your doctor.

Breast-feeding The drug passes into the breast milk and may affect the baby. Discuss with your doctor.

Infants and children Not recommended under 16 years for depression, or under 6 years for enuresis.

Over 60 Reduced dose may be necessary.

Driving and hazardous work Avoid such activities until you have learned how amitriptyline affects you because the drug may cause blurred vision and reduced alertness.

Alcohol Avoid excessive amounts. Alcohol may increase the sedative effects of this drug.

Surgery and general anaesthetics Amitriptyline treatment may need to be stopped before you have a general anaesthetic. Discuss with your doctor or dentist before any operation.

PROLONGED USE

No problems expected.

Amlodipine

Brand name Istin
Used in the following combined preparations
None

QUICK REFERENCE

Drug group Anti-angina drug (p.35), antihypertensive drug (p.36)
Overdose danger rating Medium
Dependence rating Low
Prescription needed Yes
Available as generic No

GENERAL INFORMATION

Amlodipine belongs to the group of drugs known as the calcium channel blockers, which interfere with electrical signals in the muscles of the heart and blood vessels.

Amlodipine is used in the treatment of angina to help prevent attacks of chest pain. Unlike some other anti-angina drugs (such as beta blockers), it can be used safely by asthmatics and non-insulin-dependent diabetics. Amlodipine is also used to reduce raised blood pressure (hypertension).

In common with other drugs of its class, amlodipine may cause the blood pressure to fall too low at the start of treatment, and, in rare cases, angina may become worse at the start of treatment. Amlodipine may sometimes cause mild to moderate swelling of the legs and ankles.

INFORMATION FOR USERS

Your drug prescription is tailored for you. Do not alter dosage without checking with your doctor.

How taken Tablets.

Frequency and timing of doses Once daily.

Adult dosage range 5–10mg daily.

Onset of effect 6–12 hours.

Duration of action 24 hours.

Diet advice None.

Storage Keep in a closed container in a cool, dry place out of reach of children.

Missed dose If you miss a dose and you remember it within 12 hours, take it as soon as you remember. However, if you do not remember until later, do not take the missed dose and do not double up the next one. Instead, go back to your regular schedule.

Stopping the drug Unless serious adverse effects occur (see below), do not stop taking the drug without consulting your doctor. Stopping the drug may lead to worsening of the underlying condition.

Exceeding the dose An occasional unintentional extra dose is unlikely to cause problems. Large overdoses may markedly lower blood pressure; notify your doctor immediately.

POSSIBLE ADVERSE EFFECTS

Amlodipine can cause various minor adverse effects, including leg and ankle swelling, headache, flushing, fatigue, and nausea. Dizziness may occur, especially when you stand or get up, because the muscles in the walls of blood vessels in the legs may not contract sufficiently. If palpitations develop, discuss with your doctor. If shortness of breath develops, stop taking the drug and consult your doctor. Most serious is the rare possibility of angina worsening after treatment starts; report this to your doctor immediately. If a rash occurs, stop taking the drug and seek medical advice.

INTERACTIONS

Beta blockers Amlodipine may increase the effect of these drugs and vice versa.

SPECIAL PRECAUTIONS

Be sure to tell your doctor if:
◆ You have long-term liver or kidney problems.
◆ You have heart failure.

◆ You have diabetes.
◆ You are taking other medications.

Pregnancy Safety in pregnancy not established. Discuss with your doctor.

Breast-feeding It is not known if the drug passes into the breast milk. Discuss with your doctor.

Infants and children Not recommended.

Over 60 No special problems.

Driving and hazardous work Avoid such activities until you have learned how amlodipine affects you because the drug can cause dizziness owing to lowered blood pressure.

Alcohol Keep consumption low. Alcohol may further reduce blood pressure, causing dizziness or other symptoms.

PROLONGED USE

No problems expected.

Amoxicillin

Brand names Almodan, Amix, Amoram, Amoxil, Galenamox, Rimoxallin

Used in the following combined preparations Amiclav, Augmentin, Co-amoxiclav

QUICK REFERENCE

Drug group Penicillin antibiotic (p.62)

Overdose danger rating Low

Dependence rating Low

Prescription needed Yes

Available as generic Yes

GENERAL INFORMATION

Amoxicillin is prescribed for a variety of infections, especially of the ear, nose, throat, and respiratory tract; cystitis; uncomplicated gonorrhoea; and certain skin and soft tissue infections. It is absorbed well by the body when taken orally.

The drug can cause minor stomach upset and a rash. It can also provoke a more severe allergic reaction, with fever, swelling of the mouth and tongue, itching, and breathing difficulties, suggesting penicillin allergy.

INFORMATION FOR USERS

Your drug prescription is tailored for you. Do not alter dosage without checking with your doctor.

How taken Tablets, capsules, liquid, powder (dissolved in water), injection.
Frequency and timing of doses Usually 3 x daily.
Dosage range *Adults* 750mg–1.5g daily. In some cases, a short course of up to 6g daily is given. A single dose of 3g may be given as a preventative. *Children* Reduced dose according to age and weight.
Onset of effect 1–2 hours.
Duration of action Up to 8 hours.
Diet advice None.
Storage Keep in a closed container in a cool, dry place out of reach of children.
Missed dose Take as soon as you remember, then take your next scheduled dose.
Stopping the drug Unless an allergic reaction occurs, take the full course. Even if you feel better, the original infection may still be present and symptoms may recur.
Exceeding the dose An occasional unintentional extra dose is unlikely to be a cause for concern. But if you notice any unusual symptoms, or if a large overdose has been taken, notify your doctor.

POSSIBLE ADVERSE EFFECTS

Nausea and diarrhoea are common. If a rash or joint swelling occur, consult your doctor. Wheezing, shortness of breath, an itching rash, or a fever may indicate an allergic reaction. If any of these occur, stop taking the drug and call your doctor immediately.

INTERACTIONS

Oral contraceptives Amoxicillin may reduce the pill's effectiveness and increase the risk of breakthrough bleeding.
Anticoagulant drugs Amoxicillin may alter the anticoagulant effect of these drugs, so patients may have to be monitored more closely.

SPECIAL PRECAUTIONS

Be sure to tell your doctor if:
◆ You have a long-term kidney problem.
◆ You have an allergy (for example, hay fever, asthma, or eczema).
◆ You have had a previous allergic reaction to a penicillin or cephalosporin antibiotic.
◆ You have ulcerative colitis.
◆ You have glandular fever.
◆ You have chronic leukaemia.
◆ You are taking other medications.

Pregnancy No evidence of risk.
Breast-feeding The drug passes into the breast milk, but at normal doses adverse effects on the baby are unlikely; discuss with your doctor.
Infants and children Reduced dose necessary.
Over 60 No known problems.
Driving and hazardous work No known problems.
Alcohol No known problems.

PROLONGED USE

The drug is usually given only in short courses.

Amphotericin

Brand names Abelcet, AmBisome, Amphocil, Fungilin, Fungizone
Used in the following combined preparations
None

QUICK REFERENCE

Drug group Antifungal drug (p.76
Overdose danger rating Low (oral)
Dependence rating Low
Prescription needed Yes
Available as generic Yes

GENERAL INFORMATION

Amphotericin, a highly effective and powerful antifungal drug, is given by injection to treat serious systemic fungal infections and by mouth to treat candida (thrush) of the mouth or intestines; it is not used in vaginal thrush.

Injections are supervised, usually in hospital, due to potentially serious adverse effects. A test dose for allergy may be given before a full injection. The drug's new formulations seem to be less toxic than the original injection. Adverse reactions to oral forms are rare.

INFORMATION FOR USERS

Your drug prescription is tailored for you. Do not alter dosage without checking with your doctor.
How taken Tablets, lozenges, liquid, injection.
Frequency and timing of doses Every 6 hours (by mouth). Daily, usually over a 6-hour period (by injection).
Dosage range 400–800mg daily (tablets and liquid). 40–80mg daily (lozenges). Dosage for injection is determined individually.

Onset of effect Improvement may be noticed after 2–4 days.

Duration of action 3–6 hours.

Diet advice When given by injection, this drug may reduce the levels of potassium and magnesium in the blood. To correct this, mineral supplements may be recommended.

Storage Keep in a closed container in a cool, dry place out of reach of children. Some brands of injection should be stored in the fridge.

Missed dose Take oral dose as soon as you remember, then take your next scheduled dose.

Stopping the drug Take the full course. Even if symptoms improve, the original infection may still be present and symptoms may recur if treatment is stopped too soon.

Exceeding the dose An occasional unintentional extra oral dose is unlikely to be a cause for concern. But if you notice unusual symptoms, notify your doctor.

POSSIBLE ADVERSE EFFECTS

Adverse effects are rare with oral forms. Injections are given only under close medical supervision, so problems such as headache, nausea, indigestion, and abdominal or muscle pain can be monitored and treated promptly.

INTERACTIONS (injection only)

Digitalis drugs Amphotericin may increase the toxicity of digoxin.

Diuretics Amphotericin increases the risk of low potassium levels with diuretics.

Aminoglycoside antibiotics Taken with amphotericin, these drugs increase the risk of kidney damage.

Corticosteroids These may increase loss of potassium from the body due to amphotericin.

Ciclosporin increases the likelihood of kidney damage when taken with amphotericin.

SPECIAL PRECAUTIONS

Be sure to tell your doctor if:
◆ You have a long-term kidney problem.
◆ You have previously had an allergic reaction to amphotericin.
◆ You are taking other medications.

Pregnancy There is no evidence of risk from oral forms of the drug. Injections are given only when the infection is very serious.

Breast-feeding No evidence of risk from oral forms of the drug. It is not known whether the drug passes into the breast milk when given by injection. Discuss with your doctor.

Infants and children Reduced dose may be necessary.

Over 60 No special problems.

Driving and hazardous work No known problems.

Alcohol No known problems.

PROLONGED USE

Injections of the drug may reduce blood levels of potassium and magnesium, damage the kidneys, and cause blood disorders.

Monitoring Regular blood tests to monitor liver and kidney function, potassium and magnesium levels, and blood cell counts are advised during treatment with injections.

Anastrozole

Brand name Arimidex
Used in the following combined preparations
None

QUICK REFERENCE

Drug group Anticancer drug (p.96)
Overdose danger rating Low
Dependence rating Low
Prescription needed Yes
Available as generic No

GENERAL INFORMATION

Anastrozole is used to treat breast cancers, most of which are stimulated by oestrogen. It inhibits the enzymes that manufacture estradiol (a natural oestrogen) in the body, reducing production by more than 80 per cent. Anastrozole is used to treat postmenopausal women. It has not proved effective in cancers that are not oestrogen-sensitive. It is contra-indicated in pregnancy and breast-feeding. Biochemical tests must confirm that the woman being treated is postmenopausal.

Any adverse effects of anastrozole are mainly gastrointestinal or gynaecological and are similar to menopausal symptoms.

INFORMATION FOR USERS

Your drug prescription is tailored for you. Do not alter dosage without checking with your doctor.

How taken Tablets.
Frequency and timing of doses Once daily.
Adult dosage range 1mg.
Onset of effect 30 minutes.
Duration of action 24 hours.
Diet advice None.
Storage Keep in a closed container in a cool, dry place out of reach of children.
Missed dose Take as soon as you remember. If your next dose is due within 2 hours, take a single dose now and skip the next.
Stopping the drug Do not stop the drug without consulting your doctor. Stopping the drug may lead to worsening of the underlying condition.
Exceeding the dose An occasional unintentional extra dose is unlikely to be a cause for concern. But if you notice any unusual symptoms, or if a large overdose has been taken, notify your doctor.

POSSIBLE ADVERSE EFFECTS

Anastrozole is usually well tolerated and most side effects are relatively minor. Hot flushes, headache, fatigue, and dizziness are common. Joint pain or stiffness, vaginal dryness, rash or hair thinning, and nausea and constipation may occur, but are rare. Consult your doctor if the symptoms are severe.

INTERACTIONS

Tamoxifen and oestrogens These drugs oppose the effects of anastrozole.

SPECIAL PRECAUTIONS

Be sure to tell your doctor if:
◆ You are premenopausal.
◆ You have kidney or liver problems.
◆ You are allergic to anastrozole.
◆ You are taking other medications.
Pregnancy Not prescribed in pregnancy.
Breast-feeding Not prescribed for women who are breast-feeding.
Infants and children Not recommended.
Over 60 No special problems.
Driving and hazardous work Do not drive until you know how the drug affects you. It can cause drowsiness.
Alcohol No known problems.

PROLONGED USE

No known problems.

Monitoring Women with osteoporosis or at risk of osteoporosis will have their bone mineral density assessed at the start of treatment and at regular intervals.

Apomorphine

Brand names APO-go, Uprima
Used in the following combined preparations
None

QUICK REFERENCE

Drug group Drug for parkinsonism (p.18) and drug for impotence (p.110)
Overdose danger rating High
Dependence rating Low
Prescription needed Yes
Available as generic No

GENERAL INFORMATION

Apomorphine, a derivative of morphine, has a chemical structure similar to dopamine. It stimulates the vomiting centre in the brain but is used to control the "on-off" episodes of parkinsonism. A patient will be given 2–3 days of treatment with the antiemetic drug domperidone before stopping their existing antiparkinsonism drugs to provoke an "off" period. Increasing doses of apomorphine are given by injection to find the lowest effective dose. Then the regular drug treatment is restarted. At the first sign of an "off" period, an apomorphine injection is given. Dosing is adjusted according to response.

Apomorphine is also used in the treatment of erectile dysfunction. The drug acts on the hypothalamus, a region within the brain, to improve nerve signals to the penis.

INFORMATION FOR USERS

Your drug prescription is tailored for you. Do not alter dosage without checking with your doctor.
How taken Tablets, injection.
Frequency and timing of doses *Parkinsonism* 1–10 x daily, or continuous infusion. *Erectile dysfunction* 1–3 x daily, 20 minutes before sexual activity.
Adult dosage range *Parkinsonism* 3–30mg daily, up to a maximum of 100mg. *Erectile dysfunction* 2–9mg.

Onset of effect *Parkinsonism* A few minutes. *Erectile dysfunction* 20 minutes.
Duration of action 2 hours.
Diet advice None.
Storage Keep in closed original container in a cool, dry place, out of reach of children.
Missed dose *Parkinsonism* Take as soon as you need to. *Erectile dysfunction* Take the next time you need to, but no more than 3 times in 24 hours.

OVERDOSE ACTION

An unintentional extra dose may cause vomiting. If a large overdose has been taken, seek immediate medical advice. Take emergency action if breathing problems or loss of consciousness occur.

POSSIBLE ADVERSE EFFECTS

Injections have a strong emetic effect, so the anti-emetic drug domperidone must be taken at the same time. Doses for impotence are usually lower and tend not to cause this problem. Nausea, vomiting, headache, dizziness, drowsiness and fatigue, rhinitis, sore throat, cough, sweating, hot flushes, and taste disturbance are common; if they are severe or, rarely, if fainting occurs, consult your doctor.

INTERACTIONS

Nitrates Taken with apomorphine, these drugs can cause a fall in blood pressure.

SPECIAL PRECAUTIONS

Be sure to tell your doctor if:
◆ You have an abnormality of the penis (if being treated for erectile dysfunction).
◆ You have kidney or liver problems.
◆ You have recently had heart problems.
◆ You have high or low blood pressure.
◆ You are taking other medications.
Pregnancy Safety not established. Discuss with your doctor.
Breast-feeding Safety not established. Discuss with your doctor.
Infants and children Not recommended.
Over 60 No special problems.
Driving and hazardous work Avoid until you know how the drug affects you. It can cause dizziness, lightheadedness, drowsiness, and fainting. If you have parkinsonism, driving is not allowed.

Alcohol Avoid. Alcohol can diminish sexual performance.

PROLONGED USE

No known problems.

Aspirin

Brand names Angettes, Aspro, Caprin, Disprin, Nu-Seals Aspirin, and others
Used in the following combined preparations
Anadin, Aspav, Codis, Veganin, and others

QUICK REFERENCE

Drug group Non-opioid analgesic (p.10), antiplatelet drug (p.39), and antipyretic
Overdose danger rating High
Dependence rating Low
Prescription needed No
Available as generic Yes

GENERAL INFORMATION

Aspirin relieves pain, reduces fever, and alleviates symptoms of arthritis. In low doses, it helps to prevent blood clots, particularly in atherosclerosis or angina due to coronary artery disease. It also reduces the risk of heart attacks and strokes in people with known medical problems. It is present in many medicines for colds, flu, headache, menstrual pain, and joint or muscular aches.

Aspirin may irritate the stomach and may even cause stomach ulcers or bleeding. In children, it can cause Reye's syndrome, a rare but serious brain and liver disorder. For this reason, aspirin should not be given to children under the age of 16 years, except on the advice of a doctor. Another drawback of aspirin is that it can provoke asthma attacks.

INFORMATION FOR USERS

Follow instructions on the label. Call your doctor if symptoms worsen.
How taken Tablets, SR-capsules, suppositories.
Frequency and timing of doses Every 4–6 hours, as needed, with or after food or milk (relief of pain or fever); once daily (prevention of blood clots).
Adult dosage range *Relief of pain or fever* 300–900mg per dose. *Prevention of blood clots* 75–300mg daily.

Onset of effect 30–60 minutes (tablets); 1½–8 hours (coated tablets/SR-capsules).

Duration of action
Up to 12 hours (relief of pain or fever); several days (prevention of blood clots).

Diet advice Take with or straight after food.

Storage Keep in a closed container in a cool, dry place out of reach of children.

Missed dose Take as soon as you remember. If your next dose is due within 2 hours, take a single dose now and skip the next.

Stopping the drug Taken in the short term, aspirin can be safely stopped as soon as you no longer need it. Seek medical advice before stopping long-term treatment unless severe adverse effects occur (see below).

OVERDOSE ACTION

Seek immediate medical advice. Take emergency action if restlessness, stomach pain, vomiting, or ringing in the ears occur.

POSSIBLE ADVERSE EFFECTS

Adverse effects are more likely with high doses but may be reduced by taking the drug with food or in buffered or enteric-coated forms. If indigestion, rash, or wheezing occur, stop taking aspirin. If you vomit blood, have black bowel movements, or experience ringing noises in the ears, stop taking the drug and contact your doctor urgently.

INTERACTIONS

Anticoagulants Aspirin may add to the anticoagulant effect of such drugs, leading to an increased risk of abnormal bleeding.

Drugs for gout Aspirin may reduce the effect of these drugs.

Corticosteroids These drugs may increase the risk of stomach bleeding with aspirin.

NSAIDs These drugs may increase the likelihood of stomach irritation with aspirin.

Methotrexate Aspirin may increase the toxicity of this drug.

Oral antidiabetic drugs Aspirin may increase the effect of these drugs.

SPECIAL PRECAUTIONS

Be sure to consult your doctor or pharmacist before taking this drug if:
◆ You have long-term liver or kidney problems.
◆ You have asthma.
◆ You are allergic to aspirin.
◆ You have a blood clotting disorder.
◆ You have had a stomach ulcer.
◆ You are taking other medications.

Pregnancy Not usually recommended. An alternative drug may be safer. Discuss with your doctor.

Breast-feeding The drug passes into the breast milk. Discuss with your doctor.

Infants and children Do not give to children under 16 years, except on a doctor's advice.

Over 60 Adverse effects more likely.

Driving and hazardous work No special problems.

Alcohol Keep consumption low. Alcohol increases the likelihood of stomach irritation with this drug.

Surgery and general anaesthetics Regular treatment with aspirin may need to be stopped about one week before you have surgery. Discuss with your doctor or dentist before any operation.

PROLONGED USE

Except for low doses to help prevent blood clotting, aspirin should not be taken for longer than 2 days except on your doctor's advice. Prolonged use of aspirin may worsen asthma; it may also lead to bleeding in, and ulcers of, the stomach.

Atenolol

Brand names Antipressan, Atenix, Tenormin
Used in the following combined preparations
Beta-Adalat, Co-tenidone, Kalten, Tenchlor, Tenif, Tenoret, Tenoretic, Totaretic

QUICK REFERENCE
Drug group Beta blocker (p.30)
Overdose danger rating Medium
Dependence rating Low
Prescription needed Yes
Available as generic Yes

GENERAL INFORMATION

Atenolol belongs to the group of drugs known as the beta blockers. It prevents the heart from beating too quickly and is used primarily to treat irregular heart rhythms (arrhythmias), angina, and hypertension (high blood pressure). Atenolol may also be given after a heart attack to protect the heart from suffering further damage.

Atenolol is a cardioselective beta blocker and is less likely than other beta blockers to provoke breathing difficulties. However, it should still be used with caution by people suffering from asthma, bronchitis, or other forms of respiratory disease. The drug is sometimes prescribed together with a diuretic for high blood pressure.

Atenolol does not cure heart disease but only controls the symptoms. Therefore, the drug usually has to be taken on a long-term basis.

INFORMATION FOR USERS

Your drug prescription is tailored for you. Do not alter dosage without checking with your doctor.

How taken Tablets, liquid, injection.

Frequency and timing of doses 1–2 x daily.

Adult dosage range 25–100mg daily.

Onset of effect 2–4 hours.

Duration of action 20–30 hours.

Diet advice None.

Storage Keep in a tightly closed container in a cool, dry place out of reach of children. Protect from light.

Missed dose Take as soon as you remember. If your next dose of atenolol is due within 6 hours, do not take the missed dose but take the next scheduled dose as usual.

Stopping the drug Unless you experience wheezing or difficulty in breathing, do not stop taking atenolol without consulting your doctor. Sudden withdrawal of atenolol may lead to dangerous worsening of the underlying condition; the drug should be withdrawn gradually.

Exceeding the dose An occasional unintentional extra dose is unlikely to be a cause for concern. But if you notice any unusual symptoms, or if a large overdose has been taken, notify your doctor.

POSSIBLE ADVERSE EFFECTS

Atenolol has adverse effects that are common to most beta blockers. These include aching muscles, dry eyes, and cold hands and feet. You may also suffer from dizziness or headache. Symptoms tend to diminish with long-term use. However, if the symptoms are severe, seek medical advice. If you develop a rash, wheezing or difficulty in breathing, stop taking the drug and consult your doctor without delay.

INTERACTIONS

Anti-arrhythmic drugs Used together with atenolol, these drugs may increase the risk of adverse effects on the heart.

Antidiabetic drugs Used with atenolol, these may increase the risk, and/or mask many symptoms, of low blood sugar.

Decongestants Used with atenolol, these may increase blood pressure and heart rate.

Calcium channel blockers Taken with atenolol, some of these drugs may further decrease the blood pressure and/or heart rate and may also reduce the force of the heart's pumping action.

NSAIDs These drugs may reduce the antihypertensive effect of atenolol.

SPECIAL PRECAUTIONS

Be sure to tell your doctor if:

◆ You have any other heart condition.

◆ You have a long-term kidney problem.

◆ You have diabetes.

◆ You have a lung disorder such as asthma or bronchitis.

◆ You are taking other medications.

Pregnancy Safety in pregnancy not established. Discuss with your doctor.

Breast-feeding The drug passes into the breast milk. Discuss with your doctor.

Infants and children Not recommended.

Over 60 No special problems. Reduced dose may be necessary if there is impaired kidney function.

Driving and hazardous work Avoid such activities until you have learned how atenolol affects you because the drug can cause dizziness.

Alcohol No special problems with small intake.

Surgery and general anaesthetics Atenolol may need to be stopped before you have a general anaesthetic. Discuss this with your doctor or dentist before any surgery.

PROLONGED USE

No special problems expected.

Atorvastatin

Brand name Lipitor
Used in the following combined preparations
None

QUICK REFERENCE
Drug group Lipid-lowering drug (p.37)
Overdose danger rating Low
Dependence rating Low
Prescription needed Yes
Available as generic No

GENERAL INFORMATION

Atorvastatin is a member of the statin group of lipid-lowering drugs. It is used to treat hypercholesterolaemia (high blood cholesterol levels) in patients who have not responded to other treatments, such as a special diet, and are at risk of developing heart disease.

Atorvastatin acts in the liver by blocking the action of an enzyme needed for the manufacture of cholesterol. As a result, blood levels of cholesterol are lowered, which can help to prevent coronary heart disease.

Rarely, atorvastatin can cause pain, inflammation, and damage in the muscles. The risk is increased if the drug is given with a fibrate (another kind of lipid-lowering drug).

INFORMATION FOR USERS

Your drug prescription is tailored for you. Do not alter dosage without checking with your doctor.
How taken Tablets.
Frequency and timing of doses Once daily.
Adult dosage range 10–40mg; up to 80mg (inherited hypercholesterolaemia).
Onset of effect Within 2 weeks. Full beneficial effects may not be seen for 4–6 weeks.
Duration of action 20–30 hours.
Diet advice A low-fat diet is usually recommended.
Storage Keep in a closed container in a cool, dry place out of reach of children.
Missed dose Take as soon as you remember. If your next dose is due within 8 hours, do not take the missed dose, but take the next one on schedule.
Stopping the drug Do not stop the drug without consulting your doctor. Stopping may cause the original condition to recur.

Exceeding the dose An occasional unintentional extra dose is unlikely to cause problems. Large overdoses, however, may cause liver problems; notify your doctor.

POSSIBLE ADVERSE EFFECTS

Adverse effects of atorvastatin, which include nausea, headache, and insomnia, are usually mild and transient. Muscle damage is a rare side effect. Any muscle aching or weakness, or a rash, should be reported to your doctor at once.

INTERACTIONS

Anticoagulant drugs Atorvastatin may increase the effect of anticoagulants.
Antifungal drugs Itraconazole, ketoconazole, and possibly other antifungals may increase the risk of muscle damage with atorvastatin.
Other lipid-lowering drugs Taken with atorvastatin, these drugs may increase the risk of muscle damage.
Ciclosporin and other immunosuppressant drugs Atorvastatin is not usually prescribed with these drugs because of the increased risk of muscle damage. However, if using the drugs together is unavoidable, close monitoring is advised.

SPECIAL PRECAUTIONS

Be sure to tell your doctor if:
◆ You have had liver problems.
◆ You are a heavy drinker.
◆ You are taking other medications.
Pregnancy Not usually prescribed. Safety not established. Discuss with your doctor.
Breast-feeding Safety not established. Discuss with your doctor.
Infants and children Not recommended.
Over 60 No special problems.
Driving and hazardous work No special problems.
Alcohol Avoid excessive amounts. Taken with alcohol, atorvastatin may increase the risk of liver problems developing.

PROLONGED USE

Long-term use of atorvastatin can affect liver function.
Monitoring Regular blood tests to check liver function are needed. Tests of muscle function may be carried out.

Atropine

Brand name Minims Atropine
Used in the following combined preparations
Actonorm, Co-phenotrope, Diarphen, Isopto Atropine, Lomotil, Tropergen

QUICK REFERENCE

Drug group Anticholinergic drug for irritable bowel syndrome (p.45) and mydriatic drug (p.116)
Overdose danger rating High
Dependence rating Low
Prescription needed Yes (except powder)
Available as generic Yes

GENERAL INFORMATION

Atropine is an anticholinergic drug. Because of its antispasmodic action, which relaxes the muscle wall of the intestine, the drug has been used to relieve abdominal cramps in irritable bowel syndrome. Atropine may also be prescribed in combination with diphenoxylate, an antidiarrhoeal drug, to relieve muscle spasm. This combination can be dangerous in overdosage, however, particularly in young children.

Atropine eye drops, used to enlarge the pupil during eye examinations, are part of the treatment for uveitis.

In addition, atropine may be used as part of the premedication before a general anaesthetic. It is occasionally injected to restore normal heart beat in heart block (see p34).

The drug must be used with caution in children and elderly people because these groups of people are particularly sensitive to the effects of atropine.

INFORMATION FOR USERS

Your drug prescription is tailored for you. Do not alter dosage without checking with your doctor.
How taken Tablets, injection, eye ointment, eye drops.
Frequency and timing of doses Once only, or up to 4 times daily, according to condition (eye drops); as directed (other forms).
Adult dosage range 1–2 drops as directed (eye drops); as directed (other forms).
Onset of effect Varies according to method of administration (tablets, injection, eye ointment); 30 minutes (eye drops).

Duration of action 7 days or longer (eye drops); several hours (other forms).
Diet advice None.
Storage Keep in a closed container in a cool, dry place out of reach of children. Protect from light.
Missed dose Take as soon as you remember. If your next dose is due within 2 hours, take a single dose now and skip the next.
Stopping the drug Do not stop taking the drug without consulting your doctor.

OVERDOSE ACTION

Seek immediate medical advice in all cases. Take emergency action if palpitations, tremor, delirium, fits, or loss of consciousness occur.

POSSIBLE ADVERSE EFFECTS

The use of this drug is limited by the frequency of its anticholinergic (see Autonomic nervous system, p8) effects. These commonly include blurred vision, dry mouth, and constipation. Difficulty in passing urine, palpitations, confusion, nausea and vomiting, and dizziness may also occur and should be reported to your doctor without delay. If the eye drops cause stinging, pain, and irritation, or if a rash occurs on contact, stop using them and call your doctor immediately.

INTERACTIONS

Anticholinergic drugs Atropine increases the risk of side effects from drugs that also have anticholinergic effects.
Ketoconazole Atropine reduces the absorption of ketoconazole from the digestive tract. An increased dose may be necessary.

SPECIAL PRECAUTIONS

Be sure to tell your doctor if:
◆ You have long-term liver or kidney problems.
◆ You have prostate problems.
◆ You have gastro-oesophageal reflux.
◆ You have glaucoma.
◆ You have urinary difficulties.
◆ You have ulcerative colitis.
◆ You wear contact lenses (eye drops).
◆ You have heart problems or high blood pressure.
◆ You are taking other medications.
Pregnancy Safety in pregnancy not established. Discuss with your doctor.

Breast-feeding The drug passes into the breast milk and may affect the baby. Discuss with your doctor.

Infants and children Combination with diphenoxylate not recommended under 4 years; reduced dose necessary in older children.

Over 60 Increased likelihood of adverse effects.

Driving and hazardous work Avoid such activities until you have learned how atropine affects you because the drug can cause blurred vision and may impair concentration.

Alcohol No special problems.

PROLONGED USE

No problems expected.

Azathioprine

Brand names Azamune, Immunoprin, Imuran, Oprisine
Used in the following combined preparations None

QUICK REFERENCE

Drug group Antirheumatic drug (p.52) and immunosuppressant drug (p.99)
Overdose danger rating Medium
Dependence rating Low
Prescription needed Yes
Available as generic Yes

GENERAL INFORMATION

Azathioprine is an immunosuppressant drug that is used to prevent the rejection of transplanted organs by the immune system. The drug is also given for severe rheumatoid arthritis that has failed to respond to conventional drug therapy.

Autoimmune diseases and collagen diseases (including polymyositis, systemic lupus erythematosus, myasthenia gravis, and dermatomyositis) may be treated with azathioprine, usually when corticosteroids have not been effective.

Azathioprine is administered only under close medical supervision because of the risk of serious adverse effects. These effects include suppression of the production of white blood cells, thereby increasing the risk of infection, as well as the risk of excessive or prolonged bleeding.

INFORMATION FOR USERS

Your drug prescription is tailored for you. Do not alter dosage without checking with your doctor.

How taken Tablets, injection.

Frequency and timing of doses Usually once daily with or after food.

Dosage range Initially according to bodyweight and the condition being treated and then adjusted according to response.

Onset of effect 2–4 weeks. Antirheumatic effect may not be felt for 8 weeks or more.

Duration of action The immunosuppressant effects may last for several weeks after the drug is stopped.

Diet advice None.

Storage Keep in a closed container in a cool, dry place out of reach of children. Protect from light.

Missed dose Take as soon as you remember, then return to your normal schedule. If more than 2 doses are missed, consult your doctor.

Stopping the drug Do not stop taking the drug without consulting your doctor. If azathioprine is taken to prevent graft transplant rejection, stopping treatment could provoke the rejection of the transplant.

Exceeding the dose An occasional unintentional extra dose is unlikely to cause problems. Large overdoses, however, may cause nausea, vomiting, abdominal pains, and diarrhoea; seek urgent medical advice.

POSSIBLE ADVERSE EFFECTS

The most common effects of azathioprine are nausea, loss of appetite, thinning hair, weakness, and fatigue. The drug may also have adverse effects on the blood that could lead to sore throat and fever. Unusual bleeding or bruising may be a sign of reduced levels of platelets in the blood. In either case, call your doctor urgently.

INTERACTIONS

Allopurinol Allopurinol increases the effects and toxicity of azathioprine; dosage of one or both drugs will need to be reduced.

Warfarin Azathioprine may reduce the effect of warfarin.

Co-trimoxazole and trimethoprim These drugs may increase the risk of blood problems if taken with azathioprine.

Corticosteroids These drugs may increase the risk of infections and bowel problems.

SPECIAL PRECAUTIONS

Be sure to tell your doctor if:
♦ You have long-term liver or kidney problems.
♦ You have had a previous allergic reaction to azathioprine or 6-mercaptopurine.
♦ You have recently had shingles or chickenpox.
♦ You have an infection.
♦ You have a blood disorder.
♦ You are taking other medications.

Pregnancy Azathioprine has been taken in pregnancy without problems. Discuss with your doctor.

Breast-feeding A small amount of the drug passes into the breast milk. Discuss with your doctor.

Infants and children No special problems.

Over 60 Increased likelihood of adverse effects. Reduced dose necessary.

Driving and hazardous work Avoid such activities until you have learned how azathioprine affects you because the drug can cause weakness and fatigue.

Alcohol No special problems.

PROLONGED USE

There may be a slightly increased risk of some cancers with long-term use of azathioprine. Blood changes may also occur. Avoidance of exposure to sunlight may help to prevent adverse skin effects.

Monitoring Regular checks on blood composition are usually carried out.

Baclofen

Brand names Baclospas, Balgifen, Lioresal
Used in the following combined preparations
None

QUICK REFERENCE

Drug group Muscle-relaxant drug (p.54)
Overdose danger rating Medium
Dependence rating Low
Prescription needed Yes
Available as generic Yes

GENERAL INFORMATION

Baclofen is a muscle-relaxant drug that acts on the central nervous system, including the spinal cord. The drug relieves the spasms, cramping, and rigidity of muscles caused by a variety of disorders, including multiple sclerosis and spinal cord injury. Baclofen is also used to treat the spasticity that results from brain injury, cerebral palsy, or stroke. Although the drug does not cure any of these disorders, it increases mobility, allowing other treatment, such as physiotherapy, to be carried out.

Baclofen is less likely to cause muscle weakness than similar drugs, and its side effects, such as dizziness or drowsiness, are usually temporary. Elderly people are more susceptible to side effects, however, especially during the early stages of treatment.

INFORMATION FOR USERS

Your drug prescription is tailored for you. Do not alter dosage without checking with your doctor.
How taken Tablets, liquid, injection (specialist use).
Frequency and timing of doses 3 x daily with food or milk.
Adult dosage range 15mg daily (starting dose). Daily dose may be increased by 15mg every 3 days as necessary. Maximum daily dose: 100mg.
Onset of effect Some benefits may appear after 1–3 hours, but full beneficial effects may not be felt for several weeks. A dose 1 hour before a specific task will improve mobility.
Duration of action Up to 8 hours.
Diet advice None.

Storage Keep in a closed container in a cool, dry place out of reach of children. Protect liquid from light.
Missed dose Take as soon as you remember. If your next dose is due within 2 hours, take a single dose now and skip the next.
Stopping the drug Do not stop taking the drug without consulting your doctor, who will supervise a gradual reduction in dosage. Abrupt cessation of the drug may cause hallucinations, fits, and worsening spasticity.
Exceeding the dose An occasional unintentional extra dose is unlikely to cause problems. Large overdoses, however, may cause weakness, vomiting, and severe drowsiness; notify your doctor.

POSSIBLE ADVERSE EFFECTS

Common adverse effects, such as dizziness or drowsiness, are related to the drug's sedative effects. Such effects are minimized by starting with a low dose, which is gradually increased. Nausea, muscle weakness and difficulty in passing urine may also occur. If the symptoms are severe, consult your doctor. Rare adverse effects include constipation, diarrhoea, and confusion.

INTERACTIONS

Antihypertensive and diuretic drugs Baclofen may increase the blood-pressure-lowering effect of such drugs.
Drugs for parkinsonism Some drugs used for parkinsonism may cause confusion and hallucinations if taken with baclofen.
Sedatives All drugs with a sedative effect on the central nervous system may increase the sedative properties of baclofen.
Tricyclic antidepressants may increase the effects of baclofen, leading to muscle weakness.

SPECIAL PRECAUTIONS

Be sure to tell your doctor if:
◆ You have long-term liver or kidney problems.
◆ You have difficulty in passing urine.
◆ You have had a peptic ulcer.
◆ You have had epileptic fits.
◆ You have diabetes.
◆ You suffer with breathing problems.
◆ You are taking other medications.
Pregnancy Safety in pregnancy not established. Discuss with your doctor.

Breast-feeding The drug passes into the breast milk, but at normal doses adverse effects are unlikely. Discuss with your doctor.

Infants and children Reduced dose necessary.

Over 60 Increased likelihood of adverse effects. Reduced dose may therefore be necessary.

Driving and hazardous work Avoid such activities until you have learned how baclofen affects you because the drug can cause confusion and drowsiness.

Alcohol Avoid excessive amounts. Alcohol may increase the sedative effects of this drug.

Surgery and general anaesthetics Be sure to inform your doctor or dentist that you are taking baclofen before you have a general anaesthetic.

PROLONGED USE

No problems expected.

Beclometasone

Brand names AeroBec, Asmabec, Beclazone, Becloforte, Beconase, Becotide, Filair, Nasobec, Propaderm, Qvar, and others

Used in the following combined preparation
Ventide

QUICK REFERENCE

Drug group Corticosteroid (p.80) and Topical corticosteroid (p.120)

Overdose danger rating Low

Dependence rating Low

Prescription needed No (some preparations)

Available as generic Yes

GENERAL INFORMATION

Beclometasone is a corticosteroid drug prescribed to relieve the symptoms of allergic rhinitis (as nasal spray) and to control asthma (as an inhalant). It controls nasal symptoms by reducing inflammation and mucus production in the nose. It also helps to reduce chest symptoms, such as wheezing and coughing. The drug may be taken regularly to reduce the severity and frequency of asthma attacks. Once an attack has started, however, the drug does not relieve symptoms.

Beclometasone is given primarily to treat asthma that has not responded to bronchodilators (see p.23) alone. It is also the main ingredient in some skin creams and ointments

for inflammatory conditions, particularly eczema. Being potent, it is not usually used on the face.

There are few serious adverse effects with beclometasone given topically by nasal spray or inhaler. Fungal infections causing mouth and throat irritation are a possible side effect of inhaling the drug. These can be avoided to some degree by the use of a spacer device (see p.25) and by rinsing the mouth and gargling with water after each inhalation.

INFORMATION FOR USERS

Your drug prescription is tailored for you. Do not alter dosage without checking with your doctor.

How taken Cream, ointment, inhaler, nasal spray.

Frequency and timing of doses 2–4 x daily.

Dosage range *Adults* 1–2 puffs 2–4 x daily according to preparation used (asthma); 1–2 sprays in each nostril 2–4 x daily (allergic rhinitis); as directed but usually 1–2 x daily (skin conditions). *Children* Reduced dose according to age and weight.

Onset of effect Within 1 week (asthma); 1–3 days (allergic rhinitis). Full benefit may not be felt for up to 4 weeks.

Duration of action Several days after stopping the drug.

Diet advice None.

Storage Keep in a closed container in a cool, dry place out of reach of children. Protect from light.

Missed dose Take as soon as you remember. If your next dose is due within 2 hours, take a single dose now and skip the next.

Stopping the drug Do not stop taking the drug without consulting your doctor; symptoms may recur. Sometimes a gradual reduction in dosage is recommended.

Exceeding the dose An occasional unintentional extra dose is unlikely to be a cause for concern. However, if you notice any unusual symptoms, or if a large overdose has been taken, notify your doctor. Adverse effects may occur if the recommended dose is regularly exceeded over a prolonged period.

POSSIBLE ADVERSE EFFECTS

The main side effects of the nasal spray and inhaler are irritation of the nasal passages and fungal infection of the throat and mouth, which may lead to sore throat or hoarseness. More serious side effects, such as permanent skin changes, may be seen with the ointment. Beclometasone ointment should not normally be used on the face.

INTERACTIONS
None.

SPECIAL PRECAUTIONS
Be sure to tell your doctor if:
◆ You have had tuberculosis or another nasal or respiratory infection.
◆ You have a skin infection (cream/ointment).
◆ You have varicose ulcers (cream/ointment).
◆ You are taking other medications.
Pregnancy No evidence of risk.
Breast-feeding No evidence of risk.
Infants and children Reduced dose necessary. Avoid prolonged use of ointment in infants and children.
Over 60 No known problems.
Driving and hazardous work No known problems.
Alcohol No known problems.

PROLONGED USE
No problems expected when the drug is used for asthma or rhinitis, but high doses of nasal spray can give systemic effects. Prolonged use of cream or ointment should be avoided if possible because it can cause permanent skin changes, and high doses can suppress the body's own corticosteroid production.
Monitoring Periodic checks to ensure healthy adrenal gland function may be required if large doses of beclometasone are being used.

Bendroflumethiazide

Brand names Aprinox, Neo-NaClex
Used in the following combined preparations
Corgaretic, Inderetic, Inderex, Neo-NaClex-K, Prestim

QUICK REFERENCE
Drug group Thiazide diuretic (p.32)
Overdose danger rating Low
Dependence rating Low
Prescription needed Yes
Available as generic Yes

GENERAL INFORMATION
Bendroflumethiazide (formerly known as bendrofluazide) belongs to the group of drugs known as the thiazide diuretics, which remove excess water from the body. It is frequently used as a treatment for high blood pressure (see Antihypertensive drugs, p.36). Bendroflumethiazide is also used in higher doses to reduce oedema (water retention) caused by heart conditions, and for treating premenstrual oedema.

As with all thiazides, the drug increases the loss of potassium in the urine, which can cause a variety of symptoms (see Possible adverse effects, below), and increases the likelihood of irregular heart rhythms, particularly in people taking drugs such as digoxin for heart failure. This effect is rare with low doses, but potassium supplements may be given with bendroflumethiazide as a precaution.

INFORMATION FOR USERS
Your drug prescription is tailored for you. Do not alter dosage without checking with your doctor.
How taken Tablets.
Frequency and timing of doses Once daily, early in the day. (Sometimes 1–3 x per week.)
Adult dosage range 2.5–10mg daily.
Onset of effect Within 2 hours.
Duration of action 6–12 hours.
Diet advice This drug may reduce potassium in the body, so you should eat plenty of fresh fruit and vegetables. Discuss with your doctor the advisability of reducing salt intake as a further precaution for hypertension.
Storage Keep in a closed container in a cool, dry place out of reach of children.
Missed dose No cause for concern, but take as soon as you remember. However, if it is late in the day, do not take the missed dose or you may need to get up during the night to pass urine. Take the next scheduled dose as usual.
Stopping the drug Do not stop taking the drug without consulting your doctor; symptoms may recur.
Exceeding the dose An occasional unintentional extra dose is unlikely to be a cause for concern. But if you notice any unusual symptoms, or if a large overdose has been taken, notify your doctor.

POSSIBLE ADVERSE EFFECTS

Some adverse effects, such as dizziness, which is common, and nausea, fatigue, and leg cramps, are the result of excessive loss of potassium but can usually be corrected by taking a potassium supplement. Impotence is a recognized adverse effect. Bendroflumethiazide may precipitate gout in susceptible people, and certain forms of diabetes may become more difficult to control. The blood cholesterol level may rise slightly.

INTERACTIONS

NSAIDs Non-steroidal anti-inflammatory drugs may reduce the diuretic effect of bendroflumethiazide. They also reduce the drug's effect in lowering blood pressure. Conversely, bendroflumethiazide may increase the toxic effects of NSAIDs on the kidneys.

Digoxin The effects of digoxin may be increased if excessive potassium is lost.

Anti-arrhythmic drugs Low potassium levels may increase the toxicity of these drugs.

Lithium Bendroflumethiazide may increase lithium levels in the blood.

Corticosteroids These drugs further increase the loss of potassium from the body when taken with bendroflumethiazide. Potassium supplements may be necessary.

SPECIAL PRECAUTIONS

Be sure to tell your doctor if:
◆ You have long-term liver or kidney problems.
◆ You have had gout.
◆ You have diabetes.
◆ You have Addison's disease.
◆ You have systemic lupus erythematosus (SLE).
◆ You are taking other medications.

Pregnancy Not usually prescribed. Safety in pregnancy not established. The drug may affect the baby adversely. Discuss with your doctor.

Breast-feeding The drug passes into the breast milk and may reduce your milk supply. However, the amount absorbed is usually too small to be harmful. Discuss with your doctor.

Infants and children Not usually prescribed. Reduced dose necessary.

Over 60 Reduced dose may be necessary.

Driving and hazardous work No special problems.

Alcohol No problems expected if consumption is kept low.

PROLONGED USE

Prolonged use of this drug can lead to excessive loss of potassium and imbalances of other salts.

Monitoring Blood tests may be performed periodically to check kidney function and levels of potassium and other salts.

Benzoyl peroxide

Brand names Acnecide, Brevoxyl, Panoxyl
Used in the following combined preparations
Benzamycin, Quinoderm

QUICK REFERENCE

Drug group Drug for acne (p.123) and fungal skin infections (p.76)
Overdose danger rating Low
Dependence rating Low
Prescription needed Yes (some preparations)
Available as generic No

GENERAL INFORMATION

Benzoyl peroxide is used in a variety of topical preparations for the treatment of acne and some fungal skin infections, particularly of the feet. Available over the counter, it comes in concentrations of varying strengths for moderate acne.

Benzoyl peroxide works by removing the top layer of skin and unblocking the sebaceous glands. The drug reduces inflammation of blocked hair follicles by killing bacteria that infect them.

Benzoyl peroxide may cause irritation due to its drying effect on the skin, but this generally diminishes with time. The drug should be applied to the affected areas as directed on the label. Washing the area prior to application greatly enhances the drug's beneficial effects. Side effects are less likely if treatment is started with a preparation containing a low concentration of benzoyl peroxide, and changed to a stronger preparation only if necessary. Marked dryness and peeling of the skin may occur but can usually be controlled by reducing the frequency of application. Care should be taken to avoid contact of the drug with the eyes, mouth, and mucous membranes. It is also advisable to avoid excessive exposure to sunlight. Preparations of benzoyl peroxide may bleach clothing.

INFORMATION FOR USERS

Follow instructions on the label. Call your doctor if symptoms worsen.

How taken Cream, lotion, gel.

Frequency and timing of doses 1–2 x daily.

Dosage range Apply sparingly to affected skin, as instructed on the label.

Onset of effect Reduces oiliness of the skin immediately. Acne usually improves within 4–6 weeks.

Duration of action 24–48 hours.

Diet advice None.

Storage Keep in a closed container in a cool, dry place out of reach of children.

Missed dose Apply as soon as you remember.

Stopping the drug Can safely be stopped as soon as you no longer need it.

Exceeding the dose A single extra application is unlikely to cause problems. Regular overuse, however, may result in extensive irritation, peeling, redness, and swelling.

POSSIBLE ADVERSE EFFECTS

Application of benzoyl peroxide may cause temporary burning or stinging of the skin. Redness, peeling, and swelling may result from excessive drying of the skin and usually clears up if the treatment is stopped or used less frequently. If severe burning, blistering, or crusting occur, stop using benzoyl peroxide and consult your doctor.

INTERACTIONS

Skin-drying preparations Medicated cosmetics, soaps, toiletries, and other anti-acne preparations increase the likelihood of dry, irritated skin if used with benzoyl peroxide.

SPECIAL PRECAUTIONS

Be sure to consult your doctor or pharmacist before using this drug if:
◆ You have eczema.
◆ You have sunburn.
◆ You have had a previous allergic reaction to benzoyl peroxide.

◆ You are taking other medications.

Pregnancy No evidence of risk.

Breast-feeding No evidence of risk.

Infants and children Not usually recommended under 12 years except under medical supervision.

Over 60 Not usually required.

Driving and hazardous work No known problems.

Alcohol No known problems.

PROLONGED USE

Benzoyl peroxide usually takes 4–6 weeks to produce an effect. Continuation of treatment beyond this time should be on the advice of your doctor.

Betahistine

Brand name Serc
Used in the following combined preparations
None

QUICK REFERENCE

Drug group Drug for Ménière's disease (p.22)
Overdose danger rating High
Dependence rating Low
Prescription needed Yes
Available as generic Yes

GENERAL INFORMATION

Betahistine resembles the naturally occurring substance histamine in some of its effects. The drug was introduced in the 1970s as a treatment for Ménière's disease, which is caused by the pressure of excess fluid in the inner ear.

Taken regularly, betahistine reduces the frequency and severity of the nausea and vertigo attacks that characterize this condition. It is also effective in treating tinnitus (ringing in the ears). The drug is thought to work by reducing pressure in the inner ear, possibly by improving blood flow in the small blood vessels. Drug treatment is not successful in all cases, and surgery may be needed.

INFORMATION FOR USERS

Your drug prescription is tailored for you. Do not alter dosage without checking with your doctor.

How taken Tablets.
Frequency and timing of doses 3 x daily after food.
Adult dosage range 24–48mg daily.
Onset of effect Within 1 hour.
Duration of action 6–12 hours.
Diet advice None.
Storage Keep in a closed container in a cool, dry place out of reach of children.
Missed dose Take as soon as you remember. If your next dose is due within 2 hours, take a single dose now and skip the next.
Stopping the drug Do not stop taking the drug without consulting your doctor; symptoms may recur.

OVERDOSE ACTION

Seek immediate medical advice in all cases. Large overdoses may cause collapse requiring emergency action.

POSSIBLE ADVERSE EFFECTS

Adverse effects of betahistine are minor and rarely cause problems. Nausea, indigestion, and headache may occur. If, rarely, a rash occurs, consult your doctor.

INTERACTIONS

Antihistamines Although unproven, there is a possibility that betahistine may reduce the effects of these drugs.

SPECIAL PRECAUTIONS

Be sure to tell your doctor if:
◆ You have asthma.
◆ You have a peptic ulcer.
◆ You have phaeochromocytoma.
◆ You are taking other medications.
Pregnancy Safety in pregnancy not established. Discuss with your doctor.
Breast-feeding The drug passes into the breast milk, but at normal doses adverse effects on the baby are unlikely. Discuss with your doctor.
Infants and children Not recommended.
Over 60 No special problems.
Driving and hazardous work No special problems.
Alcohol No special problems.

PROLONGED USE

No special problems.

Betamethasone

Brand names Betacap, Betnelan, Betnesol, Betnovate, Bettamousse, Diprosone, Vista-Methasone
Used in the following combined preparations Betnesol-N, Betnovate-C, Betnovate-N, Diprosalic, Fucibet, Lotriderm

QUICK REFERENCE

Drug group Corticosteroid (p80)
Overdose danger rating Low
Dependence rating Low
Prescription needed Yes
Available as generic Yes

GENERAL INFORMATION

Betamethasone is a corticosteroid drug used to treat a variety of conditions. When injected directly into the joints, it relieves joint inflammation and the pain and stiffness of rheumatoid arthritis. It is also given by mouth or injection to treat certain endocrine conditions affecting the pituitary and adrenal glands, and some blood disorders. Betamethasone is also used topically to treat skin complaints, such as eczema and psoriasis.

When betamethasone is taken for short periods in low or moderate doses, it rarely causes serious side effects. High doses or prolonged use of the drug, however, can lead to many symptoms (see below).

INFORMATION FOR USERS

Your drug prescription is tailored for you. Do not alter dosage without checking with your doctor.
How taken Tablets, injection, cream, ointment, rectal ointment, lotion, scalp solution, eye ointment, eye/ear/nose drops.
Frequency and timing of doses Usually once daily in the morning (systemic). Otherwise varies according to disorder being treated.
Dosage range Varies; follow your doctor's instructions.
Onset of effect Within 30 minutes (injection); within 48 hours (other forms).
Duration of action Up to 24 hours.
Diet advice A low-sodium and high potassium diet may be recommended when the oral form of betamethasone is prescribed for extended periods. Follow the advice of your doctor.

Storage Keep in a closed container in a cool, dry place out of reach of children. Protect from light.

Missed dose Take as soon as you remember. If your next dose is due within 2 hours, take a single dose now and skip the next.

Stopping the drug Do not stop tablets without consulting your doctor, who may supervise a gradual reduction in dosage. Stopping abruptly after long-term treatment may cause pituitary and adrenal gland problems.

Exceeding the dose An occasional unintentional extra dose is unlikely to cause problems. However, if you notice any unusual symptoms, or if a large overdose has been taken, notify your doctor.

POSSIBLE ADVERSE EFFECTS

Topical preparations of betamethasone are unlikely to cause adverse effects unless overused. Serious adverse effects usually occur only with high doses taken by mouth for long periods. They include indigestion, peptic ulcers, acne, mood changes, skin thinning, and muscle weakness.

INTERACTIONS

Insulin, antidiabetic drugs, and oral anticoagulant drugs Betamethasone may alter insulin requirements and the effects of these drugs.

Vaccines Serious reactions can occur when certain vaccinations are given during betamethasone treatment.

Antihypertensive drugs and drugs used in myasthenia gravis Betamethasone may reduce the effects of these drugs.

Anticonvulsants These drugs may reduce the effects of betamethasone.

SPECIAL PRECAUTIONS

Be sure to tell your doctor if:
◆ You suffer from a mental disorder.
◆ You have a heart condition.
◆ You have glaucoma.
◆ You have high blood pressure.
◆ You have a history of epilepsy.
◆ You have had a peptic ulcer.
◆ You have had tuberculosis.
◆ You have any infection.
◆ You have diabetes.
◆ You have liver or kidney problems.
◆ You are taking other medications.

Avoid exposure to chickenpox, measles, or shingles if you are on systemic treatment.

Pregnancy No evidence of risk with topical preparations. Low doses of tablets are unlikely to harm the baby. Discuss with your doctor.

Breast-feeding No evidence of risk with topical preparations. In normal doses taken by mouth, adverse effects on the baby are unlikely. Discuss with your doctor.

Infants and children Reduced dose necessary.

Over 60 Reduced dose may be necessary.

Driving and hazardous work No known problems.

Alcohol Keep consumption low. Betamethasone tablets increase the risk of peptic ulcers.

PROLONGED USE

People taking betamethasone tablets regularly should carry a "steroid treatment card". Prolonged use by mouth can lead to peptic ulcers, thin skin, fragile bones, muscle weakness, and adrenal gland suppression. Prolonged use of topical treatment may lead to skin thinning. Betamethasone can also retard growth in children.

Bezafibrate

Brand names Bezalip, Bezalip-Mono
Used in the following combined preparations
None

QUICK REFERENCE

Drug group Lipid-lowering drug (p.37)
Overdose danger rating Low
Dependence rating Low
Prescription needed Yes
Available as generic Yes

GENERAL INFORMATION

Bezafibrate belongs to a group of drugs, usually called fibrates, that lower lipid levels in the blood. Fibrates are particularly effective in decreasing blood levels of triglycerides; they also reduce levels of cholesterol.

Raised levels of lipids (fats) in the blood are associated with atherosclerosis (deposition of fat in blood vessel walls). This can lead to coronary heart disease (for example, angina and heart attacks) and cerebrovascular disease (for example, stroke). When bezafibrate is taken with a diet that is low in saturated fats, there is good evidence that the chances of a heart attack are reduced.

INFORMATION FOR USERS
Your drug prescription is tailored for you. Do not alter dosage without checking with your doctor.
How taken Tablets.
Frequency and timing of doses 1–3 x daily with a little liquid after a meal.
Adult dosage range 400–600mg daily.
Onset of effect A beneficial effect on blood fat levels may not occur for some weeks, and it takes months or years for fat deposits in the arteries to be reduced. Treatment should be withdrawn if no adequate response is obtained within 3–4 months.
Duration of action About 6–24 hours. This may vary according to the individual.
Diet advice A low-fat diet will have been recommended. Follow your doctor's advice.
Storage Keep in a closed container in a cool, dry place out of reach of children.
Missed dose Take as soon as you remember. If your next dose is due within 4 hours (and you take it once daily), take a single dose now and skip the next. If you take the drug 2–3 times daily, take the next dose as normal.
Stopping the drug Do not stop taking the drug without consulting your doctor.
Exceeding the dose An occasional unintentional extra dose is unlikely to be a cause for concern. But if you notice unusual symptoms, notify your doctor.

POSSIBLE ADVERSE EFFECTS
The most common adverse effects are on the gastrointestinal tract (such as loss of appetite and nausea) but normally diminish as treatment continues. If headache, muscle pain, dizziness, or rash occur, consult your doctor.

INTERACTIONS
Anticoagulants Bezafibrate may increase the effect of anticoagulants such as warfarin. Your doctor will reduce the dosage of your anticoagulant when starting you on bezafibrate.
MAOIs There is a risk of liver damage when bezafibrate is taken with an MAOI.
Antidiabetic drugs Bezafibrate may interact with these drugs to lower blood sugar levels.

Pravastatin, simvastatin, and other lipid-lowering drugs whose names end in "statin" There is an increased risk of muscle damage if bezafibrate is taken with these drugs.

SPECIAL PRECAUTIONS
Be sure to tell your doctor if:
◆ You have long-term liver or kidney problems.
◆ You have a history of gallbladder disease.
◆ You are taking other medications.
Pregnancy Safety in pregnancy not established. Discuss with your doctor.
Breast-feeding The drug may pass into the breast milk and may affect the baby. Discuss with your doctor.
Infants and children Not usually prescribed.
Over 60 No special problems expected.
Driving and hazardous work No special problems.
Alcohol Keep consumption low. Heavy intake of alcohol raises triglyceride levels, counteracting the effect of bezafibrate.

PROLONGED USE
No problems expected, but patients who have kidney disease will need special care because there is a high risk of muscle problems developing.
Monitoring Blood tests will be performed occasionally to monitor the effect of the drug on lipids in the blood.

Botulinum Toxin

Brand names Botox, Dysport, NeuroBloc
Used in the following combined preparations None

QUICK REFERENCE
Drug group Muscle relaxant (p.54)
Overdose danger rating High
Dependence rating Low
Prescription needed Yes
Available as generic No

GENERAL INFORMATION
Botulinum toxin is a neurotoxin (nerve poison) that is produced naturally by the bacterium *Clostridium botulinum*. The toxin causes botulism, a rare but serious form of food poisoning.

Research has found that there are several slightly different components in botulinum toxin. Two are used medically: botulinum A toxin and botulinum B toxin. These are used therapeutically to treat conditions in which there are painful muscle spasms – for example, spastic foot deformity, blepharospasm (spasm of the eyelids, causing them almost to close), hemifacial spasm, and spasmodic torticollis (spasms of the neck muscles, causing the head to jerk). Botulinum toxin A is also used to treat very resistant and distressing cases of hyperhidrosis (excessive sweating). The effects that are produced by the toxins may last for 2–3 months, until new nerve endings have formed.

Botulinum toxin is used cosmetically to remove facial wrinkles by paralysing the muscles under the skin. The drug is not licensed for this use in the UK, however.

INFORMATION FOR USERS

This drug is given only under medical supervision and is not for self-administration.

How taken Injection.

Frequency and timing of doses Every 2–3 months, depending on response.

Adult dosage range The dose depends on the particular condition being treated. Individual injections may range from 1.25 units to 50 units. The number of injection sites depends on the size and number of the muscles to be paralysed. Specialist judgement is necessary.

Onset of effect Within 3 days to 2 weeks.

Duration of action 2–3 months.

Diet advice None.

Storage Not applicable as the drug is not normally kept in the home.

Missed dose Attend for treatment at the next possible time.

Stopping the drug Discuss with your doctor whether you should stop receiving the drug.

Exceeding the dose Overdose is unlikely since treatment is carefully monitored, and the drug is given intravenously only under close medical supervision.

POSSIBLE ADVERSE EFFECTS

Botulinum toxin can commonly cause reduced blinking and dry eyes, painful swallowing, and pain or weakness at the site of injection. Misplaced injections may paralyse unintended muscle groups. All paralyses are likely to be long-lasting. In rare cases, botulinum toxin causes glaucoma, neck weakness, head tremor, and hypersensitivity reactions. Consult your doctor in all cases.

INTERACTIONS

None.

SPECIAL PRECAUTIONS

Be sure to tell your doctor if:

◆ You have any disorder of muscle activity, such as myasthenia gravis.

◆ You are taking an anticoagulant drug or have a bleeding disorder.

◆ You are allergic to botulinum toxin.

Pregnancy Not prescribed.

Breast-feeding Not prescribed.

Infants and children Reduced dose necessary.

Over 60 No special problems.

Driving and hazardous work Avoid such activities until you have learned how botulinum toxin affects you; the drug can cause drooping of the eyelid and dryness or watering of the eye, which could lead to double vision.

Alcohol No known problems.

PROLONGED USE

To maintain the desired effects, the drug may have to be administered at regular intervals.

Bromocriptine

Brand name Parlodel

Used in the following combined preparations None

QUICK REFERENCE

Drug group Drug for parkinsonism (p.18) and pituitary agent (p.85)

Overdose danger rating Low

Dependence rating Low

Prescription needed Yes

Available as generic Yes

GENERAL INFORMATION

By inhibiting secretion of the hormone prolactin from the pituitary gland, bromocriptine is used in the treatment of conditions that are associated with excessive prolactin production. These include some types of female infertility and occasionally male infertility and impotence. Bromocriptine is effective in treating some benign breast conditions and other symptoms of menstrual disorders. The drug may be used to suppress lactation in women who do not wish to breast-feed.

Bromocriptine also reduces the release of growth hormone, and therefore is used in the treatment of acromegaly (see p.86).

In addition, the drug is effective in relieving the symptoms of parkinsonism. It is now widely used to treat people who are in the advanced stages of parkinsonism when other drugs have failed or are unsuitable.

Serious adverse effects are uncommon with low doses of bromocriptine. The most common problems are nausea and vomiting, which can be minimized by taking the drug with meals. In rare cases, it may cause ulceration of the stomach.

INFORMATION FOR USERS

Your drug prescription is tailored for you. Do not alter dosage without checking with your doctor.

How taken Tablets, capsules.

Frequency and timing of doses 1–4 x daily with food.

Adult dosage range Dose depends on condition being treated and your response. In most cases, treatment starts with a daily dose of 1–1.25mg, gradually increased until satisfactory response is achieved.

Onset of effect Variable depending on the condition.

Duration of action About 8 hours.

Diet advice None.

Storage Keep in a closed container in a cool, dry place out of reach of children. Protect from light.

Missed dose Take as soon as you remember. If your next dose is due within 2 hours, take a single dose now and skip the next.

Stopping the drug Do not stop taking the drug without consulting your doctor; symptoms may recur.

Exceeding the dose An occasional unintentional extra dose is unlikely to be a cause for concern. However, if you notice any unusual symptoms, or if a large overdose has been taken, notify your doctor.

POSSIBLE ADVERSE EFFECTS

Adverse effects, such as nausea or vomiting and constipation, are usually dose-related. When used for parkinsonism, the drug may cause abnormal movements. If you experience dizziness, drowsiness, or headaches, consult your doctor.

INTERACTIONS

Antipsychotic drugs These drugs oppose the action of bromocriptine and increase the risk of parkinsonism.

Phenylpropanolamine, ephedrine, and pseudoephedrine These drugs are found in some over-the-counter cough and cold remedies. Use of these remedies with bromocriptine may lead to severe adverse effects.

Erythromycin and other macrolide antibiotics These drugs may produce increased levels of bromocriptine and heighten the risk of adverse effects.

Domperidone and metoclopramide These two drugs may reduce some of the effects of bromocriptine.

SPECIAL PRECAUTIONS

Be sure to tell your doctor if:
◆ You have a stomach ulcer.
◆ You have a history of psychiatric disorders.
◆ You have heart problems.
◆ You have porphyria.
◆ You have a history of lung disease.
◆ You are taking other medications.

Pregnancy Safety in pregnancy not established. Discuss with your doctor.

Breast-feeding The drug suppresses milk production, and prevents it completely if given within 12 hours of childbirth. If you wish to breast-feed, consult your doctor.

Infants and children Not usually prescribed under 15 years.

Over 60 Reduced dose may be necessary.

Driving and hazardous work Avoid such activities until you have learned how bromocriptine affects you because the drug may cause dizziness and drowsiness.

Alcohol Avoid. Alcohol increases the likelihood of confusion and reduces tolerance to bromocriptine.

PROLONGED USE

No special problems.

Monitoring Periodic blood tests may be performed to check hormone levels. Gynaecological tests may be carried out annually (or every six months in post-menopausal women). Monitoring for other, rare adverse effects (such as peptic ulcer in acromegaly) may also be carried out.

Budesonide

Brand names Budenofalk, Entocort, Pulmicort, Rhinocort Aqua
Used in the following combined preparations Symbicort

QUICK REFERENCE

Drug group Corticosteroid (p.80)
Overdose danger rating Low
Dependence rating Low
Prescription needed Yes
Available as generic Yes

GENERAL INFORMATION

Budesonide is a corticosteroid drug. It is often used as an inhaler to prevent attacks of asthma, although it will not stop an existing attack. Like other corticosteroids, budesonide is used by people whose asthma is not controlled by bronchodilators (see p.23) alone. It is also used as a nasal spray to relieve the symptoms of allergic rhinitis and for nasal polyps. In addition, it is used in the form of slow-release capsules to relieve the symptoms of Crohn's disease and as an enema to treat ulcerative colitis. Budesonide controls symptoms by reducing inflammation, whether it is in the nose, lungs, or intestine.

There are fewer, usually less serious, side effects with the inhaler or nasal spray, since the drug is absorbed in much smaller quantities than when it is taken by mouth. Fungal infections causing irritation of the mouth and throat may occur, however. These can be avoided to some degree by using a spacer device (see p.25) and by rinsing the mouth and gargling with water after each inhalation.

INFORMATION FOR USERS

Your drug prescription is tailored for you. Do not alter dosage without checking with your doctor.

How taken SR-capsules, enema, inhaler, powder for inhalation, nasal spray.
Frequency and timing of doses 1–3 x daily (capsules); once daily at bedtime (enema); twice daily (inhaler); once or twice daily (spray).
Dosage range 3–9mg (capsules); 2mg (enema); 200–1,600mcg (inhaler); 100–200mcg (spray).
Onset of effect *Asthma* Within 1 week. *Other conditions* 1–3 days.
Duration of action 12–24 hours.
Diet advice None.
Storage Keep in a closed container in a cool, dry place out of reach of children.
Missed dose Take as soon as you remember. If your next dose is due within 2 hours, take a single dose now and skip the next.
Stopping the drug Do not stop taking the drug without consulting your doctor; symptoms may recur. The SR-capsules used in Crohn's disease should be stopped gradually.
Exceeding the dose An occasional extra dose of budesonide is unlikely to be a cause for concern. However, if you notice any unusual symptoms, or if a large overdose has been taken, notify your doctor.

POSSIBLE ADVERSE EFFECTS

The main side effects of inhalers and nasal spray are confined to the nasal passages and mouth. The drug may cause nasal irritation, cough, sore throat or hoarseness, and nosebleeds. Capsules and enemas can commonly cause gastrointestinal disturbances. Rash and mood disorders may occur, but more rarely. High doses of budesonide by any route can cause weight gain and other long-term side effects associated with corticosteroids.

Contact your doctor if a nosebleed, sore throat, or a rash occur. If there is any pain in the eye, stop taking the drug and contact your doctor without delay.

INTERACTIONS

None.

SPECIAL PRECAUTIONS

Be sure to tell your doctor if:
◆ You have had tuberculosis or another respiratory infection.
◆ You are taking other medications.
Pregnancy Discuss with your doctor, especially if the drug is used for Crohn's disease.

Breast-feeding Discuss with your doctor, especially if the drug is used for Crohn's disease.
Infants and children Reduced dose necessary.
Over 60 No special problems.
Driving and hazardous work No special problems.
Alcohol No special problems.

PROLONGED USE

Prolonged use may be required for asthma prevention, but there may be a small risk of glaucoma, cataracts, and effects on bone with high doses taken by inhaler on a long-term basis. People undergoing such treatment are advised to carry a "steroid treatment card" or wear a Medic-alert bracelet.

Monitoring If the drug is being taken in large doses, periodic checks may be needed to ensure that the adrenal glands are working properly. Children using inhalers may have their growth (height) monitored regularly.

Bumetanide

Brand name Burinex
Used in the following combined preparations
Burinex A, Burinex K

QUICK REFERENCE

Drug group Loop diuretic (p.32)
Overdose danger rating Low
Dependence rating Low
Prescription needed Yes
Available as generic Yes

GENERAL INFORMATION

Bumetanide is a powerful, short-acting loop diuretic used to treat oedema (fluid accumulation in tissue spaces) due to heart failure, nephrotic syndrome, and cirrhosis of the liver. The drug is particularly useful in treating people with impaired kidney function who do not respond well to thiazide diuretics. Because it is fast-acting, it is often injected in an emergency to relieve pulmonary oedema.

Bumetanide increases potassium loss in the urine, which can result in a wide variety of symptoms (see Possible adverse effects, below). For this reason, potassium supplements or a diuretic that conserves potassium within the body are often given with the drug.

INFORMATION FOR USERS

Your drug prescription is tailored for you. Do not alter dosage without checking with your doctor.

How taken Tablets, liquid, injection.
Frequency and timing of doses Usually once daily in the morning; twice daily in some cases.
Dosage range 0.5–5mg daily. Dose may be increased if kidney function is impaired.
Onset of effect Within 30 minutes by mouth; more quickly by injection.
Duration of action 2–4 hours.
Diet advice Use of this drug may reduce potassium in the body, so eat plenty of fresh fruit and vegetables such as bananas and tomatoes.
Storage Keep in a closed container in a cool, dry place out of reach of children. Protect from light.
Missed dose No cause for concern, but take as soon as you remember. If it is late in the day, however, do not take the missed dose, or you may need to get up during the night to pass urine. Take the next scheduled dose as usual.
Stopping the drug Do not stop taking the drug without consulting your doctor; symptoms may recur.
Exceeding the dose An occasional unintentional extra dose is unlikely to be a cause for concern. But if you notice any unusual symptoms, or if a large overdose has been taken, notify your doctor.

POSSIBLE ADVERSE EFFECTS

Adverse effects are due mainly to the rapid fluid loss produced by bumetanide, which can lead to dizziness and fainting. These diminish as the body adjusts. The drug may precipitate gout in susceptible people and can affect control of diabetes. If you experience lethargy, severe muscle cramps, nausea, vomiting, or a rash, consult your doctor.

INTERACTIONS

Anti-arrhythmic drugs Low potassium levels associated with bumetanide may increase the toxicity of these drugs.
Antibacterials Bumetanide can increase the ear damage caused by some antibiotics.
Digoxin Excessive potassium loss may increase the adverse effects of digoxin.
NSAIDs These drugs may reduce the diuretic effect of bumetanide.

Lithium Bumetanide may raise levels of lithium in the blood, increasing the risk of lithium toxicity.

Pimozide Low potassium levels increase the risk of abnormal heart rhythms with this antipsychotic drug.

SPECIAL PRECAUTIONS

Be sure to tell your doctor if:
◆ You have long-term liver or kidney problems.
◆ You have diabetes.
◆ You have prostate trouble.
◆ You have gout.
◆ You are taking other medications.

Pregnancy Not usually prescribed. May cause a reduction in blood supply to the developing baby. Discuss with your doctor.

Breast-feeding Bumetanide may reduce the supply of milk. Discuss with your doctor.

Infants and children Not usually prescribed. Reduced dose necessary.

Over 60 Dosage is often reduced.

Driving and hazardous work Avoid such activities until you have learned how bumetanide affects you because the drug may cause dizziness and fainting.

Alcohol Keep consumption low. The drug increases the likelihood of dehydration and hangovers after drinking alcohol.

PROLONGED USE

Serious problems are unlikely, but the levels of certain salts in the body may occasionally become abnormal when bumetanide is taken long term.

Monitoring Regular blood tests may be performed to check kidney function and levels of body salts.

Bupropion

Brand name Zyban
Used in the following combined preparations
None

QUICK REFERENCE

Drug group Nicotine withdrawal aid
Overdose danger rating High
Dependence rating Low
Prescription needed Yes
Available as generic No

GENERAL INFORMATION

Bupropion (also known as amfebutamone) is an antidepressant, but it is chemically unrelated to other antidepressant drugs. Although it has been used to treat depression, it is generally used as an aid for people who are trying to give up tobacco-smoking. The person being treated must commit in advance to a stop date. Treatment is started while the patient is still smoking and the "target stop date" decided on within the first two weeks of treatment. Bupropion will be stopped after seven weeks if the smoker has not given up completely by then. Although the drug can be an effective aid, nicotine replacement therapy is more popular.

Bupropion should not be prescribed to people with a history of seizures or eating disorders, or to people withdrawing from benzodiazepine drugs or alcohol. The drug should also not be prescribed to people with manic depression or psychosis because there is a risk of mania developing.

INFORMATION FOR USERS

Your drug prescription is tailored for you. Do not alter dosage without checking with your doctor.

How taken SR-tablets.
Frequency and timing of doses 1–2 x daily.
Adult dosage range 150–300mg.
Onset of effect Up to 4 weeks for full effect.
Duration of action 12 hours.
Diet advice None.
Storage Keep in original closed container in a cool, dry place out of reach of children.
Missed dose Take as soon as you remember. If your next dose is due within 2 hours, take a single dose now and skip the next dose.
Stopping the drug Do not stop taking the drug without consulting your doctor. The doctor may want to taper the dose.

OVERDOSE ACTION

Seek immediate medical advice in all cases. Take emergency action if consciousness is lost.

POSSIBLE ADVERSE EFFECTS

Common adverse effects of bupropion include insomnia, poor concentration, headache, dizziness, tremor, nausea, and vomiting. Rash, fever, and depression are also common but should be discussed with your doctor in all cases. Some of these effects may be the result of nicotine withdrawal rather than the effects of bupropion. Rarely, palpitations, anxiety, or seizures may develop; seek medical advice.

INTERACTIONS

General note There is a wide range of drugs that, when taken with bupropion, increase the likelihood of seizures. Check with your doctor if you are taking other medications. .

Ritonavir, amantadine, and levodopa These drugs increase the risk of side effects with bupropion.

Anticonvulsant drugs Phenytoin and carbamazepine may reduce the blood levels and effects of bupropion. Sodium valproate may increase its blood levels and effects.

SPECIAL PRECAUTIONS

Be sure to tell your doctor if:
◆ You have had a recent head injury or have a history of seizures.
◆ You have an eating disorder.
◆ You have cancer of the nervous system.
◆ You have diabetes.
◆ You have manic depression or a psychosis.
◆ You have kidney or liver problems.
◆ You are withdrawing from alcohol or benzodiazepine dependence.
◆ You are taking other medications.

Pregnancy Safety in pregnancy not established. Giving up smoking without using drugs is recommended.

Breast-feeding Safety not established. The drug passes into the breast milk and may affect the baby adversely.

Infants and children Not recommended.

Over 60 Increased sensitivity to the effects of bupropion. Reduced dose may therefore be necessary.

Driving and hazardous work Avoid until you have learned how bupropion affects you. The drug may cause impaired concentration and dizziness.

Alcohol Avoid. Alcohol will increase any sedative effects.

PROLONGED USE

Bupropion is used for up to 9 weeks for cessation of smoking.

Monitoring Progress will be reviewed after about 3–4 weeks, and the drug continued only if it is having some effect.

Calcipotriol

Brand names Dovobet, Dovonex
Used in the following combined preparations
None

QUICK REFERENCE
Drug group Drug for psoriasis (p.124)
Overdose danger rating Low
Dependence rating Low
Prescription needed Yes
Available as generic No

GENERAL INFORMATION

Calcipotriol is used for scalp psoriasis and in the treatment of plaque psoriasis affecting up to 40 per cent of the patient's skin area.

Calcipotriol is similar to vitamin D. It is thought to work by reducing production of the skin cells that cause skin thickening and scaling, which are the most common symptoms of psoriasis. Because this drug is related to vitamin D, excessive use (total doses of more than 100g per week) can lead to a rise in calcium levels in the body; otherwise, calcipotriol is unlikely to cause any serious adverse effects.

The drug is applied to the affected areas in the form of cream, ointment, or scalp solution. It should not be used on the face, and it is important that the hands are washed after application to avoid accidentally transferring the substance to unaffected areas. Local irritation may occur during the early stages of treatment.

INFORMATION FOR USERS

Your drug prescription is tailored for you. Do not alter dosage without checking with your doctor.
How taken Cream, ointment, scalp solution.
Frequency and timing of doses 1–2 x daily.
Adult dosage range Maximum 100g per week (cream or ointment); maximum 60ml per week (scalp solution). Less if both types of preparation are used together.
Onset of effect Improvement is seen within 2 weeks.
Duration of action One application lasts for up to 12 hours. The beneficial effects are longer lasting.
Diet advice None.

Storage Store at room temperature out of reach of children.
Missed dose Apply the next dose at the scheduled time.
Stopping the drug Do not stop taking the drug without consulting your doctor; symptoms may recur.
Exceeding the dose Excessive, prolonged use of calcipotriol may lead to an increase in blood calcium levels, which can cause nausea, constipation, thirst, and frequent urination; notify your doctor.

POSSIBLE ADVERSE EFFECTS

Temporary local irritation may occur when treatment is started. Other effects, such as thirst, frequent urination, constipation, and nausea, are usually due to heavy or prolonged use, leading to high calcium levels in the blood. If you develop a rash on light-exposed areas, consult your doctor.

INTERACTIONS
None known.

SPECIAL PRECAUTIONS
Be sure to tell your doctor if:
◆ You have a metabolic disorder.
◆ You have previously had a hypersensitivity reaction to the drug.
◆ You are taking other medications.
Pregnancy Safety in pregnancy not established. Discuss with your doctor.
Breast-feeding It is not known whether the drug passes into breast milk. Discuss with your doctor.
Infants and children Not recommended under 6 years.
Over 60 No problems expected.
Driving and hazardous work No problems expected.
Alcohol No problems expected.

PROLONGED USE
No problems are expected from low doses of calcipotriol. If the effects of the preparation decline after several weeks, they may be regained by suspending use for a few weeks and then recommencing treatment.
Monitoring Regular checks on calcium levels in the blood or urine are required during prolonged or heavy use.

Captopril

Brand names Acepril, Capoten, Ecopace, Kaplon, Tensopril
Used in the following combined preparations
Acezide, Capozide, Capto-co

QUICK REFERENCE

Drug group Vasodilator (p.31) and antihypertensive drug (p.36)
Overdose danger rating Medium
Dependence rating Low
Prescription needed Yes
Available as generic Yes

GENERAL INFORMATION

Captopril belongs to the ACE (angiotensin-converting enzyme) inhibitor group of drugs. It is used to treat high blood pressure and heart failure (in which the heart is unable to deal with its workload). The drug works by relaxing the muscles in blood vessel walls, allowing the vessels to dilate (widen), which enables the blood to circulate more easily and helps to lower blood pressure. It may also be given to patients following a heart attack, and is sometimes used to prevent or delay kidney damage in patients with diabetes. Captopril is often given with a diuretic to increase its effect on high blood pressure and heart failure.

The first dose of captopril is usually very small and should be taken while lying down because there is a risk of a sudden fall in blood pressure.

A variety of minor side effects may occur with captopril; many people develop a persistent dry cough, while others experience taste disturbance, which a reduction in dose may help to minimize.

INFORMATION FOR USERS

Your drug prescription is tailored for you. Do not alter dosage without checking with your doctor.
How taken Tablets.
Frequency and timing of doses 2–3 x daily.
Adult dosage range 12.5–25mg daily initially, gradually increased to 50–150mg daily. Starting doses of 6.25mg may be used.
Onset of effect 30–60 minutes.
Duration of action 6–8 hours.

Diet advice None.
Storage Keep in a closed container in a cool, dry place out of reach of children.
Missed dose Take as soon as you remember. If your next dose is due within 2 hours, take a single dose now and skip the next.
Stopping the drug Unless severe adverse effects occur (see below), do not stop taking the drug without consulting your doctor. Stopping the drug may lead to worsening of the underlying condition.
Exceeding the dose An occasional unintentional extra dose is unlikely to cause problems. Large overdoses, however, may cause dizziness or fainting; notify your doctor.

POSSIBLE ADVERSE EFFECTS

Captopril causes a variety of minor adverse effects: primarily rashes and gastrointestinal symptoms. These usually disappear soon after treatment has started. Dizziness on standing is likely to occur after the first dose. Nausea and headache are common but are usually mild and transient. A persistent dry cough is the most common adverse effect, but this can be minimized by taking smaller, more frequent, doses; some people may have to stop taking the drug. Loss of taste, and rash and itching, are other common adverse effects. If dizziness, fainting, runny nose, sore throat, confusion and mood changes, or chest pain and palpitations occur, consult your doctor. If you develop jaundice, facial swelling, or breathing difficulties, stop taking the drug and seek urgent medical advice.

INTERACTIONS

NSAIDs Some of these drugs may reduce the effectiveness of captopril. There is also a risk of kidney damage when they are taken with it.
Lithium Blood levels of lithium may be raised by captopril.
Other vasodilators (such as nitrates) These drugs may reduce blood pressure even further.
Potassium supplements and potassium-sparing diuretics Taken with captopril, these drugs increase the risk of high blood potassium levels.
Ciclosporin This drug increases the risk of high blood potassium levels with captopril.
Diuretics Starting captopril while taking these drugs can cause a rapid fall in blood pressure, but the two drugs are often given together.

SPECIAL PRECAUTIONS

Be sure to tell your doctor if:
◆ You have suffered from severe allergies.
◆ You have long-term kidney problems.
◆ You have coronary artery disease.
◆ You have peripheral vascular disease.
◆ You are on a low-sodium diet.
◆ You are allergic to other ACE inhibitors.
◆ You are taking other medications.

Pregnancy Not usually prescribed. There is evidence of harm to the developing baby. Discuss with your doctor.

Breast-feeding The drug passes into the breast milk, but at normal doses adverse effects on the baby are unlikely. Consult your doctor.

Infants and children Not usually prescribed.

Over 60 Reduced dose may be necessary.

Driving and hazardous work Avoid until you have learned how captopril affects you because the drug can cause dizziness and fainting.

Alcohol Avoid excessive amounts. Alcohol may increase the blood-pressure-lowering and adverse effects of this drug.

Surgery and general anaesthetics Notify your doctor or dentist that you are taking captopril.

PROLONGED USE

Rarely, prolonged use can lead to changes in the blood count or kidney function.

Monitoring Periodic checks on potassium levels, white blood cell count, kidney function, and urine are usually performed.

Carbamazepine

Brand names Carbagen, Epimaz, Tegretol, Tegretol Retard, Teril Retard, Timonil Retard
Used in the following combined preparations None

QUICK REFERENCE

Drug group Anticonvulsant drug (p.16) and antimanic drug (p.16)
Overdose danger rating Medium
Dependence rating Low
Prescription needed Yes
Available as generic Yes

GENERAL INFORMATION

Carbamazepine is used to treat some forms of epilepsy as it reduces the likelihood of fits due to abnormal nerve signals in the brain.

Carbamazepine is also prescribed to relieve the intermittent severe pain caused by damage to the cranial nerves in trigeminal neuralgia. In addition, it is occasionally prescribed for manic depression and diabetes insipidus, and for pain relief in diabetic neuropathy.

To avoid side effects, the drug is usually started at a low dose and gradually increased until the required blood level is achieved.

INFORMATION FOR USERS

Your drug prescription is tailored for you. Do not alter dosage without checking with your doctor.

How taken Tablets, chewable tablets, liquid, suppositories.

Frequency and timing of doses 1–4 x daily.

Adult dosage range *Epilepsy* 100–1,200mg daily (low starting dose, slowly increased every 2 weeks). *Pain relief* 100–1,600mg daily. *Psychiatric disorders* 400–1,600mg daily.

Onset of effect Within 4 hours.

Duration of action 12–24 hours.

Diet advice None.

Storage Keep in a closed container in a cool, dry place out of reach of children.

Missed dose Take as soon as you remember. If your next dose is due within 2 hours, take a single dose now and skip the next.

Stopping the drug Unless severe adverse effects occur (see below), do not stop the drug without consulting your doctor; symptoms may recur.

Exceeding the dose An occasional unintentional extra dose is unlikely to cause problems. Large overdoses may cause tremor, convulsions, and coma; notify your doctor.

POSSIBLE ADVERSE EFFECTS

There are usually very few adverse effects with this drug. If blood levels get too high, however, adverse effects including drowsiness, dizziness, poor coordination, clumsiness, nausea, ankle swelling, and blurred vision, are common and the dose may need to be reduced. If rash, sore throat, or hoarseness develop, stop taking the drug and consult your doctor.

INTERACTIONS

General note Many drugs may increase or reduce the effects of carbamazepine. Discuss with your doctor or pharmacist before taking other medications.

Other anti-epileptic drugs Complex and variable interactions can occur between these drugs and carbamazepine.

SPECIAL PRECAUTIONS
Be sure to tell your doctor if:
♦ You have long-term liver or kidney problems.
♦ You have heart problems.
♦ You have had blood problems with other drugs.
♦ You are taking other medications.
Pregnancy May be associated with abnormalities in the unborn baby. Folic acid supplements should be taken before and during pregnancy. Discuss with your doctor.
Breast-feeding The drug passes into the breast milk, but at normal doses adverse effects on the baby are unlikely. Discuss with your doctor.
Infants and children Reduced dose necessary.
Over 60 May cause confused or agitated behaviour in elderly people. Reduced dose may be necessary.
Driving and hazardous work Your underlying condition, and the possibility of reduced alertness while you are taking the drug, may make such activities inadvisable. Discuss with your doctor.
Alcohol Avoid. Alcohol may increase the sedative effects of this drug.

PROLONGED USE
There is a slight risk of changes in liver function, or skin or blood abnormalities, occurring during prolonged use.
Monitoring Periodic blood tests may be performed to monitor levels of the drug, blood cell counts, and liver and kidney function.

Carbaryl

Brand name Carylderm
Used in the following combined preparations
None

QUICK REFERENCE
Drug group Drugs to treat skin parasites (p.122)
Overdose danger rating Low
Dependence rating Low
Prescription needed Yes
Available as generic No

GENERAL INFORMATION
Carbaryl is an insecticide used in the treatment of head and crab lice. It kills the lice by interfering with the functioning of their nervous system, causing paralysis and death.

The drug is applied topically either as water-based liquid or alcohol-based lotion. All members of a household should be treated at the same time, at the first sign of infestation. Liquid is more suitable for small children and asthmatics, who may be affected by the alcoholic fumes of lotion. In addition, lotion is unsuitable for treating crab lice because it causes genital irritation.

Lice develop resistance to insecticides, so it is possible that carbaryl (or alternatives such as malathion) may not clear them. If the drug does not work for you, consult your pharmacist or doctor.

INFORMATION FOR USERS
Your drug prescription is tailored for you. Do not alter dosage without checking with your doctor.
How taken Topical liquid, lotion.
Frequency and timing of doses Once, repeating after a week.
Adult dosage range As directed.
Onset of effect Lotion or liquid should be left on for 12 hours before being washed off.
Duration of action Until washed off.
Diet advice None.
Storage Keep in a closed container in a cool, dry place out of reach of children. Protect from light.
Missed dose If you forget the second application, use it as soon as you remember.
Stopping the drug Carbaryl is used as a single application or as a short course of treatment.
Exceeding the dose An occasional unintentional extra application is unlikely to be a cause for concern. Take emergency action if the drug is accidentally swallowed.

POSSIBLE ADVERSE EFFECTS
Used correctly, carbaryl is unlikely to cause adverse effects, although skin irritation may occur. Some lotions give off alcoholic fumes that may cause wheezing in asthmatics.

INTERACTIONS
None.

SPECIAL PRECAUTIONS
Be sure to tell your doctor if:
◆ You have asthma.
Pregnancy No evidence of risk. It is unlikely that enough carbaryl would be absorbed to affect the developing baby.
Breast-feeding No evidence of risk. It is unlikely that enough carbaryl would be absorbed to affect the baby, but discuss with your doctor or pharmacist before use.
Infants and children No special problems.
Over 60 No special problems.
Driving and hazardous work No special problems.
Alcohol No special problems.

PROLONGED USE
Carbaryl is intended for intermittent use only. The treatment should not be used for prolonged periods.

Carbimazole

Brand name Neo-Mercazole
Used in the following combined preparations
None

QUICK REFERENCE
Drug group Drug for thyroid disorders (p.84)
Overdose danger rating Medium
Dependence rating Low
Prescription needed Yes
Available as generic No

GENERAL INFORMATION
Carbimazole is an antithyroid drug used to suppress the formation of thyroid hormones in people who have an overactive thyroid gland (hyperthyroidism). In some people, particularly those with Graves' disease (the most common form of hyperthyroidism), drug treatment alone may relieve the disorder.

Carbimazole is also used in more serious cases. If the thyroid gland is to be partially removed by surgery, the drug may be given beforehand to restore the gland's normal function. If radioactive iodine is used to destroy some of the thyroid cells, carbimazole is given to intensify its absorption. The drug also prevents the harmful release of thyroid hormone that can sometimes follow the use of radioactive iodine. Because the full benefits of this medication are not felt for several weeks, beta blockers may be given during this period to help control symptoms.

Maintenance treatment may be continued for as long as 18 months unless surgery or radioactive iodine are used. Occasionally, the dose of carbimazole is kept high (often around 30mg per day), and thyroxine is also prescribed as thyroid function diminishes. This approach may be more effective and may prevent a goitre from developing.

INFORMATION FOR USERS
Your drug prescription is tailored for you. Do not alter dosage without checking with your doctor.
How taken Tablets.
Frequency and timing of doses 2–3 x daily.
Adult dosage range 15–40mg daily (occasionally a larger dose may be needed). Once control is achieved, dosage is reduced gradually to a maintenance dose of 5–15mg for about 18 months.
Onset of effect Some improvement is usually felt within 1–3 weeks. Full beneficial effects usually take 4–8 weeks.
Duration of action 12–24 hours.
Diet advice Your doctor may advise you to avoid foods that are high in iodine, such as cod and mackerel.
Storage Keep in a closed container in a cool, dry place out of reach of children.
Missed dose Take as soon as you remember. If your next dose is due, take both of the doses together.
Stopping the drug Do not stop taking the drug without consulting your doctor; symptoms may recur.
Exceeding the dose An occasional unintentional extra dose is unlikely to cause problems. Large overdoses may cause nausea, vomiting, and headache; notify your doctor.

POSSIBLE ADVERSE EFFECTS
Headache, dizziness, nausea, and joint pain are common. Serious side effects are rare. A sore throat or mouth ulcers may indicate adverse effects on the blood, requiring prompt medical attention. If hair loss, rash or itching, occur consult your doctor. If jaundice develops, seek medical advice without delay.

INTERACTIONS
None.

SPECIAL PRECAUTIONS
Be sure to tell your doctor if:
◆ You have long-term liver or kidney problems.
◆ You are taking other medications.
Pregnancy The drug may be associated with defects in the developing baby. Discuss with your doctor.
Breast-feeding The drug passes into breast milk, but mothers may breast-feed as long as the lowest effective dose is used and the baby carefully monitored. Discuss with your doctor.
Infants and children Reduced dose necessary.
Over 60 No special problems.
Driving and hazardous work Usually no problems, but carbimazole may cause dizziness.
Alcohol No known problems.

PROLONGED USE
Carbimazole may stop or reduce the production of blood cells by the bone marrow. For this reason, it is very important to report to your doctor immediately any symptoms, such as a sore throat, that suggest an infection.
Monitoring Blood cell counts are carried out, and periodic tests of thyroid function are usually required.

Cefalexin

Brand names Ceporex, Keflex, Kiflone, Tenkorex
Used in the following combined preparations
None

QUICK REFERENCE
Drug group Cephalosporin antibiotic (p.62)
Overdose danger rating Low
Dependence rating Low
Prescription needed Yes
Available as generic Yes

GENERAL INFORMATION
Cefalexin is a cephalosporin antibiotic that is prescribed for a variety of mild to moderate infections. It does not have such a wide range of uses as some other antibiotics, but it is helpful in treating cystitis, and certain skin and soft tissue infections. In some cases it is prescribed as follow-up treatment for severe infections after a more powerful cephalosporin has been given by injection.

Diarrhoea is the most common side effect of cefalexin, although it tends to be less severe than with other cephalosporin antibiotics. In addition, some people may find that they are allergic to this drug, especially if they are sensitive to penicillin.

INFORMATION FOR USERS
Your drug prescription is tailored for you. Do not alter dosage without checking with your doctor.
How taken Tablets, capsules, liquid.
Frequency and timing of doses 2–4 x daily.
Dosage range *Adults* 1–2g daily, up to a maximum of 6g. *Children* Reduced dose according to age and weight.
Onset of effect Within 1 hour.
Duration of action 6–12 hours.
Diet advice None.
Storage Keep tablets and capsules in a closed container in a cool, dry place out of reach of children. Keep liquid refrigerated, but do not freeze, and keep for no longer than 10 days. Protect from light.
Missed dose Take as soon as you remember. If your next dose is due at this time, take both doses together.
Stopping the drug Take the full course. Even if you feel better, the original infection may still be present and may recur if treatment is stopped too soon.
Exceeding the dose An occasional unintentional extra dose is unlikely to be a cause for concern. But if you notice any unusual symptoms, or if a large overdose has been taken, notify your doctor.

POSSIBLE ADVERSE EFFECTS
Most people suffer no serious adverse effects. Diarrhoea is common but tends not to be severe. Nausea and abdominal pain may occur. Rare effects, such as rash, itching, and wheezing, are usually due to an allergic reaction; in these cases, the drug may have to be stopped.

INTERACTIONS
Probenecid This drug increases the level of cefalexin in the blood; the dosage of cefalexin may need to be adjusted accordingly.

Oral contraceptives Cefalexin may reduce the contraceptive effect of these drugs. Discuss with your doctor.

SPECIAL PRECAUTIONS
Be sure to tell your doctor if:
◆ You have a long-term kidney problem.
◆ You have had a previous allergic reaction to a penicillin or cephalosporin antibiotic.
◆ You have a history of blood disorders.
◆ You are taking other medications.
Pregnancy No evidence of risk to the developing baby.
Breast-feeding The drug passes into the breast milk, but at normal doses adverse effects on the baby are unlikely. Discuss with your doctor.
Infants and children Reduced dose necessary.
Over 60 No special problems.
Driving and hazardous work No known problems.
Alcohol No known problems.

PROLONGED USE
Cefalexin is usually given only for short courses of treatment.

Celecoxib

Brand name Celebrex
Used in the following combined preparations
None

QUICK REFERENCE
Drug group Analgesic (p.9) and non-steroidal anti-inflammatory drug (p.50)
Overdose danger rating Medium
Dependence rating Low
Prescription needed Yes
Available as generic No

GENERAL INFORMATION
Celecoxib is a type of NSAID known as a COX-2 inhibitor (see p.51). These drugs provide the benefits of other NSAIDs but with less risk of causing gastrointestinal problems such as stomach ulcers.

Celecoxib reduces pain, inflammation, and stiffness and is used to relieve the symptoms of both osteoarthritis and rheumatoid arthritis. Elderly patients and those of Afro-Caribbean origin are usually prescribed a low dose at first because they may be more sensitive to the drug's effects. Unlike aspirin and some other NSAIDs, celecoxib does not protect against coronary heart disease.

INFORMATION FOR USERS
Your drug prescription is tailored for you. Do not alter dosage without checking with your doctor.
How taken Capsules.
Frequency and timing of doses 1–2 x daily.
Adult dosage range 200–400mg daily.
Onset of effect 1 hour.
Duration of action 8 hours.
Diet advice None.
Storage Keep in a cool, dry place out of reach of children.
Missed dose Take as soon as you remember. If your next dose is due within 4 hours, take a single dose now and skip the next.
Stopping the drug If being used short term, the drug can safely be stopped as soon as you no longer need it. If prescribed for long-term use, do not stop taking the drug without consulting your doctor.
Exceeding the dose An occasional unintentional extra dose is unlikely to cause problems. Large overdoses can cause stomach and intestinal pain and damage; notify your doctor.

POSSIBLE ADVERSE EFFECTS
Gastrointestinal, nervous, and respiratory symptoms are the most likely adverse effects. Rash and swollen ankles are also common. If these or severe indigestion, abdominal pain, diarrhoea, flatulence, dizziness, or insomnia occur, consult your doctor. Stop taking the drug and seek urgent medical advice if palpitations, breathing difficulties, and black or bloodstained vomit and faeces occur.

INTERACTIONS
Anticoagulants The effects of warfarin are increased by celecoxib.
ACE inhibitors Taken with celecoxib, these drugs increase the risk of renal failure.
Antihypertensives and diuretics The blood-pressure-lowering effects of these drugs may be reduced by celecoxib.
Lithium Celecoxib increases the levels and effects of this drug.

Ciclosporin and tacrolimus These drugs may increase the risk of renal toxicity with celecoxib.
Methotrexate NSAIDs (possibly including celecoxib) slow excretion of this drug, increasing toxicity.
Carbamazepine, fluconazole, rifampicin, and barbiturates These drugs reduce the effect of celecoxib.

SPECIAL PRECAUTIONS
Be sure to tell your doctor if:
◆ You have asthma.
◆ You have angina/coronary heart disease.
◆ You are allergic to aspirin or celecoxib.
◆ You are allergic to sulphonamides.
◆ You have a peptic ulcer or gastrointestinal bleeding.
◆ You have inflammatory bowel disease.
◆ You have congestive heart failure.
◆ You are taking other medicines.
Pregnancy Not prescribed.
Breast-feeding Not prescribed.
Infants and children Not recommended.
Over 60 Elderly may be more sensitive to the drug's effects. Lower doses may be necessary.
Driving and hazardous work Avoid until you have learned how the drug affects you. It can cause dizziness, vertigo, and sleepiness.
Alcohol Alcohol may increase drowsiness and the risk of stomach irritation.

PROLONGED USE
No problems expected as the drug is intended for long-term use.
Monitoring Periodic tests of kidney function may be performed.

Cetirizine/Levocetirizine

Brand names Benadryl, Piriteze, Xyzal, Zirtek, Zirtek Allergy
Used in the following combined preparations None

QUICK REFERENCE
Drug group Antihistamine (p.58)
Overdose danger rating Medium
Dependence rating Low
Prescription needed Yes (some tablets and all liquid preparations)
Available as generic No

GENERAL INFORMATION
Cetirizine and levocetirizine are long-acting antihistamines. The drugs' main use is in the treatment of allergic rhinitis, particularly hay fever. Cetirizine is also used to treat allergic skin conditions, such as urticaria (hives).

The main difference between these and traditional antihistamines such as amine is that they are less sedating and may therefore be suitable for people when they need to avoid sleepiness – for example, when they are driving or at work. However, because cetirizine and levocetirizine can cause drowsiness in some people, you should learn how the drugs affect you before you undertake any activities that require concentration.

INFORMATION FOR USERS
Follow instructions on the label. Call your doctor if symptoms worsen.
How taken Tablets, liquid.
Frequency and timing of doses 1–2 x daily.
Adult dosage range *Cetirizine* 10mg daily. *Levocetirizine* 5mg daily.
Onset of effect 1–3 hours. Some effect may not be felt for 1–2 days.
Duration of action Up to 24 hours.
Diet advice None.
Storage Keep in a closed container in a cool, dry place out of reach of children.
Missed dose No cause for concern, but take as soon as you remember. If your next dose is due within 8 hours, take a single dose now and skip the next.
Stopping the drug Can be safely stopped as soon as you no longer need it.
Exceeding the dose An occasional unintentional extra dose is unlikely to cause problems. Large overdoses, however, may cause nausea or drowsiness and have adverse effects on the heart; notify your doctor.

POSSIBLE ADVERSE EFFECTS
The most common effects are dry mouth and fatigue; drowsiness is rare. Taking 5mg twice a day can reduce the side effects.

INTERACTIONS
Anticholinergic drugs All drugs with anticholinergic effects, including antipsychotics and tricyclic antidepressants, can increase the anticholinergic effects cetirizine and levocetirizine.

Sedatives Cetirizine and levocetirizine may increase the sedative effects of anti-anxiety drugs, sleeping drugs, antidepressants, and antipsychotics.

Allergy tests Antihistamines should be discontinued approximately 48 hours before allergy skin testing.

SPECIAL PRECAUTIONS

Be sure to consult your doctor or pharmacist before taking this drug if:
◆ You have long-term liver or kidney problems.
◆ You have glaucoma.
◆ You are taking other medications.

Pregnancy Safety in pregnancy not established. Discuss with your doctor.

Breast-feeding The drug passes into the breast milk. Discuss with your doctor.

Infants and children Not recommended under 2 years, but may be prescribed for special use under 6 years.

Over 60 No problems expected.

Driving and hazardous work Avoid such activities until you have learned how cetirizine and levocetirizine affect you because the drugs can cause drowsiness in some people.

Alcohol Keep consumption low.

PROLONGED USE

No problems expected.

Chloramphenicol

Brand names Chloromycetin, Kemicetine, Minims Chloramphenicol
Used in the following combined preparation Actinac

QUICK REFERENCE

Drug group Antibiotic (p.62)
Overdose danger rating Low
Dependence rating Low
Prescription needed Yes
Available as generic Yes

GENERAL INFORMATION

Chloramphenicol is an antibiotic drug used topically to treat eye and ear infections. Given by mouth or injection, the drug is used in the treatment of meningitis and brain abscesses. Chloramphenicol is also effective in treating acute infections such as typhoid, pneumonia, epiglottitis, or meningitis caused by bacteria that is resistant to other antibiotics.

Most people experience few adverse effects since not enough of the drug is absorbed to cause harm when applied topically. However, it occasionally causes serious or even fatal blood disorders and, for this reason, chloramphenicol by mouth or injection is normally only given to treat life-threatening infections that do not respond to safer drugs.

INFORMATION FOR USERS

Your drug prescription is tailored for you. Do not alter dosage without checking with your doctor.

How taken Capsules, liquid, injection, cream, eye and ear drops, eye ointment.

Frequency and timing of doses Every 6 hours (by mouth or injection); every 2–6 hours (eye preparations); 3 x daily (ear drops).

Adult dosage range Varies according to preparation and condition. Follow your doctor's instructions.

Onset of effect 1–3 days, depending on the condition and preparation.

Duration of action 6–8 hours.

Diet advice None.

Storage Keep in a closed container in a cool, dry place out of reach of children. Protect from light.

Missed dose Take as soon as you remember (capsules, liquid). If your next dose is due, double the dose to make up the missed dose. For skin, eye, and ear preparations, apply as soon as you remember.

Stopping the drug Unless severe adverse effects occur (see below), take the full course. Even if you feel better, the infection may still be present and may recur if treatment is stopped too soon.

Exceeding the dose An occasional unintentional extra dose is unlikely to be a cause for concern. But if you notice any unusual symptoms, or if a large overdose has been taken, notify your doctor.

POSSIBLE ADVERSE EFFECTS

Transient irritation may occur with eye or ear drops. If you are receiving the drug by mouth or injection, and numbness in the hands or feet, blurred vision, or rash occur, stop taking the drug and consult your doctor. Sore throat, fever, and unusual tiredness with any form of the drug may be signs of blood abnormalities and should be reported to your doctor without delay, even if treatment has been stopped.

INTERACTIONS

General note Chloramphenicol by mouth or injection may increase the effect of certain other drugs, including phenytoin, oral anticoagulants, and oral antidiabetics. Phenobarbital or rifampicin may reduce the effect of chloramphenicol.

Antidiabetic drugs Chloramphenicol by mouth or injection may increase the effect of antidiabetic drugs.

Ciclosporin, tacrolimus, and sirolimus The blood levels of these drugs may rise if they are given at the same time as chloramphenicol capsules, liquid, or injection.

SPECIAL PRECAUTIONS

Be sure to tell your doctor if:
◆ You have long-term liver or kidney problems.
◆ You have a blood disorder.
◆ You are taking other medications.

Pregnancy No evidence of risk with eye or ear preparations. Safety in pregnancy not established in other methods of administration. Discuss with your doctor.

Breast-feeding No evidence of risk with eye or ear preparations. Taken by mouth, the drug passes into the breast milk and may increase the risk of blood disorders in the baby. Discuss with your doctor.

Infants and children Reduced dose necessary.

Over 60 No problems expected.

Driving and hazardous work No known problems.

Alcohol No known problems.

PROLONGED USE

Prolonged use of chloramphenicol may increase the risk of serious blood disorders and eye damage.

Monitoring Periodic blood-cell counts and eye tests may be performed. Blood levels of the drug are usually monitored in infants given chloramphenicol by mouth or injection.

Chlordiazepoxide

Brand names Librium, Tropium
Used in the following combined preparations
None

QUICK REFERENCE

Drug group Benzodiazepine anti-anxiety drug (p.13)
Overdose danger rating Medium
Dependence rating Medium
Prescription needed Yes
Available as generic Yes

GENERAL INFORMATION

Introduced in the mid-1960s, chlordiazepoxide belongs to the group of anti-anxiety drugs known as the benzodiazepines. These drugs are used to help relieve tension and nervousness, relax muscles, and encourage sleep.

Prescribed primarily to treat anxiety, chlordiazepoxide is also used to relieve the symptoms of alcohol withdrawal.

Chlordiazepoxide may lead to dependence and withdrawal symptoms if taken regularly over a long period, and it may also lose effectiveness with time. For these reasons, courses of treatment are usually limited to between two and four weeks.

INFORMATION FOR USERS

Your drug prescription is tailored for you. Do not alter dosage without checking with your doctor.

How taken Tablets, capsules.

Frequency and timing of doses 1–3 x daily.

Adult dosage range 10–100mg daily. Dosage varies considerably from person to person.

Onset of effect 1–2 hours.

Duration of action 12–24 hours, but some effects may last up to 4 days.

Diet advice None.

Storage Keep in a closed container in a cool, dry place out of reach of children.

Missed dose No cause for concern, but take when you remember. If your next dose is due within 2 hours, take a single dose now and skip the next.

Stopping the drug If you have been taking the drug for less than 2 weeks, it can be safely stopped as soon as you feel you no longer need it. However, if you have been taking the drug for longer, consult your doctor, who may supervise a gradual reduction in dosage. Stopping abruptly may lead to withdrawal symptoms.

Exceeding the dose An occasional unintentional extra dose is unlikely to cause problems. Large overdoses may cause excessive drowsiness or coma; notify your doctor.

POSSIBLE ADVERSE EFFECTS

The principal adverse effects of chlordiazepoxide are related to its sedative properties and include drowsiness, dizziness, and forgetfulness. These effects normally diminish after the first few days of treatment.

INTERACTIONS

Anticonvulsant drugs Chlordiazepoxide may increase or decrease the effects of some anticonvulsant drugs.

Sedatives All drugs that have a sedative effect are likely to increase the sedative properties of chlordiazepoxide. Such drugs include anti-anxiety and sleeping drugs, antihistamines, opioid analgesics, antidepressants, and antipsychotics.

SPECIAL PRECAUTIONS

Be sure to tell your doctor if:
◆ You have long-term liver or kidney problems.
◆ You have a history of breathing problems.
◆ You have had problems with alcohol or drug abuse.
◆ You are taking other medications.

Pregnancy Safety in pregnancy not established. Discuss with your doctor.

Breast-feeding The drug passes into the breast milk and may affect the baby. Discuss with your doctor.

Infants and children Not recommended.

Over 60 Reduced dose may be necessary.

Driving and hazardous work Avoid such activities until you have learned how chlordiazepoxide affects you because the drug can cause reduced alertness and slowed reactions.

Alcohol Avoid. Alcohol may increase the sedative effects of this drug.

PROLONGED USE

Regular use of chlordiazepoxide over several weeks can lead to a reduction in its effect as the body adapts to it. The drug may also be habit-forming when taken for extended periods, especially if it is taken in doses that are larger than average.

Chloroquine

Brand names Avloclor, Nivaquine
Used in the following combined preparation
Paludrine/Avloclor

QUICK REFERENCE

Drug group Antimalarial drug (p.75) and antirheumatic drug (p.52)
Overdose danger rating High
Dependence rating Low
Prescription needed No (malaria prevention); Yes (other uses)
Available as generic Yes

GENERAL INFORMATION

Chloroquine was introduced for the prevention and treatment of malaria. It usually clears an attack of the disease within three days. Injections of the drug may be given when an attack is severe. As a preventative treatment, a low dose is given once weekly, starting one week before visiting a high-risk area and continuing for four weeks after leaving. Chloroquine is not suitable for use in all parts of the world because resistance to the drug has developed in some areas. The drug's other main use is in the treatment of autoimmune diseases, such as rheumatoid arthritis and lupus erythematosus.

Common side effects include nausea, headache, diarrhoea, and abdominal cramps. Occasionally a rash develops. More seriously, the drug can damage the retina during prolonged treatment, causing blurred vision that sometimes progresses to blindness. Regular eye checks are needed to detect early changes.

INFORMATION FOR USERS

Follow instructions on the label. Call your doctor if symptoms worsen.

How taken Tablets, liquid, injection.

Frequency and timing of doses *Prevention of malaria* 1 x weekly (by mouth); *treatment of malaria* 1–4 x daily (by mouth). *Arthritis* 1 x daily.

Adult dosage range *Prevention of malaria* 300mg (2 tablets) as a single dose on the same day each week. Start 1 week before entering endemic area, and continue for 4 weeks after leaving. *Treatment of malaria* Initial dose 600mg (4 tablets) and following doses 300mg. *Rheumatoid arthritis* 150mg (1 tablet) per day.

Onset of effect 2–3 days. In rheumatoid arthritis, full effect may not be felt for up to 6 months.

Duration of action Up to 1 week.

Diet advice None.

Storage Keep in a closed container in a cool, dry, place out of reach of children. Protect from light.

Missed dose Take as soon as you remember, but if your next dose is due within 24 hours (1 x weekly schedule), or 6 hours (1–2 x daily schedule), take a single dose now and skip the next.

Stopping the drug Unless severe adverse effects occur (see below), do not stop taking the drug without consulting your doctor.

OVERDOSE ACTION

Seek immediate medical advice in all cases. Take emergency action if breathing difficulties, fits, or loss of consciousness occur.

POSSIBLE ADVERSE EFFECTS

Side effects such as nausea, diarrhoea, and abdominal pain are common and might be avoided by taking chloroquine with food. Rarely, headache and dizziness, hearing disorders, and mood changes, may occur. If a rash or any changes in vision develop, stop taking the drug and consult your doctor without delay.

INTERACTIONS

Anti-epileptic drugs Chloroquine may reduce the effect of these drugs.

Digoxin The level of digoxin in the blood may be increased by chloroquine.

Ciclosporin Chloroquine increases the blood level of ciclosporin.

Amiodarone Chloroquine may increase the risk of abnormal heart rhythms if taken with this drug.

SPECIAL PRECAUTIONS

Be sure to consult your doctor or pharmacist before taking this drug if:

◆ You have liver or kidney problems.

◆ You have glucose-6-phosphate dehydrogenase (G6PD) deficiency.

◆ You have eye or vision problems.

◆ You have psoriasis.

◆ You have a history of epilepsy.

◆ You suffer from porphyria.

◆ You are taking other medications.

Pregnancy No evidence of risk with low doses. High doses may affect the baby. Discuss with your doctor.

Breast-feeding The drug may pass into breast milk in small amounts. At normal doses effects on the baby are unlikely. Discuss with your doctor.

Infants and children Reduced dose necessary.

Over 60 No special problems, except that it may be difficult to tell between changes in eyesight due to aging and those that are drug-induced.

Driving and hazardous work Avoid such activities until you have learned how chloroquine affects you because the drug may cause dizziness.

Alcohol Keep consumption low.

PROLONGED USE

Prolonged use of chloroquine may cause eye damage and blood disorders.

Monitoring Periodic eye tests (which are often self-tests) and blood counts must be carried out.

Chlorphenamine

Brand names Calimal, Piriton
Used in the following combined preparations
Contac 400, Dristan, Expulin, Galpseud Plus, Haymine, Tixylix Cough and Cold

QUICK REFERENCE

Drug group Antihistamine (p.58)
Overdose danger rating Medium
Dependence rating Low
Prescription needed No (tablets and liquid); yes (injection)
Available as generic Yes

GENERAL INFORMATION

Chlorphenamine has been used for more than 30 years to treat allergies such as allergic rhinitis (hay fever), allergic conjunctivitis, urticaria (hives), insect bites and stings, and angioedema (allergic swellings). Chlorphenamine is also included in several over-the-counter cold remedies (see p.27).

Like other antihistamines, chlorphenamine relieves allergic skin symptoms such as itching, swelling, and redness. It also reduces sneezing and the runny nose and itching eyes of hay fever. In addition, it has a mild anticholinergic (see Autonomic nervous system, p.8) action, which suppresses mucus secretion.

Chlorphenamine may also be administered by a doctor to prevent or treat allergic reactions to blood transfusions or X-ray contrast material, and can be given with epinephrine (adrenaline) injections to treat acute allergic shock (anaphylaxis).

INFORMATION FOR USERS

Follow instructions on the label. Call your doctor if symptoms worsen.

How taken Tablets, liquid, injection.

Frequency and timing of doses 4–6 x daily (tablets, liquid); single dose as needed (injection).

Dosage range *Adults* 12–24mg daily (by mouth); up to 40mg daily (injection). *Children* Reduced dose according to age and weight.

Onset of effect Within 60 minutes (by mouth); within 20 minutes (injection).

Duration of action 4–6 hours (tablets, liquid, injection).

Diet advice None.

Storage Keep in a closed container in a cool, dry place out of reach of children.

Missed dose Take as soon as you remember. If your next dose is due within 2 hours, take a single dose now and skip the next.

Stopping the drug Can be safely stopped as soon as you no longer need it.

Exceeding the dose An occasional unintentional extra dose is unlikely to cause problems. Large overdoses, however, may cause drowsiness or agitation; notify your doctor.

POSSIBLE ADVERSE EFFECTS

Drowsiness is the most common adverse effect of chlorphenamine. Dizziness may also occur. Other adverse effects are rare. Some of these effects, such as dryness of the mouth, blurred vision, and difficulty passing urine, are due to its anticholinergic effects. Children taking the drug may become excitable.

Gastrointestinal irritation may occur, but this problem can be reduced by taking the tablets or liquid with food or drink. If you develop a rash, stop taking the drug and consult your doctor.

INTERACTIONS

Sedatives All drugs that have a sedative effect are likely to increase the sedative properties of chlorphenamine.

Phenytoin The effects of phenytoin may be enhanced by chlorphenamine.

MAOIs and tricyclic antidepressants These drugs may increase the adverse effects of chlorphenamine.

Anticholinergic drugs All drugs that have an anticholinergic effect, including certain drugs for treating parkinsonism, are likely to add to the anticholinergic effect of chlorphenamine.

SPECIAL PRECAUTIONS

Be sure to consult your doctor or pharmacist before taking this drug if:
◆ You have a long-term liver problem.
◆ You have had epileptic fits.
◆ You have glaucoma.
◆ You have urinary difficulties.
◆ You are taking other medications.

Pregnancy Safety in pregnancy not established. Discuss with your doctor.

Breast-feeding The drug passes into the breast milk, but at normal doses adverse effects on the baby are unlikely. Discuss with your doctor.

Infants and children Reduced dose necessary.

Over 60 Increased likelihood of adverse effects. Reduced dose may therefore be necessary.

Driving and hazardous work Avoid such activities until you have learned how chlorphenamine affects you because the drug can cause drowsiness, dizziness, and blurred vision.

Alcohol Avoid. Alcohol may increase the sedative effects of this drug.

PROLONGED USE

The effect of chlorphenamine may become weaker with prolonged use over a period of weeks or months as the body adapts to the treatment. Changing to a different antihistamine may be recommended.

Chlorpromazine

Brand names Chloractil, Largactil
Used in the following combined preparations
None

QUICK REFERENCE

Drug group Phenothiazine antipsychotic (p.15) and
anti-emetic drug (p.21)
Overdose danger rating Medium
Dependence rating Low
Prescription needed Yes
Available as generic Yes

GENERAL INFORMATION

Chlorpromazine was the first antipsychotic
drug to be marketed and it is still used today.
It has a tranquillizing effect that is useful in
the short-term treatment of anxiety, agitation, and aggressive behaviour.

Chlorpromazine is prescribed for the
treatment of schizophrenia, mania, and
other disorders where confused, aggressive,
or abnormal behaviour may occur and a
degree of sedation is beneficial. Other uses
of this drug include the treatment of nausea
and vomiting, especially when caused by
drug or radiation treatment; and treating
severe, prolonged hiccoughs.

Chlorpromazine can produce a number of
adverse effects, some of which may be serious.
After continuous use of chlorpromazine over
several years, eye changes and skin discoloration may occur, particularly in women.

INFORMATION FOR USERS

Your drug prescription is tailored for you.
Do not alter dosage without checking with
your doctor.
How taken Tablets, liquid, injection, suppositories.
Frequency and timing of doses 1–4 x daily.
Adult dosage range *Mental illness* 75–300mg
daily; dose is started low and gradually increased. Some patients may need up to
1,000mg daily. *Nausea and vomiting* 40–150mg
daily.
Onset of effect 30–60 minutes (by mouth);
15–20 minutes (injection); up to 30 minutes
(suppository).
Duration of action 8–12 hours (by mouth or
injection); 3–4 hours (suppository); some

effects may persist for up to 3 weeks when
the drug is stopped after regular use.
Diet advice None.
Storage Keep in a closed container in a cool,
dry place out of reach of children. Protect
from light.
Missed dose Take as soon as you remember. If
your next dose is due within 2 hours, do not
take the missed dose. Take your next scheduled dose as usual.
Stopping the drug Unless severe adverse effects
occur (see below), do not stop taking the
drug without consulting your doctor; symptoms may recur.
Exceeding the dose An occasional unintentional extra dose is unlikely to cause
problems. Larger overdoses may cause unusual drowsiness, fainting, abnormal heart
rhythms, muscle rigidity, and agitation.
Notify your doctor.

POSSIBLE ADVERSE EFFECTS

Chlorpromazine commonly causes mild
drowsiness and has an anticholinergic (see
Autonomic nervous system, p.8) effect,
which can cause symptoms such as blurring
of vision. It may also cause dizziness or fainting and infrequent periods. The most significant adverse effect is parkinsonism. If you
develop jaundice, or a rash on areas of skin
exposed to light, stop taking the drug and
consult your doctor urgently.

INTERACTIONS

Drugs for parkinsonism Chlorpromazine may
reduce the effect of these drugs.
Anticholinergic drugs These drugs may intensify the anticholinergic properties of
chlorpromazine.
Sedatives All drugs that have a sedative effect
on the central nervous system are likely to
increase chlorpromazine's sedative properties.

SPECIAL PRECAUTIONS

Be sure to tell your doctor if:
◆ You have long-term liver or kidney problems.
◆ You have had heart problems.
◆ You have had epileptic fits.
◆ You have thyroid disease.
◆ You have Parkinson's disease.
◆ You have glaucoma.
◆ You are taking other medications.

Pregnancy Not usually prescribed. If taken near the time of delivery, it can prolong labour and may cause drowsiness in the newborn baby. Discuss with your doctor.

Breast-feeding The drug passes into the breast milk and may affect the baby. Discuss with your doctor.

Infants and children Not recommended for infants under 1 year. Reduced dose necessary for older children.

Over 60 Initial dosage is low; it may be increased if there are no adverse reactions (such as abnormal limb movements or low blood pressure).

Driving and hazardous work Avoid such activities until you have learned how chlorpromazine affects you as the drug can cause drowsiness and slowed reactions.

Alcohol Avoid excessive amounts. Alcohol may increase the sedative effects of this drug.

Surgery and general anaesthetics Chlorpromazine treatment may need to be stopped before you have a general anaesthetic. Discuss this with your doctor or dentist before any operation.

PROLONGED USE
If used for more than a few months, chlorpromazine may cause movement disorders. Occasionally, jaundice may occur due to an allergic effect of the drug.

Chorionic gonadotrophin

Brand names Choragon, Pregnyl, Profasi
Used in the following combined preparations
None

QUICK REFERENCE
Drug group Drug for infertility (p.109)
Overdose danger rating Low
Dependence rating Low
Prescription needed Yes
Available as generic No

GENERAL INFORMATION
Produced by the placenta, human chorionic gonadotrophin (HCG) is a hormone that stimulates the ovaries to produce two other hormones, oestrogen and progesterone, that are essential to the conception and early growth of the fetus. The hormone is extracted from the urine of pregnant women and has several medical purposes.

The principal value is in the treatment of female infertility. Given by injection, usually with another hormone, HCG encourages the ovaries to release an egg (ovulation) so that it can be fertilized. Ovulation usually occurs 18 hours after injection, and intercourse should follow within 48 hours. The likelihood of multiple births increases because several eggs may be released by the ovaries at once.

In rare cases the drug is also given to young boys to treat undescended testes.

The drug is occasionally given to men to improve sperm production; treatment may take as long as 6 to 9 months.

INFORMATION FOR USERS
This drug is given only under medical supervision and is not for self-administration.

How taken Injection.
Frequency and timing of doses 1–3 x per week.
Dosage range Dosage varies from person to person, and may need adjustment during treatment.
Onset of effect *Female infertility* 1–8 days. *Male infertility* 6–9 months.
Duration of action 2–3 days.
Diet advice None.
Storage Not applicable. This drug is not kept in the home.
Missed dose Arrange to receive the missed dose as soon as possible. More than 24 hours' delay may reduce the chance of conception.
Stopping the drug Complete the course of treatment as directed. Stopping the drug prematurely reduces the chance of conception.
Exceeding the dose The drug is always injected under close medical supervision. Overdose is unlikely.

POSSIBLE ADVERSE EFFECTS
When HCG is taken for fertility problems, the more common adverse effects, including headache, tiredness, and mood changes, are rarely severe and tend to diminish with time. Women who take large doses may experience abdominal pain or swelling due to overstimulation of the ovaries. Men may experience breast enlargement and swollen ankles and should consult their doctor.

INTERACTIONS
None.

SPECIAL PRECAUTIONS
Be sure to tell your doctor if:
◆ You have a long-term kidney problem.
◆ You have asthma.
◆ You have had epileptic fits.
◆ You suffer from migraine.
◆ You have a heart disorder.
◆ You have had a previous allergic reaction to this drug.
◆ You have prostate trouble.
◆ You are taking other medications.

Pregnancy Not prescribed.

Breast-feeding Not prescribed.

Infants and children HCG is safely prescribed to treat undescended testes in boys.

Over 60 Not usually required.

Driving and hazardous work Usually no problems, but the drug can cause tiredness.

Alcohol Avoid excessive amounts. Alcohol increases tiredness and, if taken in excess, may reduce fertility.

PROLONGED USE
No special problems.

Monitoring Women taking HCG to improve fertility usually have regular pelvic examinations and checks on cervical mucus to confirm that ovulation is taking place. Men are given regular sperm counts.

Ciclosporin

Brand names Neoral, Sandimmun, SangCya
Used in the following combined preparations None

QUICK REFERENCE
Drug group Immunosuppressant drug (p.99)
Overdose danger rating Medium
Dependence rating Low
Prescription needed Yes
Available as generic No

GENERAL INFORMATION
Introduced in 1984, ciclosporin is one of the immunosuppressants, a group of drugs that suppress the body's natural defences against infection and foreign cells. This action is of particular use following organ transplants, when the recipient's immune system may reject the transplanted organ unless the immune system is controlled.

Ciclosporin is widely used following many types of transplant, such as those of the heart, bone marrow, kidney, liver, and pancreas. The drug's use has considerably reduced the risk of rejection. Ciclosporin is also sometimes used to treat rheumatoid arthritis, some severe types of dermatitis, and severe psoriasis when other treatments have failed.

Because ciclosporin reduces the immune system's effectiveness, people taking it are more susceptible than usual to infections. The drug can also cause high blood pressure and kidney damage.

Different brands of ciclosporin may reach different levels in your blood. It is important to know which brand you are taking. Do not try to make dose changes on your own. Ask your pharmacist for a patient information leaflet on the product you are taking.

INFORMATION FOR USERS
Your drug prescription is tailored for you. Do not alter dosage without checking with your doctor.

How taken Capsules, liquid, injection.

Frequency and timing of doses 1–2 x daily. The liquid can be mixed with water, apple juice, or orange juice just before taking. Do not mix with grapefruit juice.

Dosage range Dosage is calculated on an individual basis according to age and weight.

Onset of effect Within 12 hours.

Duration of action Up to 3 days.

Diet advice Avoid high-potassium foods, such as bananas and tomatoes, and potassium supplements. Avoid grapefruit juice.

Storage Capsules should be left in the blister pack until required. Keep in a closed container in a cool, dry place out of reach of children. Do not refrigerate.

Missed dose Take as soon as you remember. If your dose is more than 36 hours late, consult your doctor.

Stopping the drug Do not stop taking the drug without consulting your doctor. Stopping the drug may lead to transplant rejection.

Exceeding the dose An occasional unintentional extra dose is unlikely to cause any problems. Large overdoses, however, may cause vomiting and diarrhoea and may affect kidney function; notify your doctor.

POSSIBLE ADVERSE EFFECTS

The most common adverse effects are gum swelling, excessive growth of body hair, nausea and vomiting, tremor, and high blood pressure. Headache and muscle cramps may also occur. Less common effects are diarrhoea, facial swelling, flushing, "pins and needles" sensation, rash, and itching.

INTERACTIONS

General note Ciclosporin may interact with a large number of drugs. Check with your doctor or pharmacist before taking any new prescription or over-the-counter medications. Grapefuit juice can increase blood levels of ciclosporin. Avoid grapefruit flesh and juice for 1 hour before taking ciclosporin.

SPECIAL PRECAUTIONS

Ciclosporin is prescribed only under close medical supervision, taking account of your present condition and medical history.

Pregnancy Not usually prescribed. Safety in pregnancy not established. Discuss with your doctor.

Breast-feeding Not recommended. Safety in breast-feeding not established. The drug passes into the breast milk and may affect the baby. Discuss with your doctor.

Infants and children Safety not established. The drug is used only with great caution to treat infants and children.

Over 60 Reduced dose may be necessary.

Driving and hazardous work No known problems.

Alcohol No known problems.

Sunlight Avoid prolonged, unprotected exposure to sunlight.

PROLONGED USE

Long-term use, especially in high doses, can affect kidney and/or liver function. It may reduce numbers of white blood cells, thus increasing susceptibility to infection.

Monitoring Regular blood tests should be carried out as well as tests for liver and kidney function. Blood levels of ciclosporin should also be checked regularly.

Cimetidine

Brand names Acid-Eze, Acitak, Dyspamet, Galenamet, Peptimax, Tagamet, Zita
Used in the following combined preparations
None

QUICK REFERENCE

Drug group Anti-ulcer drug (p.43)
Overdose danger rating Low
Dependence rating Low
Prescription needed No (some preparations)
Available as generic Yes

GENERAL INFORMATION

Introduced in the 1970s, cimetidine was the first of a new group of anti-ulcer drugs. It reduces secretion of gastric acid and pepsin, an enzyme that helps in the digestion of protein. By reducing levels of acid and pepsin, it promotes ulcer healing in the stomach and duodenum. It is also used for reflux oesophagitis, in which acid stomach contents may flow up the oesophagus. Treatment is usually given in four- to eight-week courses, with further short courses if symptoms recur.

Cimetidine also affects the actions of certain enzymes in the liver, where many drugs are broken down. It is therefore prescribed with caution to people who are receiving other drugs, particularly anticoagulants and anticonvulsants, whose levels need to be carefully controlled. Since cimetidine promotes healing of the stomach lining, it may mask the symptoms of stomach cancer and delay diagnosis. It is therefore prescribed with caution if symptoms persist.

INFORMATION FOR USERS

Follow instructions on the label. Call your doctor if symptoms worsen.

How taken Tablets, liquid, injection.
Frequency and timing of doses 1–4 x daily (after meals and at bedtime).
Adult dosage range 800–1,600mg daily (occasionally increased to 2,400mg daily).
Onset of effect Within 90 minutes.
Duration of action 2–6 hours.
Diet advice None.
Storage Keep in a closed container in a cool, dry place out of reach of children. Protect from light.

Missed dose Do not take the missed dose. Take your next dose as usual.

Stopping the drug If cimetidine has been prescribed by your doctor, do not stop taking the drug without consulting him or her, unless a rash occurs; if you stop, symptoms may recur.

Exceeding the dose An occasional unintentional extra dose is unlikely to be a cause for concern. But if you notice any unusual symptoms, or if a large overdose has been taken, notify your doctor.

POSSIBLE ADVERSE EFFECTS

Adverse effects of cimetidine are uncommon but include diarrhoea and dizziness, confusion and tiredness. They are usually related to dosage level and almost always disappear when the drug is stopped. Muscle pain may occur. Men may suffer from impotence and breast enlargement. If any of these symptoms occur, seek medical advice. If you develop a rash, stop taking the drug and consult your doctor.

INTERACTIONS

Benzodiazepines Cimetidine may increase the blood levels of some of these drugs, increasing the risk of adverse effects.

Theophylline/aminophylline Cimetidine may increase the blood levels of theophylline/aminophylline, and their dose may need to be reduced.

Sildenafil Cimetidine may increase the blood level of this drug.

Beta blockers and anti-arrhythmic drugs Cimetidine may increase the blood levels of these drugs.

Anticonvulsant drugs Cimetidine may increase the blood levels of these drugs, and their dose may need to be reduced.

Anticoagulant drugs Cimetidine may increase the effect of anticoagulants, and their dose may need to be reduced.

SPECIAL PRECAUTIONS

Be sure to consult your doctor or pharmacist before taking this drug if:
◆ You have long-term liver or kidney problems.
◆ You are taking other medications.
Pregnancy Safety in pregnancy not established. Discuss with your doctor.

Breast-feeding The drug passes into the breast milk, but at normal doses adverse effects on the baby are unlikely. Discuss with your doctor.

Infants and children Reduced dose necessary.

Over 60 No special problems unless kidney function is reduced. Risk of stomach cancer is higher in elderly people and must be excluded before cimetidine is prescribed.

Driving and hazardous work No special problems.

Alcohol Avoid. Alcohol may aggravate the underlying condition and counter the beneficial effects of cimetidine.

PROLONGED USE

Courses of longer than 8 weeks are not usually necessary.

Cinnarizine

Brand names Cinaziere, Stugeron, Stugeron Forte
Used in the following combined preparations None

QUICK REFERENCE

Drug group Antihistamine anti-emetic drug (p.21)
Overdose danger rating Medium
Dependence rating Low
Prescription needed No
Available as generic Yes

GENERAL INFORMATION

Introduced in the 1970s, cinnarizine is an antihistamine drug used mainly to control nausea and vomiting, especially motion sickness. It is also used to control the symptoms (nausea and vertigo) of inner ear disorders such as labyrinthitis and Ménière's disease.

Taken in high doses, cinnarizine has a vasodilator effect and is used to improve circulation in Raynaud's disease and peripheral vascular disease.

Cinnarizine has adverse effects similar to those of most other antihistamines. Drowsiness, the most common problem, is usually less severe than with other antihistamines.

INFORMATION FOR USERS

Follow instructions on the label. Call your doctor if symptoms worsen.

How taken Tablets, capsules.

Frequency and timing of doses 2–3 x daily. For the prevention of motion sickness, the first dose should be taken 2 hours before you are due to travel.

Dosage range *Adults* 45–90mg daily (nausea/vomiting); 150–225mg daily (circulatory disorders); 30mg, then 15mg every 8 hours as needed (motion sickness). *Children aged 5–12* 15mg, then 7.5mg every 8 hours as needed (motion sickness).

Onset of effect Within 30 minutes. Several weeks (circulation diseases).

Duration of action Up to 8 hours.

Diet advice None.

Storage Keep in a closed container in a cool, dry place out of reach of children.

Missed dose Take as soon as you remember. If your next dose is due within 2 hours, take a single dose now and skip the next.

Stopping the drug If you are taking cinnarizine for an inner ear disorder or circulatory condition, do not stop taking it without consulting your doctor, unless a rash occurs; symptoms may recur. When taken for motion sickness, the drug can be safely stopped as soon as you no longer need it.

Exceeding the dose An occasional unintentional extra dose is unlikely to cause problems. Large overdoses, however, may cause drowsiness or agitation; notify your doctor.

POSSIBLE ADVERSE EFFECTS

Drowsiness or lethargy are the main adverse effects of cinnarizine. Anticholinergic (see Autonomic nervous system, p.8) effects, such as blurred vision and dry mouth, may also occur occasionally. If you develop a rash, stop taking the drug and consult your doctor.

INTERACTIONS

General note All drugs that have a sedative effect on the central nervous system, including sleeping drugs, antidepressants, antianxiety drugs, and opioid analgesics, may increase cinnarizine's sedative properties.

SPECIAL PRECAUTIONS

Be sure to consult your doctor or pharmacist before taking this drug if:
◆ You have low blood pressure.
◆ You have porphyria.
◆ You have glaucoma.
◆ You have an enlarged prostate.
◆ You are taking other medications.

Pregnancy Safety in pregnancy not established. Discuss with your doctor.

Breast-feeding Safety not established. Discuss with your doctor.

Infants and children Reduced dose necessary.

Over 60 No special problems.

Driving and hazardous work Avoid such activities until you have learned how cinnarizine affects you because the drug can cause drowsiness.

Alcohol Avoid. Alcohol may increase the sedative effects of this drug.

PROLONGED USE

Development or aggravation of extrapyramidal symptoms (abnormal movements) may occur, rarely, in elderly people after prolonged use of cinnarizine.

Ciprofibrate

Brand name Modalim
Used in the following combined preparations
None

QUICK REFERENCE

Drug group Lipid-lowering drug (p.37)
Overdose danger rating Low
Dependence rating Low
Prescription needed Yes
Available as generic No

GENERAL INFORMATION

Ciprofibrate belongs to a group of drugs called fibrates, which are used to treat high lipid (fat) levels in the blood (hyperlipidaemia). These drugs are particularly effective in reducing the level of triglycerides in the blood, and they also lower cholesterol levels.

Hyperlipidaemia is associated with atherosclerosis (deposition of fat in the walls of blood vessels. This can lead to coronary heart disease (for example, angina and heart attacks) and cerebrovascular disease (for example, stroke). When ciprofibrate is combined with a diet that is low in saturated fats, there is good evidence that the risk of coronary heart disease is reduced.

INFORMATION FOR USERS

Your drug prescription is tailored for you. Do not alter dosage without checking with your doctor.

How taken Tablets.

Frequency and timing of doses Once daily.

Adult dosage range 100mg daily.

Onset of effect A reduction in blood lipid levels occurs within 4 weeks of starting treatment.

Duration of action Several days.

Diet advice A low-fat diet may be recommended. Follow the advice of your doctor or dietitian.

Storage Keep in a closed container in a cool dry place out of the reach of children.

Missed dose Do not take the missed dose. Take your next dose at the usual time.

Stopping the drug Do not stop the drug without consulting your doctor.

Exceeding the dose An occasional unintentional extra dose is unlikely to be a cause for concern. But if you notice unusual symptoms, notify your doctor.

POSSIBLE ADVERSE EFFECTS

The most common adverse effects are those involving the gastrointestinal system, such as nausea, vomiting, diarrhoea, and indigestion. These effects are usually mild and tend to diminish as treatment continues. If the symptoms are severe, seek medical advice. If you develop a rash or headache, consult your doctor. If muscle pain, weakness, or cramps develop, seek medical attention without delay.

INTERACTIONS

Anticoagulants Ciprofibrate may increase the effect of anticoagulants such as warfarin.

Lipid-lowering drugs Use of these drugs with ciprofibrate may increase the risk of muscle problems.

Antidiabetic drugs Ciprofibrate may interact with antidiabetic drugs to lower blood glucose levels.

SPECIAL PRECAUTIONS

Be sure to tell your doctor if:
◆ You have long-term liver or kidney problems.
◆ You have thyroid problems.
◆ You are taking other medications.

Pregnancy Safety in pregnancy not established. Discuss with your doctor.

Breast-feeding Safety in breast-feeding not established. Discuss with your doctor.

Infants and children Not recommended.

Over 60 No special problems, but poor kidney function may require dose adjustment.

Driving and hazardous work No special problems.

Alcohol No special problems.

PROLONGED USE

No problems expected, but patients with kidney disease will need special care as there is a high risk of muscle problems developing.

Monitoring Blood tests will be carried out to monitor the effect of the drug on lipid levels in the blood and also to check liver function.

Ciprofloxacin

Brand name Ciproxin
Used in the following combined preparations
None

QUICK REFERENCE

Drug group Antibacterial (p.66)
Overdose danger rating Medium
Dependence rating Low
Prescription needed Yes
Available as generic Yes

GENERAL INFORMATION

Ciprofloxacin, a quinolone antibacterial, is used to treat several types of bacteria resistant to other commonly used antibiotics. It is especially useful for intestine and urinary tract infections and is also used to treat gonorrhoea.

When it is taken by mouth, ciprofloxacin is well absorbed by the body and works quickly and effectively. In more severe systemic bacterial infections, however, it may be necessary to administer the drug by injection. Ciprofloxacin has a long duration of action and needs to be taken only once or twice daily.

INFORMATION FOR USERS

Your drug prescription is tailored for you. Do not alter dosage without checking with your doctor.

How taken Tablets, liquid, injection.

Frequency and timing of doses 2 x daily with plenty of fluids.

Adult dosage range 500mg–1.5g daily (tablets); 200–400mg daily (injection).

Onset of effect Within a few hours; full beneficial effect may not be felt for several days.

Duration of action About 12 hours.

Diet advice Do not get dehydrated; ensure that you drink fluids regularly.

Storage Keep in a closed container in a cool, dry place out of reach of children. The injection must be protected from light.

Missed dose Take as soon as you remember, and take your next dose as usual.

Stopping the drug Unless severe adverse effects occur (see below), take the full course. Even if you feel better the original infection may still be present, and symptoms may recur if treatment is stopped too soon.

Exceeding the dose An occasional unintentional extra dose is unlikely to cause problems. Large overdoses, however, may cause mental disturbance and fits; notify your doctor.

POSSIBLE ADVERSE EFFECTS

Ciprofloxacin commonly causes nausea, vomiting, abdominal pain, diarrhoea, rash, and itching. Other side effects are less common, except when very high doses are given. These include dizziness, confusion, sleep disturbance, and photosensitivity. Convulsions and painful or inflamed tendons should be reported to your doctor at once, the drug stopped, and the affected limbs rested.

INTERACTIONS

Oral iron preparations and antacids containing magnesium or aluminium hydroxide interfere with absorption of ciprofloxacin. Do not take antacids within 2 hours of taking ciprofloxacin tablets.

Anticoagulants and oral antidiabetics Ciprofloxacin may increase blood levels of these drugs; their dosage may need to be adjusted.

Theophylline Ciprofloxacin may increase the blood levels of this drug; its dose may need to be adjusted and its blood levels monitored.

Phenytoin Ciprofloxacin may increase blood levels of this drug.

NSAIDs Taken with ciprofloxacin, these drugs increase the risk of epileptic fits.

SPECIAL PRECAUTIONS

Be sure to tell your doctor if:

◆ You have long-term liver or kidney problems.

◆ You have had epileptic fits.

◆ You have glucose-6-phosphate dehydrogenase (G6PD) deficiency.

◆ You are taking other medications.

Pregnancy Safety in pregnancy not established. Discuss with your doctor.

Breast-feeding The drug passes into the breast milk and may affect the baby adversely. Discuss with your doctor.

Infants and children Ciprofloxacin is not usually recommended.

Over 60 The drug may make elderly people more susceptible to tendinitis.

Driving and hazardous work Avoid such activities until you have learned how ciprofloxacin affects you because it can cause dizziness.

Alcohol Avoid. Alcohol may increase the sedative effects of this drug.

Sunlight Avoid excessive exposure.

PROLONGED USE

No problems expected.

Monitoring Blood tests may be necessary to monitor kidney and liver function.

Cisplatin

Brand names None
Used in the following combined preparations None

QUICK REFERENCE

Drug group Anticancer drug (p.96)
Overdose danger rating High
Dependence rating Low
Prescription needed Yes
Available as generic Yes

GENERAL INFORMATION

Cisplatin is one of the most effective drugs available to treat a wide variety of cancers including those of the ovaries, testes, head, neck, bladder, cervix, and lung. The drug is also used in the treatment of certain children's cancers and some cancers of the blood. It is usually given together with other anticancer drugs.

The most common and serious adverse effect of cisplatin is impaired kidney function.

To reduce the risk of permanent kidney damage, the drug is usually given only once every three weeks, which allows the kidneys time to recover between courses of treatment. Nausea and vomiting may occur following administration. These symptoms usually start within an hour and last for up to 24 hours. In some cases, they can persist for up to a week, and because they may be quite severe, antiemetic drugs are given to reduce them.

Damage to hearing is common and may be more severe in children. Use of cisplatin may also increase the risk of anaemia, blood clotting disorders, and infection during treatment. Some of the drug's unwanted effects may be avoided by using carboplatin instead.

INFORMATION FOR USERS

This drug is given only under medical supervision and is not for self-administration.

How taken Injection.

Frequency and timing of doses Every 3 weeks for up to 5 days; it may be given alone or in combination with other anticancer drugs.

Adult dosage range Dosage is determined individually according to body height, weight, and response.

Onset of effect Some adverse effects, such as nausea and vomiting, may appear within 1 hour of starting treatment.

Duration of action Some adverse effects may last up to 1 week after treatment has stopped.

Diet advice Prior to treatment it is important that the body is well hydrated. Therefore, 1–2 litres of fluid are usually given by infusion over 8–12 hours.

Storage Not applicable. The drug is not normally kept in the home.

Missed dose Not applicable. Cisplatin is given only in hospital under medical supervision.

Stopping the drug Not applicable. The drug will be stopped under medical supervision.

Exceeding the dose Overdosage is unlikely since treatment is carefully monitored, and the drug is only given intravenously.

POSSIBLE ADVERSE EFFECTS

Most adverse effects, such as nausea, vomiting, loss of appetite or taste, ringing in the ears, and hearing loss, appear within a few hours of injection and will be carefully monitored in hospital after each dose. Some wear off within 24 hours. Nausea and appetite loss may last for up to a week. Your doctor will monitor you for effects causing hearing loss, rash, wheezing, or abnormal sensations.

INTERACTIONS

General note Several drugs (for example, antibacterials such as gentamicin) increase the adverse effects of cisplatin. Because cisplatin is given only under close medical supervision, these interactions are carefully monitored and the dosage is adjusted accordingly.

SPECIAL PRECAUTIONS

Cisplatin is prescribed only under close medical supervision, taking account of your present condition and your medical history.

Pregnancy Not usually prescribed. Cisplatin may cause birth defects or premature birth. Discuss with your doctor.

Breast-feeding Not advised. The drug passes into the breast milk and may affect the baby adversely. Discuss with your doctor.

Infants and children The risk of hearing loss is increased. Reduced dose used.

Over 60 A reduced dose may be needed. There is an increased likelihood of adverse effects.

Driving and hazardous work No known problems.

Alcohol No known problems.

PROLONGED USE

Prolonged use increases the risk of damage to the kidneys, nerves, and bone marrow, and to the hearing.

Monitoring Hearing tests and blood checks to monitor kidney function and bone marrow activity are carried out regularly.

Citalopram

Brand name Cipramil
Used in the following combined preparations
None

QUICK REFERENCE
Drug group Antidepressant drug (p.14)
Overdose danger rating Medium
Dependence rating Low
Prescription needed Yes
Available as generic No

GENERAL INFORMATION

Citalopram is a member of the selective sero-tonin re-uptake inhibitor (SSRI) group of antidepressant drugs. It is used for depressive illness and panic disorder. The drug gradually improves mood, increases physical activity, and restores interest in everyday activities.

Citalopram is generally well tolerated. It may sometimes produce gastrointestinal adverse effects, such as nausea, vomiting, or diarrhoea, but these effects are related to the dose and usually diminish with continued use of the drug.

Like other SSRIs, citalopram causes fewer anticholinergic (see Autonomic nervous system, p.8) side effects, and it is less sedating, than the tricyclic antidepressants. It is also less likely to be harmful if it is taken in overdose. The drug can, however, cause drowsiness and can impair the performance of tasks such as driving.

INFORMATION FOR USERS

Your drug prescription is tailored for you. Do not alter dosage without checking with your doctor.

How taken Tablets, oral drops.

Frequency and timing of doses Once daily in the morning or evening.

Adult dosage range *Depressive illness* 20–60mg. *Panic attacks* 10mg (starting dose); 20–30mg (usual range).

Onset of effect Some benefit may appear within 7 days, but full benefits may not be felt for 2–4 weeks.

Duration of action Antidepressant effect may persist for some weeks following prolonged treatment.

Diet advice None.

Storage Keep in a closed container in a cool, dry place out of reach of children.

Missed dose Take as soon as you remember. If your next dose is due within 8 hours, take a single dose now and skip the next.

Stopping the drug Unless severe adverse effects occur (see below), do not stop taking citalopram without consulting your doctor. Stopping the drug abruptly can cause withdrawal symptoms.

Exceeding the dose An occasional unintentional extra dose is unlikely to be a cause for concern. But if you notice any unusual symptoms, or if a large overdose has been taken, notify your doctor.

POSSIBLE ADVERSE EFFECTS

Common adverse effects, such as nausea, vomiting, indigestion, and diarrhoea, usually diminish with a reduction in dosage. Some people may experience a dry mouth, sweating, anxiety, insomnia, headache, tremor, or drowsiness. If palpitations or rapid heart rate, confusion, convulsions, or rash occur, however, stop taking the drug and consult your doctor urgently.

INTERACTIONS

Sumatriptan and other 5HT$_1$ agonists, and lithium There is an increased risk of adverse effects when citalopram is taken with these drugs.

Terfenadine The risk of arrhythmias (abnormal heart rhythms) is increased when this drug is taken with citalopram.

MAOIs These drugs may cause a severe reaction if taken with citalopram; avoid citalopram if MAOIs have been taken in the last 14 days.

Anticoagulants The effect of these drugs may be increased by citalopram.

SPECIAL PRECAUTIONS

Be sure to tell your doctor if:
◆ You have epilepsy.
◆ You have liver or kidney problems.
◆ You have had a manic-depressive illness.
◆ You have had heart problems.
◆ You have been taking MAOIs or other antidepressants.
◆ You are taking other medications.

Pregnancy Safety in pregnancy not established. Discuss with your doctor.

Breast-feeding The drug may pass into breast milk and may affect the baby. Discuss with your doctor.

Infants and children Not recommended.

Over 60 Reduced dose necessary.

Driving and hazardous work Avoid such activities until you have learned how citalopram affects you because it can cause drowsiness.

Alcohol No special problems.

PROLONGED USE

No problems expected. However, mild withdrawal symptoms may occur if the drug is not stopped gradually.

Clarithromycin

Brand names Klaricid, Klaricid XL
Used in the following combined preparations
None

QUICK REFERENCE

Drug group Antibiotic (p.62)
Overdose danger rating Low
Dependence rating Low
Prescription needed Yes
Available as generic No

GENERAL INFORMATION

Clarithromycin is a macrolide antibiotic drug that is similar to erythromycin (see p.235), from which it is derived. It has similar actions and uses to erythromycin, but is slightly more active.

Clarithromycin is used to treat upper respiratory tract infections, such as middle ear infections, sinusitis, and pharyngitis, and lower respiratory tract infections, including whooping cough, bronchitis, and pneumonia. It is also used to treat skin and soft tissue infections, including gonorrhoea. In addition, given with anti-ulcer drugs (see p.43) and other antibiotics, clarithromycin is used to eradicate *Helicobacter pylori*, the bacterium that causes many peptic ulcers.

INFORMATION FOR USERS

Your drug prescription is tailored for you. Do not alter dosage without checking with your doctor.
How taken Tablets, liquid, granules, injection.
Frequency and timing of doses 2 x daily, up to 14 days.
Adult dosage range 500mg–1g daily.
Onset of effect 1–4 hours.
Duration of action 1–12 hours.
Diet advice None.
Storage Keep in a closed container in a cool, dry place out of the reach of children. Protect from light.
Missed dose Take as soon as you remember. If your next dose is due within 2 hours, take a single dose now and skip the next.
Stopping the drug Take the full course. Even if you feel better, the infection may still be present and symptoms may recur if treatment is stopped too soon.

Exceeding the dose An occasional unintentional extra dose is unlikely to be a cause for concern. But if you notice any unusual symptoms, or if a large overdose has been taken, notify your doctor.

POSSIBLE ADVERSE EFFECTS

Clarithromycin is generally well tolerated. Gastrointestinal disturbances such as indigestion nausea, vomiting, and diarrhoea are the most common problems, along with headache, and joint and muscle pain. Rash is also common but should always be discussed with your doctor. Hearing loss is a rare possibility, but it is usually reversible on stopping the drug. If there are signs of an altered sense of taste or smell, anxiety and insomnia, confusion and hallucinations, consult your doctor. If you show signs of jaundice, stop taking the drug and seek immediate medical advice.

INTERACTIONS

Warfarin, midazolam, disopyramide, rifabutin, phenytoin, ciclosporin, and tacrolimus Blood levels and effects of these drugs are increased by clarithromycin.
Carbamazepine, theophylline, and digoxin The blood levels and toxicity of these drugs are increased by clarithromycin.
Zidovudine Blood levels of zidovudine are reduced if this drug is taken at the same time as clarithromycin.
Ergot derivatives There is an increased risk of ergot toxicity if these drugs are taken with clarithromycin.
Pimozide and terfenadine These drugs may cause cardiac arrhythmias (abnormal heart rhythms) if taken with clarithromycin.
Lipid-lowering drugs whose names end in "statin" If these drugs are taken with clarithromycin, there is a risk of rhabdomyolysis (muscle damage).

SPECIAL PRECAUTIONS

Be sure to tell your doctor if:
◆ You have liver or kidney problems.
◆ You have had an allergic reaction to erythromycin or clarithromycin.
◆ You have a heart problem.
◆ You have porphyria.
◆ You are taking other medications.

Pregnancy Safety in pregnancy not established. Discuss with your doctor.

Breast-feeding Clarithromycin passes into the breast milk and may affect the baby. Discuss with your doctor.

Infants and children Reduced dose necessary.

Over 60 No special problems.

Driving and hazardous work No known problems.

Alcohol No known problems.

PROLONGED USE

Prolonged use of clarithromycin is not usually necessary. In courses of over 14 days, there is a risk of developing antibiotic-resistant infections.

Clobetasol

Brand name Dermovate
Used in the following combined preparation
Dermovate-NN

QUICK REFERENCE

Drug group Topical corticosteroid (p.120)
Overdose danger rating Low
Dependence rating Low
Prescription needed Yes
Available as generic No

GENERAL INFORMATION

Clobetasol is a corticosteroid drug (see p.80) used in the short-term treatment of severe skin conditions such as discoid lupus erythematosus, lichen planus and lichen simplex, eczema, and psoriasis. The drug is generally considered the strongest topical corticosteroid and is therefore used only when the disorder has not responded to treatment with another topical corticosteroid.

It is important to apply clobetasol thinly and sparingly to affected areas because it can cause systemic adverse effects such as pituitary and adrenal gland suppression and Cushing's syndrome. Other effects include irreversible structural changes to the skin in treated areas. In addition, the drug can exacerbate eczema infected with a virus such as herpes simplex.

Treatment of psoriasis with clobetasol must only be carried out with specialist care and supervision.

INFORMATION FOR USERS

Your drug prescription is tailored for you. Do not alter dosage without checking with your doctor.

How taken Cream, ointment, scalp application.

Frequency and timing of doses 1 x 2 times daily. If treating the face, use for no more than 5 days.

Dosage range No more than 50g weekly.

Onset of effect 12 hours. Full beneficial effect after 48 hours.

Duration of action Up to 24 hours.

Diet advice None.

Storage Keep in a closed container, in a cool, dry place out of reach of children.

Missed dose Use as soon as you remember. If your next application is due within 8 hours, apply the usual amount now and skip the next application.

Stopping the drug Do not stop using the drug without consulting your doctor; symptoms may recur.

Exceeding the dose An occasional unintentional extra application is unlikely to cause problems. But if you notice any unusual symptoms, notify your doctor.

POSSIBLE ADVERSE EFFECTS

Most people who use clobetasol as directed have no problems. Adverse effects, including thinning of the skin, stretch marks, and loss of pigmentation, mainly affect the skin when high doses are used; some cannot be reversed. Mood changes, high blood pressure, and weight gain may occur if the drug is used in high doses and is absorbed through the skin.

INTERACTIONS

None.

SPECIAL PRECAUTIONS

Be sure to tell your doctor if:
◆ You have a cold sore or chickenpox.
◆ You have any other infection.
◆ You have psoriasis.
◆ You have acne or rosacea.
◆ You are taking other medications.

Pregnancy Safety in pregnancy not established. Discuss with your doctor.

Breast-feeding The drug passes into the breast milk and may affect the baby. Discuss with your doctor.

Infants and children Not recommended for infants under 1 year. Used only with great caution for short periods in older children because overuse can slow growth.
Over 60 No special problems.
Driving and hazardous work No special problems.
Alcohol No special problems.

PROLONGED USE

Clobetasol is not normally used for more than 4 weeks. If the condition has not improved in 2 to 4 weeks, notify your doctor.

Clomifene

Brand name Clomid
Used in the following combined preparations
None

QUICK REFERENCE

Drug group Drug for infertility (p.109)
Overdose danger rating Low
Dependence rating Low
Prescription needed Yes
Available as generic Yes

GENERAL INFORMATION

Clomifene increases the output of hormones by the pituitary gland, thereby stimulating ovulation (egg release) in women. If hormone levels in the blood fail to rise after clomifene is taken, the pituitary gland is not working as it should.

For the treatment of female infertility, tablets are taken within about 5 days of the onset of each menstrual cycle. This stimulates ovulation. If the drug has not stimulated ovulation after several months, other drugs may be prescribed.

Multiple pregnancies (usually twins) occur more commonly in women treated with clomifene than in those who have not been treated. Adverse effects include an increased risk of ovarian cysts and ectopic pregnancy.

INFORMATION FOR USERS

Your drug prescription is tailored for you. Do not alter dosage without checking with your doctor.
How taken Tablets.

Frequency and timing of doses Once daily for 5 days during each menstrual cycle.
Dosage range 50mg daily initially; dose may be increased up to 100mg daily.
Onset of effect Ovulation occurs 4–10 days after the last dose in any cycle. However, ovulation may not occur for several months.
Duration of action 5 days.
Diet advice None.
Storage Keep in a closed container in a cool, dry place out of reach of children. Protect from light.
Missed dose Take as soon as you remember. If your next dose is due, take the missed dose and the next scheduled dose together.
Stopping the drug Unless severe adverse effects occur (see below), take as directed by your doctor. Stopping the drug will reduce the chances of conception.
Exceeding the dose An occasional unintentional extra dose is unlikely to be a cause for concern. But if you notice any unusual symptoms, or if a large overdose has been taken, notify your doctor.

POSSIBLE ADVERSE EFFECTS

Most side effects are dose-related. These include hot flushes, nausea, vomiting, "breakthrough" bleeding, abdominal discomfort and bloating, dizziness, and breast tenderness. Ovarian enlargement and cyst formation can occur, but this usually resolves within a few weeks of stopping the drug. If blurred vision, severe pain in the chest or abdomen, or convulsions occur, or a rash develops, stop taking the drug and consult your doctor.

INTERACTIONS

None.

SPECIAL PRECAUTIONS

Be sure to tell your doctor if:
◆ You have a long-term liver problem.
◆ You are taking other medications.
Pregnancy Not prescribed. The drug will be stopped as soon as pregnancy occurs.
Breast-feeding Not prescribed.
Infants and children Not prescribed.
Over 60 Not prescribed.
Driving and hazardous work No special problems.
Alcohol Keep consumption low.

PROLONGED USE

Prolonged use of clomifene may cause visual impairment. No more than 6 courses of treatment are recommended since further courses may lead to an increased risk of ovarian cancer.

Monitoring Eye tests may be recommended if symptoms of visual impairment are noticed. Monitoring of body temperature and blood or urine hormone levels is performed to detect signs of ovulation and pregnancy.

Clomipramine

Brand names Anafranil, Anafranil SR
Used in the following combined preparations
None

QUICK REFERENCE

Drug group Tricyclic antidepressant (p.14)
Overdose danger rating High
Dependence rating Low
Prescription needed Yes
Available as generic Yes

GENERAL INFORMATION

Clomipramine belongs to the class of antidepressant drugs known as the tricyclics. It is used mainly in the long-term treatment of depression. It elevates the patient's mood, improves appetite, increases physical activity, and restores interest in everyday activities.

Clomipramine is particularly useful in the treatment of obsessive and phobic disorders. In this case, the drug has to be taken for many weeks to achieve its full effect.

This drug has the same adverse effects as other tricyclic drugs, such as drowsiness, dizziness, dry mouth, and constipation. In overdose, clomipramine may cause coma and dangerously abnormal heart rhythms.

INFORMATION FOR USERS

Your drug prescription is tailored for you. Do not alter dosage without checking with your doctor.
How taken SR-tablets, capsules.
Frequency and timing of doses 1–4 x daily.
Adult dosage range 10–250mg daily.
Onset of effect Some effects may be felt within a few days, but full antidepressant effect may not be felt for up to 4 weeks. For phobic and obsessional disorders, full effect may take up to 12 week.
Duration of action Antidepressant effect may last up to 2 weeks (prolonged treatment).
Diet advice None.
Storage Keep in a closed container in a cool, dry place out of reach of children.
Missed dose Take as soon as you remember. If your next dose is due within 3 hours, take a single dose now and skip the next.
Stopping the drug Stopping the drug abruptly can cause withdrawal symptoms and recurrence of the original trouble. Consult your doctor, who may supervise a gradual reduction in dosage.

OVERDOSE ACTION

Seek immediate medical advice in all cases. Take emergency action if palpitations are noted or consciousness is lost.

POSSIBLE ADVERSE EFFECTS

Adverse effects are mainly due to the drug's anticholinergic (see Autonomic nervous system, p8) action, and include drowsiness and dizziness, dry mouth, constipation, blurred vision, and urinary difficulties. If you experience palpitations, consult your doctor urgently.

INTERACTIONS

Sedatives All drugs that have a sedative effect may intensify those of clomipramine.
Antihypertensives Clomipramine may enhance the effect of some of these drugs.
Anticonvulsants Clomipramine may reduce the effects of these drugs and vice versa.
MAOIs A serious reaction may occur if these drugs are given with clomipramine.
Quinidine Taken with clomipramine, this drug increases the risk of abnormal heart rhythms.

SPECIAL PRECAUTIONS

Be sure to tell your doctor if:
◆ You have heart problems.
◆ You have had epileptic fits.
◆ You have long-term liver or kidney problems.
◆ You have had glaucoma.
◆ You have thyroid disease.
◆ You have had prostate trouble.
◆ You have had mania or a psychotic illness.
◆ You are taking other medications.

Pregnancy Safety in pregnancy not established. Discuss with your doctor.

Breast-feeding The drug passes into the breast milk and may affect the baby. Discuss with your doctor.

Infants and children Not recommended.

Driving and hazardous work Avoid such activities until you have learned how clomipramine affects you because the drug may cause blurred vision, drowsiness, and dizziness.

Alcohol Avoid. Alcohol may increase the sedative effects of this drug.

Surgery and general anaesthetics Clomipramine treatment may need to be stopped before you have a general anaesthetic. Discuss this with your doctor or dentist before any operation.

PROLONGED USE

No problems expected.

Monitoring Regular checks on heart and liver function are recommended.

Clonazepam

Brand name Rivotril
Used in the following combined preparations
None

QUICK REFERENCE

Drug group Benzodiazepine anticonvulsant drug (p.16)

Overdose danger rating Medium

Dependence rating Medium

Prescription needed Yes

Available as generic No

GENERAL INFORMATION

Clonazepam belongs to a group of drugs known as the benzodiazepines. These drugs are mainly used as anti-anxiety drugs (see p.13) and sleeping drugs (see p.11). However, clonazepam is used almost exclusively as an anticonvulsant drug to prevent and treat epileptic fits.

The drug is particularly useful for the prevention of brief muscle spasms (myoclonus) and absence seizures (petit mal) in children, but other forms of epilepsy, such as sudden flaccidity or fits induced by flashing lights, also respond to clonazepam treatment. Being a benzodiazepine, the drug also has tranquillizing and sedative effects.

Clonazepam is used either alone or together with other anticonvulsant drugs. Its anticonvulsant effect may begin to wear off after some months.

INFORMATION FOR USERS

Your drug prescription is tailored for you. Do not alter dosage without checking with your doctor.

How taken Tablets, injection.

Frequency and timing of doses 1–3 x daily.

Dosage range *Adults* 1mg daily (starting dose), increased gradually to 4–8 mg daily (maintenance dose).
Children Reduced dose according to age and weight.

Onset of effect Within 1 hour.

Duration of action Approximately 30 hours.

Diet advice None.

Storage Keep in a closed container in a cool, dry place out of reach of children.

Missed dose No cause for concern, but take as soon as you remember. Take your next dose when it is due.

Stopping the drug Do not stop taking the drug without consulting your doctor because withdrawal symptoms may occur, and your illness may recur.

Exceeding the dose An occasional unintentional extra dose is unlikely to cause problems. Larger overdoses may cause unusual drowsiness and confusion; notify your doctor.

POSSIBLE ADVERSE EFFECTS

The principal adverse effects of this drug are related to its sedative and tranquillizing properties and include drowsiness, dizziness, forgetfulness, and muscle weakness. Increased salivation may also occur. These effects normally diminish after the first few days of treatment and can often be reduced by medically supervised adjustment of dosage.

INTERACTIONS

Sedatives All drugs that have a sedative effect on the central nervous system are likely to add to the sedative properties of clonazepam. Such drugs include anti-anxiety and sleeping drugs, antihistamines, opioid analgesics, antidepressants, and antipsychotics.

Other anticonvulsants Clonazepam may alter the effects of other anticonvulsants you are taking, or they may alter the effect of clonazepam. Adjustment in dosage or change of drug may be necessary.

SPECIAL PRECAUTIONS

Be sure to tell your doctor if:
◆ You have severe respiratory disease.
◆ You have long-term liver or kidney problems.
◆ You are taking other medications.
◆ You have had problems with drug or alcohol abuse.

Pregnancy Safety in pregnancy not established. Discuss with your doctor.

Breast-feeding The drug passes into the breast milk and may affect the baby adversely. Discuss with your doctor.

Infants and children Reduced dose necessary.

Over 60 Reduced dose may be necessary.

Driving and hazardous work Your underlying condition, as well as the possibility of drowsiness while taking clonazepam, may make such activities inadvisable. Discuss with your doctor.

Alcohol Avoid. Alcohol may increase the sedative effects of this drug.

PROLONGED USE

Both beneficial and adverse effects of clonazepam may become less marked during prolonged treatment with clonazepam as the body adapts to the drug.

Clopidogrel

Brand name Plavix
Used in the following combined preparations
None

QUICK REFERENCE

Drug group Antiplatelet drug (p.39)
Overdose danger rating Medium
Dependence rating Low
Prescription needed Yes
Available as generic No

GENERAL INFORMATION

Clopidogrel is an antiplatelet drug that is used to prevent blood clots from forming. It is prescribed to patients who have a tendency to develop clots in the fast-flowing blood of the arteries and heart, or those who have had a stroke or a heart attack.

Clopidogrel may be suitable for people who cannot take aspirin for its antiplatelet effects. The drug reduces the tendency of platelets to stick together when blood flow is disrupted. However, this can lead to abnormal bleeding. You should, therefore, report any unusual bleeding to your doctor immediately, and, if you require dental treatment, you should tell your dentist that you are taking clopidogrel.

Adverse effects are not common; they are usually associated with bleeding.

INFORMATION FOR USERS

Your drug prescription is tailored for you. Do not alter dosage without checking with your doctor.

How taken Tablets.
Frequency and timing of doses Once daily.
Dosage range 75mg.
Onset of effect 1 hour.
Duration of action 24 hours.
Diet advice None.
Storage Keep in a closed container in a cool, dry place out of reach of children.
Missed dose Take as soon as you remember. If your next dose is due within 4 hours, take a single dose now and skip the next.
Stopping the drug Unless you develop a sore throat or a bleeding problem, do not stop the drug without consulting your doctor.
Exceeding the dose An occasional unintentional extra dose is unlikely to be a cause for concern. But if you notice any unusual symptoms, or if a large overdose has been taken, notify your doctor.

POSSIBLE ADVERSE EFFECTS

The main adverse effects of clopidogrel are bruising and bleeding, such as nosebleeds, bleeding from a stomach ulcer, or blood in the urine. Report any unusual bleeding or bruising to your doctor without delay. Nausea, vomiting, abdominal pain, and diarrhoea are less common. Headache and dizziness may also occur. If you experience a rash or itching, seek medical advice. If you develop a sore throat, stop taking the drug and consult your doctor urgently.

INTERACTIONS

Aspirin and other NSAIDs Clopidogrel increases the effect of aspirin on platelets. The risk of gastrointestinal bleeding is increased when clopidogrel is used with NSAIDs.

Anticoagulant drugs (such as warfarin) The anticoagulant effect of these drugs is increased if they are taken with clopidogrel.

SPECIAL PRECAUTIONS

Be sure to tell your doctor if:
◆ You have liver or kidney problems.
◆ You have a condition, such as a peptic ulcer, that makes you more likely to bleed.
◆ You are taking other medications.
Pregnancy Safety in pregnancy not established. Discuss with your doctor.
Breast-feeding The drug passes into the breast milk and may affect the baby. Discuss with your doctor.
Infants and children Not recommended.
Over 60 No special problems.
Driving and hazardous work No special problems.
Alcohol Excessive alcohol intake may irritate the stomach and increase the risk of bleeding.
Surgery and general anaesthetics Clopidogrel may need to be stopped a week before surgery. Discuss with your doctor or dentist.

PROLONGED USE

No special problems.

Clotrimazole

Brand names Abtrim, Canesten, Candiden, Masnoderm
Used in the following combined preparations
Canesten HC, Lotriderm

QUICK REFERENCE

Drug group Antifungal drug (p.76)
Overdose danger rating Low
Dependence rating Low
Prescription needed Yes (for combined preparations)
Available as generic Yes

GENERAL INFORMATION

Clotrimazole is an antifungal drug commonly used to treat fungal and yeast infections. It is used for tinea (ringworm) of the skin, and candida (thrush) of the mouth, vagina, or penis. The drug is applied as a cream, spray, topical solution, or dusting powder on affected areas of skin and as pessaries or cream for vaginal conditions such as candida.

Adverse effects are very rare, but some people may experience burning and irritation of the skin at the site of application.

INFORMATION FOR USERS

Follow instructions on the label. Call your doctor if symptoms worsen.
How taken Pessaries, cream, spray, dusting powder, topical solution.
Frequency and timing of doses 2–3 x daily (skin cream, spray, solution); once daily at bedtime (pessaries); 1–2 x daily (vaginal cream).
Dosage range *Vaginal infections* One applicatorful (5g) per dose (vaginal cream); 100–500mg per dose (pessaries). *Skin infections* (skin cream, spray, solution) As directed.
Onset of effect Within 2–3 days.
Duration of action Up to 12 hours.
Diet advice None.
Storage Keep in a closed container in a cool, dry place out of reach of children.
Missed dose No cause for concern, but make up the missed dose or application as soon as you remember.
Stopping the drug Unless a rash occurs, apply the full course. Even if symptoms disappear, the original infection may still be present and may recur if treatment is stopped too soon.
Exceeding the dose An occasional unintentional extra dose is unlikely to cause problems. But if you notice unusual symptoms or if a large amount has been swallowed, notify your doctor.

POSSIBLE ADVERSE EFFECTS

Clotrimazole rarely causes adverse effects. However, skin and vaginal preparations may occasionally cause localized stinging or irritation. If a rash develops, stop using the drug.

INTERACTIONS

None known.

SPECIAL PRECAUTIONS

Be sure to tell your doctor or pharmacist if:
◆ You are taking other medications.
Pregnancy No evidence of risk to the developing baby, but use only on your doctor's advice.

Breast-feeding No evidence of risk.
Infants and children No special problems, but use of pessaries is not recommended.
Over 60 No special problems.
Driving and hazardous work No known problems.
Alcohol No known problems.

PROLONGED USE

No problems expected.

Clozapine

Brand name Clozaril
Used in the following combined preparations
None

QUICK REFERENCE

Drug group Antipsychotic drug (p.15)
Overdose danger rating Medium
Dependence rating Low
Prescription needed Yes
Available as generic No

GENERAL INFORMATION

Clozapine is an antipsychotic drug used to treat schizophrenia. It is prescribed only for patients who have not responded to other treatments or those who have experienced intolerable side effects with other drugs. Clozapine helps to control severe resistant schizophrenia, helping the patient to re-establish a more normal lifestyle. The improvement is gradual, and relief of severe symptoms can take more than 3 weeks.

All treatment is started and supervised by a hospital, because all patients must be registered with the Clozaril Patient Monitoring Service (CPMS). The drug can cause a very serious side effect: agranulocytosis (a large decrease in the number of white blood cells). Blood tests are done before treatment and regularly thereafter; the drug is supplied only if results are normal.

Clozapine is less likely than other antipsychotics to cause parkinsonism.

INFORMATION FOR USERS

This drug is given only under strict medical supervision and continual monitoring.
How taken Tablets.

Frequency and timing of doses 1–3 x daily; a larger dose may be given at night.
Adult dosage range 25–900mg daily.
Onset of effect Gradual. Some effect may appear within 3–5 days, but the full beneficial effect may not be felt for over 3 weeks.
Duration of action Up to 16 hours.
Diet advice None.
Storage Keep in a closed container in a cool, dry place out of reach of children.
Missed dose Take as soon as you remember. If your next dose is due within 2 hours, take a single dose now and skip the next. If you miss more than 2 days' tablets, notify your doctor; you may need to restart at a lower dose.
Stopping the drug Do not stop taking the drug without consulting your doctor; symptoms may recur.
Exceeding the dose An occasional unintentional extra dose is unlikely to cause problems. Large overdoses may cause unusual drowsiness, fits, and agitation; notify your doctor.

POSSIBLE ADVERSE EFFECTS

Clozapine is less likely to cause the parkinsonian side effects (tremor and stiffness) that occur with other antipsychotic drugs. The most serious adverse effect is agranulocytosis, and strict monitoring of the white blood cell count is necessary.

Common effects include drowsiness, tiredness, dry mouth, weight gain, and a fast heartbeat. The drug can also cause dizziness, fainting, and constipation. More unusual effects are blurred vision, tremor and muscle rigidity, and fever and sore throat. Clozapine may, rarely, cause epileptic fits. Drowsiness or tiredness may signal the onset of a fit; if they occur, seek urgent medical advice.

INTERACTIONS

General note A number of drugs increase the risk of adverse effects on the blood. Do not take other medication without checking with your doctor or pharmacist.
Sedatives All drugs that have a sedative effect on the central nervous system are likely to increase the sedative properties of clozapine.

SPECIAL PRECAUTIONS

Be sure to tell your doctor if:
◆ You have long-term liver or kidney problems.

◆ You have a history of blood disorders.
◆ You have had epileptic fits.
◆ You have heart problems.
◆ You have colon problems or have had bowel surgery.
◆ You have diabetes.
◆ You have glaucoma.
◆ You have prostate problems.
◆ You are taking other medications.

Pregnancy Not usually prescribed. Safety in pregnancy not established. Discuss with your doctor.

Breast-feeding The drug passes into the breast milk and may affect the baby adversely. Discuss with your doctor.

Infants and children Not prescribed.

Over 60 Adverse effects are more likely. Initial dose is low and is slowly increased.

Driving and hazardous work Avoid such activities until you have learned how clozapine affects you because the drug can cause drowsiness, dizziness, and blurred vision.

Alcohol Avoid. Alcohol may increase the sedative effects of this drug.

PROLONGED USE

There is a risk of agranulocytosis (see Introduction, above), and occasionally liver function may be upset. Significant weight gain may also occur.

Monitoring Tests to measure the white blood cell count are carried out weekly for the first 18 weeks, fortnightly until the end of the first year, and, if blood counts are stable, at four-weekly intervals thereafter. Liver function tests may also be performed.

Codeine

Used in the following combined preparations
Benylin with Codeine, Co-codamol, Codafen Continus, Codis, Diarrest, Migraleve, Panadol Ultra, Solpadeine, Solpadol, Syndol, Terpoin, Tylex, Veganin, and others

QUICK REFERENCE

Drug group Opioid analgesic (p.9), antidiarrhoeal drug (p.44), and cough suppressant (p.27)
Overdose danger rating High
Dependence rating Medium
Prescription needed Yes (some preparations)
Available as generic Yes

GENERAL INFORMATION

Codeine is a mild opioid analgesic that is similar to, but weaker than, morphine. It has been in common medical use since the beginning of the twentieth century.

Codeine is prescribed primarily to relieve mild to moderate pain and is often combined with a non-opioid analgesic such as paracetamol. The drug is also an effective cough suppressant and, for this reason, is included as an ingredient in many non-prescription cough syrups and cold relief preparations.

Like the other opioid drugs, codeine commonly produces constipation. This effect sometimes makes it useful in the short-term control of diarrhoea.

Although codeine is habit-forming, addiction seldom occurs if the drug is used for a limited period of time and at the recommended dosage.

Other rare, adverse effects of treatment with codeine include a rash, hives, wheezing, and breathing difficulties. If these effects occur, they should be reported to your doctor without delay.

INFORMATION FOR USERS

Your drug prescription is tailored for you. Do not alter dosage without checking with your doctor.

How taken Tablets, liquid, injection.

Frequency and timing of doses *Pain* 4–6 x daily. *Cough* 3–4 x daily when necessary. *Diarrhoea* every 4–6 hours when necessary.

Adult dosage range *Pain* 120–240mg daily. *Cough* 45–120mg daily. *Diarrhoea* 30–180mg daily.

Onset of effect 30–60 minutes.

Duration of action 4–6 hours.

Diet advice None.

Storage Keep in a closed container in a cool, dry place out of reach of children. Protect from light.

Missed dose Take as soon as you remember if the drug is needed for the relief of symptoms. If it is not needed, do not take the missed dose, and return to your normal dosing schedule when necessary.

Stopping the drug Treatment with codeine can be safely stopped as soon as you no longer need it.

OVERDOSE ACTION

Seek immediate medical advice in all cases. Take emergency action if there are symptoms such as slow or irregular breathing, severe drowsiness, or loss of consciousness.

POSSIBLE ADVERSE EFFECTS

Serious adverse effects are rare with codeine. Constipation occurs, especially with prolonged use, but other side effects such as nausea, vomiting, dizziness, and drowsiness are not usually troublesome when the drug is taken at recommended doses, and usually disappear if the dose is reduced. If you experience agitation or restlessness, stop taking the drug. If you develop a rash, hives, wheezing, or breathlessness, stop taking it and seek urgent medical attention.

INTERACTIONS

Sedatives All drugs that have a sedative effect on the central nervous system are likely to increase sedation with codeine. Such drugs include sleeping drugs, antidepressants, antihistamines, and alcohol.

SPECIAL PRECAUTIONS

Be sure tell your doctor if:
◆ You have long-term liver or kidney problems.
◆ You have a lung disorder such as asthma or bronchitis.
◆ You are taking other medications.
Pregnancy No evidence of risk, but codeine may adversely affect the baby's breathing if taken during labour.
Breast-feeding The drug passes into the breast milk, but at normal doses adverse effects on the baby are unlikely. Discuss with your doctor.
Infants and children Reduced dose necessary.
Over 60 Reduced dose may be necessary.
Driving and hazardous work Avoid these activities until you have learned how codeine affects you because the drug may cause dizziness and drowsiness.
Alcohol Avoid. Alcohol may increase the sedative effects of codeine.

PROLONGED USE

Codeine is normally used only for short-term relief of symptoms. It can be habit-forming if taken for extended periods, especially if higher-than-average doses are taken.

Colchicine

Brand names None
Used in the following combined preparations
None

QUICK REFERENCE

Drug group Drug for gout (p.53)
Overdose danger rating High
Dependence rating Low
Prescription needed Yes
Available as generic Yes

GENERAL INFORMATION

Colchicine, a drug originally extracted from the autumn crocus flower and later synthesized, has been used since the 18th century for gout. Although it has now, to some extent, been superseded by newer drugs, it is still often used to relieve joint pain and inflammation in flare-ups of gout. Colchicine is most effective when taken at the first sign of symptoms, and almost always produces an improvement. The drug is also often given during the first few months of treatment with allopurinol or probenecid (other drugs used for treating gout), because it may at first increase the frequency of gout attacks.

In addition, colchicine is prescribed for the relief of the symptoms of familial Mediterranean fever (a rare congenital condition).

INFORMATION FOR USERS

Your drug prescription is tailored for you. Do not alter dosage without checking with your doctor.
How taken Tablets.
Frequency and timing of doses *Prevention of gout attacks* 2–3 x daily. *Relief of gout attacks* Every 2–3 hours.
Adult dosage range *Prevention of gout attacks* 1–1.5mg daily. *Relief of gout attacks* 1mg initially, followed by 0.5mg every 2–3 hours, until relief of pain, vomiting, or diarrhoea occurs, or until a total dose of 6mg is reached. This course must not be repeated within 3 days.
Onset of effect *Prevention of gout attacks* Several days before full effect is felt. *Relief of gout attacks* 6–24 hours.
Duration of action Up to 2 hours. Some effects may last longer.

Diet advice Certain foods are known to make gout worse. Discuss with your doctor.

Storage Keep in a closed container in a cool, dry place out of reach of children. Protect from light.

Missed dose Take as soon as you remember. If your next dose is due within 30 minutes, take a single dose now and skip the next.

Stopping the drug When taking colchicine frequently during an acute gout attack, stop if diarrhoea or abdominal pain develop.

OVERDOSE ACTION

Seek immediate medical advice in all cases. Some reactions can be fatal. Take emergency action if severe nausea, vomiting, bloody diarrhoea, severe abdominal pain, or loss of consciousness occur.

POSSIBLE ADVERSE EFFECTS

The most common adverse effects of colchicine include nausea, vomiting, diarrhoea, and abdominal pain; less common effects are numbness and tingling, unusual bleeding or bruising, and a rash. The appearance of any symptom that may be an adverse effect of colchicine is a sign that you should stop taking the drug until you have received further medical advice.

INTERACTIONS

Ciclosporin Taking ciclosporin with colchicine may produce adverse effects on the kidneys.

SPECIAL PRECAUTIONS

Be sure to tell your doctor if:
◆ You have long-term liver or kidney problems.
◆ You have heart problems.
◆ You have a blood disorder.
◆ You have stomach ulcers.
◆ You suffer from chronic inflammation of the bowel.
◆ You are taking other medications.

Pregnancy Not usually prescribed. Colchicine may cause defects in the developing baby. Discuss with your doctor.

Breast-feeding The drug passes into the breast milk and may affect the baby. Discuss with your doctor.

Infants and children Not recommended.

Over 60 Increased likelihood of adverse effects.

Driving and hazardous work No special problems.

Alcohol Avoid. Alcohol may increase stomach irritation caused by colchicine.

PROLONGED USE

Prolonged use of this drug may lead to hair loss, rash, tingling in the hands and feet, muscle pain and weakness, and blood disorders.

Monitoring Periodic blood checks are usually required.

Colestyramine

Brand names Questran, Questran Light
Used in the following combined preparations
None

QUICK REFERENCE

Drug group Lipid-lowering drug (p.37)
Overdose danger rating Low
Dependence rating Low
Prescription needed Yes
Available as generic Yes

GENERAL INFORMATION

Colestyramine is a resin that binds bile acids in the intestine, preventing their reabsorption. Cholesterol in the body is normally manufactured from bile acids; therefore, colestyramine reduces cholesterol levels in the blood. The drug is used to treat hyperlipidaemia (high levels of fat in the blood) in people who have not responded to dietary changes.

In liver disorders such as primary biliary cirrhosis, bile salts sometimes accumulate in the bloodstream and cause itching. Colestyramine may be prescribed to alleviate this problem. Its action on the bile acids makes bowel movements bulkier, producing an antidiarrhoeal effect.

Taken in large doses, the drug often causes bloating, mild nausea, and constipation. It may also interfere with the body's ability to absorb fat and certain fat-soluble vitamins, causing pale, bulky, foul-smelling faeces.

INFORMATION FOR USERS

Your drug prescription is tailored for you. Do not alter dosage without checking with your doctor.

How taken Powder mixed with water, juice, or soft food.

Frequency and timing of doses 1–4 x daily before meals and at bedtime.

Adult dosage range 4–36g daily.

Onset of effect May take several weeks for full beneficial effects to be felt.

Duration of action 12–24 hours.

Diet advice A low-fat, low-calorie diet may be advised for patients who are overweight. Use of this drug may deplete levels of certain vitamins. Supplements may be advised.

Storage Keep in a closed container in a cool, dry place out of reach of children.

Missed dose Take as soon as you remember.

Stopping the drug Do not stop taking the drug without consulting your doctor.

Exceeding the dose An occasional unintentional extra dose is unlikely to cause problems. But if you notice any unusual symptoms, or if a large overdose has been taken, notify your doctor.

POSSIBLE ADVERSE EFFECTS

Adverse effects are more likely if large doses are taken by people over 60. Minor effects such as indigestion and abdominal discomfort are rarely a cause for concern. Nausea, vomiting, and constipation may also occur. High doses may cause diarrhoea. More serious effects, such as bruising or increased bleeding, are usually due to vitamin deficiency.

INTERACTIONS

General note Colestyramine reduces the body's ability to absorb other drugs. If you are taking other medicines, you should tell your doctor or pharmacist so that they can discuss with you the best way to take all your drugs. To avoid problems, take other drugs at least 1 hour before, or 4–6 hours after, taking colestyramine. The dosage of other drugs may need to be adjusted.

SPECIAL PRECAUTIONS

Be sure to tell your doctor if:
◆ You have jaundice.
◆ You have a peptic ulcer.
◆ You suffer from haemorrhoids.
◆ You are taking other medications.

Pregnancy Safety in pregnancy not established. Discuss with your doctor.

Breast-feeding Safety not established. The drug may cause vitamin deficiency in the baby. Discuss with your doctor.

Infants and children Not recommended under 6 years. Reduced dose necessary in older children.

Over 60 Increased likelihood of adverse effects.

Driving and hazardous work No special problems.

Alcohol Although this drug does not interact with alcohol, your underlying condition may make it inadvisable to take alcohol.

PROLONGED USE

As this drug reduces vitamin absorption, supplements of vitamins A, D, and K may be advised.

Monitoring Periodic blood checks are usually required to monitor blood cholesterol levels.

Conjugated oestrogens

Brand name Premarin
Used in the following combined preparation Premique, Prempak-C

QUICK REFERENCE

Drug group Female sex hormone (p.88)
Overdose danger rating Low
Dependence rating Low
Prescription needed Yes
Available as generic Yes

GENERAL INFORMATION

Preparations of conjugated oestrogens consist of naturally occurring oestrogens derived from the urine of pregnant mares. In tablet form, they are prescribed as part of hormone replacement therapy (see HRT p.89), to relieve menopausal symptoms such as hot flushes and sweating. Conjugated oestrogens are usually taken on a cyclic dosing schedule, usually in conjunction with a progestogen, to simulate the hormonal changes that occur in a normal menstrual cycle.

The drugs may also be used in the form of vaginal cream to relieve pain and dryness of the vagina or vulva after the menopause.

Conjugated oestrogens do not provide contraception. A woman can still become pregnant up to 2 years after her last period (if she is under 50 years) or up to 1 year after the end of menstruation (if she is over 50 years). Taken alone, the preparations are associated with an increased risk of cancer of the uterus. For this reason, they are usually combined with a progestogen to reduce the risk; they are usually used alone in women who have had a hysterectomy.

INFORMATION FOR USERS

Your drug prescription is tailored for you. Do not alter dosage without checking with your doctor.

How taken Tablets, cream.

Frequency and timing of doses Once daily.

Adult dosage range *Hormone replacement therapy* 0.625–1.25mg daily (tablets); 1–2g daily (cream).

Onset of effect 5–20 days.

Duration of action 1–2 days.

Diet advice None.

Storage Keep in a closed container in a cool, dry place out of reach of children.

Missed dose Take as soon as you remember.

Stopping the drug Do not stop without consulting your doctor as symptoms may recur.

Exceeding the dose An occasional unintentional extra dose is unlikely to be a cause for concern. But if you notice any unusual symptoms, or if a large overdose has been taken, notify your doctor.

POSSIBLE ADVERSE EFFECTS

The most common adverse effects of conjugated oestrogens are symptoms like those in the early stages of pregnancy, such as nausea, vomiting, weight increase or decrease, and breast swelling or tenderness. These generally diminish or disappear after 2–3 months of treatment. The drugs may also reduce sex drive. Women on a cyclic schedule will menstruate towards the end of each cycle. Discuss any depression or vaginal bleeding with your doctor. Sudden, sharp pain in the chest, groin, or legs may indicate an abnormal blood clot; stop taking the drug and seek urgent medical attention.

INTERACTIONS

Tobacco-smoking Smoking increases the risk of serious adverse effects on the heart and circulation with conjugated oestrogens.

Oral anticoagulant drugs Conjugated oestrogens reduce the anticoagulant effect of these drugs.

SPECIAL PRECAUTIONS

Be sure to tell your doctor if:
◆ You have heart failure or hypertension (high blood pressure).
◆ You have had blood clots or a stroke.
◆ You have a history of breast disease.
◆ You have had fibroids in the uterus.
◆ You suffer from migraine or epilepsy.
◆ You have long-term liver or kidney problems.
◆ You are taking other medications.

Pregnancy Not prescribed. May adversely affect the developing baby. Discuss with your doctor.

Breast-feeding Not prescribed. The drug passes into the breast milk and may inhibit the flow of milk. Discuss with your doctor.

Infants and children Not prescribed.

Over 60 No special problems.

Driving and hazardous work No known problems.

Alcohol No known problems.

Surgery and general anaesthetics The drug may need to be stopped several weeks before surgery. Discuss with your doctor.

PROLONGED USE

HRT is usually only advised for short-term use around the menopause and is no longer normally recommended for long-term use or for the treatment of osteoporosis because of the increased risk of disorders such as breast cancer, stroke, and thromboembolism.

Monitoring Regular physical examinations (such as mammograms) and blood-pressure checks are advised.

Co-phenotrope

Brand names Diarphen, Lomotil, Tropergen
Used in the following combined preparations
(Co-phenotrope is a combination of two drugs)

QUICK REFERENCE

Drug group Opioid antidiarrhoeal drug (p.44)
Overdose danger rating Medium
Dependence rating Medium
Prescription needed Yes
Available as generic Yes

GENERAL INFORMATION

Co-phenotrope is an antidiarrhoeal drug that contains a combination of diphenoxylate and atropine. It reduces the muscular contractions of the bowel and, therefore, the fluidity and frequency of bowel movements. Co-phenotrope is prescribed for the relief of sudden or recurrent bouts of diarrhoea.

Co-phenotrope is not suitable for treating diarrhoea due to infection, poisons, or antibiotics because it may delay recovery by slowing the expulsion of harmful substances from the bowel. Co-phenotrope can cause toxic megacolon, a dangerous dilation of the bowel that shuts off the blood supply to the wall of the bowel and increases the risk of perforation (the development of a hole in the bowel wall).

At recommended doses, co-phenotrope rarely has serious adverse effects. If the drug is taken in excessive amounts, the atropine will cause highly unpleasant anticholinergic (see Autonomic nervous system, p.8) effects. This drug is especially dangerous for young children and must be stored out of their reach.

INFORMATION FOR USERS

Your drug prescription is tailored for you. Do not alter dosage without checking with your doctor.

How taken Tablets.

Frequency and timing of doses 3–4 x daily.

Dosage range *Adults* 10mg initially, followed by 5mg every 6 hours until diarrhoea is controlled. *Children* Reduced dose necessary according to age. Not recommended under 4 years.

Onset of effect Within 1 hour. Control of diarrhoea may take some hours.

Duration of action Up to 24 hours.

Diet advice Always drink plenty of water during an attack of diarrhoea.

Storage Keep in a closed container in a cool, dry place out of the reach of children. Protect from light.

Missed dose Take as soon as you remember. If your next dose is due within 3 hours, take a single dose now and skip the next.

Stopping the drug Can be safely stopped as soon as you no longer need it.

Exceeding the dose An occasional unintentional extra dose is unlikely to cause problems.

Large overdoses may cause unusual drowsiness, dry mouth and skin, restlessness, and, in extreme cases, loss of consciousness. Symptoms of overdose may be delayed. Notify your doctor.

POSSIBLE ADVERSE EFFECTS

Drowsiness is a common adverse effect of co-phenotrope. Other adverse effects, such as restlessness, headache, rash, itching, and dizziness, occur infrequently. If nausea, vomiting, or abdominal pain or discomfort occur, stop taking the drug and notify your doctor immediately.

INTERACTIONS

Sedatives All drugs that have a sedative effect on the central nervous system may increase the sedative effect of co-phenotrope. These include anti-anxiety drugs, sleeping drugs, antihistamines, opioid analgesics, antidepressants, and antipsychotics.

MAOIs There is a risk of a dangerous rise in blood pressure if MAOIs are taken together with co-phenotrope.

SPECIAL PRECAUTIONS

Be sure to tell your doctor if:
◆ You have a long-term liver problem.
◆ You have severe abdominal pain.
◆ You have bloodstained diarrhoea.
◆ You have recently taken antibiotics.
◆ You have ulcerative colitis.
◆ You have recently travelled abroad.
◆ You are taking other medications.

Pregnancy Safety in pregnancy not established. Discuss with your doctor.

Breast-feeding The drug passes into the breast milk and may cause drowsiness in the baby. Discuss with your doctor.

Infants and children Not recommended under 4 years. Reduced dose necessary for older children.

Over 60 Reduced dose may be necessary.

Driving and hazardous work Avoid all such activities until you have learned how co-phenotrope affects you because the drug may cause drowsiness and dizziness.

Alcohol Avoid. Alcohol may increase the sedative effects of this drug.

PROLONGED USE

Not usually recommended.

Co-proxamol

Brand names Cosalgesic, Distalgesic
Used in the following combined preparations
(Co-proxamol is a combination of two drugs)

QUICK REFERENCE

Drug group Opioid analgesic (p.9)
Overdose danger rating High
Dependence rating Medium
Prescription needed Yes
Available as generic Yes

GENERAL INFORMATION

Co-proxamol is the generic name for a combination of the non-opioid analgesic drug paracetamol and a mild opioid analgesic, dextropropoxyphene. Co-proxamol is widely used for the relief of mild to moderate pain, but research does not show it to be more effective than paracetamol alone.

Because the drug contains an opioid, it can cause a variety of side effects common to drugs of that group: dizziness, mild euphoria, nausea, and constipation. Co-proxamol may also be habit-forming if it is taken regularly for an extended period. Overdose with this drug is dangerous because dextropropoxyphene may interfere with breathing if it is taken in excess, and overdose of paracetamol may cause irreversible damage to the liver and kidneys.

INFORMATION FOR USERS

Your drug prescription is tailored for you. Do not alter dosage without checking with your doctor.
How taken Tablets.
Frequency and timing of doses 3–4 x daily as necessary.
Adult dosage range 2 tablets per dose, up to a maximum of 8 tablets daily.
Onset of effect 30–60 minutes.
Duration of action 6 hours.
Diet advice None.
Storage Keep in a closed container in a cool, dry place out of reach of children.
Missed dose Take as soon as you remember if needed for the relief of pain. Do not take doses less than 4 hours apart.
Stopping the drug If you have been taking the drug regularly for less than 4 weeks, it can be safely stopped as soon as you no longer need it. If you have been taking the drug regularly for longer than this, your doctor may recommend a gradual reduction in dosage.

OVERDOSE ACTION

Seek immediate medical advice in all cases. Take emergency action if irregular breathing, drowsiness or loss of consciousness occur.

POSSIBLE ADVERSE EFFECTS

Serious adverse effects are rare with this drug. However, dizziness, drowsiness, nausea, vomiting, and constipation occur in some people. If you become euphoric or you develop hallucinations, stop taking the drug. If you develop a rash, stop taking it and consult your doctor.

INTERACTIONS

General note All drugs that have a sedative effect are likely to increase the sedative properties of co-proxamol. These include sleeping drugs, anti-anxiety drugs, antidepressants, and alcohol.
Carbamazepine Co-proxamol can enhance the effects of carbamazepine.
Oral anticoagulant drugs Co-proxamol may increase the anticoagulant effect of these drugs.

SPECIAL PRECAUTIONS

Be sure to tell your doctor if:
◆ You have long-term liver or kidney problems.
◆ You have had problems with drug or alcohol abuse.
◆ You have a lung disorder such as asthma or bronchitis.
◆ You suffer from depression.
◆ You are taking other medications.
Pregnancy Safety in pregnancy not established. Discuss with your doctor.
Breast-feeding The drug passes into the breast milk and may affect the baby. Discuss with your doctor.
Infants and children Not recommended.
Over 60 Reduced dose necessary.
Driving and hazardous work Avoid such activities until you have learned how co-proxamol affects you because the drug can cause drowsiness and dizziness.

Alcohol Avoid. Alcohol will dangerously increase the toxicity of this drug.

PROLONGED USE
Co-proxamol is not usually prescribed for long-term use. It can be habit-forming if taken for extended periods, and a higher dose may be needed to produce the same effect as your body adapts to the drug.

Co-trimoxazole

Brand names Fectrim, Septrin
Used in the following combined preparations
(Co-trimoxazole is a combination of two drugs)

QUICK REFERENCE
Drug group Antibacterial drug (p.66)
Overdose danger rating Medium
Dependence rating Low
Prescription needed Yes
Available as generic Yes

GENERAL INFORMATION
Co-trimoxazole is a combination of the two antibacterial drugs trimethoprim and sulfamethoxazole. It is prescribed for the treatment of serious respiratory and urinary tract infections only when they cannot be treated with other drugs. Co-trimoxazole is also used to prevent and treat pneumocystis pneumonia and to treat toxoplasmosis and the fungal infection nocardiasis. In addition, the drug may be used to treat otitis media in children if no safer drug is suitable. Although co-trimoxazole was widely prescribed in the past, its use has now greatly declined with the introduction of new, more effective, and safer drugs.

Co-trimoxazole may produce certain rare but serious adverse effects. Such effects include skin rashes, blood disorders, and liver or kidney damage.

INFORMATION FOR USERS
Your drug prescription is tailored for you. Do not alter dosage without checking with your doctor.
How taken Tablets, liquid, injection.
Frequency and timing of doses Normally 2 x daily, preferably with food.

Adult dosage range Usually 4 tablets daily (a standard tablet is 480mg). Higher doses may be used for the treatment of pneumocystis pneumonia, toxoplasmosis, and nocardiasis.
Onset of effect 1–4 hours.
Duration of action 12 hours.
Diet advice Drink plenty of fluids, particularly in warm weather.
Storage Keep in a closed container in a cool, dry place out of reach of children. Protect from light.
Missed dose Take as soon as you remember. If your normal dose is 480mg, double this; if it is more than 480mg, take one dose only.
Stopping the drug Unless severe adverse effects occur (see below), take the full course. Even if you feel better, the original infection may still be present and symptoms may recur if treatment is stopped too soon.
Exceeding the dose An occasional unintentional extra dose is unlikely to be a cause for concern. Large overdoses, however, may cause nausea, vomiting, dizziness, and confusion; notify your doctor.

POSSIBLE ADVERSE EFFECTS
Adverse effects can be caused by either the trimethoprim or the sulfamethoxazole ingredient of this preparation. The most common problem is rash or itching; if this occurs, stop taking the drug and consult your doctor without delay. Nausea or vomiting, diarrhoea, a sore tongue, and headache are less common and should also be discussed with your doctor. If you become jaundiced, stop taking the drug and seek urgent medical attention because some types of adverse effects are potentially serious.

INTERACTIONS
Warfarin Co-trimoxazole may increase the anticoagulant effect of this drug; the dose of warfarin may have to be reduced. Blood-clotting status may have to be checked.
Phenytoin Co-trimoxazole may cause a build-up of phenytoin in the body; the dose of phenytoin may have to be reduced.
Oral antidiabetic drugs Co-trimoxazole may increase the blood-sugar-lowering effect of these drugs.
Ciclosporin Taking ciclosporin together with co-trimoxazole can impair kidney function.

SPECIAL PRECAUTIONS

Be sure to tell your doctor if:

◆ You have long-term liver or kidney problems.
◆ You have a blood disorder.
◆ You have glucose-6-phosphate dehydrogenase (G6PD) deficiency.
◆ You are allergic to sulphonamide drugs.
◆ You suffer from porphyria.
◆ You are taking other medications.

Pregnancy Not usually prescribed. The drug may cause defects in the developing baby. Discuss with your doctor.

Breast-feeding The drug passes into the breast milk, but at normal levels adverse effects on the baby are unlikely. Discuss with your doctor.

Infants and children Not recommended in infants under 6 weeks old. Reduced dose necessary in older children.

Over 60 Side effects are more likely. Used only when necessary, often in reduced dosage.

Driving and hazardous work No known problems.

Alcohol No known problems.

PROLONGED USE

Long-term use of co-trimoxazole may lead to folic acid deficiency, which can cause anaemia. Folic acid supplements may be needed.

Monitoring Regular blood tests are recommended.

Cyclophosphamide

Brand name Endoxana
Used in the following combined preparations
None

QUICK REFERENCE

Drug group Anticancer drug (p.96)
Overdose danger rating Medium
Dependence rating Low
Prescription needed Yes
Available as generic Yes

GENERAL INFORMATION

Cyclophosphamide belongs to a group of anticancer drugs known as alkylating agents. It is used for a wide range of cancers, including lymphomas (lymph gland cancers), leukaemias, and solid tumours, particularly of the breast and lung. It is commonly given together with radiotherapy or other drugs. Cyclophosphamide has also been used for autoimmune diseases (see Immunosuppressant drugs, p.99).

The drug causes nausea, vomiting, and hair loss, and can affect the heart, lungs, and liver. It can also cause bladder damage in susceptible people because it produces a toxic substance called acrolein. To reduce toxicity, people considered to be at risk may be given a drug called mesna before and after each dose of cyclophosphamide. In addition, because the drug often reduces production of blood cells, it may lead to abnormal bleeding and an increased risk of infection, and to reduced fertility in men.

INFORMATION FOR USERS

Your drug prescription is tailored for you. Do not alter dosage without checking with your doctor.

How taken Tablets, injection.

Frequency and timing of doses Varies from once daily to every 3 weeks, depending on the condition being treated.

Dosage range Dosage is determined individually according to the nature of the condition, body weight, and response.

Onset of effect Some effects may appear within hours of starting treatment. Full beneficial effects, however, may not be felt for many weeks.

Duration of action Several weeks.

Diet advice High fluid intake with frequent bladder emptying is recommended. This will usually prevent the drug from causing bladder irritation.

Storage Keep in a closed container in a cool, dry place out of reach of children. Protect from light.

Missed dose Injections are given only in hospital. If you are taking tablets, take the missed dose as soon as you remember. If your next dose is due within 6 hours, take a single dose now and skip the next. Tell your doctor that you missed a dose.

Stopping the drug The drug will be stopped under medical supervision (injection). Do not stop taking the drug without consulting your doctor (tablets). Stopping the drug may lead to worsening of the underlying condition.

Exceeding the dose An occasional unintentional extra dose is unlikely to be a cause for concern. Large overdoses, however, may cause nausea and vomiting and may damage the bladder; notify your doctor.

POSSIBLE ADVERSE EFFECTS

Cyclophosphamide often causes nausea and vomiting, which usually diminish as your body adjusts. Hair loss is a common sign that the drug is having an effect on growing cells. Mouth ulcers may also occur, and women often experience irregular periods. Cloudy or bloodstained urine may be a sign of bladder damage and requires prompt medical attention. Those people thought to be at risk of bladder damage may be given mesna before and after doses of cyclophosphamide.

INTERACTIONS

None.

SPECIAL PRECAUTIONS

Cyclophosphamide is prescribed only under close medical supervision, taking account of your present condition and medical history.
Pregnancy Not usually prescribed. May cause birth defects. Discuss with your doctor.
Breast-feeding Not advised. The drug passes into the breast milk and may affect the baby adversely. Discuss with your doctor.
Infants and children Reduced dose necessary.
Over 60 No special problems.
Driving and hazardous work No known problems.
Alcohol No problems expected, but avoid excessive amounts.

PROLONGED USE

Prolonged use of this drug may reduce the production of blood cells.
Monitoring Periodic checks on blood composition and on all effects of the drug are usually required.

Danazol

Brand name Danol
Used in the following combined preparations
None

QUICK REFERENCE

Drug group Drug for menstrual disorders (p.104)
Overdose danger rating Low
Dependence rating Low
Prescription needed Yes
Available as generic Yes

GENERAL INFORMATION

Danazol is a synthetic steroid hormone that inhibits hormones called pituitary gonadotrophins. It is used in a range of conditions, including endometriosis (fragments of endometrial tissue growing outside the uterus) and menorrhagia (very heavy menstrual periods), and, in men, to reduce gynaecomastia (breast swelling). It has also been used as long-term treatment for hereditary angioedema (a rare allergic disorder that causes facial swelling). In addition, danazol is used to relieve pain, tenderness, and lumpiness in the breasts caused by fibrocystic disease.

Treatment commonly disrupts normal menstrual periods, and in some cases periods may cease altogether. Women taking high doses of the drug may notice unusual hair growth and deepening of the voice.

INFORMATION FOR USERS

Your drug prescription is tailored for you. Do not alter dosage without checking with your doctor.
How taken Capsules.
Frequency and timing of doses 1–4 x daily.
Dosage range 200–800mg daily, depending on the condition being treated, its severity, and the response to the drug.
Onset of effect Some effects occur after a few days. Full beneficial effects may take some months.
Duration of action 1–2 days.
Diet advice None.
Storage Keep in a closed container in a cool, dry place out of reach of children.
Missed dose Take as soon as you remember. If your next dose is due within 2 hours, take a single dose now and skip the next.

Stopping the drug Do not stop taking the drug without consulting your doctor; symptoms may recur.
Exceeding the dose An occasional unintentional extra dose is unlikely to cause problems. But if you notice any unusual symptoms, or if a large overdose has been taken, notify your doctor.

POSSIBLE ADVERSE EFFECTS

In low doses, danazol rarely causes adverse effects. Higher doses may produce effects including acne, weight gain, ankle swelling, muscle cramps, and nausea, due to hormonal changes. Reduced breast size, voice changes, and unusual hair growth in women may also occur but are largely reversed after treatment. If blurred vision or headaches develop, consult your doctor.

INTERACTIONS

Oral anticoagulant drugs Danazol may increase the effects of these drugs.
Immunosuppressants Danazol may increase the effects of ciclosporin and tacrolimus.
Oral antidiabetic drugs Danazol may reduce the effects of these drugs.
Anticonvulsant drugs Danazol may increase the effects of carbamazepine, and possibly other antiepileptic drugs.

SPECIAL PRECAUTIONS

Be sure to tell your doctor if:
◆ You have any long-term liver or kidney problems.
◆ You have heart disease.
◆ You have had epileptic fits.
◆ You suffer from migraine.
◆ You have unexplained vaginal bleeding.
◆ You have diabetes mellitus.
◆ You are taking other medications.
Pregnancy Not prescribed. May cause masculine characteristics in a female baby. Nonhormonal methods of contraception should be used for women of childbearing age; and pregnancy should be avoided for 3 months after the end of treatment.
Breast-feeding The drug passes into the breast milk and may affect the baby. Discuss with your doctor.
Infants and children Not recommended.
Over 60 Unlikely to be required.

Driving and hazardous work No known problems.
Alcohol No known problems.

PROLONGED USE

The drug is normally taken for 3–9 months, depending on the condition being treated. There is a slight risk of liver damage.
Monitoring Periodic liver function tests may be carried out.

Desmopressin

Brand names DDAVP, Desmospray, Desmotabs, Nocutil
Used in the following combined preparations None

QUICK REFERENCE

Drug group Drug for diabetes insipidus (p.82)
Overdose danger rating Medium
Dependence rating Low
Prescription needed Yes
Available as generic Yes

GENERAL INFORMATION

Desmopressin is a synthetic form of the hormone vasopressin. Low levels of vasopressin in the body can lead to diabetes insipidus, which causes frequent urination and continual thirst. Desmopressin can be used to correct this deficiency.

The drug is also used to test for diabetes insipidus, to check kidney function, and to treat nocturnal enuresis (bedwetting) in both children and adults. When given by injection, desmopressin helps to boost clotting factors in haemophilia.

Side effects include low blood sodium and fluid retention (which may require control of the amount of fluid consumed and, sometimes, monitoring of body weight and blood pressure to check the body's water balance).

Desmopressin should not be taken during an episode of vomiting and diarrhoea because the body's fluid balance may be upset.

INFORMATION FOR USERS

Your drug prescription is tailored for you. Do not alter dosage without checking with your doctor.

How taken Tablets, injection, nasal solution, nasal spray.
Frequency and timing of doses *Diabetes insipidus* 3 x daily (tablets); 1–2 x daily (nasal spray/solution). *Nocturnal enuresis* At bedtime (tablets, nasal spray/solution). The patient should avoid fluids from 1 hour before bedtime to 8 hours afterwards.
Dosage range *Diabetes insipidus* Adults: 300–600mcg daily (tablets); 1–4 puffs (nasal spray); 10–40mcg daily (nasal solution). Children: 300–600mcg daily (tablets); up to 2 puffs (nasal spray); 20mcg (nasal solution). *Nocturnal enuresis* 200–400mcg for children over 5 years only (tablets); 20–40mcg (nasal solution); 2–4 puffs (nasal spray).
Onset of effect Begins within a few minutes, with full effects developing in a few hours (injection, nasal solution, and nasal spray);. 30–90 minutes (tablets).
Duration of action 8 hours (tablets); 8–12 hours (injection and nasal solutions); 10–12 hours (nasal spray).
Diet advice Your doctor may advise you to monitor your fluid intake.
Storage Keep in a cool, dry place (tablets) or in a refrigerator, without freezing (nasal solution and nasal spray), out of reach of children. Protect from light.
Missed dose Take as soon as you remember. If your next dose is due within 2 hours, take a single dose now and skip the next.
Stopping the drug Unless vomiting or diarrhoea occur, do not stop taking the drug without consulting your doctor; symptoms of diabetes insipidus may recur.
Exceeding the dose An occasional unintentional extra dose is unlikely to cause problems. Large overdoses may prevent the kidneys from eliminating fluid, with ensuing problems including convulsions. Notify your doctor immediately.

POSSIBLE ADVERSE EFFECTS

Desmopressin can cause fluid retention and low blood sodium, especially if fluid intake is too high. In serious cases, this problem can lead to confusion and convulsions. Headache, nausea, vomiting, and epistaxis (nosebleeds) may also occur. If vomiting or diarrhoea occur, stop taking the drug and consult your doctor.

INTERACTIONS

Antidepressants, chlorpropamide, and carbamazepine These drugs may increase the body's response to desmopressin.

Indometacin This anti-inflammatory drug may increase the body's response to desmopressin.

SPECIAL PRECAUTIONS

Be sure to tell your doctor if:
◆ You have heart problems.
◆ You have high blood pressure.
◆ You have kidney problems.
◆ You have cystic fibrosis.
◆ You have asthma or allergic rhinitis.
◆ You have epilepsy.
◆ You are taking other medications.

Pregnancy Used with caution in pregnancy.

Breast-feeding The drug passes into breast milk, in small amounts, but at normal doses adverse effects on the baby are unlikely.

Infants and children No special problems in children; infants may need monitoring to ensure that fluid balance is correct.

Over 60 May need monitoring to ensure that fluid balance is correct.

Driving and hazardous work No known problems.

Alcohol Your doctor may advise on your fluid intake.

PROLONGED USE

Diabetes insipidus No problems expected.

Nocturnal enuresis The drug will be withdrawn for at least a week after 3 months of use, so that doctors can assess the need to continue treatment.

Dexamethasone

Brand name Decadron
Used in the following combined preparations
Dexa-Rhinaspray, Maxidex, Maxitrol, Otomize, Sofradex, and others

QUICK REFERENCE

Drug group Corticosteroid (p.80)
Overdose danger rating Low
Dependence rating Low
Prescription needed Yes
Available as generic Yes

GENERAL INFORMATION

Dexamethasone is a long-acting corticosteroid drug. It is prescribed to suppress inflammatory and allergic disorders, such as rheumatoid arthritis, shock, and brain swelling (due to injury or tumour).

The drug is also used in conjunction with other drugs to alleviate nausea and vomiting associated with chemotherapy. It is available in different forms, including tablets, oral solution, injection, and eye and ear drops.

Low doses taken for short periods rarely cause serious side effects. But, as with other corticosteroids, long-term treatment with high doses can cause unpleasant or dangerous side effects. Some infections, such as chickenpox, may be more severe in people taking dexamethasone.

INFORMATION FOR USERS

Your drug prescription is tailored for you. Do not alter dosage without checking with your doctor.

How taken Tablets, injection, eye drops, ear drops/spray.

Frequency and timing of doses 1–4 x daily with food (by mouth); 1–6 hourly (eye drops).

Dosage range Usually 0.5–10mg daily (by mouth).

Onset of effect 1–4 days.

Duration of action Some effects may last for several days.

Diet advice None.

Storage Keep in a closed container in a cool, dry place out of reach of children. Protect from light.

Missed dose Take as soon as you remember. If your next dose is due within 2 hours, take a single dose now and skip the next.

Stopping the drug Do not stop taking the drug without consulting your doctor, who will supervise a gradual reduction in dosage.

Exceeding the dose An occasional unintentional extra dose is unlikely to be a cause for concern. But if you notice any unusual symptoms, or if a large overdose has been taken, notify your doctor.

POSSIBLE ADVERSE EFFECTS

Indigestion and weight gain are common. More serious adverse effects of dexamethasone only occur with high doses taken for long periods. These effects, including acne and skin thinning, raised blood pressure, muscle weakness, and mood changes, will be carefully monitored during prolonged treatment.

INTERACTIONS

Antidiabetic drugs Dexamethasone reduces the action of antidiabetics. The dosage of these drugs may need to be adjusted accordingly to prevent abnormally high blood glucose.

Barbiturates, phenytoin, rifampicin, and carbamazepine These drugs may reduce the effectiveness of dexamethasone. The dosage may need to be adjusted accordingly.

Oral anticoagulant drugs Dexamethasone may increase the effects of these drugs.

NSAIDs These drugs may increase the likelihood of indigestion from dexamethasone.

Antacids These drugs may reduce the effectiveness of dexamethasone, and should be taken at least 2 hours apart from it.

Vaccines Dexamethasone can interact with some vaccines. Discuss with your doctor before having any vaccinations.

SPECIAL PRECAUTIONS

Be sure to tell your doctor if:
◆ You have had a peptic ulcer.
◆ You have glaucoma.
◆ You have had tuberculosis.
◆ You have had depression or mental illness.
◆ You have a herpes infection.
◆ You are taking other medications.

Avoid exposure to people with chickenpox or shingles if you are on systemic treatment (tablets or injection).

Pregnancy Safety in pregnancy not established. Discuss with your doctor.

Breast-feeding The drug passes into the breast milk, but at normal doses adverse effects on the baby are unlikely. Consult your doctor.

Infants and children Reduced dose necessary.

Over 60 No known problems.

Driving and hazardous work No known problems.

Alcohol Avoid. Alcohol may increase the risk of peptic ulcer with this drug.

PROLONGED USE

Prolonged use of dexamethasone can lead to glaucoma, cataracts, diabetes, mental disturbances, muscle wasting, fragile bones, and thin skin, and can retard growth in children. If you are receiving long-term treatment, you are advised to carry a "steroid treatment" card, which can be obtained from your doctor or pharmacist.

Diazepam

Brand names Diazemuls, Diazepam Rectubes, Rimapam, Stesolid, Tensium, Valclair
Used in the following combined preparations
None

QUICK REFERENCE

Drug group Benzodiazepine anti-anxiety drug (p.13), muscle relaxant (p.54), and anticonvulsant (p.16)
Overdose danger rating Medium
Dependence rating High
Prescription needed Yes
Available as generic Yes

GENERAL INFORMATION

Introduced in the early 1960s, diazepam is the best known and most widely used of the benzodiazepine group of drugs. The benzodiazepines help relieve tension and nervousness, relax muscles, and encourage sleep. Their actions and adverse effects are described more fully on page 13.

Diazepam has a wide range of uses. Besides being commonly used in the treatment of anxiety and anxiety-related insomnia, it is prescribed as a muscle relaxant, in the treatment of alcohol withdrawal, and for the relief of epileptic fits. Given intravenously, diazepam is used to sedate people who are undergoing certain uncomfortable medical procedures.

Diazepam can be habit-forming if it is taken regularly over a long period of time. The effects of the drug may also diminish with time. For these reasons, courses of treatment with diazepam are limited to two weeks whenever possible.

INFORMATION FOR USERS

Your drug prescription is tailored for you. Do not alter dosage without checking with your doctor.

How taken Tablets, liquid, injection, suppositories, rectal solution.

Frequency and timing of doses 1–4 x daily.
Adult dosage range *Anxiety* 6–30mg daily. *Muscle spasm* 2–60mg daily.
Onset of effect Immediate effect (injection, rectal solution); 30 minutes–2 hours (other methods of administration).
Duration of action Up to 24 hours. Some effect may last up to 4 days.
Diet advice None.
Storage Keep in a closed container in a cool, dry place out of reach of children.
Missed dose Take as soon as you remember. If your next dose is due within 2 hours, take a single dose now and skip the next.
Stopping the drug If you have been taking the drug continuously for less than 2 weeks, it can be safely stopped as soon as you no longer need it. But if you have been taking it for longer, consult your doctor, who will supervise gradual dosage reduction. Stopping abruptly may lead to withdrawal symptoms.
Exceeding the dose An occasional unintentional extra dose is unlikely to cause problems. Larger overdoses may cause excessive drowsiness; notify your doctor.

POSSIBLE ADVERSE EFFECTS

Diazepam's main adverse effects are related to its sedative properties. They include daytime drowsiness, dizziness or unsteadiness, headache, blurred vision, and forgetfulness or confusion. These normally diminish after a few days and can often be reduced by dosage adjustment. If a rash develops, consult your doctor.

INTERACTIONS

Sedatives All drugs that have a sedative effect on the central nervous system can increase the sedative properties of diazepam. These drug include anti-anxiety drugs and sleeping drugs, antihistamines, opioid analgesics, antidepressants, and antipsychotics.
Cimetidine, isoniazid, ritonavir, and amprenavir These drugs may inhibit the breakdown of diazepam, leading to increased levels in the blood and a risk of adverse effects.

SPECIAL PRECAUTIONS

Be sure to tell your doctor if:
◆ You have severe respiratory disease.
◆ You have long-term liver or kidney problems.

◆ You have had problems with alcohol or drug abuse.
◆ You are taking other medications.
Pregnancy Safety in pregnancy not established. Discuss with your doctor.
Breast-feeding The drug passes into the breast milk and may affect the baby. Discuss with your doctor.
Infants and children Reduced dose necessary.
Over 60 Reduced dose may be necessary. Increased likelihood of adverse effects.
Driving and hazardous work Avoid such activities until you have learned how diazepam affects you because the drug can cause reduced alertness, slowed reactions, and increased aggression.
Alcohol Avoid. Alcohol may increase the sedative effects of this drug.

PROLONGED USE

Regular use of this drug over several weeks can lead to a reduction in its effect as the body adapts. Diazepam may also be habit-forming when taken for extended periods, and severe withdrawal reactions can occur on stopping the drug suddenly.

Diclofenac

Brand names Diclomax SR, Motifene, Rhumalgan, Volraman, Voltarol, and others
Used in the following combined preparation Arthrotec

QUICK REFERENCE

Drug group Non-steroidal anti-inflammatory drug (p.50), analgesic (p.9), and drug for gout (p.53)
Overdose danger rating Low
Dependence rating Low
Prescription needed Yes
Available as generic Yes

GENERAL INFORMATION

Taken as a single dose, diclofenac has analgesic properties similar to those of paracetamol. It is taken to relieve mild to moderate headache, menstrual pain, and pain following minor surgery. Diclofenac given regularly over a long period has an anti-inflammatory effect and is used to relieve the pain and stiffness associated with rheumatoid arthritis and advanced osteoarthritis. Some formulations are slow-release (SR) and can be taken less frequently, while still relieving pain effectively. Diclofenac may also be prescribed to treat acute attacks of gout.

The combined preparation Arthrotec contains diclofenac (see p.212) and misoprostol (see p.321). Misoprostol helps to prevent gastroduodenal ulceration, which is sometimes caused by diclofenac, and may be particularly useful in those patients who are at risk of developing this problem.

INFORMATION FOR USERS

Your drug prescription is tailored for you. Do not alter dosage without checking with your doctor.

How taken Tablets, dispersible tablets, SR-tablets, capsules, SR-capsules, injection, suppositories, gel.

Frequency and timing of doses 1–3 x daily with food.

Adult dosage range 75–150mg daily.

Onset of effect Approximately 1 hour (pain relief). The full anti-inflammatory effect may take 2 weeks to develop.

Duration of action Up to 12 hours; up to 24 hours (SR-preparations).

Diet advice None.

Storage Keep in a closed container in a cool, dry place out of reach of children.

Missed dose Take as soon as you remember. If your next dose is due within 2 hours, take a single dose now and skip the next.

Stopping the drug When taken for short-term pain relief, diclofenac can be safely stopped as soon as you no longer need it. Seek medical advice before stopping long-term treatment of arthritis unless serious adverse effects occur (see below).

Exceeding the dose An occasional unintentional extra dose is unlikely to be a cause for concern. But if you notice any unusual symptoms or if a large overdose has been taken, notify your doctor.

POSSIBLE ADVERSE EFFECTS

The most common adverse effects are gastrointestinal disturbances. If symptoms such as abdominal pain and swollen feet or ankles occur, discuss them with your doctor. If you develop a rash, wheezing or breathlessness, bruising, bleeding, vomiting, or bloodstained or black bowel movements, stop taking the drug and call your doctor without delay.

INTERACTIONS

General note Diclofenac interacts with many drugs, including other NSAIDs, oral anticoagulants, and corticosteroids, to increase the risk of bleeding and/or ulcers.

Antihypertensive drugs and diuretics The beneficial effects of these drugs may be reduced with diclofenac.

Ciclosporin Diclofenac may increase the risk of kidney problems.

Lithium, digoxin, and methotrexate Diclofenac may increase the blood levels of these drugs to an undesirable extent.

Indigestion remedies Some diclofenac preparations are enteric-coated, so that they will pass through the stomach before dissolving. Indigestion remedies may disrupt this coating, so they should be taken 2 hours before or 2 hours after diclofenac.

SPECIAL PRECAUTIONS

Be sure to tell your doctor if:
◆ You have long-term liver or kidney problems.
◆ You have a bleeding disorder.
◆ You have had a peptic ulcer or oesophagitis.
◆ You have porphyria.
◆ You suffer from indigestion.
◆ You are allergic to aspirin.
◆ You suffer from asthma.
◆ You have heart problems or hypertension (high blood pressure).
◆ You are taking other medications.

Pregnancy Not usually prescribed in the last 3 months of pregnancy. Diclofenac may increase the risk of adverse effects on the baby's heart and may prolong labour. Discuss with your doctor.

Breast-feeding Small amounts of the drug pass into the breast milk, but adverse effects on the baby are unlikely. Discuss with your doctor.

Infants and children Reduced dose necessary.

Over 60 Increased risk of adverse effects. Reduced dose may therefore be necessary.

Driving and hazardous work No problems expected.

Alcohol Keep consumption low. Alcohol may increase the risk of stomach irritation.

Surgery and general anaesthetics Discuss with your doctor or dentist before any surgery.

PROLONGED USE

There is an increased risk of bleeding from peptic ulcers and in the bowel with prolonged use of diclofenac.

Dicycloverine

Brand name Merbentyl
Used in the following combined preparation
Kolanticon

QUICK REFERENCE

Drug group Drug for irritable bowel syndrome (p.45)
Overdose danger rating Medium
Dependence rating Low
Prescription needed No (doses of 10mg or less);
Yes (doses of more than 10mg)
Available as generic No

GENERAL INFORMATION

Dicycloverine is a mild anticholinergic (see Autonomic nervous system, p.8) antispasmodic drug that relieves painful abdominal cramps in the gastrointestinal tract. It is used to treat irritable bowel syndrome, indigestion that is not associated with ulcers, and colicky conditions in babies (over 6 months only).

Because dicycloverine has anticholinergic properties, it may also be combined with other drugs used to treat flatulence, indigestion, and diarrhoea. It relieves symptoms but does not cure the underlying condition. Additional treatment with further drugs, and self-help measures such as dietary changes, may be recommended by your doctor.

Side effects with dicycloverine are rare, but they include headaches, constipation, urinary difficulties, and palpitations.

INFORMATION FOR USERS

Follow instructions on the label. Call your doctor if symptoms worsen.
How taken Tablets, liquid.
Frequency and timing of doses 3–4 x daily before or after meals.
Dosage range *Adults* 30–60mg daily. *Children* Reduced dose according to age and weight.
Onset of effect Within 1–2 hours.

Duration of action 4–6 hours.
Diet advice None.
Storage Keep in a closed container in a cool, dry place out of reach of children. Protect from light.
Missed dose Take as soon as you remember. If your next dose is due within 2 hours, take a single dose now and skip the next.
Stopping the drug The drug can be stopped without causing problems when it is no longer needed.
Exceeding the dose An occasional unintentional extra dose is unlikely to cause problems. Large overdoses, however, may cause drowsiness, dizziness, and difficulty in swallowing; notify your doctor.

POSSIBLE ADVERSE EFFECTS

Most people notice no adverse effects. Those effects that do occur are related to dicycloverine's anticholinergic properties; they include drowsiness, dry mouth, and constipation. These effects may be overcome by adjusting the dosage, or may disappear after a few days as your body adjusts. If you experience severe headache or blurred vision, or have palpitations or difficulty in passing urine, consult your doctor.

INTERACTIONS

Sedatives All drugs that have a sedative effect on the central nervous system may increase the sedative properties of dicycloverine.
Anticholinergic drugs These drugs may increase the adverse effects of dicycloverine.

SPECIAL PRECAUTIONS

Be sure to consult your doctor or pharmacist before taking this drug if:
◆ You have glaucoma.
◆ You have urinary problems.
◆ You have hiatus hernia.
◆ You are taking other medications.
Pregnancy No evidence of risk.
Breast-feeding The drug passes into the breast milk, but at normal doses adverse effects on the baby are unlikely. Discuss with your doctor.
Infants and children Reduced dose necessary.
Over 60 Reduced dose necessary. Elderly people are more susceptible to the drug's anticholinergic side effects.

Driving and hazardous work Avoid such activities until you have learned how dicycloverine affects you because the drug can cause drowsiness and blurred vision.
Alcohol Avoid. Alcohol may increase the sedative effects of this drug.

PROLONGED USE
No problems expected.

Digoxin

Brand name Lanoxin
Used in the following combined preparations
None

QUICK REFERENCE
Drug group Digitalis drug (p.29)
Overdose danger rating High
Dependence rating Low
Prescription needed Yes
Available as generic Yes

GENERAL INFORMATION
Digoxin is the most widely used form of digitalis, a compound obtained from the leaves of the foxglove plant. It is sometimes given in the treatment of congestive heart failure and certain alterations of heart rhythm. Digoxin increases the force of the heartbeat, making it more effective in pumping blood around the body. This, in turn, helps to control breathlessness, fluid retention, and tiredness.

The effective dose of digoxin can be close to the toxic dose; therefore, treatment needs to be monitored carefully to prevent toxic doses from being reached. Adverse effects are not infrequent, and their occurrence may suggest that the dose should be reduced. Consult your doctor, who can check the level of digoxin in your blood and find the correct dose for you.

INFORMATION FOR USERS
Your drug prescription is tailored for you. Do not alter dosage without checking with your doctor.
How taken Tablets, liquid, injection.
Frequency and timing of doses Up to 3 x daily (starting dose); once daily, or divided to reduce nausea (maintenance dose).

Adult dosage range 62.5–250mcg daily (by mouth).
Onset of effect Within a few minutes (injection); within 1–2 hours (by mouth).
Duration of action Up to 4 days.
Diet advice Digoxin may be more toxic if potassium levels are depleted, so your diet should include fresh fruit and vegetables, such as bananas and tomatoes.
Storage Keep in a closed container in a cool, dry place out of reach of children. Protect from light.
Missed dose Take as soon as you remember. If your next dose is due within 8 hours, take a dose now and skip the next.
Stopping the drug Unless palpitations occur, do not stop taking the drug without consulting your doctor. Stopping the drug may lead to worsening of the underlying condition.

OVERDOSE ACTION
Seek immediate medical advice in all cases. Take emergency action if palpitations, severe weakness, chest pain, or loss of consciousness occur.

POSSIBLE ADVERSE EFFECTS
The possible adverse effects are usually due to increased blood levels of the drug. Common effects include tiredness, loss of appetite, and nausea. More rarely, confusion, visual disturbance, or nausea may occur; these effects should be reported to your doctor. The drug is often given for disorders in which palpitations are experienced. If palpitations accompanied by breathlessness, chest pain, or lightheadedness or collapse occur, stop taking the drug and seek medical attention without delay.

INTERACTIONS
General note Many drugs interact with digoxin. Do not take any other medication unless on the advice of your doctor or pharmacist.
Diuretics These drugs may increase the risk of adverse effects from digoxin.
Antacids These may reduce the effects of digoxin. The effect of digoxin may increase when such drugs are stopped.
Anti-arrhythmic drugs These drugs may increase blood levels of digoxin.

SPECIAL PRECAUTIONS

Be sure to tell your doctor if:
◆ You have a long-term liver problem.
◆ You have thyroid trouble.
◆ You are taking other medications.
Pregnancy No evidence of risk, but adjustment in dose may be necessary.
Breast-feeding The drug passes into the breast milk, but at normal doses adverse effects on the baby are unlikely. Discuss with your doctor.
Infants and children Reduced dose necessary.
Over 60 Reduced dose may be necessary. Increased likelihood of adverse effects.
Driving and hazardous work Special problems are unlikely, but do not undertake these activities until you know how digoxin affects you.
Alcohol No special problems.

PROLONGED USE

No problems expected.
Monitoring Periodic checks on blood levels of digoxin and body salts may be advised.

Dihydrocodeine

Brand names DF118 Forte, DHC Continus
Used in the following combined preparations
Co-dydramol, Galake, Remedeine

QUICK REFERENCE

Drug group Opioid analgesic (p.9)
Overdose danger rating High
Dependence rating Medium
Prescription needed Yes
Available as generic Yes

GENERAL INFORMATION

Dihydrocodeine is an opioid analgesic related to codeine (see p.198) and of similar potency. Primarily used for the relief of mild to moderate pain, it has also been used as a cough suppressant. As with codeine, the possible side effects limit the dose that can be taken. Dihydrocodeine causes constipation, nausea, and vomiting.

The drug is also used in combination with paracetamol; in this way, a lower dose of the opioid can be used to give pain relief with fewer side effects. A combined preparation containing dihydrocodeine and paracetamol is available under the name co-dydramol.

INFORMATION FOR USERS

Your drug prescription is tailored for you. Do not alter dosage without checking with your doctor.
How taken Tablets, SR-tablets, liquid, injection.
Frequency and timing of doses 4–6 x daily.
Adult dosage range 120–240mg daily.
Onset of effect 30–60 minutes.
Duration of action 4–6 hours.
Diet advice None.
Storage Keep in a closed container in a cool, dry place out of the reach of children.
Missed dose Take as soon as you remember if using it for relief of symptoms. If not needed, do not take the missed dose; return to your normal dosage schedule when necessary.
Stopping the drug Can be safely stopped as soon as you no longer need it.

OVERDOSE ACTION

Seek immediate medical advice in all cases. Take emergency action if slow or irregular breathing, severe drowsiness, or loss of consciousness occur.

POSSIBLE ADVERSE EFFECTS

The most common adverse effects are constipation, nausea, vomiting, headache, drowsiness or dizziness, and vertigo. Abdominal pain and a rash or itching occur more rarely. Seek medical advice if confusion or hallucinations occur. If you have breathing difficulties, stop taking the drug and consult your doctor. Tolerance and dependence may occur.

INTERACTIONS

Sedatives All drugs that have a sedative effect on the central nervous system increase the sedative properties of dihydrocodeine. Such drugs include other opioid analgesics, sleeping drugs, antihistamines, antipsychotics, and antidepressants.
MAOIs These may cause a dangerous rise in blood pressure. Avoid using together and for 14 days after stopping MAOI treatment.

SPECIAL PRECAUTIONS

Be sure to tell your doctor if:
◆ You have liver or kidney problems.
◆ You have phaeochromocytoma.
◆ You have a lung disorder such as asthma or bronchitis.

◆ You have a problem with alcohol abuse.
◆ You have an enlarged prostate.
◆ You have low blood pressure.
◆ You have an underactive thyroid.
◆ You are taking other medications.

Pregnancy No evidence of risk, but it may affect the baby's breathing in labour.

Breast-feeding Safety not established. Discuss with your doctor.

Infants and children Not recommended under 4 years. Reduced dose necessary for older children.

Over 60 Reduced dose necessary.

Driving and hazardous work Avoid such activities until you have learned how dihydrocodeine affects you because the drug can cause drowsiness, dizziness, and nausea.

Alcohol Avoid. Alcohol may increase the sedative effects of dihydrocodeine.

PROLONGED USE

Dihydrocodeine is generally only used in the short term since it can be habit-forming if used long-term.

Diltiazem

Brand names Adizem, Calcicard, Dilzem, Slozem, Tildiem, and others
Used in the following combined preparations
None

QUICK REFERENCE

Drug group Anti-angina drug (p.35) and antihypertensive drug (p.36)
Overdose danger rating Medium
Dependence rating Low
Prescription needed Yes
Available as generic Yes

GENERAL INFORMATION

Diltiazem belongs to a group of drugs known as calcium channel blockers. These drugs interfere with the conduction of electrical signals in the muscles of the heart and blood vessels.

Diltiazem is used in the treatment of angina. When taken regularly, it reduces the frequency of angina attacks. However, it does not work quickly enough to reduce the pain of an angina attack that is already in progress. Longer-acting formulations are used to treat high blood pressure. Diltiazem does not adversely affect breathing, and it is of particular value for people with asthma, for whom other anti-angina drugs may not be suitable.

Different brands may not be equivalent, so you should always take the same brand.

INFORMATION FOR USERS

Your drug prescription is tailored for you. Do not alter dosage without checking with your doctor.

How taken Tablets, SR-tablets, capsules, SR-capsules.

Frequency and timing of doses 3 x daily (tablets/capsules); 1–2 x daily (SR-tablets/SR-capsules).

Adult dosage range 180–480mg daily.

Onset of effect 2–3 hours.

Duration of action 6–8 hours.

Diet advice None.

Storage Keep in a closed container in a cool, dry place out of reach of children.

Missed dose Take as soon as you remember. If your next dose is due within 2 hours, take a single dose now and skip the next.

Stopping the drug Unless a rash occurs, do not stop taking the drug without consulting your doctor; symptoms may recur. Stopping suddenly may worsen angina.

Exceeding the dose An occasional unintentional extra dose is unlikely to cause problems. Large overdoses may cause dizziness or collapse; notify your doctor urgently.

POSSIBLE ADVERSE EFFECTS

Diltiazem can cause various minor symptoms that are common to all calcium channel blockers, including headache, nausea, and dry mouth. If you develop swelling of the legs or ankles, consult your doctor. The most serious effect is the possibility of a slowed heart beat, which may cause tiredness or dizziness. These effects can sometimes be controlled by dosage adjustment. If you develop a rash, stop taking the drug and seek immediate medical advice.

INTERACTIONS

Antihypertensive drugs Diltiazem increases the effects of these drugs, further reducing blood pressure, but this interaction is often desired for better control of blood pressure.

Anticonvulsant drugs Levels of these drugs may be altered by diltiazem.

Anti-arrhythmic drugs There is a risk of side effects on the heart if these drugs are taken with diltiazem.

Digoxin Blood levels and adverse effects of this drug may be increased if it is taken with diltiazem. The dosage of digoxin may need to be reduced.

Theophylline/aminophylline Diltiazem may increase the levels of this drug.

Beta blockers These drugs increase the risk of the heart rate slowing.

SPECIAL PRECAUTIONS

Be sure to tell your doctor if:

◆ You have long-term liver or kidney problems.

◆ You have heart failure.

◆ You are taking other medications.

Pregnancy Not usually prescribed. Discuss with your doctor.

Breast-feeding The drug passes into the breast milk and may affect the baby. Discuss with your doctor.

Infants and children Not recommended.

Over 60 Reduced dose may be necessary. Increased likelihood of adverse effects.

Driving and hazardous work Avoid such activities until you have learned how diltiazem affects you because the drug can cause dizziness due to lowered blood pressure.

Alcohol Avoid excessive amounts. Alcohol may lower blood pressure, causing dizziness.

PROLONGED USE

No problems expected.

Dipyridamole

Brand name Persantin
Used in the following combined preparation
Asasantin Retard

QUICK REFERENCE

Drug group Antiplatelet drug (p.39)
Overdose danger rating Medium
Dependence rating Low
Prescription needed Yes
Available as generic Yes

GENERAL INFORMATION

Dipyridamole was introduced in the late 1970s as an anti-angina drug, to improve the ability of people with angina to take exercise. More effective drugs are now available, but dipyridamole is still prescribed as an anti-platelet drug. It acts by "thinning" the blood, which reduces the likelihood of clots forming in the bloodstream. This is especially important in people who have had a stroke or have undergone heart valve replacement surgery.

Dipyridamole is usually given together with other drugs such as warfarin or aspirin. It can also be given by injection during certain types of diagnostic test on the heart.

Side effects may occur, especially in the early days of treatment. If they persist, your doctor may advise a reduction in dosage.

INFORMATION FOR USERS

Your drug prescription is tailored for you. Do not alter dosage without checking with your doctor.

How taken Tablets, capsules, MR-capsules, liquid, injection (for diagnostic tests only).

Frequency and timing of doses 3–4 x daily, 1 hour before meals (tablets, capsules, liquid); 2 x daily with food (MR-capsules).

Adult dosage range 300–600mg daily.

Onset of effect Within 1 hour. Full therapeutic effect may not be felt for 2–3 weeks.

Duration of action Up to 8 hours. Up to 12 hours (MR-capsules).

Diet advice None.

Storage Keep in a closed container in a cool, dry place out of reach of children. Protect from light.

Missed dose Take as soon as you remember. If your next dose is due within 2 hours, take a single dose now and skip the next.

Stopping the drug Unless severe adverse effects occur (see below), do not stop taking the drug without consulting your doctor; withdrawal could lead to abnormal blood clotting.

Exceeding the dose An occasional unintentional extra dose is unlikely to be a cause for concern. Large overdoses may cause dizziness or vomiting; notify your doctor.

POSSIBLE ADVERSE EFFECTS

Adverse effects are rare. Dizziness, headache, fainting, and stomach upsets including nausea and diarrhoea may occur. If symptoms are severe, consult your doctor. If a rash develops, stop taking the drug and seek urgent medical advice. Occasionally, dipyridamole may aggravate angina.

INTERACTIONS

Anticoagulants Dipyridamole may add to the effects of these drugs, increasing the risk of uncontrolled bleeding. The dosage of the anticoagulant should be reduced.

Antacids These may reduce the effectiveness of dipyridamole.

SPECIAL PRECAUTIONS

Be sure to tell your doctor if:

◆ You have low blood pressure.

◆ You suffer from migraine.

◆ You have angina.

◆ You have had a recent heart attack.

◆ You are taking other medications.

Pregnancy Safety in pregnancy not established. Discuss with your doctor.

Breast-feeding The drug passes into the breast milk but at normal doses adverse effects on the baby are unlikely. Discuss with your doctor.

Infants and children Reduced dose necessary.

Over 60 No special problems.

Driving and hazardous work No problems expected.

Alcohol No known problems.

PROLONGED USE

No known problems.

Disulfiram

Brand name Antabuse
Used in the following combined preparations None

QUICK REFERENCE

Drug group Alcohol abuse deterrent
Overdose danger rating Medium
Dependence rating Low
Prescription needed Yes
Available as generic No

GENERAL INFORMATION

Disulfiram is used to help alcoholics abstain from alcohol. It does not cure alcoholism but provides a powerful deterrent to drinking.

If you are taking disulfiram and drink even a small amount of alcohol, very unpleasant reactions follow. These are due to high levels of acetaldehyde, a chemical formed by the partial breakdown of alcohol in the body, because disulfiram prevents this chemical from being broken down further into harmless substances. Effects include flushing, a throbbing headache, nausea, thirst, breathlessness, palpitations, dizziness, and fainting. Such reactions may last from 30 minutes to several hours, leaving you feeling drowsy. The reactions can also include loss of consciousness, so it is wise to carry a card naming a person to be notified in an emergency.

It is important not to drink any alcohol for at least 24 hours before starting treatment with disulfiram, and for at least a week after stopping. Any foods, medicines, and even toiletries that contain alcohol should also be avoided.

INFORMATION FOR USERS

Your drug prescription is tailored for you. Do not alter dosage without checking with your doctor.

How taken Tablets.

Frequency and timing of doses Once daily.

Adult dosage range 800mg initially, gradually reduced over 5 days to 100–200mg (maintenance dose).

Onset of effect Interaction with alcohol occurs within a few minutes of taking alcohol.

Duration of action Interaction with alcohol can occur for up to 6 days after the last dose of disulfiram.

Diet advice Avoid all alcoholic drinks, even in very small amounts. Food, fermented vinegar, medicines, mouthwashes, and lotions containing alcohol should also be avoided.

Storage Keep in a closed container in a cool, dry place out of reach of children. Protect from light.

Missed dose Take as soon as you remember. If your next dose is due within 2 hours, take a single dose now and skip the next.

Stopping the drug Do not stop taking the drug without consulting your doctor.

Exceeding the dose An occasional unintentional extra dose is unlikely to cause problems. Large overdoses may cause a temporary increase in adverse effects; notify your doctor.

POSSIBLE ADVERSE EFFECTS

Adverse effects, such as drowsiness, nausea or vomiting, and reduced libido, may occur but usually disappear with continued treatment. If they persist or become severe, the dosage may need to be adjusted. The most potentially severe effects are due to interaction with alcohol (see General information, above).

INTERACTIONS

General note A number of drugs can produce an adverse reaction when taken with disulfiram. Check with your doctor or pharmacist before taking any other medication.

Phenytoin Disulfiram increases the blood levels of this drug.

Anticoagulant drugs Disulfiram increases the effect of these drugs.

Metronidazole A severe reaction can occur if this drug is taken with disulfiram.

Theophylline Disulfiram may increase the toxic effects of this drug.

SPECIAL PRECAUTIONS

Be sure to tell your doctor if:
◆ You have long-term liver or kidney problems.
◆ You have heart problems, coronary artery disease, or high blood pressure.
◆ You have had epileptic fits.
◆ You have diabetes.
◆ You have breathing problems.
◆ You are taking other medications.

Pregnancy Safety in pregnancy not established. Discuss with your doctor.

Breast-feeding The drug passes into the breast milk and may affect the baby adversely. Discuss with your doctor.

Over 60 Reduced dose may be necessary.

Driving and hazardous work Avoid such activities until you have learned how disulfiram affects you because the drug can cause drowsiness and dizziness.

Alcohol Disulfiram may interact dangerously with alcohol. Never drink alcohol while under treatment with disulfiram, and avoid all foods, medicines, and toiletries containing alcohol.

PROLONGED USE

Not usually given for longer than 6 months without review. It is wise to carry a card stating that you are taking disulfiram and naming someone to be notified in an emergency.

Domperidone

Brand name Motilium
Used in the following combined preparations
Domperamol

QUICK REFERENCE

Drug group Anti-emetic drug (p.21)
Overdose danger rating Medium
Dependence rating Low
Prescription needed No
Available as generic No

GENERAL INFORMATION

Domperidone is an anti-emetic drug that was first introduced in the early 1980s. It is particularly effective for treating nausea and vomiting caused by gastroenteritis, chemotherapy, or radiotherapy. Domperidone is not effective for motion sickness or nausea that is caused by inner ear disorders such as Ménière's disease.

The main advantage of domperidone over other anti-emetics is that it does not usually cause drowsiness or other adverse effects (such as abnormal movement). However, the drug is not suitable for long-term treatment of gastrointestinal disorders, for which alternative drug treatment is often prescribed.

Domperidone may also be used to relieve dyspepsia (indigestion and heartburn); and, in combination with paracetamol, it is sometimes used to treat acute attacks of migraine.

INFORMATION FOR USERS

Follow instructions on the label. Call your doctor if symptoms worsen.

How taken Tablets, liquid, suppositories.
Frequency and timing of doses *Nausea/vomiting* Every 4–8 hours as required. *Dyspepsia* 3 x daily with water before meals and at night (tablets only).
Adult dosage range *Nausea/vomiting* 10–20mg (by mouth); 30–60mg (rectally).
Onset of effect Within 1 hour. The effects of the drug may be delayed if taken after the onset of nausea.
Duration of action Approximately 6 hours.
Diet advice None.
Storage Keep in a closed container in a cool, dry place out of reach of children. Protect from light.

Missed dose Take as soon as you remember for dyspepsia. If your next dose is due within 4 hours, take a single dose now and skip the next. Then return to your normal dosing schedule.

Stopping the drug Can be safely stopped as soon as you no longer need it.

Exceeding the dose An occasional unintentional extra dose is unlikely to cause problems. Large overdoses may cause dizziness; notify your doctor.

POSSIBLE ADVERSE EFFECTS

Adverse effects from this drug are rare. However, if you begin to experience muscle spasms or tremors, breast enlargement or milk secretion, or reduced libido, or if you develop a rash, consult your doctor.

INTERACTIONS

Anticholinergic drugs These may reduce the beneficial effects of domperidone.

Opioid analgesics These may reduce the beneficial effects of domperidone.

Bromocriptine and cabergoline Domperidone may reduce the effects of these drugs in some people.

SPECIAL PRECAUTIONS

Be sure to tell your doctor if:
◆ You have a long-term kidney problem.
◆ You have thyroid disease.
◆ You are taking other medications.

Pregnancy Safety in pregnancy not established. Discuss with your doctor.

Breast-feeding The drug may pass into the breast milk, but at normal doses adverse effects on the baby are unlikely. Discuss with your doctor.

Infants and children Prescribed only to treat nausea and vomiting caused by anticancer drugs or radiation therapy. Reduced dose necessary.

Over 60 No special problems.

Driving and hazardous work No special problems.

Alcohol No special problems, but alcohol is best avoided in cases of nausea and vomiting.

PROLONGED USE

Not prescribed for longer than 12 weeks.

Donepezil

Brand name Aricept
Used in the following combined preparations
None

QUICK REFERENCE

Drug group Drug for dementia (p.19)
Overdose danger rating Medium
Dependence rating Low
Prescription needed Yes
Available as generic No

GENERAL INFORMATION

Donepezil is an inhibitor of the enzyme acetylcholinesterase. This enzyme breaks down the natural neurotransmitter acetylcholine to limit its effects. Blocking the enzyme raises the levels of acetylcholine in the brain, which increases alertness. Donepezil has been found to reduce the progression of dementia due to Alzheimer's disease in up to half of the patients given the drug, and it is used to diminish deterioration in that disease. It is not currently recommended for dementia due to other causes.

It is usual for an expert to start you on the treatment and assess you after about three months to decide whether the drug is helping and whether it is worth continuing treatment. Side effects may include bladder outflow obstruction and psychiatric problems, such as agitation and aggression, which might be thought due to the disease.

INFORMATION FOR USERS

Your drug prescription is tailored for you. Do not alter dosage without checking with your doctor.

How taken Tablets.

Frequency and timing of doses Once daily at bedtime.

Adult dosage range 5–10mg.

Onset of effect 1 hour. Full effects might take up to 3 months.

Duration of action 1–2 days.

Diet advice None.

Storage Keep in a closed container in a cool, dry place out of reach of children.

Missed dose Take as soon as you remember. A carer should be overseeing the taking of the tablets.

Stopping the drug Do not stop taking the drug without consulting your doctor; symptoms may recur.

Exceeding the dose An occasional unintentional extra dose is unlikely to be a cause for concern. But if you notice any unusual symptoms, or if a large overdose has been taken, notify your doctor.

POSSIBLE ADVERSE EFFECTS

Adverse effects of donepezil include agitation, fatigue, insomnia, and problems such as accidents. (Such problems, however, are common in people with dementia, even those who are not being treated.) Other adverse effects include nausea, vomiting, diarrhoea, muscle cramps, and headache. If you experience dizziness or fainting, or you have palpitations or difficulty in passing urine, consult your doctor urgently.

INTERACTIONS

General note This drug is relatively new and interactions with other drugs are not fully established. If changes in the effect of donepezil are noticed when other drugs are taken or removed, discuss with your doctor.

Muscle relaxants used in surgery Donepezil may increase the effect of some muscle relaxants, but it may also block some others.

SPECIAL PRECAUTIONS

Be sure to tell your doctor if:
◆ You have a heart problem.
◆ You have asthma or respiratory problems.
◆ You have had a gastric or duodenal ulcer.
◆ You are taking an NSAID regularly.
◆ You are taking other medications.

Pregnancy Safety in pregnancy not established. Discuss with your doctor.

Breast-feeding Not recommended.

Infants and children Not recommended.

Over 60 No special problems.

Driving and hazardous work Your underlying condition may make such activities inadvisable. Discuss with your doctor.

Alcohol Avoid. Alcohol may reduce the effect of donepezil.

Surgery and general anaesthetics Donepezil treatment may need to be stopped before you have a general anaesthetic. Discuss with your doctor or dentist before any operation.

PROLONGED USE

Treatment may be continued for as long as there is benefit. Stopping the drug leads to a gradual loss of the improvements.

Monitoring Periodic checks may be performed to determine whether the drug is still providing some benefit.

Dorzolamide

Brand name Trusopt
Used in the following combined preparation Cosopt

QUICK REFERENCE

Drug group Drug for Glaucoma (p.114)
Overdose danger rating Low
Dependence rating Low
Prescription needed Yes
Available as generic No

GENERAL INFORMATION

Dorzolamide is a carbonic anhydrase inhibitor (a kind of diuretic drug) used, in the form of eye drops only, to treat glaucoma and for ocular hypertension (high blood pressure inside the eye). The drug relieves the pressure by reducing production of aqueous humour, the clear fluid in the front chamber of the eye.

Dorzolamide may be used, either alone or combined with a beta blocker, by people who are resistant to the effects of beta blockers or for whom these drugs are unsuitable.

Most of the side effects of dorzolamide are local to the eye, but systemic effects may occur if enough of the drug is absorbed into the body.

INFORMATION FOR USERS

Your drug prescription is tailored for you. Do not alter dosage without checking with your doctor.

How taken Eye drops.

Frequency and timing of doses 3 x daily (on its own); 2 x daily (combined preparation).

Adult dosage range 1 drop in the affected eye(s) or as directed.

Onset of effect 15–30 minutes.

Duration of action 4–8 hours.

Diet advice None.

Storage Keep in a closed container in a cool, dry place out of reach of children. Protect from light. Discard eye drops 4 weeks after opening them.

Missed dose Use as soon as you remember. If your next dose is due, skip the missed dose then go back to your normal dosing schedule.

Stopping the drug Unless severe adverse effects occur (see below), do not stop taking the drug without consulting your doctor; symptoms may recur.

Exceeding the dose An occasional unintentional extra application is unlikely to cause problems. Excessive use may provoke side effects as described below.

POSSIBLE ADVERSE EFFECTS

Local side effects include conjunctivitis and keratitis (inflammation of the cornea, the transparent part of the eye). This may lead to burning, stinging, or runny eyes; inflammation or soreness of the eyes or blurred vision; or a bitter taste in the mouth. Systemic side effects, such as nausea, dizziness, tiredness, and headache may also occur. If you develop a rash or breathing difficulties, stop taking the drug and consult your doctor urgently.

INTERACTIONS

General note Dorzolamide may interact with the following drugs, but there appear to be no published reports of problems. Consult your doctor.

Thiazide diuretics When these drugs are taken with dorzolamide, excessive loss of potassium may occur.

Aspirin This drug may increase dorzolamide levels and also the risk of adverse effects.

Lithium Dorzolamide may reduce blood levels of lithium.

SPECIAL PRECAUTIONS

Be sure to tell your doctor if:
◆ You have liver or kidney problems.
◆ You are allergic to sulphonamide drugs.
◆ You are allergic to benzalkonium chloride.
◆ You are taking other medications.

Pregnancy Not prescribed. Discuss with your doctor.

Breast-feeding Not recommended. Discuss with your doctor.

Infants and children Not recommended.

Over 60 No special problems.

Driving and hazardous work Avoid such activities until you have learned how dorzolamide affects you because the drug can cause dizziness and blurred vision.

Alcohol No special problems.

PROLONGED USE

No special problems.

Dosulepin

Brand names Dothapax, Prepadine, Prothiaden
Used in the following combined preparations
None

QUICK REFERENCE

Drug group Tricyclic antidepressant drug (p.14)
Overdose danger rating High
Dependence rating Low
Prescription needed Yes
Available as generic Yes

GENERAL INFORMATION

Dosulepin belongs to a class of antidepressant drugs known as the the tricyclics and is used in the long-term treatment of depression. The drug is particularly useful when the depression is accompanied by anxiety and insomnia. Dosulepin has a number of effects; it elevates mood, increases physical activity, improves the appetite, and restores the individual's interest in everyday activities. Taken at night, the drug encourages sleep and helps to eliminate the need for additional sleeping drugs.

Dosulepin takes several weeks to achieve its full antidepressant effect. It has adverse effects that are common to all tricyclic antidepressants. These include a risk of the drug causing dangerous heart rhythms, fits, and coma if its levels build up in the body or if it is taken in overdose.

INFORMATION FOR USERS

Your drug prescription is tailored for you. Do not alter dosage without checking with your doctor.

How taken Tablets, capsules.
Frequency and timing of doses 2–3 x daily or once at night.

Adult dosage range 75–150mg daily (maximum of 225mg in some circumstances).

Onset of effect Full antidepressant effect may not be felt for 2–4 weeks, but adverse effects may be noticed within a day or two.

Duration of action Several days.

Diet advice None.

Storage Keep in a closed container in a cool, dry place out of reach of children.

Missed dose Take as soon as you remember. If your next dose is due within 2 hours, take a single dose now and skip the next.

Stopping the drug Unless severe adverse effects occur (see below), do not stop taking the drug without consulting your doctor, who may supervise a gradual reduction in dosage. Abrupt cessation may cause withdrawal symptoms and a recurrence of the original problem.

OVERDOSE ACTION

Seek immediate medical advice in all cases. Take emergency action if palpitations or loss of consciousness occur.

POSSIBLE ADVERSE EFFECTS

The adverse effects of dosulepin are mainly due to its anticholinergic (see Autonomic nervous system, p.8) action. They include drowsiness, dry mouth, sweating, and blurred vision and are more common in the early days of treatment. The drug can also affect normal heart rhythm. If dizziness, fainting, rash, difficulty in passing urine, palpitations, or loss of consciousness occur, stop taking the drug and consult your doctor urgently.

INTERACTIONS

Sedatives All drugs that have a sedative effect on the central nervous system increase the sedative properties of dosulepin.

Heavy smoking This may reduce the antidepressant effect of dosulepin.

Antiarrhythmic drugs Dosulepin should be avoided by patients taking amiodarone (see p.138), sotalol (see p.389), and other medications that can affect heart rhythms.

MAOIs In the rare cases where these drugs are given with dosulepin, serious interactions may occur.

Antiepileptic drugs Dosulepin may reduce the effectiveness of these drugs.

SPECIAL PRECAUTIONS

Be sure to tell your doctor if:
◆ You have heart problems.
◆ You have had epileptic fits.
◆ You have any long-term liver or kidney problems.
◆ You have glaucoma.
◆ You have prostate trouble.
◆ You have had mania or a psychotic illness.
◆ You are taking other medications.

Pregnancy Safety in pregnancy not established. Discuss with your doctor.

Breast-feeding The drug passes into the breast milk, but effects on the baby are unlikely. Discuss with your doctor.

Infants and children Not recommended.

Over 60 This age group has a greater risk of adverse effects.

Driving and hazardous work Avoid all such activities until you have learned how dosulepin affects you because the drug can reduce alertness and may cause blurred vision, dizziness, and drowsiness.

Alcohol Avoid. Alcohol may increase the sedative effects of this drug.

Surgery and general anaesthetics Dosulepin treatment may need to be stopped before you have a general anaesthetic. Discuss this with your doctor or dentist before you have any surgery.

PROLONGED USE

No problems expected.

Monitoring Any person experiencing drowsiness, confusion, muscle cramps, or convulsions should be monitored for low blood sodium levels.

Doxazosin

Brand name Cardura, Cardura XL
Used in the following combined preparations
None

QUICK REFERENCE

Drug group Vasodilator (p.31), antihypertensive drug (p.36), and drug for urinary disorders (p.112)
Overdose danger rating Medium
Dependence rating Low
Prescription needed Yes
Available as generic No

GENERAL INFORMATION

Doxazosin is an antihypertensive vasodilator drug that relieves hypertension (high blood pressure). The drug works by relaxing the muscles in the blood vessel walls, which allows them to dilate and thereby eases the flow of blood. Because it is eliminated slowly from the body, it is usually given only once daily. Doxazosin may be administered together with other antihypertensive drugs, including beta blockers, because its effects on blood pressure are increased when it is combined with most other antihypertensives.

Doxazosin can also be given to patients who have an enlarged prostate gland. It relaxes the muscles around the bladder exit and prostate gland, allowing urine to flow out more easily.

Dizziness and fainting may occur at the onset of treatment with doxazosin, because the first dose may cause a marked fall in blood pressure. For this reason, the initial dose is usually low. It should be taken at home, preferably just before bedtime.

INFORMATION FOR USERS

Your drug prescription is tailored for you. Do not alter dosage without checking with your doctor.

How taken MR-tablets.

Frequency and timing of doses Once daily, at the same time each day.

Adult dosage range *Hypertension* 1mg (starting dose), increased gradually as necessary up to 16mg. *Enlarged prostate* 1mg (starting dose), increased gradually at 1–2-week intervals up to 8mg.

Onset of effect Within 2 hours.

Duration of action 24 hours.

Diet advice None.

Storage Keep in a closed container in a cool, dry place out of reach of children.

Missed dose If you forget to take a tablet, skip that dose completely but carry on as normal the following day.

Stopping the drug Do not stop taking the drug without consulting your doctor. Stopping the drug may lead to a rise in blood pressure.

Exceeding the dose An occasional unintentional extra dose is unlikely to be a cause for concern. Larger overdoses may cause dizziness or fainting; notify your doctor.

POSSIBLE ADVERSE EFFECTS

Nausea, a stuffy or runny nose, headache, drowsiness, and weakness are common adverse effects of doxazosin. The main problem, however, is that the drug may cause dizziness or fainting when you stand up. Urinary incontinence may occur in women. Consult your doctor if you develop a rash. If, rarely, palpitations or chest pain occur, seek urgent medical advice.

INTERACTIONS

Antihypertensive drugs Any drugs that can reduce the blood pressure are likely to have an increased effect when taken with doxazosin. These include diuretics, beta blockers, ACE inhibitors, nitrates, calcium channel blockers, and some antipsychotics and antidepressants.

SPECIAL PRECAUTIONS

Be sure to tell your doctor if:
◆ You have any long-term liver or kidney problems.
◆ You have had an allergic reaction to doxazosin in the past.
◆ You are taking other medications.

Pregnancy Safety in pregnancy not established. Discuss with your doctor.

Breast-feeding The drug passes into the breast milk and may affect the baby. Discuss with your doctor.

Infants and children Not recommended.

Over 60 Reduced dose may be necessary. Take extra care when standing up until you have learned how doxazosin affects you.

Driving and hazardous work Avoid such activities until you have learned how doxazosin affects you because the drug can cause drowsiness, dizziness, and fainting.

Alcohol Avoid excessive amounts. Alcohol may increase some of the adverse effects of doxazosin, such as dizziness, drowsiness, and fainting.

Surgery and general anaesthetics A general anaesthetic may increase the blood-pressure-lowering effect of doxazosin. Discuss this with your doctor or dentist before having any surgery.

PROLONGED USE

No known problems.

Doxorubicin

Brand names Caelyx, Myocet
Used in the following combined preparations
None

QUICK REFERENCE

Drug group Cytotoxic anticancer drug (p.96)
Overdose danger rating Medium
Dependence rating Low
Prescription needed Yes
Available as generic Yes

GENERAL INFORMATION

Doxorubicin is one of the most effective anticancer drugs. It is prescribed for a wide variety of cancers, usually in conjunction with other anticancer drugs. Doxorubicin is used in the treatment of acute leukaemia and cancer of the lymph nodes (Hodgkin's disease), lung, breast, bladder, stomach, thyroid, and reproductive organs. It is also used to treat Kaposi's sarcoma in AIDS patients.

Nausea and vomiting after injection are the most common side effects of this drug. Although these symptoms are unpleasant, they tend to become less severe as the body adjusts to the treatment. Doxorubicin may stain the urine bright red, but this effect is not harmful. More seriously, because the drug interferes with the production of blood cells, blood clotting disorders, anaemia, and infections may occur. Therefore, effects on the blood will be carefully monitored. Hair loss is also a common side effect of the treatment. Heart rhythm disturbance and heart failure are rare, dose-dependent side effects that may also occur.

INFORMATION FOR USERS

This drug is given only under medical supervision and is not for self-administration.
How taken Injection, bladder instillation.
Frequency and timing of doses Every 1–3 weeks.
Adult dosage range Dosage is determined individually according to body height, weight, and response.
Onset of effect Some adverse effects may appear within 1 hour, but the full beneficial effects may not be felt for up to 4 weeks.
Duration of action Adverse effects can persist for up to 2 weeks after treatment has stopped.

Diet advice None.
Storage Not applicable. The drug is not normally kept in the home.
Missed dose The drug is administered in hospital under close medical supervision. If for some reason you skip your dose, contact your doctor as soon as you can.
Stopping the drug Do not stop taking the drug without consulting your doctor. Stopping abruptly may lead to a worsening of the underlying condition.
Exceeding the dose Overdosage is unlikely since treatment is carefully monitored and supervised.

POSSIBLE ADVERSE EFFECTS

Nausea and vomiting generally occur within an hour of injection. Hair loss, loss of appetite, and diarrhoea are common. Mouth ulcers and skin irritation or ulcers may also occur. Palpitations may indicate that the drug is having an adverse effect on the heart. Since treatment is closely supervised in hospital, all adverse effects are monitored.

INTERACTIONS

Ciclosporin Administration of ciclosporin while you are receiving doxorubicin can lead to adverse effects on the nervous system.

SPECIAL PRECAUTIONS

Doxorubicin is prescribed only under close medical supervision, taking account of your present condition and medical history.
Pregnancy Not usually prescribed. The drug may cause birth defects or premature birth. Discuss with your doctor.
Breast-feeding Not advised. The drug passes into the breast milk and may affect the baby adversely. Discuss with your doctor.
Infants and children Reduced dose necessary.
Over 60 Increased risk of adverse effects. Reduced dose may be necessary.
Driving and hazardous work No known problems.
Alcohol No known problems.

PROLONGED USE

Prolonged use of doxorubicin may reduce the activity of the bone marrow, leading to reduced production of all types of blood cell. It may also affect the heart adversely.

Monitoring Periodic checks on blood composition are usually required. Regular heart examinations are also carried out.

Doxycycline

Brand names Demix, Doxylar, Vibramycin, Vibramycin-D
Used in the following combined preparations None

QUICK REFERENCE

Drug group Tetracycline antibiotic (p.62)
Overdose danger rating Low
Dependence rating Low
Prescription needed Yes
Available as generic Yes

GENERAL INFORMATION

Doxycycline is a type of antibiotic drug known as a tetracycline. It is used to treat infections of the urinary, respiratory, and gastrointestinal tracts. It is also prescribed for treatment of some sexually transmitted diseases, skin, eye, and prostate infections, acne, and malaria prevention (see p.75).

Doxycycline is less likely than other tetracyclines to cause diarrhoea as a side effect, and its absorption is not significantly impaired by milk and food. The drug can therefore be taken with meals to reduce side effects such as nausea or indigestion. Unlike most other tetracyclines, doxycycline is also safe for people whose kidney function is impaired.

Like other tetracyclines, however, the drug can stain developing teeth and may affect bone development. It is therefore usually avoided in young children or pregnant women.

INFORMATION FOR USERS

Your drug prescription is tailored for you. Do not alter dosage without checking with your doctor.
How taken Tablets, capsules.
Frequency and timing of doses 1–2 x daily with water, or with or after food, in sitting or standing position, and well before going to bed, to avoid the risk of throat irritation.
Dosage range 100–200mg daily.
Onset of effect 4–12 hours; several weeks for acne.

Duration of action Up to 24 hours; for acne, several weeks.
Diet advice None.
Storage Keep in a closed container in a cool, dry place out of reach of children.
Missed dose Take as soon as you remember. If your next dose is due within 6 hours, take a single dose now and skip the next.
Stopping the drug Take the full course. Even if you feel better, the original infection may still be present and symptoms may recur if treatment is stopped too soon.
Exceeding the dose An occasional unintentional extra dose is unlikely to be a cause for concern. But if you notice any unusual symptoms, or if a large overdose has been taken, notify your doctor.

POSSIBLE ADVERSE EFFECTS

Adverse effects are rare, but some people may experience nausea, vomiting, or diarrhoea. Other possible adverse effects include rash, itching, and increased sensitivity of the skin to sunlight. If you experience headaches or visual disturbances, stop taking the drug and consult your doctor without delay.

INTERACTIONS

Penicillin antibiotics Doxycycline interferes with the antibacterial action of these drugs.
Oral anticoagulant drugs Doxycycline may increase the anticoagulant action of these drugs.
Barbiturates, carbamazepine, and phenytoin All of these drugs reduce the effectiveness of doxycycline; therefore, doxycycline dosage may need to be increased.
Oral contraceptives A slight risk exists of doxycycline reducing the effectiveness of oral contraceptives. Discuss with your doctor.
Antacids and preparations containing iron, calcium, or magnesium These may impair absorption of this drug. Do not take within 2–3 hours of doxycycline.
Ciclosporin, digoxin, and lithium Doxycycline may increase the blood levels of this drug.

SPECIAL PRECAUTIONS

Be sure to tell your doctor if:
◆ You have a long-term liver problem.
◆ You have previously suffered an allergic reaction to a tetracycline antibiotic.

◆ You have porphyria.
◆ You have systemic lupus erythematosus.
◆ You have myasthenia gravis.
◆ You are taking other medications.

Pregnancy Not used in pregnancy. It may discolour the teeth of the developing baby.

Breast-feeding The drug passes into the breast milk. It may lead to discoloration of the baby's teeth and may also have other adverse effects. Discuss with your doctor.

Infants and children Not recommended under 12 years. Reduced dose necessary for older children.

Over 60 No special problems. Dispersible tablets should be used as they are less likely to cause oesophageal irritation or ulceration.

Driving and hazardous work No known problems.

Alcohol Excessive amounts may decrease the effectiveness of doxycycline.

Surgery and general anaesthetics Notify your doctor or dentist that you are taking doxycycline before any operation.

Sunlight Avoid excessive exposure.

PROLONGED USE

Not usually prescribed in the long term, except for acne.

Dydrogesterone

Brand names Duphaston, Duphaston HRT
Used in the following combined preparations
Femoston, Femapak

QUICK REFERENCE

Drug group Female sex hormone (p.88)
Overdose danger rating Low
Dependence rating Low
Prescription needed Yes
Available as generic No

GENERAL INFORMATION

Dydrogesterone is a progestogen, a synthetic hormone similar to the natural female sex hormone progesterone. The drug is widely used to treat a variety of menstrual disorders that are thought to result from a deficiency of progesterone. These include premenstrual syndrome and absent, irregular, or painful periods (see p.104).

Dydrogesterone is also prescribed together with an oestrogen as part of hormone replacement therapy (HRT) following the menopause. It may be prescribed for endometriosis (p.100), and is also given to prevent miscarriage in women who have had repeated miscarriages.

Dydrogesterone is usually taken on selected days during the menstrual cycle, depending on the disorder that is being treated.

INFORMATION FOR USERS

Your drug prescription is tailored for you. Do not alter dosage without checking with your doctor.

How taken Tablets, patches.

Frequency and timing of doses 1–3 x daily. In many conditions, this drug is taken at certain times in the menstrual cycle.

Adult dosage range 10–30mg daily.

Onset of effect Beneficial effects of this drug may not be felt for several months.

Duration of action 12 hours.

Diet advice None.

Storage Keep in a closed container in a cool, dry place out of reach of children. Protect from light.

Missed dose Take as soon as you remember. If your next dose is due within 2 hours, take a single dose now and skip the next.

Stopping the drug Do not stop taking the drug without consulting your doctor; symptoms may recur.

Exceeding the dose An occasional unintentional extra dose is unlikely to be a cause for concern. But if you notice any unusual symptoms, or if a large overdose has been taken, notify your doctor.

POSSIBLE ADVERSE EFFECTS

Irregular periods and "breakthrough" bleeding are the most common adverse effects but may be helped by dosage adjustment. Fluid retention (leading to swollen feet or ankles), weight gain, nausea or vomiting, breast tenderness, headache, or dizziness may also occur. Consult your doctor if any of these become severe or if you develop a rash.

INTERACTIONS

Ciclosporin Dydrogesterone increases the effects of this drug.

SPECIAL PRECAUTIONS

Be sure to tell your doctor if:

◆ You have long-term liver or kidney problems.

◆ You have heart or circulatory problems.

◆ You have diabetes.

◆ You have high blood pressure.

◆ You have porphyria.

◆ You or a family member have had breast cancer.

◆ You are taking other medications.

Pregnancy No evidence of risk at normal dosage. The drug is used to prevent miscarriage.

Breast-feeding The drug passes into the breast milk, but at normal doses adverse effects on the baby are unlikely. High doses may suppress milk production.

Infants and children Not prescribed.

Over 60 No special problems.

Driving and hazardous work Avoid such activities until you have learned how dydrogesterone affects you because the drug may, rarely, cause dizziness.

Alcohol No special problems.

PROLONGED USE

No special problems.

Efavirenz

Brand name Sustiva
Used in the following combined preparations
None

QUICK REFERENCE

Drug group Drug for HIV and immune deficiency
(p.100)
Overdose danger rating Medium
Dependence rating Low
Prescription needed Yes
Available as generic No

GENERAL INFORMATION

Efavirenz is a reverse transcriptase inhibitor, which is a type of antiretroviral drug used to treat HIV infection. It is given together with other antiretrovirals – for example, two other reverse transcriptase inhibitors – as combination therapy to slow down the production of the virus. The aim of this treatment is to reduce the damage done to the immune system by the virus. Combination antiretroviral therapy is not a cure for HIV. If the drugs are taken regularly on a long-term basis, they can reduce the level of the virus in the body and improve the outlook for the HIV patient. However, the patient will remain infectious, and will suffer a relapse if treatment is stopped.

INFORMATION FOR USERS

Your drug prescription is tailored for you. Do not alter dosage without checking with your doctor.
How taken Tablets, capsules, liquid.
Frequency and timing of doses Once daily, usually at night to minimize adverse effects.
Adult dosage range 600mg, but may be reduced according to body weight.
Onset of effect 1 hour.
Duration of action 24 hours.
Diet advice None.
Storage Keep in the original container in a cool, dry place out of the reach of children.
Missed dose Take as soon as you remember. If your next dose is due within 2 hours, take a single dose now and skip the next. It is very important not to miss doses on a regular basis as this could lead to the development of drug-resistant HIV.

Stopping the drug Do not stop taking the drug without consulting your doctor. It may be necessary to withdraw all your drugs gradually, starting with efavirenz.
Exceeding the dose An occasional unintentional extra dose is unlikely to cause problems. However, if you notice any unusual symptoms, or if a large overdose has been taken, notify your doctor.

POSSIBLE ADVERSE EFFECTS

Gastrointestinal upset, including nausea, vomiting and diarrhoea, and rash are the most common adverse effects. Efavirenz can cause vivid dreams and changes in sleep patterns, but these tend to wear off with time. If any of the symptoms are severe, or mood changes occur, seek medical advice. If you develop a rash, contact your doctor without delay.

INTERACTIONS

General note A wide range of drugs may interact with efavirenz, causing either an increase in adverse effects or a reduction in the effect of the antiretroviral drugs. Check with your doctor or pharmacist before taking any new drugs, including those from the dentist and supermarket, and herbal medicines.

SPECIAL PRECAUTIONS

Be sure to tell your doctor if:
◆ You have liver or kidney problems.
◆ You have an infection such as hepatitis B or C.
◆ You are pregnant or planning pregnancy.
◆ You are taking other medications.
Pregnancy Should not be used during pregnancy except on strict medical advice. Pregnancy should be avoided by using barrier, in addition to other, methods of contraception.
Breast-feeding Safety in breast-feeding not established. Breast-feeding is not recommended for HIV-positive mothers as the virus may be passed to the baby.
Infants and children Not prescribed to children under 3 years. Reduced dose necessary in older children.
Over 60 Reduced dose may be necessary to minimize adverse effects.
Driving and hazardous work Avoid such activities until you have learned how efavirenz affects you because the drug can cause dizziness.

Alcohol No known problems, although some people may find the effects of alcohol are more pronounced while taking efavirenz.

PROLONGED USE
No known problems.
Monitoring Regular blood samples are taken to check the drug's effects on the virus and for changes in lipid, cholesterol, and glucose levels.

Enalapril

Brand names Enacard, Ednyt, Innovace, Pralenal
Used in the following combined preparation
Innozide

QUICK REFERENCE
Drug group Vasodilator (p.31)
Overdose danger rating Medium
Dependence rating Low
Prescription needed Yes
Available as generic Yes

GENERAL INFORMATION
Enalapril is an ACE (angiotensin-converting enzyme) inhibitor used to treat high blood pressure (see p.36) and heart failure (in which the heart is unable to deal with its workload). It may also be given to patients following a heart attack and is sometimes used to prevent or delay kidney damage in patients with diabetes. It is often given with a diuretic to increase its effect on high blood pressure and heart failure. Enalapril relaxes the muscles in blood vessel walls, dilating (widening) them, which enables the blood to circulate more easily and helps to lower blood pressure. The drug is long-acting and is taken once or twice daily. The first dose may cause a sudden drop in blood pressure, especially in patients taking a diuretic. For this reason, you should lie down for 2–3 hours afterwards.

Enalapril may cause a variety of minor side effects, such as a persistent dry cough and taste disturbance, which a reduction in dose may help to minimize.

INFORMATION FOR USERS
Your drug prescription is tailored for you. Do not alter dosage without checking with your doctor.

How taken Tablets.
Frequency and timing of doses 1–2 x daily.
Adult dosage range 2.5–5mg daily (starting dose), increased to 10–40mg daily (maintenance dose).
Onset of effect Within 1 hour.
Duration of action 24 hours.
Diet advice None.
Storage Keep in a closed container in a dry place below 25°C, out of reach of children. Protect from light.
Missed dose Take as soon as you remember. If your next dose is due within 8 hours, take a single dose now and skip the next.
Stopping the drug Unless severe adverse effects occur (see below), do not stop taking the drug without consulting your doctor. Stopping the drug may lead to worsening of the underlying condition.
Exceeding the dose An occasional unintentional extra dose is unlikely to be a cause for concern. Large overdoses may cause dizziness or fainting; notify your doctor.

POSSIBLE ADVERSE EFFECTS
Common adverse effects such as dizziness and headache usually diminish with long-term treatment. Less common problems may also diminish in time, but dosage adjustment may be necessary. A rash may occur, but usually disappears when the drug is stopped. A persistent dry cough is the most common effect, but this can be minimized by taking smaller, more frequent, doses. Consult your doctor if you develop a cough, rash, fainting, or muscle cramps. If you suffer from wheezing or breathing difficulties, and swelling, stop taking the drug and seek urgent medical advice.

INTERACTIONS
Antihypertensive drugs and NSAIDs These drugs are likely to enhance the blood-pressure-lowering effect of enalapril.
Lithium Enalapril increases the levels of lithium in the blood, and serious adverse effects from lithium excess may occur.
Ciclosporin Taken with enalapril, this drug may increase blood levels of potassium.
Potassium supplements and potassium-sparing diuretics Enalapril may add to the effect of these drugs, leading to raised levels of potassium in the blood.

NSAIDs Some of these drugs may reduce the effectiveness of enalapril. There is also risk of kidney damage when they are taken with it.

SPECIAL PRECAUTIONS
Be sure to tell your doctor if:
◆ You have suffered from severe allergies.
◆ You have long-term kidney problems.
◆ You have coronary artery disease.
◆ You have angioedema.
◆ You have peripheral vascular disease.
◆ You are on a low-sodium diet.
◆ You are allergic to other ACE inhibitors.
◆ You are taking other medications.

Pregnancy Not prescribed. May cause defects in the developing baby.

Breast-feeding The drug passes into the breast milk, but at normal doses adverse effects on the baby are unlikely. Discuss with your doctor.

Infants and children Not usually prescribed.

Over 60 Reduced dose may be necessary.

Driving and hazardous work Avoid such activities until you have learned how enalapril affects you because the drug can cause dizziness and fainting.

Alcohol Avoid excessive amounts. Alcohol may increase the blood-pressure-lowering and adverse effects of this drug.

Surgery and general anaesthetics Notify your doctor or dentist that you are taking enalapril.

PROLONGED USE
No problems expected.

Monitoring Periodic tests on blood and urine should be performed.

Ephedrine

Brand name None
Used in the following combined preparations
Do-Do Chesteze, Franol, Franol Plus, Haymine, and others

QUICK REFERENCE
Drug group Bronchodilator (p.23) and decongestant (p.26)
Overdose danger rating Medium
Dependence rating Low
Prescription needed No
Available as generic Yes

GENERAL INFORMATION
In use for more than 50 years, ephedrine is a drug that promotes the release of nor-ephedrine, a neurotransmitter. It was once widely prescribed as a bronchodilator to relax the muscles surrounding the airways, easing the breathing difficulty caused by asthma, and to help some patients suffering from chronic bronchitis or emphysema. Newer, more effective drugs have largely replaced ephedrine for these purposes. Its main use now is as a decongestant in nasal drops and cough preparations. In addition, ephedrine injections may be used as a method of restoring normal blood pressure after anaesthetic procedures.

Adverse effects are unusual with nasal drops used in moderation, but taken by mouth the drug may stimulate the heart and central nervous system, causing palpitations and anxiety. It is not recommended for elderly people, who are more sensitive to ephedrine's effects on the heart, and the drug may also cause urinary retention in elderly men.

INFORMATION FOR USERS
Follow instructions on the label. Call your doctor if symptoms worsen.

How taken Tablets, syrup, injection, nasal drops.

Frequency and timing of doses 3 x daily (by mouth); 3–4 x daily (nasal drops).

Dosage range *Adults* 45–180mg daily (by mouth); 1–2 drops into each nostril per dose (drops); 3–6mg every 3–4 minutes to maximum of 30mg (injection). *Children* Reduced dose according to age and weight.

Onset of effect Within 15–60 minutes.

Duration of action 3–6 hours.

Diet advice None.

Storage Keep in a closed container in a cool, dry place out of reach of children. Protect from light.

Missed dose Do not take the missed dose. Take your next dose as usual.

Stopping the drug Can be safely stopped as soon as you no longer need it.

Exceeding the dose An occasional unintentional extra dose is unlikely to cause problems. Large overdoses may cause shortness of breath, high fever, fits, or loss of consciousness; notify your doctor immediately.

POSSIBLE ADVERSE EFFECTS

Adverse effects from ephedrine nasal drops are uncommon, although local irritation can occur. When taken by mouth, the drug may affect the central nervous system, causing insomnia and anxiety; however, taking the last dose before 4 pm may prevent insomnia. It may also affect the cardiovascular system, causing palpitations or chest pain, which need urgent medical attention. Other adverse effects include cold extremities, tremor, a dry mouth, and urinary difficulties. If you develop palpitations or chest pain, stop taking the drug and consult your doctor without delay.

INTERACTIONS

MAOIs Ephedrine may interact with these drugs to cause a dangerous rise in blood pressure.

Beta blockers Ephedrine may interact with these drugs to cause a dangerous rise in blood pressure.

Antihypertensive drugs Ephedrine may counteract the effects of some of these drugs.

SPECIAL PRECAUTIONS

Be sure to consult your doctor or pharmacist before taking this drug if:
◆ You have a long-term kidney problem.
◆ You have heart disease.
◆ You have high blood pressure.
◆ You have diabetes.
◆ You have an overactive thyroid gland.
◆ You have had glaucoma.
◆ You have urinary difficulties.
◆ You are taking other medications.

Pregnancy Safety in pregnancy not established. Discuss with your doctor.

Breast-feeding The drug passes into the breast milk and may affect the baby. Discuss with your doctor.

Infants and children Reduced dose necessary.

Over 60 Not usually prescribed.

Driving and hazardous work Avoid such activities until you have learned how ephedrine affects you. There are no special problems with nasal drops.

Alcohol No special problems.

Surgery and general anaesthetics Ephedrine may need to be stopped before you have a general anaesthetic. Discuss this with your doctor or dentist before surgery.

PROLONGED USE

Not recommended except on medical advice. Decongestant effects may lessen with nasal drops, and rebound congestion may occur.

Epinephrine (Adrenaline)

Brand names Ana-Guard, Anapen, EpiPen, Eppy, Minijet Adrenaline
Used in the following combined preparations Ganda, several local anaesthetics (e.g. Xylocaine)

QUICK REFERENCE

Drug group Drug for glaucoma (p.114) and drug for cardiac resuscitation and anaphylaxis
Overdose danger rating High
Dependence rating Low
Prescription needed Yes
Available as generic Yes

GENERAL INFORMATION

Epinephrine is a neurotransmitter produced in the centre (medulla) of the adrenal glands. Synthetic forms have existed since 1900. It is given in an emergency to stimulate heart activity and raise blood pressure. It also narrows blood vessels in the skin and intestine.

Epinephrine is injected to counteract cardiac arrest or relieve severe allergic reactions (anaphylaxis). For those at risk of anaphylaxis, pre-filled syringes are available for immediate self-injection at the start of an attack.

Given as eye drops, epinephrine lowers the pressure within the eye, making it useful in glaucoma and eye surgery. Because it constricts blood vessels, it is also used to control bleeding and to slow the dispersal, and thereby prolong the effect, of local anaesthetics.

INFORMATION FOR USERS

Your drug prescription is tailored for you. Do not alter dosage without checking with your doctor.

How taken Injection, eye drops.
Frequency and timing of doses As directed according to method of administration and underlying disorder.
Dosage range As directed according to method of administration and underlying disorder.
Onset of effect Within 5 minutes (injection); within 1 hour (eye drops).

Duration of action Up to 4 hours (injection); up to 24 hours (eye drops).
Diet advice None.
Storage Keep in a closed container in a cool, dry place out of reach of children. Protect from light.
Missed dose Do not take the missed dose. Take the next dose as usual.
Stopping the drug Do not stop using the eye drops without consulting your doctor; stopping the drug may lead to worsening of the underlying condition.

OVERDOSE ACTION

Seek immediate medical advice in all cases. Take emergency action if palpitations, breathing difficulties, or loss of consciousness occur.

POSSIBLE ADVERSE EFFECTS

The drug's main adverse effects are related to its stimulant action on the heart and central nervous system. Nervousness, restlessness, dry mouth, nausea, vomiting, and cold extremities are common. If headache, blurred vision or palpitations occur, consult your doctor. Eye drops may cause burning or inflammation.

INTERACTIONS

General note A variety of drugs interact with epinephrine to increase the risk of palpitations and/or high blood pressure. Such drugs include MAOIs and tricyclic antidepressants.
Beta blockers Epinephrine can produce a dangerous rise in blood pressure with certain beta blockers, such as propranolol.
Antidiabetic drugs Epinephrine may reduce the effectiveness of these drugs.

SPECIAL PRECAUTIONS

Be sure to tell your doctor if:
◆ You have a heart problem.
◆ You have diabetes.
◆ You have an overactive thyroid gland.
◆ You have a nervous system problem.
◆ You have high blood pressure.
◆ You are taking other medications.
Pregnancy Not usually prescribed. May cause defects in the developing baby and prolong labour. Discuss with your doctor.
Breast-feeding Adverse effects on the baby are unlikely. Discuss with your doctor.

Infants and children Reduced dose necessary.
Over 60 Reduced dose may be necessary. Increased likelihood of adverse effects.
Driving and hazardous work No known problems.
Alcohol No known problems.
Surgery and general anaesthetics Epinephrine may need to be stopped before you have a general anaesthetic. Discuss this with your doctor or dentist before any surgery.

PROLONGED USE

Long-term use of epinephrine eye drops with soft contact lenses is not recommended.

Ergotamine

Brand names None
Used in the following combined preparations Cafergot, Migril

QUICK REFERENCE

Drug group Drug used for migraine (p.20)
Overdose danger rating Medium
Dependence rating Medium
Prescription needed Yes
Available as generic Yes

GENERAL INFORMATION

Ergotamine is used to treat migraine but its use has largely been superseded by newer agents with fewer adverse effects. The drug may also be used in the prevention of cluster headaches. Its use in migraine should be restricted to occasions when other analgesics are ineffective. It should be taken at the first sign of migraine (the "aura"). Later use may be ineffective and cause stomach upset.

Ergotamine causes temporary narrowing of blood vessels and, therefore, should not be used by people with poor circulation. If taken too frequently, the drug can dangerously reduce circulation to the hands and feet; it should never be taken regularly. Frequent migraine attacks may indicate the need for a drug to prevent migraine.

INFORMATION FOR USERS

Your drug prescription is tailored for you. Do not alter dosage without checking with your doctor.

How taken Tablets, suppositories.

Frequency and timing of doses Once at the onset (all forms), repeated if needed after 30 minutes (tablets) or 5 minutes (inhaler), up to the maximum dose (see below).

Adult dosage range Varies according to product. Generally 1–2mg per dose. Take no more than 4mg in 24 hours or 8mg in 1 week. Treatment should not be repeated within 4 days or more than twice a month.

Onset of effect 15–30 minutes.

Duration of action Up to 24 hours.

Diet advice Changes in diet are unlikely to affect this drug's action, but certain foods may provoke migraine attacks in some people.

Storage Keep in a closed container in a cool, dry place out of reach of children. Protect from light.

Missed dose Regular doses of this drug are not necessary and may be dangerous. Take only when you have symptoms of migraine.

Stopping the drug Can be safely stopped as soon as you no longer need it.

Exceeding the dose An occasional unintentional extra dose is unlikely to cause problems. Large overdoses may cause vomiting, dizziness, fits, or coma; notify your doctor immediately.

POSSIBLE ADVERSE EFFECTS

Digestive disturbance, abdominal pain, muscle cramps, and nausea (for which an antiemetic may be given) are common. Diarrhoea and muscle pain and stiffness may also occur. Cold or numb fingers and toes are rare but serious effects that may result from arterial spasm. If these symptoms or chest pain, leg pain, or groin pain occur, stop taking the drug and seek immediate medical advice.

INTERACTIONS

Beta blockers These drugs may increase circulatory problems with ergotamine.

Sumatriptan and related drugs The risk of adverse effects on blood circulation is increased if ergotamine is used with these drugs.

Erythromycin and related antibiotics and antivirals Taken with ergotamine, these drugs increase the likelihood of adverse effects.

Oral contraceptives There is an increased risk of blood clotting in women taking these drugs with ergotamine.

SPECIAL PRECAUTIONS

Be sure to tell your doctor if:

◆ You have long-term liver or kidney problems.

◆ You have heart problems.

◆ You have poor circulation.

◆ You have high blood pressure.

◆ You have had a recent stroke.

◆ You have an overactive thyroid gland.

◆ You are taking other medications.

Pregnancy Not usually prescribed. Ergotamine can cause contractions of the uterus.

Breast-feeding Not recommended. The drug passes into breast milk and may affect the baby. It may also reduce your milk supply.

Infants and children Not usually prescribed.

Over 60 Use with caution. Hidden heart or circulatory problems may be aggravated.

Driving and hazardous work Avoid such activities until you have learned how ergotamine affects you because it can cause vertigo.

Alcohol No special problems, but some spirits may provoke migraine in some people.

Surgery and general anaesthetics Notify your doctor if you have used ergotamine within 48 hours prior to surgery.

PROLONGED USE

Reduced circulation to the hands and feet may result if doses near to the maximum are taken for too long. Do not exceed the recommended dosage and length of treatment; a "rebound" headache may occur.

Erythromycin

Brand names Eryacne, Erymax, Erythrocin, Erythroped, Rommix, Stiemycin, Tiloryth

Used in the following combined preparation Zineryt

QUICK REFERENCE

Drug group Antibiotic (p.62)

Overdose danger rating Low

Dependence rating Low

Prescription needed Yes

Available as generic Yes

GENERAL INFORMATION

One of the safest and most widely used antibiotics, erythromycin is effective against many bacteria. The drug is commonly used as an alternative for people who are allergic to penicillin and related antibiotics.

Erythromycin is used to treat infections of the throat, middle ear, and chest (including some rare types of pneumonia, such as Legionnaires' disease). The drug is also used to treat sexually transmitted diseases such as chlamydial infections; some forms of gastro-enteritis; and some bone and joint infections.

In addition, erythromycin may be included as part of the treatment for diphtheria and is sometimes given to treat, and reduce the likelihood of infecting others with, per-tussis (whooping cough).

When taken by mouth, erythromycin may sometimes cause nausea and vomiting. Other possible adverse effects include a rash as well as a rare risk of liver disorders. Oral administration or topical application of erythromycin is sometimes helpful in the treatment of acne.

INFORMATION FOR USERS

Your drug prescription is tailored for you. Do not alter dosage without consulting your doctor.

How taken Tablets, capsules, liquid, injection, topical solution.

Frequency and timing of doses Every 6–12 hours before or with meals.

Dosage range 1–4g daily.

Onset of effect 1–4 hours.

Duration of action 6–12 hours.

Diet advice None.

Storage Keep in a closed container in a cool, dry place out of reach of children.

Missed dose Take as soon as you remember. If your next dose is due within 2 hours, take a single dose now and skip the next.

Stopping the drug Take the full course. Even if you feel better, the original infection may still be present and symptoms may recur if treatment is stopped too soon.

Exceeding the dose An occasional unintentional extra dose is unlikely to be a cause for concern. But if you notice any unusual symptoms, or if a large overdose has been taken, notify your doctor.

POSSIBLE ADVERSE EFFECTS

Nausea and vomiting are the most common adverse effects of treatment with erythro-mycin and are most likely to occur when large doses are taken by mouth. Diarrhoea is also common. Deafness is a rare adverse effect that may occur with high doses in people who have poor kidney function. Symptoms such as fever, rash, and jaundice may be a sign of a liver disorder and should always be reported to your doctor.

INTERACTIONS

General note Erythromycin interacts with a number of other drugs, particularly the following.

Warfarin Erythromycin increases the risk of bleeding with warfarin.

Terfenadine and mizolastine Erythromycin increases the risk of adverse effects on the heart with these drugs.

Ergotamine Erythromycin increases the risk of side effects with this drug.

Carbamazepine, digoxin, and some immunosuppressants Erythromycin may increase blood levels of these drugs.

Theophylline/aminophylline Erythromycin increases the risk of adverse effects with these drugs.

Lipid-lowering drugs ending in -statin Erythromycin may increase the risk of muscular aches and pains with statins.

SPECIAL PRECAUTIONS

Be sure to tell your doctor if:
◆ You have long-term liver or kidney problems.
◆ You have had a previous allergic reaction to erythromycin.
◆ You have porphyria.
◆ You are taking other medications.

Pregnancy There is no evidence of risk to the developing baby.

Breast-feeding The drug passes into the breast milk, but at normal doses adverse effects on the baby are unlikely. Discuss with your doctor.

Infants and children Reduced dose necessary.

Over 60 No special problems.

Driving and hazardous work No known problems.

Alcohol No known problems.

PROLONGED USE

Courses of longer than 14 days may increase the risk of liver damage.

Erythropoietin (Epoetin, Darbepoetin)

Brand names Aranesp, Eprex, NeoRecormon
Used in the following combined preparations
None

QUICK REFERENCE

Drug group Kidney hormone
Overdose danger rating Low
Dependence rating Low
Prescription needed Yes
Available as generic No

GENERAL INFORMATION

Erythropoietin is a naturally occurring hormone produced by the kidneys; it stimulates the body to produce red blood cells. Epoetin and darbepoetin are manufactured forms of erythropoietin that are used to treat anaemia associated with chronic kidney disease.

Epoetin is available in two forms (alpha and beta), both of which may also be used to treat anaemia caused by certain cancer treatments. They are also used to boost the level of red blood cells before surgery. Patients donate blood before surgery, and this is used during or after the surgery. In addition, epoetin may be used as an alternative to blood transfusions in major orthopaedic (bone) surgery.

Darbepoetin is a derivative of epoetin and it has a longer duration of action. It can, therefore, be given less frequently.

Both epoetin and darbepoetin have been used by athletes to enhance their performance. However, this is not a recognized use and the drugs are banned by sport governing bodies.

INFORMATION FOR USERS

Your drug prescription is tailored for you. Do not alter dosage without checking with your doctor.
How taken Injection.
Frequency and timing of doses 1–3 x weekly, depending on the product and condition being treated.
Dosage range Dosage is calculated on an individual basis according to bodyweight. The dosage also varies depending on the product and condition being treated.

Onset of effect The drug is active inside the body within 4 hours, but effects may not be noted for 2–3 months.
Duration of action Some effects may persist for several days.
Diet advice None. However, if you have kidney failure, you may have to follow a special diet.
Storage Store at 2–8°C, out of reach of children. Do not freeze or shake the liquid. Protect from light.
Missed dose Do not make up any missed doses.
Stopping the drug Discuss with your doctor.
Exceeding the dose A single excessive dose is unlikely to be a cause for concern. However, too high a dose over a long period can increase the likelihood of adverse effects.

POSSIBLE ADVERSE EFFECTS

The most common effects are increased blood pressure and problems at the site of the injection. All unusual symptoms should be discussed with your doctor immediately.

INTERACTIONS

ACE inhibitor drugs These drugs may increase the level of potassium in the blood, and epoetin may enhance their blood-pressure-lowering effect.
Iron supplements These may increase the effect of epoetin if you have a low level of iron in your blood.

SPECIAL PRECAUTIONS

Be sure to tell your doctor if:
◆ You have high blood pressure.
◆ You have a long-term liver problem.
◆ You have previously suffered allergic reactions to any drugs.
◆ You have peripheral vascular disease.
◆ You have had epileptic fits.
◆ You are taking other medications.
Pregnancy Not usually prescribed. Safety in pregnancy not established. Discuss with your doctor.
Breast-feeding Safety not established. Discuss with your doctor.
Infants and children Reduced dose necessary.
Over 60 No known problems.
Driving and hazardous work Not applicable.
Alcohol Follow your doctor's advice regarding alcohol.

PROLONGED USE

The long-term effects of the drug are still under investigation, but problems are unlikely if treatment is carefully monitored.
Monitoring Regular blood tests to monitor blood composition and blood pressure monitoring are required.

Estradiol

Brand names Aerodiol, Climaval, Estraderm, FemSeven, Menorest, Oestrogel, Progynova, Zumenon, and others
Used in the following combined preparations
Climagest, Climesse, Estracombi, Femapak, Trisequens, and others

QUICK REFERENCE

Drug group Female sex hormone (p.88)
Overdose danger rating Low
Dependence rating Low
Prescription needed Yes
Available as generic No

GENERAL INFORMATION

Estradiol is a naturally occurring oestrogen (female sex hormone). It is used mainly as hormone replacement therapy (HRT) for menopausal and post-menopausal symptoms such as hot flushes, night sweats, and vaginal atrophy. Estradiol is often given with a progestogen, either as separate drugs or as a combined product. In certain cases, treatment is for a specific number of days each month; follow your doctor's instructions carefully.

Taken alone, estradiol is associated with an increased risk of cancer of the uterus. For this reason, is is usually combined with a progestogen to reduce the risk; it is usually used alone in women who have had a hysterectomy.

Estradiol is available in a variety of forms, including implants and skin patches. Skin patches may cause a local rash and itching at the site of application.

INFORMATION FOR USERS

Your drug prescription is tailored for you. Do not alter dosage without checking with your doctor.
How taken Tablets, pessaries, vaginal rings, skin gel, patches, implants, nasal spray.

Frequency and timing of doses Once daily (tablets, gel); every 1–7 day (skin patches); every 4–8 months (implants); every 1–7 days (pessaries); every 3 months (vaginal ring); 1–4 sprays daily (nasal spray).
Adult dosage range 1–2mg daily (tablets); 2–4 measures daily (skin gel); 25–100mcg daily (skin patches); 25–100mg per dose (implants); 25mcg per dose (pessaries); 7.5mcg daily (vaginal ring).
Onset of effect 10–20 days.
Duration of action Up to 24 hours; some effects may be longer lasting.
Diet advice None.
Storage Keep in a closed container in a cool, dry place out of reach of children.
Missed dose Take as soon as you remember. If your next daily treatment is due within 4 hours, take one dose now and skip the next.
Stopping the drug Do not stop taking the drug without consulting your doctor; symptoms may recur.
Exceeding the dose An occasional unintentional extra dose is unlikely to be a cause for concern. But if you notice any unusual symptoms, or if a large overdose has been taken, notify your doctor.

POSSIBLE ADVERSE EFFECTS

The most common adverse effects are similar to symptoms in the early stages of pregnancy and generally diminish with time. They include nausea or vomiting, breast swelling or tenderness, and weight gain. Headache and symptoms of depression may also occur. Swelling or pain in the leg, or a sudden sharp pain in the chest, may indicate an abnormal blood clot that needs urgent attention.

INTERACTIONS

Tobacco smoking This increases the risk of serious adverse effects on the heart and circulation with estradiol.
St John's wort This substance may reduce the effects of estradiol.
Rifampicin This drug may reduce the effects of estradiol.
Anticonvulsants The effects of estradiol are reduced by carbamazepine, phenytoin, and phenobarbital.
Anticoagulant drugs The effects of these drugs are reduced by estradiol.

SPECIAL PRECAUTIONS

Be sure to tell your doctor if:
◆ You have a long-term liver problem.
◆ You have heart or circulation problems.
◆ You have porphyria.
◆ You have had blood clots or a stroke.
◆ You have diabetes.
◆ You are a smoker.
◆ You suffer from migraine or epilepsy.
◆ You are taking other medications.

Pregnancy Not prescribed.

Breast-feeding Not prescribed. The drug passes into breast milk and may inhibit its flow. Discuss with your doctor.

Infants and children Not usually prescribed.

Over 60 No special problems.

Driving and hazardous work No problems expected.

Alcohol No known problems.

Surgery and general anaesthetics You may need to stop taking estradiol several weeks before major surgery. Discuss with your doctor.

PROLONGED USE

HRT is usually only advised for short-term use around the menopause and is no longer normally recommended for long-term use or for the treatment of osteoporosis because of the increased risk of disorders such as breast cancer, stroke, and thromboembolism.

Monitoring Blood-pressure checks and physical examinations, including regular mammograms, may be performed.

Ethambutol

Brand name None
Used in the following combined preparations
None

QUICK REFERENCE

Drug group Antituberculous drug (p.67)
Overdose danger rating Medium
Dependence rating Low
Prescription needed Yes
Available as generic Yes

GENERAL INFORMATION

Ethambutol is an antibiotic used in treating tuberculosis. It is combined with other antituberculous drugs to enhance its effect and reduce the risk of the infection becoming drug resistant. Ethambutol is not used in all cases. It is more likely to be used in people with a history of tuberculosis; those with a low immune status; and those in whom the infection may be caused by a resistant organism.

Although the drug has few common adverse effects, it may occasionally cause optic neuritis, a type of eye damage that leads to blurring and fading of vision. As a result, ethambutol is not usually prescribed for children under six years of age or for other patients who are unable to communicate their symptoms adequately. Before starting treatment, a full ophthalmic examination is recommended.

INFORMATION FOR USERS

Your drug prescription is tailored for you. Do not alter dosage without checking with your doctor.

How taken Tablets.

Frequency and timing of doses Once daily.

Adult dosage range According to bodyweight.

Onset of effect It may take several days for symptoms to improve.

Duration of action Up to 24 hours.

Diet advice None.

Storage Keep in a closed container in a cool, dry place out of reach of children.

Missed dose Take as soon as you remember. If your next dose is due within 6 hours, take a single dose now and skip the next.

Stopping the drug Take the full course. Even if you feel better, the original infection may still be present and may recur (and be more difficult to treat) if treatment is stopped too soon.

Exceeding the dose An occasional unintentional extra dose is unlikely to cause problems. Large overdoses may cause headache and abdominal pain. Notify your doctor.

POSSIBLE ADVERSE EFFECTS

Side effects are uncommon but are more likely after prolonged treatment at high doses. They include nausea or vomiting, dizziness, and numbness and tingling of the hands or feet. If a rash or itching develop, stop taking the drug and consult your doctor. Blurred vision, loss of colour vision, and eye pain require prompt medical attention.

INTERACTIONS

Antacids Those containing aluminium salts may decrease levels of ethambutol and should be taken at least 2 hours before or after ethambutol.

SPECIAL PRECAUTIONS

Be sure to tell your doctor if:
◆ You have a kidney problem.
◆ You have cataracts or other eye problems.
◆ You have gout.
◆ You have had a previous allergic reaction to this drug.
◆ You are taking other medications.
Pregnancy Safety in pregnancy not established. Discuss with your doctor.
Breast-feeding The drug passes into breast milk, but at normal doses adverse effects on the baby are unlikely. Discuss with your doctor.
Infants and children Not generally prescribed under 6 years, and often not under 13 years.
Over 60 Increased likelihood of adverse effects. Reduced dose may therefore be needed.
Driving and hazardous work Avoid such activities until you have learned how ethambutol affects you because it can cause dizziness.
Alcohol No known problems.

PROLONGED USE

Prolonged use of ethambutol may increase the risk of eye damage.
Monitoring Periodic eye tests are usually needed.

Ethinylestradiol

Used in the following combined preparations
Combined oral contraceptives (e.g. Brevinor, Eugynon 30, Femodene, Loestrin, Microgynon 30, Norimin, Ovranette, Ovysmen), Dianette

QUICK REFERENCE

Drug group Female sex hormone (p.88) and oral contraceptive (p.105)
Overdose danger rating Low
Dependence rating Low
Prescription needed Yes
Available as generic Yes

GENERAL INFORMATION

Ethinylestradiol is a synthetic oestrogen similar to estradiol, a natural female sex hormone. It is widely used in oral contraceptives, in combination with a synthetic progestogen.

Ethinylestradiol is occasionally given to control abnormally heavy bleeding from the uterus and to treat delayed sexual development (hypogonadism) in females. Certain breast and prostate cancers also respond to it. It is used in conjunction with cyproterone to treat severe acne in women. High doses are sometimes given as postcoital contraception (see p.109).

Women taking an oral contraceptive containing ethinylestradiol are at increased risk of developing thrombosis (a blood clot). The risk increases in overweight women and smokers.

INFORMATION FOR USERS

Your drug prescription is tailored for you. Do not alter dosage without checking with your doctor.
How taken Tablets.
Frequency and timing of doses Once daily. Often at certain times of the menstrual cycle.
Adult dosage range *Menopausal symptoms* 10–20mcg daily. *Hormone deficiency* 10–50mcg daily. *Combined contraceptive pill* 20–40mcg daily, depending on preparation. *Acne* 35mcg daily. *Breast cancer* 1–3mg daily.
Onset of effect 10–20 days. Contraceptive protection is effective after 7 days in most cases.
Duration of action 1–2 days.
Diet advice None.
Storage Keep in a closed container in a cool, dry place out of reach of children.
Missed dose Take as soon as you remember. If your next dose is due within 4 hours, take a single dose now and skip the next. If you are taking the drug for contraceptive purposes, see What to do if you miss a pill (p.109).
Stopping the drug Do not stop taking the drug without consulting your doctor. Contraceptive protection is lost unless an alternative method is used.
Exceeding the dose An occasional unintentional extra dose is unlikely to be a cause for concern. But if you notice any unusual symptoms, or if a large overdose has been taken, notify your doctor.

POSSIBLE ADVERSE EFFECTS

The most common effects are similar to symptoms in the early stages of pregnancy and generally diminish with time. They include nausea or vomiting, breast swelling or tenderness, and weight gain. Headache, bleeding between periods, and depression may also occur.

Swelling or pain in the leg, or a sudden sharp pain in the chest, may indicate an abnormal blood clot that needs attention. If these or sudden breathlessness, itching or jaundice occur, stop taking the drug and seek urgent medical advice.

INTERACTIONS
Tobacco smoking This increases the risk of serious adverse effects on the heart and circulation with ethinylestradiol.
Rifampicin and anticonvulsant drugs These drugs significantly reduce the effectiveness of oral contraceptives containing ethinylestradiol, for which a higher dose will be needed.
Antihypertensive drugs and diuretics Ethinylestradiol may reduce the effectiveness of these drugs.
Antibiotics and St. John's wort These preparations may reduce the effectiveness of oral contraceptives containing ethinylestradiol.

SPECIAL PRECAUTIONS
Be sure to tell your doctor if:
◆ You have heart failure or hypertension (high blood pressure).
◆ You or a close relative have had blood clots or a stroke.
◆ You have a long-term liver problem.
◆ You have had breast or endometrial cancer.
◆ You have sickle cell anaemia.
◆ You have porphyria.
◆ You are a smoker.
◆ You have diabetes.
◆ You suffer from migraine or epilepsy.
◆ You are taking other medications.
Pregnancy Not prescribed. High doses may adversely affect the developing baby. Discuss with your doctor.
Breast-feeding The drug passes into the breast milk and may affect the baby; it may also inhibit milk flow. Discuss with your doctor.
Infants and children Not usually prescribed.
Over 60 No special problems.
Driving and hazardous work No known problems.
Alcohol No known problems.
Surgery and general anaesthetics Ethinylestradiol may need to be stopped several weeks before you have major surgery. Discuss this with your doctor.

PROLONGED USE
There is a possible small increased risk of breast cancer with long-term use of ethinylestradiol, but this should be weighed against the benefits of protection from cancers of the ovary and endometrium.
Monitoring Physical examinations and periodic blood-pressure checks may be performed.

Etidronate

Brand names Didronel, Didronel PMO
Used in the following combined preparations
None

QUICK REFERENCE
Drug group Drug for bone disorders (p.56)
Overdose danger rating Medium
Dependence rating Low
Prescription needed Yes
Available as generic No

GENERAL INFORMATION
Etidronate is given to treat bone disorders such as Paget's disease. It acts only on bones, reducing the activity of bone cells, which stops the progress of the disease. This action also stops calcium being released from the bones into the bloodstream, thus reducing the amount of calcium in the blood. In addition, it is used with calcium tablets to treat osteoporosis in postmenopausal women and to prevent and treat steroid-induced osteoporosis.

Generally, the side effects are mild. The most common, diarrhoea, is more likely to occur with higher doses. If taken at high doses (20mg/kg body weight daily), the drug stops new bone being formed properly, which can lead to bone thinning and fractures. High doses must, therefore, be carefully monitored and used for as short a time as possible. The effect is reversed on stopping the drug.

INFORMATION FOR USERS
Your drug prescription is tailored for you. Do not alter dosage without checking with your doctor.
How taken Tablets.

Frequency and timing of doses Once daily on an empty stomach, 2 hours before or after food.

Dosage range *Paget's disease* 5–20mg/kg bodyweight daily for a maximum of 3–6 months. Courses may be repeated after a break of at least 3 months.

Osteoporosis 400mg daily for 2 weeks, repeated every 3 months.

Onset of effect *Paget's disease/osteoporosis* Beneficial effects from etidronate may not be felt for several months.

Duration of action Some effects may persist for several weeks or months.

Diet advice Absorption of etidronate is reduced by foods, especially those containing calcium (such as dairy products), so the drug should be taken on an empty stomach. The diet must contain adequate calcium and vitamin D; supplements may be given.

Storage Keep in a closed container in a dry place below 30°C, out of reach of children. Protect from light.

Missed dose Take as soon as you remember. If your next dose is due within 6 hours, take a single dose now and skip the next.

Stopping the drug Do not stop taking the drug without consulting your doctor. Stopping the drug may lead to worsening of the underlying condition.

Exceeding the dose An occasional unintentional extra dose is unlikely to cause problems. Large overdoses may cause numbness and muscle spasm; notify your doctor.

POSSIBLE ADVERSE EFFECTS

The most common side effect is diarrhoea, which is more likely to occur if the dosage is increased above 5mg/kg daily. Other effects include headache, nausea, constipation, abdominal pain, and rash or itching. In some patients with Paget's disease, bone pain and bruising may increase initially but usually disappear with further treatment. If they persist or if fever or a sore throat develop, contact your doctor without delay.

INTERACTIONS

Antacids, and products containing calcium, magnesium, or iron These products should be given at least 2 hours before or after etidronate to minimize the risk that they will reduce the absorption of etidronate.

SPECIAL PRECAUTIONS

Be sure to tell your doctor if:
◆ You have a long-term kidney problem.
◆ You have osteomalacia.
◆ You have had a previous allergic reaction to etidronate or other bisphosphonates.
◆ You have colitis.
◆ You are taking other medications.

Pregnancy Safety in pregnancy not established. Discuss with your doctor.

Breast-feeding Safety in breast-feeding not established. Discuss with your doctor.

Infants and children Not recommended.

Over 60 No special problems.

Driving and hazardous work No special problems.

Alcohol No special problems.

PROLONGED USE

Courses of treatment longer than 3 to 6 months are not usually prescribed, but repeat courses are commonly given. Continuous use of etidronate is not recommended because it may lead to an increased risk of bone fractures.

Monitoring Blood and urine tests may be carried out.

Filgrastim

Brand name Neupogen
Used in the following combined preparations
None

QUICK REFERENCE

Drug group Blood stimulant
Overdose danger rating Medium
Dependence rating High
Prescription needed Yes
Available as generic No

GENERAL INFORMATION

Filgrastim is a synthetic form of G-CSF (granulocyte-colony stimulating factor), a naturally occurring protein responsible for the manufacture of white blood cells, which fight infection. Deficiency of G-CSF, therefore, increases the risk of infection. Filgrastim acts by stimulating the bone marrow to produce white blood cells. It also causes bone marrow cells to move into the bloodstream, where they can be collected for use in treating bone marrow disease, or to replace bone marrow that is lost during intensive cancer treatment.

Filgrastim is used to treat people with congenital neutropenia (G-CSF deficiency from birth), some AIDS patients, and people who have recently received high doses of chemo- or radiotherapy during bone-marrow transplantation or cancer treatment. Such patients are prone to frequent and severe infections.

Bone pain is a common adverse effect of filgrastim treatment but can be controlled with painkillers. There is an increased risk of leukaemia (cancer of white blood cells) if filgrastim is given to patients with certain rare blood disorders.

INFORMATION FOR USERS

The drug is given only under medical supervision and is not for self-administration.
How taken Injection.
Frequency and timing of doses Once daily.
Adult dosage range 0.5–1.2 million units/kg bodyweight, depending upon condition being treated and response to treatment.
Onset of effect 24 hours (increase); several weeks (recovery of normal numbers of white blood cells).

Duration of action Approximately 2 days.
Diet advice None.
Storage Not applicable. The drug is not normally kept in the home.
Missed dose Not applicable. The drug is given only in hospital under medical supervision.
Stopping the drug Do not stop the drug without consulting your doctor; stopping may lead to worsening of the underlying condition.
Exceeding the dose Overdose is unlikely since the drug is given only under close supervision and treatment is carefully monitored.

POSSIBLE ADVERSE EFFECTS

Adverse effects are unusual with short courses. Most common is bone pain, probably linked to the drug's stimulant effect on bone marrow. If a skin rash or difficulty in, or pain on, passing urine occur, seek medical advice.

INTERACTIONS

Cytotoxic chemotherapy or radiotherapy should not be administered within 24 hours of taking filgrastim because of the risk of increasing damage on bone marrow.

SPECIAL PRECAUTIONS

Be sure to tell your doctor if:
◆ You suffer from any blood disorders.
◆ You are taking other medications.
Pregnancy Safety in pregnancy not established. Discuss with your doctor.
Breast-feeding Safety in breast-feeding not established. Discuss with your doctor.
Infants and children No special problems.
Over 60 No special problems.
Driving and hazardous work No known problems.
Alcohol No known problems.

PROLONGED USE

Prolonged use may lead to a slightly increased risk of certain leukaemias. Cutaneous vasculitis (inflammation of blood vessels of the skin), osteoporosis (bone weakening), hair thinning, enlargement of the spleen and liver, and bleeding due to a reduction in platelet numbers may also occur.
Monitoring Blood checks and regular physical examinations are performed. X-rays or bone scans may also be carried out to check for bone thinning.

Finasteride

Brand name Propecia, Proscar
Used in the following combined preparations
None

QUICK REFERENCE

Drug group Drug used for urinary disorders (p.112)
Overdose danger rating Low
Dependence rating Low
Prescription needed Yes
Available as generic No

GENERAL INFORMATION

Finasteride is an an anti-androgen drug (see Male sex hormones, p.87) used to treat benign prostatic hyperplasia (BPH), in which an enlarged prostate gland impedes urine flow. The drug gradually shrinks the prostate, improving urine flow and other obstructive symptoms such as difficulty in starting urination.

Because the drug is excreted in semen and can feminize a male foetus, you should use a condom if your sexual partner may be, or is likely to become, pregnant. Also, women of childbearing age should not handle broken or crushed tablets because small quantities of the drug are absorbed through the skin.

The symptoms of BPH are similar to those of prostate cancer, so the drug is used only when the possibility of cancer has been ruled out.

Low doses are used to reverse male-pattern baldness by preventing the hair follicles from becoming inactive. Noticeable improvements may take about three months but disappear within a year of cessation of treatment.

INFORMATION FOR USERS

Your drug prescription is tailored for you. Do not alter dosage without checking with your doctor.
How taken Tablets.
Frequency and timing of doses Once daily.
Adult dosage range *Prostate disease* 5mg. *Male-pattern baldness* 1mg.
Onset of effect Within 1 hour, but full beneficial effects may take several months.
Duration of action 24 hours.
Diet advice None.
Storage Keep in a closed container, in a cool, dry place out of reach of children. Protect from light.

Missed dose Do not take the missed dose, but take your next scheduled dose as usual.
Stopping the drug Do not stop taking the drug without consulting your doctor. Stopping the drug may lead to worsening of the underlying condition.
Exceeding the dose An occasional unintentional extra dose is unlikely to cause problems. But if you notice any unusual symptoms, or if a large overdose has been taken, notify your doctor.

POSSIBLE ADVERSE EFFECTS

Most people experience very few adverse effects; decreased libido, impotence, and reduced ejaculate volume are the most common. Breast swelling or tenderness occur more rarely. If a blotchy rash, swollen lips, or wheezing develop, seek urgent medical attention.

INTERACTIONS

None.

SPECIAL PRECAUTIONS

Be sure to tell your doctor if:
◆ You are taking other medications.
Pregnancy Not prescribed.
Breast-feeding Not applicable.
Infants and children Not prescribed.
Over 60 No special problems.
Driving and hazardous work No special problems.
Alcohol No special problems.

PROLONGED USE

Treatment is reviewed after about 6 months to see if the drug has been effective.

Flucloxacillin

Brand names Floxapen, Fluclomix, Galfloxin, Ladropen
Used in the following combined preparations
Co-Fluampicil, Flu-Amp, Magnapen

QUICK REFERENCE

Drug group Penicillin antibiotic (p.62)
Overdose danger rating Low
Dependence rating Low
Prescription needed Yes
Available as generic Yes

GENERAL INFORMATION

Flucloxacillin is a penicillin antibiotic developed to deal with Staphylococcus bacteria that are resistant to other antibiotics. Such bacteria make enzymes (penicillinases) that neutralize the antibiotics; flucloxacillin is not inactivated by penicillinases and is therefore effective in treating penicillin-resistant staphylococcal infections. The drug is used to treat ear infections, pneumonia, impetigo, cellulitis, osteomyelitis, and endocarditis.

When combined in equal parts with ampicillin, flucloxacillin is known as co-fluampicil. This drug is used to treat mixed infections of penicillinase-producing organisms.

Staphylococci have evolved to the extent that some strains are now also resistant to flucloxacillin. These strains are the so-called methicillin-resistant *Staphylococcus aureus* (MRSA) infections. Only a few antibiotics held in reserve can deal with them.

INFORMATION FOR USERS

Your drug prescription is tailored for you. Do not alter dosage without checking with your doctor.

How taken Capsules, liquid, injection.
Frequency and timing of doses 4 x daily.
Adult dosage range 1–2g daily (oral); 1–8g daily (injection); 12g daily (for endocarditis).
Onset of effect 30 minutes.
Duration of action 4–6 hours.
Diet advice None.
Storage Keep in a closed container in a cool, dry place out of reach of children.
Missed dose Take as soon as you remember. Take your next dose at the scheduled time.
Stopping the drug Take the full course. Even if you feel better, the original infection may still be present and symptoms may recur if treatment is stopped too soon.
Exceeding the dose An occasional unintentional extra dose is unlikely to be a cause for concern. But if you notice any unusual symptoms, or if a large overdose has been taken, notify your doctor.

POSSIBLE ADVERSE EFFECTS

The most common adverse effects are diarrhoea, nausea, and abdominal pain. If bruising, sore throat, or fever occur; if you develop a rash, itching, and swollen joints (signs of an allergic reaction); or if jaundice occurs weeks or even months after finishing treatment, consult your doctor. If breathing difficulties occur, stop taking the drug and call your doctor immediately.

INTERACTIONS

Probenecid This drug reduces the excretion of flucloxacillin, thereby prolonging its effects.

SPECIAL PRECAUTIONS

Be sure to tell your doctor if:
◆ You are allergic to penicillin antibiotics.
◆ You have a history of allergy.
◆ You have liver or kidney problems.
◆ You are taking other medications.
Pregnancy No evidence of risk.
Breast-feeding No evidence of risk.
Infants and children Reduced dose necessary.
Over 60 No known problems.
Driving and hazardous work No known problems.
Alcohol No known problems.

PROLONGED USE

Although the drug is not normally necessary for long-term use, osteomyelitis and endocarditis may require longer than usual courses of treatment.
Monitoring Regular tests of liver and kidney function will be performed if a longer course of treatment is prescribed.

Fluconazole

Brand name Diflucan
Used in the following combined preparations
None

QUICK REFERENCE

Drug group Antifungal drug (p.76)
Overdose danger rating Medium
Dependence rating Low
Prescription needed Yes (except for vaginal infection preparations)
Available as generic No

GENERAL INFORMATION

Fluconazole is an antifungal drug that is used to treat local candida infections ("thrush") affecting the vagina, mouth, and skin as well as systemic or more widespread candida infections. It is also used to treat more unusual fungal infections, including cryptococcal meningitis. In addition, it may be used to prevent fungal infections in people with defective immunity. Dosage and length of course depend on the condition being treated.

The drug is generally well tolerated, but side effects such as nausea and vomiting, diarrhoea, and abdominal discomfort are common.

INFORMATION FOR USERS

Your drug prescription is tailored for you. Do not alter dosage without checking with your doctor.

How taken Capsules, liquid, injection.
Frequency and timing of doses Once daily.
Adult dosage range 50–400mg daily.
Onset of effect Within a few hours, but full beneficial effects may take several days.
Duration of action Up to 24 hours.
Diet advice None.
Storage Keep in a closed container in a cool, dry place out of reach of children. Store liquid in a refrigerator (do not freeze) for no longer than 14 days.
Missed dose Take as soon as you remember. If your next dose is due within 6 hours, take a single dose now and skip the next.
Stopping the drug Take the full course. Even if you feel better, the original infection may still be present and may recur if treatment is stopped too soon.
Exceeding the dose An occasional unintentional extra dose is unlikely to be a cause for concern. But if you notice any unusual symptoms, or if a large overdose has been taken, notify your doctor.

POSSIBLE ADVERSE EFFECTS

Fluconazole is generally well tolerated. Most problems affect the gastrointestinal tract and include flatulence, abdominal discomfort, nausea or vomiting, and diarrhoea. If, rarely, a rash occurs, it should be reported to your doctor without delay.

INTERACTIONS

General note Most interactions with other drugs relate to multiple doses of fluconazole. The relevance of a single dose of fluconazole is not established.

Anticoagulants Fluconazole may increase the effect of oral anticoagulants such as warfarin.
Oral antidiabetic drugs Fluconazole may increase the risk of hypoglycaemia with oral sulphonylureas such as gliclazide, glibenclamide, chlorpropamide, and tolbutamide.
Phenytoin, theophylline/aminophylline, ciclosporin, tacrolimus, and zidovudine Fluconazole may increase the blood levels of these drugs.
Rifampicin The effect of fluconazole may be reduced by rifampicin.
Terfenadine When this antihistamine is taken with fluconazole there is an increased risk of adverse effects on the heart.

SPECIAL PRECAUTIONS

Be sure to tell your doctor if:
◆ You have long-term liver or kidney problems.
◆ You have previously had an allergic reaction to antifungal drugs.
◆ You are taking other medications.
Pregnancy Safety in pregnancy not established. Discuss with your doctor.
Breast-feeding Not recommended. The drug passes into the breast milk. Discuss with your doctor.
Infants and children Reduced dose necessary.
Over 60 Normal dose used as long as kidney function is not impaired.
Driving and hazardous work No known problems.
Alcohol No known problems.

PROLONGED USE

Fluconazole is usually given in short courses. However, to prevent relapse of cryptococcal meningitis in patients with defective immunity, the drug may be given indefinitely.

Fluoxetine

Brand name Prozac
Used in the following combined preparations
None

QUICK REFERENCE

Drug group Antidepressant (p.14)
Overdose danger rating Medium
Dependence rating Low
Prescription needed Yes
Available as generic No

GENERAL INFORMATION

Fluoxetine belongs to a group of antidepressants called selective serotonin reuptake inhibitors (SSRIs). These drugs tend to cause less sedation than, and have different side effects to, older antidepressants. Fluoxetine elevates mood, increases physical activity, and restores interest in everyday activities.

Fluoxetine is broken down slowly and remains in the body for several weeks after treatment is stopped. It is used to treat depression, to reduce binge eating and purging activity (bulimia nervosa), and to treat obsessive-compulsive disorder. Fluoxetine is also used to treat premenstrual dysphoric disorder.

INFORMATION FOR USERS

Your drug prescription is tailored for you. Do not alter dosage without checking with your doctor.

How taken Capsules, liquid.

Frequency and timing of doses Once daily in the morning.

Adult dosage range 20–60mg daily.

Onset of effect Some benefits may appear within 14 days, but full benefits may not be felt for 4 weeks or more.

Duration of action Beneficial effects may last for up to 6 weeks following prolonged treatment. Adverse effects may wear off within a few days.

Diet advice None.

Storage Keep in a closed container in a cool, dry place out of reach of children.

Missed dose Take as soon as you remember. If your next dose is due within 8 hours, take a single dose now and skip the next.

Stopping the drug Unless a rash occurs, do not stop taking the drug without consulting your doctor, who may supervise a gradual reduction in dosage.

Exceeding the dose An occasional unintentional extra dose is unlikely to cause problems. Large overdoses, however, may cause adverse effects; notify your doctor.

POSSIBLE ADVERSE EFFECTS

The most common adverse effects of fluoxetine are restlessness, insomnia, headache, and intestinal irregularities such as nausea and diarrhoea. There are fewer anticholinergic (see Autonomic nervous system, p.8) side effects than with tricyclics. Although weight loss is a symptom of depression, fluoxetine can also cause this problem. Drowsiness and sexual dysfunction may occur. If you develop a rash, stop taking the drug and seek immediate medical advice.

INTERACTIONS

Sedatives All drugs that have a sedative effect may increase fluoxetine's sedative effects.

MAOIs Fluoxetine treatment should not be started less than 14 days after stopping an MAOI (except moclobemide) because serious adverse effects can occur. An MAOI should not be started less than 5 weeks after stopping fluoxetine.

Tricyclic antidepressants Fluoxetine reduces the breakdown of tricyclics and may increase the toxicity of these drugs.

Lithium Fluoxetine increases blood levels and toxicity of lithium.

Other antidepressants Fluoxetine reduces the breakdown of tricyclics and may result in sedation, dry mouth, and constipation.

Tryptophan Taken together, tryptophan and fluoxetine may produce agitation, restlessness, and gastric distress.

Anticoagulants Fluoxetine can increase the effect of warfarin; the dose of warfarin may need adjustment.

SPECIAL PRECAUTIONS

Be sure to tell your doctor if:

◆ You have long-term liver or kidney problems.

◆ You have heart problems.

◆ You have diabetes.

◆ You have had epileptic fits.

◆ You have previously had an allergic reaction to fluoxetine or other SSRIs.

◆ You are taking other medications.

Pregnancy Safety in pregnancy not established. Discuss with your doctor.

Breast-feeding The drug passes into the breast milk. Discuss with your doctor.

Infants and children Safety and effectiveness have not been established.

Over 60 No special problems.

Driving and hazardous work Avoid such activities until you have learned how fluoxetine affects you because the drug can cause drowsiness and can affect your judgment and coordination.

Alcohol No special problems.

PROLONGED USE
No problems expected. Side effects tend to decrease with time.

Flupentixol

Brand names Depixol, Fluanxol
Used in the following combined preparations
None

QUICK REFERENCE
Drug group Antipsychotic drug (p.15)
Overdose danger rating Medium
Dependence rating Low
Prescription needed Yes
Available as generic No

GENERAL INFORMATION
Flupentixol is an antipsychotic drug used to treat schizophrenia and similar illnesses. It is also used as an antidepressant for mild to moderate depression. Flupentixol's side effects are similar to those of phenothiazines, but it is less sedating. It is not suitable for patients with mania as it may worsen symptoms.

The drug has fewer anticholinergic (see Autonomic nervous system, p.8) effects than phenothiazines but is more likely to cause side effects such as parkinsonism. Control of severe symptoms may take up to six months, after which a lower maintenance dose is prescribed.

INFORMATION FOR USERS
Your drug prescription is tailored for you. Do not alter dosage without checking with your doctor.
How taken Tablets, injection.
Frequency and timing of doses 1–2 x daily no later than 4 pm (tablets); every 2–4 weeks (injection).
Adult dosage range *Schizophrenia and other psychoses* 6–18mg daily (tablets); from 20mg every 4 weeks to maximum of 400mg weekly (injection). *Depression* 1–3mg daily (tablets).
Onset of effect 10 days, but side effects may appear much sooner.
Duration of action Up to 12 hours (tablets); 2–4 weeks (injection).

Diet advice None.
Storage Store at room temperature out of reach of children. Protect injections from light.
Missed dose Take as soon as you remember. If your next dose is due within 2 hours, do not take the missed dose, but take your next scheduled dose as usual.
Stopping the drug Unless severe adverse effects occur (see below), do not stop taking the drug without consulting your doctor, who will supervise a gradual reduction in dosage. Abrupt cessation of the drug may cause withdrawal symptoms and a recurrence of the original problem.
Exceeding the dose An occasional unintentional extra dose is unlikely to cause problems. Larger overdoses may cause severe drowsiness, fits, low blood pressure, high or low body temperature, or shock; notify your doctor.

POSSIBLE ADVERSE EFFECTS
The possible adverse effects of this drug are mainly the result of its anticholinergic action. These include blurred vision, rapid heartbeat, dry mouth, and difficulty in passing urine. Drowsiness, nausea, weight gain, and parkinsonism or tremor may also occur. If dizziness, fainting, confusion, epileptic fits, persistent infection or sore throat, jaundice, or rash occur, stop taking the drug and seek urgent medical attention.

INTERACTIONS
Anti-arrhythmic drugs Taken with these drugs, flupentixol may increase the risk of arrhythmias (abnormal heart rhythms).
Anticholinergic drugs Flupentixol may increase the effects of these drugs.
Anticonvulsant drugs Flupentixol may reduce the effects of these drugs.
Sedatives Flupentixol enhances the effect of all sedative drugs.

SPECIAL PRECAUTIONS
Be sure to tell your doctor if:
◆ You have long-term liver or kidney problems.
◆ You have heart problems.
◆ You have porphyria.
◆ You have had epileptic fits.
◆ You have thyroid disease.
◆ You have Parkinson's disease.

◆ You have glaucoma.

◆ You are taking other medications.

Pregnancy Not usually prescribed. May cause lethargy in the baby during labour. Discuss with your doctor.

Breast-feeding The drug passes into the breast milk and may affect the baby. Discuss with your doctor.

Infants and children Not recommended.

Over 60 Reduced dose necessary. Increased risk of tardive dyskinesia (abnormal movements of the face, mouth, and tongue) or confusion.

Driving and hazardous work Avoid such activities until you have learned how flupentixol affects you because the drug can cause drowsiness and slowed reactions.

Alcohol Avoid excessive amounts. Flupentixol enhances the sedative effect of alcohol.

Surgery and general anaesthetics Flupentixol may need to be stopped before any surgery. Discuss this with your doctor or dentist.

PROLONGED USE

The risk of tardive dyskinesia increases as treatment continues. Blood disorders, as well as liver disorders, are seen occasionally.

Monitoring Blood tests may be performed, particularly if there is persistent infection.'

Flutamide

Brand names Chimax, Drogenil
Used in the following combined preparations
None

QUICK REFERENCE

Drug group Anticancer drug (p.96)
Overdose danger rating Medium
Dependence rating Low
Prescription needed Yes
Available as generic Yes

GENERAL INFORMATION

Flutamide is an anti-androgen drug used in the treatment of advanced prostate cancer, often together with drugs such as goserelin (see p.259) that control production of the male sex hormones (androgens). Both drugs are effective because the cancer is dependent on androgens for its continued development.

Treatment with goserelin-type drugs initially increases the release of testosterone, leading to a growth spurt of the cancer ("tumour flare"); flutamide is prescribed to stop this effect. In the UK, flutamide treatment is begun three days before the goserelin-type drug. Flutamide is also used to treat prostate cancer when goserelin-type drugs are not prescribed.

Flutamide may colour the urine amber or yellow-green, but this is harmless. However, you should notify your doctor straight away if your urine becomes dark-coloured, because this may be an indication of liver damage.

INFORMATION FOR USERS

Your drug prescription is tailored for you. Do not alter dosage without checking with your doctor.

How taken Tablets.

Frequency and timing of doses 3 x daily, starting 3 days before the goserelin-type drug and continuing for 3 weeks.

Adult dosage range 250mg.

Onset of effect 1 hour.

Duration of action 8 hours.

Diet advice None.

Storage Keep in a closed container in a cool, dry place out of reach of children.

Missed dose Take as soon as you remember. If your next dose is due within 2 hours, take a single dose now and skip the next.

Stopping the drug Unless you develop jaundice or pass dark urine, do not stop taking the drug without consulting your doctor because the condition may worsen rapidly.

Exceeding the dose An occasional unintentional extra dose is unlikely to be a cause for concern. But if you notice any unusual symptoms, or if a large overdose has been taken, notify your doctor.

POSSIBLE ADVERSE EFFECTS

Nausea and tiredness are common. Breast swelling also occurs when the drug is given in an effective dose; this is usually reversible when treatment stops or dosage is reduced. Other common effects include insomnia, tiredness, and headache. Dizziness, blurred vision, and skin reactions occur more rarely. If you develop jaundice or start to pass dark urine, stop taking the drug and consult your doctor urgently.

INTERACTIONS

Warfarin Flutamide increases the effects of this drug.

SPECIAL PRECAUTIONS

Be sure to tell your doctor if:
◆ You have heart problems.
◆ You have liver problems.
◆ You are taking other medications.
Pregnancy Not prescribed.
Breast-feeding Not prescribed.
Infants and children Not prescribed.
Over 60 No special problems.
Driving and hazardous work Do not undertake such activities until you have learned how flutamide affects you because the drug can cause blurred vision and dizziness.
Alcohol No special problems, but excessive consumption should be avoided.

PROLONGED USE

Prolonged use of flutamide may cause liver damage. Because it is an anti-androgen, the drug also reduces sperm count.
Monitoring Periodic liver function tests are usually performed.

Fluticasone

Brand names Cutivate, Flixonase, Flixotide
Used in the following combined preparation Seretide

QUICK REFERENCE

Drug group Corticosteroid (p.80
Overdose danger rating Low
Dependence rating Low
Prescription needed No
Available as generic No

GENERAL INFORMATION

Fluticasone is a corticosteroid drug used to control inflammation in asthma and allergic rhinitis. Because the drug does not produce relief immediately, it is important to take it regularly. For allergic rhinitis, treatment with nasal spray needs to begin 2 to 3 weeks before the hay fever season commences. People with asthma should take fluticasone regularly by inhaler to prevent attacks. Proper instruction is essential to ensure that the inhaler is used correctly. Fluticasone ointment or cream is used to treat dermatitis and eczema (see Topical corticosteroids, p.120).

There are few serious adverse effects with fluticasone because it is administered directly into the lungs (by inhaler) or the nasal mucosa (by spray). Candida ("thrush"), causing irritation of the mouth and throat, is a possible side effect of the inhaled form but can be minimized by certain simple measures (see Possible adverse effects, below).

INFORMATION FOR USERS

Your drug prescription is tailored for you. Do not alter dosage without checking with your doctor.
How taken Ointment, cream, inhaler, nasal spray.
Frequency and timing of doses *Allergic rhinitis* 1–2 x daily. *Asthma* 2 x daily.
Adult dosage range *Allergic rhinitis* 2 sprays into each nostril per dose. *Asthma* 100–1,000mcg per dose.
Onset of effect *Allergic rhinitis* 3–4 days. *Asthma* 4–7 days.
Duration of action The effects can last for several days after stopping the drug.
Diet advice None.
Storage Keep in a cool, dry place out of reach of children.
Missed dose Take as soon as you remember.
Stopping the drug Do not stop taking the drug without consulting your doctor; symptoms may recur.
Exceeding the dose An occasional unintentional extra dose is unlikely to be a cause for concern. Adverse effects may occur, however, if the recommended dose is regularly exceeded over a prolonged period.

POSSIBLE ADVERSE EFFECTS

The main side effects are irritation of the nasal passages or, rarely, nosebleeds (spray), and sore throat or mouth or hoarseness, usually due to candida infection of the throat and mouth (inhaler); this can be minimized by thoroughly rinsing the mouth, brushing the teeth, or gargling with water. Skin changes (ointment/cream) and disturbances in taste or smell may also occur. If a rash or facial swelling, breathing difficulties, or wheezing develop, consult your doctor urgently.

INTERACTIONS
None.

SPECIAL PRECAUTIONS
Be sure to tell your doctor if:
◆ You have chronic sinusitis.
◆ You have had nasal ulcers or surgery.
◆ You have had tuberculosis or another respiratory infection.
◆ You are taking other medications.
Pregnancy Safety in pregnancy not established. Discuss with your doctor.
Breast-feeding Safety in breast-feeding not established. However, fluticasone is unlikely to pass into breast milk. Discuss with your doctor.
Infants and children Not recommended under 4 years. Reduced dose necessary in older children. Avoid prolonged use of ointment in children.
Over 60 No known problems.
Driving and hazardous work No known problems.
Alcohol No known problems.

PROLONGED USE
Long-term use of high doses of fluticasone may, rarely, lead to suppression of adrenal gland function. Skin changes may also occur, particularly on the face, and prolonged use should be avoided. Patients who are undergoing long-term treatment with fluticasone should carry a steroid card or wear a Medic-alert bracelet.
Monitoring Periodic checks on adrenal gland function may be required if large doses are being taken.

Furosemide

Brand names Froop, Frusol, Lasix
Used in the following combined preparations Co-Amilofruse, Fru-Co, Frumil, Lasikal, and others

QUICK REFERENCE
Drug group Loop diuretic (p.32) and antihypertensive drug (p.36)
Overdose danger rating Low
Dependence rating Low
Prescription needed Yes
Available as generic Yes

GENERAL INFORMATION
Furosemide, in use for over 20 years, is a powerful, short-acting loop diuretic. Like other diuretics, it is used to treat oedema (accumulation of fluid in tissue spaces) caused by heart failure, and to treat certain lung, liver, and kidney disorders.

Because it is fast-acting, furosemide is often used in emergencies to relieve pulmonary oedema (fluid in the lungs). Furosemide is particularly useful for people who have impaired kidney function because they do not respond well to thiazide diuretics (see p.320).

Because furosemide increases potassium loss, potassium supplements or a potassium-sparing diuretic are often given with it.

INFORMATION FOR USERS
Your drug prescription is tailored for you. Do not alter dosage without checking with your doctor.
How taken Tablets, liquid, injection.
Frequency and timing of doses Once daily, usually in the morning; 4–6 x hourly (high dose therapy).
Adult dosage range 20–80mg daily. Dose may be increased to a maximum of 2g daily if kidney function is impaired.
Onset of effect Within 1 hour (by mouth); within 5 minutes (injection).
Duration of action Up to 6 hours.
Diet advice Use of this drug may reduce potassium in the body. Eat plenty of potassium-rich fresh fruits and vegetables, such as bananas and tomatoes.
Storage Keep in a closed container in a cool, dry place out of reach of children. Protect from light.
Missed dose No cause for concern, but take as soon as you remember. however, if it is late in the day, do not take the missed dose, or you may need to get up during the night to pass urine. Take the next scheduled dose as usual.
Stopping the drug Do not stop taking the drug without consulting your doctor; symptoms may recur.
Exceeding the dose An occasional unintentional extra dose is unlikely to be a cause for concern. But if you notice any unusual symptoms, or if a large overdose has been taken, notify your doctor.

POSSIBLE ADVERSE EFFECTS

Adverse effects of furosemide, which include dizziness, nausea, and lethargy, are caused mainly by the rapid fluid loss that is produced by furosemide. These effects tend to diminish as the body adjusts to the drug. The disturbance in body salts and water balance can also result in muscle cramps, headaches, and dizziness. If you develop a rash (which may be more marked in light-exposed areas of skin), or experience palpitations, stop taking the drug and consult your doctor urgently. Ringing in the ears may occur with high doses given by injection.

INTERACTIONS

NSAIDs Some of these drugs may reduce the diuretic effect of furosemide.

Lithium Furosemide may increase blood levels of lithium, leading to an increased risk of lithium poisoning.

Digoxin Although this drug is often prescribed with furosemide, loss of potassium may lead to digoxin toxicity when the drugs are taken together.

Aminoglycoside antibiotics The risk of hearing and kidney problems may be increased when these drugs are taken with high doses of furosemide.

Angiotensin-converting enzyme inhibitors Low blood pressure may occur when these drugs are taken with furosemide. This interaction, however, is often desired for better control of blood pressure.

SPECIAL PRECAUTIONS

Be sure to tell your doctor if:
◆ You have long-term liver problems.
◆ You have gout.
◆ You have diabetes.
◆ You have previously had an allergic reaction to furosemide or sulphonamides.
◆ You have prostate trouble.
◆ You are taking laxatives.
◆ You are taking other medications.

Pregnancy Safety in pregnancy not established. Discuss with your doctor.

Breast-feeding The drug may reduce milk supply, but the amount of it in the breast milk is unlikely to affect the baby. Discuss with your doctor.

Infants and children Reduced dose necessary.

Over 60 Reduced dose may be necessary.

Driving and hazardous work No problems expected.

Alcohol Keep consumption low. Furosemide increases the likelihood of dehydration and hangovers after alcohol consumption.

PROLONGED USE

Serious problems are unlikely, but levels of salts such as potassium, sodium, and calcium may become depleted. Low blood pressure, palpitations, headaches, difficulty in passing urine, or muscle cramps may develop, particularly in elderly people.

Monitoring Periodic tests may be performed to check on kidney function and levels of body salts.

Gabapentin

Brand name Neurontin
Used in the following combined preparations
None

QUICK REFERENCE

Drug group Anticonvulsant drug (p.16)
Overdose danger rating Medium
Dependence rating Low
Prescription needed Yes
Available as generic No

GENERAL INFORMATION

Gabapentin is an antiepileptic drug that is used to treat partial seizures. It is often prescribed in combination with other drugs when epilepsy is not being satisfactorily controlled with these drugs alone. Unlike with some other antiepileptics, blood levels of gabapentin do not need to be monitored. In addition, the drug does not interact with other anticonvulsants.

Gabapentin is also used for the relief of neuropathic pain, such as the pain that follows shingles.

Patients with impaired kidney function should be given smaller doses, and diabetic patients taking gabapentin may notice fluctuations in their blood glucose levels.

INFORMATION FOR USERS

Your drug prescription is tailored for you. Do not alter dosage without checking with your doctor.

How taken Tablets, capsules.
Frequency and timing of doses 2 x daily initially, up to 3 x daily (maintenance dose). No more than 12 hours to elapse between doses.
Adult dosage range *Epilepsy* 900–2,400mg daily; maintenance dose reached gradually over a few days. *Neuropathic pain* 1,800mg daily (maximum), reached gradually over a few days.
Onset of effect The full antiepileptic effect may not be seen for 48 hours.
Duration of action 6–8 hours.
Diet advice None.
Storage Keep in a cool, dry place out of reach of children.
Missed dose Take as soon as you remember. If your next dose is due within 4 hours, take a single dose now and skip the next.

Stopping the drug Treatment should not be stopped abruptly. Gradual withdrawal over at least 7 days is advised to reduce the risk of seizures in people being treated for epilepsy.
Exceeding the dose An occasional unintentional extra dose is unlikely to be a cause for concern. Large overdoses, however, may lead to dizziness, double vision, and slurred speech; notify your doctor.

POSSIBLE ADVERSE EFFECTS

The most common adverse effects of gabapentin are drowsiness, dizziness, fatigue, and muscle tremor. Vision disturbances, indigestion, or weight gain are less common. If these occur, seek medical advice. The most unusual effects are mood change, hallucinations, and a rash, which require urgent medical attention.

INTERACTIONS

Antacids containing aluminium or magnesium These may reduce the effect of gabapentin and should not be taken within 2 hours of it.
Urinary protein tests for diabetics False-positive readings have been recorded with some tests. Special procedures are required for diabetic people taking gabapentin.

SPECIAL PRECAUTIONS

Be sure to tell your doctor if:
◆ You have a kidney problem.
◆ You have diabetes.
◆ You have a history of psychiatric illness.
◆ You are taking any other medications.
Pregnancy The drug is likely to reach the developing baby and its effects are unknown. Discuss with your doctor.
Breast-feeding The drug passes into the breast milk, and the effects on the baby are unknown. Discuss with your doctor.
Infants and children Not recommended under 6 years. Reduced doses based on bodyweight necessary for children under 12 years.
Over 60 Doses may have to be adjusted to allow for decreased kidney function.
Driving and hazardous work Avoid such activities until you have learned how gabapentin affects because the drug can cause drowsiness or dizziness.
Alcohol Alcohol may increase the sedative effects of gabapentin.

PROLONGED USE
No problems expected.

Gentamicin

Brand names Cidomycin, Garamycin, Genticin, Minims gentamicin
Used in the following combined preparations Gentisone HC

QUICK REFERENCE

Drug group Aminoglycoside antibiotic (p.62)
Overdose danger rating Low
Dependence rating Low
Prescription needed Yes
Available as generic Yes

GENERAL INFORMATION

Gentamicin is one of the aminoglycoside antibiotics. The injectable form of the drug is usually reserved for treatment, in hospital, of serious or complicated infections. These include infections of the lungs, urinary tract, bones, and joints; wound infections; and peritonitis, septicaemia, and meningitis. The injectable form is also used together with a penicillin for the prevention and treatment of heart valve infections (endocarditis). In the form of drops, gentamicin is used to treat eye and ear infections.

Gentamicin given by injection can have serious adverse effects on the ears, which may lead to damage to the balance mechanism and deafness; it can also have serious adverse effects on the kidneys. Courses of treatment are therefore limited to the shortest duration necessary and monitoring of blood levels is usually required. Treatment is monitored with particular care when high doses are needed or when kidney function is poor.

INFORMATION FOR USERS

Your drug prescription is tailored for you. Do not alter dosage without checking with your doctor.
How taken Injection, eye and ear drops.
Frequency and timing of doses 1–3 x daily (injection); 3–4 x daily or as directed (ear drops); every 2 hours or as directed (eye drops).

Adult dosage range According to condition and response (injection); according to your doctor's instructions (eye and ear drops).
Onset of effect Within 1–2 hours.
Duration of action 8–12 hours.
Diet advice None.
Storage Keep in a closed container in a cool, dry place out of reach of children.
Missed dose Apply skin, eye, and ear preparations as soon as you remember.
Stopping the drug Complete the course. Even if you feel better, the original infection may still be present and may recur if treatment is stopped too soon.
Exceeding the dose Overdose of gentamicin by injection is dangerous but is unlikely to occur because treatment is carefully monitored. For other preparations, an occasional unintentional extra dose is unlikely to be a cause for concern. But if you notice any unusual symptoms, notify your doctor.

POSSIBLE ADVERSE EFFECTS

Adverse effects are rare with gentamicin, but those that occur with the injectable form of the drug can be serious. Dizziness, loss of balance (vertigo), ringing in the ears (tinnitus), impaired hearing, and changes in the urine should be reported promptly. Nausea or vomiting may also occur. If the ointment or cream is applied to large areas, the drug may be absorbed and could cause hearing loss. Allergic reactions, including rash and itching, may occur with all preparations that contain gentamicin. Blurred vision or eye irritation may occur with the eye preparations and should be reported to your doctor.

INTERACTIONS

General note A wide range of drugs, including furosemide, vancomycin, and cephalosporins, increase the risk of hearing loss and/or kidney failure developing with gentamicin injections.

SPECIAL PRECAUTIONS

Be sure to tell your doctor if:
◆ You have a long-term kidney problem.
◆ You have a hearing disorder.
◆ You have myasthenia gravis.
◆ You have Parkinson's disease.

◆ You have previously had an allergic reaction to aminoglycosides.

◆ You are taking other medications.

Pregnancy No evidence of risk with eye or ear drops. Injections are not prescribed, because they may cause hearing defects in the baby. Discuss with your doctor.

Breast-feeding No evidence of risk with eye or ear preparations. Given by injection, the drug may pass into the breast milk. Discuss with your doctor.

Infants and children Reduced dose necessary for injections.

Over 60 Increased likelihood of adverse effects. Reduced dose may therefore be necessary.

Driving and hazardous work No known problems from preparations for the eye and ear.

Alcohol No known problems.

PROLONGED USE

Gentamicin is not usually given for longer than 7 days. When it is given by injection, there is a risk of adverse effects on hearing and balance.

Monitoring Blood levels of gentamicin are usually checked if the drug is given by injection. Tests on kidney function are also usually carried out.

Glibenclamide

Brand names Daonil, Euglucon, Semi-Daonil
Used in the following combined preparations
None

QUICK REFERENCE

Drug group Oral antidiabetic drug (p.82)
Overdose danger rating High
Dependence rating Low
Prescription needed Yes
Available as generic Yes

GENERAL INFORMATION

Glibenclamide is a sulphonylurea oral antidiabetic drug. Like other drugs of this type, it stimulates the production and secretion of insulin from the islet cells in the pancreas and promotes the uptake of glucose into body cells, thereby lowering the level of glucose in the blood.

This drug is used in the treatment of adult (maturity-onset) diabetes mellitus, in conjunction with a diabetic diet that is low in fat and refined carbohydrate.

In conditions of severe illness, injury, or stress, glibenclamide may lose its effectiveness, making insulin injections necessary. Adverse effects of glibenclamide are generally mild, but symptoms of poor diabetic control occur if the dosage of the drug is not appropriate.

INFORMATION FOR USERS

Your drug prescription is tailored for you. Do not alter dosage without checking with your doctor.

How taken Tablets.

Frequency and timing of doses Once daily in the morning with breakfast.

Adult dosage range 5–15mg daily.

Onset of effect Within 3 hours.

Duration of action 10–15 hours.

Diet advice An individualized, low-carbohydrate, low-fat diet must be maintained in order for the drug to be fully effective. Follow the advice of your doctor.

Storage Keep in a closed container in a cool, dry place out of reach of children. Protect from light.

Missed dose Take with your next meal; do not double the dose to account for the missed dose.

Stopping the drug Do not stop taking the drug without consulting your doctor. Stopping the drug may lead to worsening of your diabetes.

OVERDOSE ACTION

Seek immediate medical advice in all cases. If any early warning symptoms of excessively low blood glucose (such as fainting, sweating, trembling, confusion, or headache) occur, eat or drink something sugary. Take emergency action if fits or loss of consciousness occur.

POSSIBLE ADVERSE EFFECTS

Serious adverse effects are rare with glibenclamide. Symptoms such as fainting or confusion, weakness or tremor, sweating, and constipation and diarrhoea may be signs of low blood glucose levels resulting from lack of food or too high a dose of the drug; if any of these symptoms occur, eat or drink something sugary immediately and seek medical assistance. Other adverse effects include nausea or vomiting, rash and itching, and weight changes. If you show signs of jaundice, consult your doctor without delay.

INTERACTIONS

General note A variety of drugs may reduce the effect of glibenclamide and may raise blood glucose levels. These include corticosteroids, oestrogens, diuretics, and rifampicin. Others increase the risk of low blood glucose. These include warfarin, sulphonamides and other antibacterials, antifungals, aspirin, beta blockers, and ACE inhibitors.

SPECIAL PRECAUTIONS

Be sure to tell your doctor if:

◆ You have long-term liver or kidney problems.

◆ You are allergic to sulphonylurea drugs.

◆ You have thyroid problems.

◆ You have porphyria.

◆ You have ever had problems with your adrenal glands.

◆ You are taking other medications.

Pregnancy Not usually prescribed. May cause abnormally low blood glucose levels in the newborn baby. Insulin is generally substituted because it gives better diabetic control.

Breast-feeding The drug passes into the breast milk and may affect the baby. Discuss with your doctor.

Infants and children Not prescribed.

Over 60 Greater likelihood of low blood glucose with glibenclamide. Reduced dose may be necessary.

Driving and hazardous work Usually no problems, but avoid such activities if you have warning signs of low blood glucose.

Alcohol Avoid. Alcohol may upset diabetic control, increasing the risk of hypoglycaemia.

Surgery and general anaesthetics Notify your doctor or dentist that you are diabetic before undergoing any type of surgery.

PROLONGED USE

No problems expected.

Monitoring Regular monitoring of glucose levels in the urine or blood is required. Periodic assessment of the eyes, heart, and kidneys may also be advised.

Gliclazide

Brand name DIAGLYK, Diamicron, Diamicron MR
Used in the following combined preparations
None

QUICK REFERENCE

Drug group Oral antidiabetic drug (p.82)
Overdose danger rating High
Dependence rating Low
Prescription needed Yes
Available as generic Yes

GENERAL INFORMATION

Gliclazide is a sulphonylurea oral antidiabetic drug. It stimulates the production and secretion of insulin from the islet cells in the pancreas. This promotes the uptake of glucose into body cells, thereby lowering the level of glucose in the blood.

Gliclazide is used to treat adult (maturity-onset) diabetes mellitus in conjunction with a diabetic diet that is low in refined carbohydrates and fats.

During severe illness, injury, stress, or surgery, gliclazide may lose its effectiveness, necessitating the use of insulin injections. Adverse effects are generally mild. However, symptoms of poor diabetic control occur if dosage of the drug is not appropriate.

INFORMATION FOR USERS

Your drug prescription is tailored for you. Do not alter dosage without checking with your doctor.

How taken Tablets, MR-Tablets.

Frequency and timing of doses 1–2 x daily (in the morning and evening with a meal).

Dosage range 40–320mg daily (doses above 160mg are divided into two doses).

Onset of effect Within 1 hour.

Duration of action 12–24 hours.

Diet advice An individualized, low-fat, low-carbohydrate diet must be maintained for the drug to be fully effective. Follow the advice of your doctor.

Storage Keep in a closed container in a cool, dry place out of reach of children.

Missed dose Take as soon as you remember with the next meal.

Stopping the drug Do not stop taking the drug without consulting your doctor. Stopping the drug may lead to worsening of the underlying condition.

OVERDOSE ACTION

Seek immediate medical advice in all cases. If early warning symptoms of excessively low blood glucose such as fainting, sweating, trembling, confusion, or headache occur, eat or drink something sugary at once. Take emergency action if fits or loss of consciousness occur.

POSSIBLE ADVERSE EFFECTS

Serious adverse effects are rare. Symptoms such as fainting or confusion, weakness or tremor, and sweating may be signs of low blood glucose due to lack of food or too high a dose of the drug. You should eat or drink something sugary immediately and seek urgent medical advice. Constipation or diarrhoea may also occur. Other, more rare, adverse effects include nausea or vomiting, a rash and itching, and weight changes. If you develop jaundice, consult your doctor without delay.

INTERACTIONS

General note A variety of drugs may reduce the effect of gliclazide and may, therefore, raise blood glucose levels. These drugs include corticosteroid drugs, oestrogens, diuretics, and rifampicin.

Other drugs increase the risk of low blood glucose. These include warfarin, sulphonamides and other antibacterial drugs, aspirin, beta blockers, ACE inhibitors, and antifungal drugs, particularly miconazole.

SPECIAL PRECAUTIONS

Be sure to tell your doctor if:
◆ You have long-term liver or kidney problems.
◆ You are allergic to sulphonylurea drugs.
◆ You have thyroid problems.
◆ You have porphyria.
◆ You have ever had problems with your adrenal glands.
◆ You are taking other medications.
Pregnancy Not recommended. Gliclazide may cause abnormally low blood glucose levels in the newborn baby. Insulin is generally substituted during pregnancy because it gives better diabetic control.

Breast-feeding The drug passes into the breast milk and may affect the baby. Discuss with your doctor.
Infants and children Not prescribed.
Over 60 Signs of low blood glucose may be more difficult to recognize. Reduced dose may be necessary.
Driving and hazardous work Avoid all such activities until you have learned how gliclazide affects you because the drug can produce dizziness, drowsiness, and confusion.
Alcohol Avoid. Alcohol may upset diabetic control, increasing the risk of hypoglycaemia.
Surgery and general anaesthetics Notify your doctor or dentist that you are diabetic before undergoing any type of surgery.

PROLONGED USE

No problems expected.
Monitoring Regular testing of the level of glucose in the blood and/or urine is required. Periodic assessment of the eyes, heart, and kidneys may also be advised.

Glyceryl trinitrate

Brand names Coro-Nitro, Deponit, Minitran, Nitro-Dur, Nitrolingual, Suscard, Sustac, Transiderm-Nitro, and others
Used in the following combined preparations None

QUICK REFERENCE

Drug group Anti-angina drug (p.35)
Overdose danger rating Medium
Dependence rating Low
Prescription needed No (most preparations); yes (injections)
Available as generic Yes

GENERAL INFORMATION

Introduced in the late 1800s, glyceryl trinitrate is one of the oldest drugs in continual use. It belongs to a group of vasodilator drugs known as nitrates, which are used to relieve the pain of angina attacks. Glyceryl trinitrate is available in short-acting forms (sublingual or buccal tablets and spray), which act very quickly to relieve angina, and in long-acting forms (slow-release tablets and skin patches). It is also given by injection in hospital for severe angina and for controlling blood pressure.

Glyceryl trinitrate may cause a variety of minor symptoms, such as flushing and headache, most of which can be controlled by adjustment of the dosage. The drug is best taken for the first time while you are sitting, as fainting may follow the drop in blood pressure caused by this medication. If the drug fails to relieve angina, and the attack lasts for more than 20 minutes, this may be a sign of a heart attack and requires urgent medical assistance.

An ointment preparation may be used for the specialist treatment of anal fissures.

INFORMATION FOR USERS
Your drug prescription is tailored for you. Do not alter dosage without checking with your doctor.

How taken SR-tablets, buccal tablets, sublingual tablets, injection, ointment, skin patches, spray.

Frequency and timing of doses *Prevention* 3 x daily (buccal and SR-tablets); once daily (patches); every 3–4 hours (ointment).
Relief Use buccal or sublingual tablets or spray at the onset of an attack or immediately prior to exercise. Dose may be repeated within 5 minutes if further relief is required.

Adult dosage range *Prevention* 7.8–30mg daily (SR-tablets); 3–15mg daily (buccal tablets); 5–15mg daily (patches); as directed (ointment).
Relief 0.3–1mg per dose (sublingual tablets); 1–3mg per dose (buccal tablets); 1–2 sprays per dose (spray).

Onset of effect Within minutes (buccal and sublingual tablets and spray); 1–3 hours (SR-tablets, patches, and ointment).

Duration of action 20–30 minutes (sublingual tablets and spray); 3–5 hours (buccal tablets and ointment); 8–12 hours (SR-tablets); up to 24 hours (patches).

Diet advice None.

Storage Keep buccal and sublingual tablets in a tightly closed glass container fitted with a foil-lined, screw-on cap in a cool, dry place out of reach of children. Protect from light. Do not expose to heat. Discard tablets within 8 weeks of opening. Check label of other preparations for storage conditions.

Missed dose Take as soon as you remember, or when needed. If your next dose is due within 2 hours, take one dose now and skip the next.

Stopping the drug Do not stop taking the drug without consulting your doctor.

Exceeding the dose An occasional unintentional extra dose is unlikely to cause problems. Large overdoses may cause dizziness, vomiting, severe headache, fits, or loss of consciousness. Notify your doctor.

POSSIBLE ADVERSE EFFECTS
The most serious effect is lowered blood pressure, which may cause dizziness. Other effects, such as headache and flushing, usually decrease in severity with regular use but can also be controlled by dosage adjustment.

INTERACTIONS
Antihypertensive drugs These drugs, which are often used by patients who also need to take glyceryl trinitrate, increase the possibility of lowered blood pressure or fainting when the two drugs are taken together.

Sildenafil The blood-pressure-lowering effect of glyceryl trinitrate is increased significantly by sildenafil. The two drugs should not be used together.

SPECIAL PRECAUTIONS
Be sure to tell your doctor if:
◆ You have any other heart condition.
◆ You have a lung condition.
◆ You have long-term liver or kidney problems.
◆ You have any blood disorders.
◆ You have glaucoma.
◆ You have thyroid disease.
◆ You are taking other medications.

Pregnancy Safety in pregnancy not established. Discuss with your doctor.

Breast-feeding It is not known whether the drug passes into the breast milk. Discuss with your doctor.

Infants and children Not usually prescribed.

Over 60 No special problems.

Driving and hazardous work Avoid such activities until you have learned how glyceryl trinitrate affects you because the drug can cause dizziness.

Alcohol Avoid excessive intake. Alcohol may increase dizziness as a result of lowered blood pressure.

PROLONGED USE

The effects of glyceryl trinitrate usually become slightly weaker during prolonged use as the body adapts. Timing of the doses may be changed to prevent this.

Monitoring Periodic checks on blood pressure are usually required.

Goserelin

Brand name Zoladex, Zoladex LA
Used in the following combined preparations
None

QUICK REFERENCE

Drug group Anticancer drug (p.96)
Overdose danger rating Low
Dependence rating Low
Prescription needed Yes
Available as generic No

GENERAL INFORMATION

Goserelin is a synthetic drug that is chemically related to the hormone gonadorelin. Like gonadorelin, it stimulates the release of hormones from the pituitary gland; these hormones, in turn, control production of the sex hormones.

Goserelin is used to suppress production of sex hormones in cancers of the breast and prostate. At the start of prostate cancer treatment, it is often given with an anti-androgen drug such as flutamide (see p.249) to control an initial growth spurt of the tumour.

The drug is also used in the management of fibroids, infertility, and endometriosis. The first dose is normally given during menstruation to avoid the possibility that the patient may be pregnant. In addition, it is advisable for women of childbearing age to use barrier methods of contraception during treatment. This is because the drug may adversely affect a developing baby.

The injections are usually given by a general practitioner or district nurse.

Loss of bone density is an important side effect of treatment with goserelin in women. Therefore, repeat courses of the drug are given only for cancerous conditions. Treatment with goserelin may also, rarely, cause ovarian cysts.

INFORMATION FOR USERS

Your drug prescription is tailored for you. Do not alter dosage without checking with your doctor

How taken Implant injection, long-acting (LA) implant injection.

Frequency and timing of doses *Endometriosis* Every 28 days; maximum of a single 6-month treatment course only (implant). *Fibroids* Implant every 28 days, maximum 3 months' treatment. *Breast and prostate cancer* Every 12 weeks (LA implant).

Adult dosage range 3.6mg every 28 days (endometriosis/fibroids/breast cancer); 10.8mg every 3 months (prostate).

Onset of effect Within 24 hours (endometriosis/fibroids); 1–2 weeks after tumour flare (prostate).

Duration of action 28 days (implant); 12 weeks (long-acting implant).

Diet advice None.

Storage Not applicable. The drug is not kept in the home.

Missed dose No cause for concern. Treatment can be resumed when possible.

Stopping the drug Do not stop treatment without consulting your doctor.

Exceeding the dose Overdosage is unlikely since treatment is not self-administered.

POSSIBLE ADVERSE EFFECTS

Symptoms similar to those of the menopause (such as hot flushes and changes in breast size), headache, and bleeding on stopping goserelin are common. Rare adverse effects include dizziness or fainting, rash or wheezing, and reaction at the injection site; if these occur, they should be reported to your doctor straight away.

INTERACTIONS

None.

SPECIAL PRECAUTIONS

Be sure to tell your doctor if:
◆ You have osteoporosis.
◆ You have previously been treated with goserelin (or another gonadorelin analogue) for endometriosis or fibroids.
◆ You have polycystic ovarian disease.
◆ You are allergic to gonadorelin analogues.
◆ You are taking other medications.

Pregnancy Not prescribed.
Breast-feeding Not recommended. Discuss with your doctor.
Infants and children Not recommended.
Over 60 No special problems.
Driving and hazardous work No special problems.
Alcohol No special problems.

PROLONGED USE

Goserelin is only used in the long term for treatment of prostate or breast cancer. Bone density is lost over time in women taking the drug, but this may be partly recoverable once treatment stops.
Monitoring Women may be monitored for changes in bone density.

Haloperidol

Brand names Dozic, Haldol, Serenace
Used in the following combined preparations
None

QUICK REFERENCE

Drug group Antipsychotic drug (p.15)
Overdose danger rating Medium
Dependence rating Low
Prescription needed Yes
Available as generic Yes

GENERAL INFORMATION

Haloperidol is used to reduce the violent, aggressive manifestations of mental illnesses such as schizophrenia, mania, dementia, and other disorders in which hallucinations are experienced. Haloperidol is also used as a short-term treatment for severe anxiety. It does not cure the underlying disorder but relieves the distressing symptoms. In addition, it is used in the control of Tourette's syndrome and may be of benefit to children with severe behavioural problems for which other drugs are ineffective.

The main drawback of the drug is that it may produce abnormal, involuntary movements and stiffness of the face and limbs.

INFORMATION FOR USERS

Your drug prescription is tailored for you. Do not alter dosage without checking with your doctor.
How taken Tablets, capsules, liquid, injection, depot injection.
Frequency and timing of doses 2–4 x daily.
Adult dosage range *Mental illness* 3–10mg daily, initially, up to maximum of 30mg daily. *Severe anxiety* 1mg daily.
Onset of effect 2–3 hours (by mouth); 20–30 minutes (injection).
Duration of action 6–24 hours (by mouth) 2–4 hours (injection); up to 4 weeks (depot injection).
Diet advice None.
Storage Keep in a closed container in a cool, dry place out of reach of children.
Missed dose Take as soon as you remember. If your next dose is due within 3 hours, take a single dose now and skip the next.
Stopping the drug Unless severe adverse effects occur (see below), do not stop taking the drug without consulting your doctor; symptoms may recur.
Exceeding the dose An occasional unintentional extra dose is unlikely to cause problems. Larger overdoses, however, may cause unusual drowsiness, muscle weakness or rigidity, and/or faintness; notify your doctor.

POSSIBLE ADVERSE EFFECTS

Various minor anticholinergic symptoms, such as dry mouth, blurred vision, and difficulty in passing urine, can occur but often become less marked with time. Appetite loss, drowsiness or lethargy, and dizziness or fainting may also occur. If stiffness of the tongue, neck, or limbs occurs after the first dose, or a rash develops, seek medical advice. If high fever, confusion, or muscle stiffness develops, stop taking the drug and consult your doctor urgently. The most significant effect, parkinsonism (abnormal face and limb movements), can be controlled by dosage adjustment.

INTERACTIONS

Sedatives Sedatives are likely to increase the sedative properties of haloperidol.
Rifampicin and anticonvulsants These drugs may reduce the effects of haloperidol, the dosage of which may need to be increased.
Lithium This drug may increase the risk of parkinsonism and effects on the nerves.
Methyldopa This drug may increase the risk of parkinsonism and low blood pressure.
Anticholinergic drugs Haloperidol may increase the side effects of these drugs.
Terfenadine This drug may have adverse effects on the heart if taken with haloperidol.

SPECIAL PRECAUTIONS

Be sure to tell your doctor if:
◆ You have long-term liver or kidney problems.
◆ You have heart or circulation problems.
◆ You have had epileptic fits.
◆ You have an overactive thyroid gland.
◆ You have Parkinson's disease.
◆ You have had glaucoma.
◆ You have asthma, bronchitis, or another lung disorder.
◆ You have had phaeochromocytoma.
◆ You are taking other medications.
Pregnancy Safety in pregnancy not established. Discuss with your doctor.

Breast-feeding The drug passes into the breast milk and may affect the baby. Discuss with your doctor.

Infants and children Rarely required. Reduced dose necessary.

Over 60 Reduced dose may be necessary.

Driving and hazardous work Avoid such activities until you have learned how haloperidol affects you because the drug may cause drowsiness and slowed reactions.

Alcohol Avoid. Alcohol may increase the sedative effect of this drug.

PROLONGED USE

Use of this drug for more than a few months may lead to tardive dyskinesia (abnormal, involuntary movements of the eyes, face, and tongue). Occasionally, jaundice may occur.

Heparin

Brand names Calciparine, Monoparin, Multiparin, Uniparin; [LMWH] Alphaparin, Clexane, Clivarine, Fragmin, Innohep

Used in the following combined preparations
None

QUICK REFERENCE

Drug group Drug that affects blood clotting (p.38)

Overdose danger rating High

Dependence rating Low

Prescription needed Yes

Available as generic Yes (heparin); no (LMWH)

GENERAL INFORMATION

Heparin is an anticoagulant drug used to prevent the formation of blood clots and aid the dispersion of existing clots. Because it acts quickly, it is particularly useful in emergencies – for example, to prevent further clotting when a clot has already reached the lungs or brain. People undergoing open heart surgery or kidney dialysis are also given heparin. A low dose of the drug is sometimes given following surgery to prevent deep vein thrombosis (clots forming in the leg veins). Heparin is often given in conjunction with other, slower-acting anticoagulants such as warfarin. It is also used to treat unstable angina.

Certoparin, dalteparin, enoxaparin, and tinzaparin are new forms of heparin called "low molecular weight heparins" (LMWH). They are now widely used and do not have to be given in hospital.

The most serious adverse effect of heparin, as with all anticoagulants, is the risk of excessive bleeding, so the ability of the blood to clot is watched very carefully. Bruising may occur around the site of the injection.

INFORMATION FOR USERS

This drug is normally given only under medical supervision and is only rarely for self-administration.

How taken Injection.

Frequency and timing of doses Every 8–12 hours or continuous intravenous infusion. LMWH forms: once daily.

Dosage range Dosage is determined by nature of condition being treated or prevented.

Onset of effect Within 15 minutes.

Duration of action 4–12 hours after treatment is stopped. LMWH forms: 24 hours after end of treatment.

Diet advice None.

Storage Keep in a cool, dry place out of reach of children.

Missed dose Notify your doctor.

Stopping the drug Do not stop taking the drug without consulting your doctor. Stopping the drug may lead to clotting of the blood.

OVERDOSE ACTION

Seek immediate medical advice in all cases. Take emergency action if bleeding, severe headache, or loss of consciousness occur. Overdose can be reversed under medical supervision by a drug called protamine.

POSSIBLE ADVERSE EFFECTS

As with all anticoagulants, bleeding is the most common adverse effect. The less common effects may occur with long-term treatment.

INTERACTIONS

Clopidogrel, ticlopidine, and dipyridamole The anticoagulant effect of heparin may be increased when it is taken with these drugs. The dosage of heparin may need to be adjusted accordingly.

Aspirin The anticoagulant effect of heparin may be increased by aspirin, and the drugs may be given together for this reason.

SPECIAL PRECAUTIONS

Be sure to tell your doctor if:

◆ You have long-term liver or kidney problems.
◆ You have high blood pressure.
◆ You bleed easily.
◆ You have any allergies.
◆ You have stomach ulcers.
◆ You are taking other medications.

Pregnancy The drug needs careful monitoring; taken near delivery, it may cause the mother to bleed excessively. Discuss with your doctor.

Breast-feeding No evidence of risk.

Infants and children Reduced dose necessary according to age and weight.

Over 60 No special problems.

Driving and hazardous work Avoid any risk of injury because excessive bruising and bleeding could occur.

Alcohol No special problems.

Surgery and general anaesthetics Heparin treatment may need to be stopped before you have surgery. Discuss this with your doctor or dentist before any operation.

PROLONGED USE

Osteoporosis and hair loss may occur very rarely; tolerance to heparin may develop.

Monitoring Periodic blood and liver function tests will be required.

Hydrochlorothiazide

Brand name None
Used in the following combined preparations
Acezide, Capozide, Co-Betaloc, Dyazide, Moducren, Moduretic, and others

QUICK REFERENCE

Drug group Thiazide diuretic (p.32)
Overdose danger rating Low
Dependence rating Low
Prescription needed Yes
Available as generic No

GENERAL INFORMATION

Hydrochlorothiazide belongs to the thiazide group of diuretic drugs, which remove excess water from the body and reduce oedema (fluid retention) in people with congestive heart failure, kidney disorders, cirrhosis of the liver, and premenstrual syndrome. This drug is used to treat high blood pressure (see Antihypertensive drugs, p.36).

Hydrochlorothiazide increases potassium loss in the urine. This can cause a variety of symptoms (see Possible adverse effects, be low), and increases the likelihood of irregular heart rhythms, particularly in patients taking drugs such as digoxin. For this reason, potassium supplements are often given with hydrochlorothiazide.

INFORMATION FOR USERS

Your drug prescription is tailored for you. Do not alter dosage without checking with your doctor.

How taken Tablets.

Frequency and timing of doses Once daily, or every 2 days, early in the day.

Adult dosage range 25–50mg daily.

Onset of effect Within 2 hours.

Duration of action 6–12 hours.

Diet advice Use of hydrochlorothiazide may reduce potassium in the body. Eat plenty of fresh fruit and vegetables, and discuss with your doctor the advisability of reducing your salt intake.

Storage Keep in a closed container in a cool, dry place out of reach of children. Protect from light.

Missed dose No cause for concern, but take as soon as you remember. If it is late in the day, however, do not take the missed dose, or you may have to get up during the night to pass urine. Take the next scheduled dose as usual.

Stopping the drug Unless a rash occurs, do not stop taking the drug without consulting your doctor; symptoms may recur.

Exceeding the dose An occasional unintentional extra dose is unlikely to be a cause for concern. But if you notice any unusual symptoms, or if a large overdose has been taken, notify your doctor.

POSSIBLE ADVERSE EFFECTS

The most common problem is muscle cramps, which often occur at night. Lethargy, dizziness, digestive disturbances, and impotence may also occur. Some effects are due to excessive potassium loss. This can sometimes be put right by taking a potassium supplement. Rarely, gout may occur in susceptible people, and certain forms of diabetes may become more difficult to control. If a rash occurs, stop taking the drug and consult your doctor.

INTERACTIONS

NSAIDs Some NSAIDs may reduce the diuretic effect of hydrochlorothiazide, the dosage of which may need to be adjusted.

Digoxin Adverse effects may be increased if excessive potassium is lost.

Corticosteroids These drugs further increase loss of potassium from the body when taken with hydrochlorothiazide.

Lithium Hydrochlorothiazide may raise lithium levels in the blood, leading to a risk of serious adverse effects.

SPECIAL PRECAUTIONS

Be sure to tell your doctor if:
◆ You have long-term liver or kidney problems.
◆ You have had gout.
◆ You have diabetes.
◆ You have porphyria.
◆ You have Addison's disease or systemic lupus erythematosus.
◆ You are taking other medications.

Pregnancy Not usually prescribed. May cause jaundice in the newborn baby. Discuss with your doctor.

Breast-feeding The drug passes into the breast milk, but at normal doses adverse effects on the baby are unlikely. Discuss with your doctor.

Infants and children Not usually prescribed. Reduced dose necessary.

Over 60 Increased likelihood of adverse effects.

Driving and hazardous work Avoid such activities until you have learned how hydrochlorothiazide affects you because the drug may reduce mental alertness and cause dizziness.

Alcohol Keep consumption low. Hydrochlorothiazide increases the likelihood of dehydration and hangovers after consumption of alcohol.

PROLONGED USE

Excessive loss of potassium and imbalances of other salts may result.

Monitoring Blood tests may be performed periodically to check kidney function and levels of potassium and other salts.

Hydrocortisone

Brand names Colifoam, Corlan, Dioderm, Efcortelan, Efcortesol, Hydrocortistab, Hydrocortone, Solu-Cortef
Used in the following combined preparations Alphaderm, Xyloproct, and many others

QUICK REFERENCE

Drug group Corticosteroid (p.80) and topical corticosteroid (p.120)
Overdose danger rating Low
Dependence rating Low
Prescription needed Yes (except for some topical preparations)
Available as generic Yes

GENERAL INFORMATION

Hydrocortisone is chemically identical to the hormone cortisol, produced by the adrenal glands. For this reason, the drug is prescribed to replace natural hormones in adrenal insufficiency (Addison's disease). The dose given replaces the body's production of hormone, and side effects should be minimal.

Hydrocortisone is used mainly in the treatment of various allergic and inflammatory conditions, however. Used topically, it provides prompt relief from inflammation of the skin, eye, and outer ear. In oral form, it relieves asthma, inflammatory bowel disease, and many rheumatic and allergic disorders. Injected directly into the joints, hydrocortisone relieves pain and stiffness (see p.53). Injections may also be given to relieve severe attacks of asthma.

Overuse of skin preparations can lead to permanent thinning of the skin. Taken by mouth, long-term treatment with high doses may cause serious side effects.

INFORMATION FOR USERS

Your drug prescription is tailored for you. Do not alter dosage without checking with your doctor.

How taken Tablets, lozenges, injection, rectal foam, cream, ointment, eye/ear ointment or drops.

Frequency and timing of doses Varies according to the condition.

Dosage range Varies according to the condition, but should be increased to cover serious injury or surgery.

Onset of effect 4 hours to several days, depending on the condition.

Duration of action Up to 12 hours.

Diet advice Salt intake may need to be restricted when the drug is taken by mouth. Potassium supplements may also be necessary.

Storage Keep in a closed container in a cool, dry place out of reach of children.

Missed dose Take as soon as you remember. If your next dose is due within 2 hours, take a single dose now and skip the next.

Stopping the drug Do not stop taking the drug without consulting your doctor. Gradual dosage reduction is required following prolonged treatment with oral hydrocortisone.

Exceeding the dose An occasional unintentional extra dose is unlikely to be a cause for concern. But if you notice any unusual symptoms, or if a large overdose has been taken, notify your doctor.

POSSIBLE ADVERSE EFFECTS

Taken by mouth, hydrocortisone may cause indigestion, weight gain, acne, fluid retention, and high blood pressure. High doses may lead to muscle weakness and mood changes; if these occur, consult your doctor. The most serious adverse effects only occur when hydrocortisone is taken by mouth in high doses for long periods of time (see Prolonged use, below). These are carefully monitored during treatment.

INTERACTIONS

Barbiturates, anticonvulsants, and rifampicin These drugs reduce the effectiveness of hydrocortisone.

Antidiabetic drugs Hydrocortisone reduces the action of these drugs.

Antihypertensive drugs Hydrocortisone reduces the effects of these drugs.

Vaccines Severe reactions can occur if certain vaccines are given during hydrocortisone treatment.

SPECIAL PRECAUTIONS

Be sure to tell your doctor if:
◆ You have liver or kidney problems.
◆ You have had a peptic ulcer.
◆ You have had a mental illness or epilepsy.
◆ You have glaucoma.
◆ You have had tuberculosis.

◆ You have diabetes or heart problems.
◆ You are taking other medications.
Avoid exposure to chickenpox, shingles, or measles if you are on systemic treatment.

Pregnancy No evidence of risk with topical preparations. Oral doses may adversely affect the developing baby. Discuss with your doctor.

Breast-feeding The drug passes into the breast milk and may affect the baby. Discuss with your doctor.

Infants and children Reduced dose necessary.

Over 60 Reduced dose may be necessary.

Driving and hazardous work No special problems.

Alcohol Avoid. Alcohol may increase the risk of peptic ulcer when the drug is taken by mouth.

PROLONGED USE

Depending on the method of administration, prolonged high doses may cause diabetes, glaucoma, fragile bones, and thin skin, and may retard growth in children. People having long-term treatment are advised to carry a "steroid treatment" card.

Monitoring Periodic checks on blood pressure are usually necessary when the drug is taken by mouth.

Hyoscine

Brand names Buscopan, Joy-Rides, Kwells, Scopoderm TTS, Travel Calm
Used in the following combined preparation Papaveretum and hyoscine

QUICK REFERENCE

Drug group Drug for irritable bowel syndrome (p.45), drug affecting the pupil (p.116), and anti-emetic (p.21)
Overdose danger rating Medium
Dependence rating Low
Prescription needed No (for most preparations)
Available as generic Yes

GENERAL INFORMATION

Originally derived from the henbane plant, hyoscine is an anticholinergic (see Autonomic nervous system, p.8) drug that has both an antispasmodic effect on the intestine and a calming action on the nerve pathways that control nausea and vomiting. By its anticholinergic action, it also dilates the pupil.

The drug has two forms: hyoscine butylbromide, which is prescribed to reduce spasm of the gastrointestinal tract in irritable bowel syndrome, and hyoscine hydrobromide, which is used to control motion sickness and giddiness and nausea due to inner-ear disturbances such as vertigo and Ménière's disease (see p.22) and can be administered as skin patches as well as in tablets. This form is also used as a premedication to dry secretions before operations. Eye drops containing the hydrobromide form are used to dilate the pupil during eye examinations and eye surgery.

INFORMATION FOR USERS

Follow instructions on the label. Call your doctor if symptoms worsen.

How taken Tablets, injection, skin patches.

Frequency and timing of doses As required up to 4 x daily by mouth (irritable bowel syndrome) or up to 3 x daily (nausea and vomiting); every 3 days (patches).

Adult dosage range *Irritable bowel syndrome* 80mg (hyoscine butylbromide) daily. *Nausea and vomiting* 0.3mg (hyoscine hydrobromide) per dose.

Onset of effect Within 1 hour.

Duration of action Up to 6 hours (by mouth); up to 72 hours (patches).

Diet advice None.

Storage Keep in a closed container in a cool, dry place out of reach of children. Protect from light.

Missed dose Take as soon as you remember, and adjust the timing of your next dose accordingly.

Stopping the drug Can be safely stopped as soon as you no longer need it.

Exceeding the dose An occasional unintentional extra dose is unlikely to cause problems. Large overdoses may cause drowsiness or agitation; notify your doctor.

POSSIBLE ADVERSE EFFECTS

Taken by mouth or by injection, hyoscine has a strong anticholinergic effect on the body, causing a variety of minor symptoms, such as dry mouth and drowsiness. These can sometimes be minimized by a reduction in dosage. If you experience blurred vision, difficulty in passing urine, or a fast heart rate, however, consult your doctor.

INTERACTIONS

Sedatives All drugs that have a sedative effect on the central nervous system are likely to increase the sedative properties of hyoscine. Such drugs include anti-anxiety and sleeping drugs, antidepressants, opioid analgesics, and antipsychotics.

Anticholinergic drugs Many drugs have anticholinergic, or antimuscarinic, effects. These are drugs that have side effects such as dry mouth, difficulty passing urine, and constipation. Using hyoscine with these drugs increases the risk of such side effects.

SPECIAL PRECAUTIONS

Be sure to consult your doctor or pharmacist before taking this drug if:

◆ You have long-term liver or kidney problems.

◆ You have heart problems.

◆ You have myasthenia gravis.

◆ You have megacolon or intestinal obstruction problems.

◆ You have had glaucoma.

◆ You have prostate trouble or urinary retention.

◆ You have porphyria.

◆ You are taking other medications.

Pregnancy Safety in pregnancy not established. Discuss with your doctor.

Breast-feeding No evidence of risk. Discuss with your doctor.

Infants and children Not recommended for children under 4 years for motion sickness. Patches not recommended for those under 10 years. Other uses not recommended for children under 6 years. Reduced dose necessary in older children.

Over 60 Reduced dose may be necessary.

Driving and hazardous work Avoid such activities until you have learned how hyoscine affects you because the drug can cause drowsiness and blurred vision.

Alcohol Avoid. Alcohol may increase the sedative effect of this drug.

PROLONGED USE

Use of this drug for longer than a few days is unlikely to be necessary.

Ibuprofen

Brand names Arthrofen, Brufen, Ebufac, Fenbid, Ibugel, Ibuleve, Ibumousse, Inoven, Motrin, Nurofen, and many others
Used in the following combined preparation
Codafen

QUICK REFERENCE

Drug group Analgesic (p.9) and non-steroidal anti-inflammatory drug (p.50)
Overdose danger rating Low
Dependence rating Low
Prescription needed No (some preparations)
Available as generic Yes

GENERAL INFORMATION

Ibuprofen is a non-steroidal anti-inflammatory drug (NSAID) which, like other NSAIDs, reduces pain, stiffness, and inflammation. It is an effective treatment for the symptoms of osteoarthritis, rheumatoid arthritis, and gout; in the treatment of rheumatoid arthritis, it may be prescribed with slower-acting drugs. Ibuprofen is also used to relieve mild to moderate headache, menstrual and dental pain, pain resulting from soft tissue injuries, or the pain that may follow an operation.

Ibuprofen has fewer side effects than many of the other NSAIDs. It rarely causes bleeding in the stomach and seems to be safer than aspirin in this respect. The drug is also available as a cream or gel that can be applied to the skin for muscular aches and sprains.

INFORMATION FOR USERS

Follow instructions on the label. Call your doctor if symptoms worsen.
How taken Tablets, SR-tablets, capsules, SR-capsules, liquid, granules, cream, mousse, gel.
Frequency and timing of doses 1–2 x daily (SR-preparations) or 4–6 x daily (general pain relief); 3–4 x daily with food (arthritis).
Adult dosage range *General pain relief* 600mg–1.8g daily. *Arthritis* 1.2–2.4g daily.
Onset of effect Pain relief begins in 1–2 hours. The full anti-inflammatory effect in arthritic conditions may not be felt for up to 2 weeks.
Duration of action 5–10 hours.
Diet advice None.

Storage Keep in a closed container in a cool, dry place out of reach of children.
Missed dose Take as soon as you remember. If your next dose is due within 2 hours, take a single dose now and skip the next.
Stopping the drug When taken for short-term pain relief, the drug can be safely stopped as soon as you no longer need it. If prescribed for the long-term treatment of arthritis, you should seek medical advice before stopping the drug unless a rash, wheezing, or breathlessness occur.
Exceeding the dose An occasional unintentional extra dose is unlikely to be a cause for concern. But if you notice any unusual symptoms, or if a large overdose has been taken, notify your doctor.

POSSIBLE ADVERSE EFFECTS

The most common adverse effects are those resulting from gastrointestinal disturbances, such as heartburn, indigestion, nausea, and vomiting. Swollen feet or ankles and ringing in the ears are uncommon adverse effects normally associated with too high a dose.

Black or bloodstained faeces should be reported to your doctor without delay. If you develop a rash, wheezing, or breathlessness, stop taking the drug and consult your doctor immediately.

INTERACTIONS

General note Ibuprofen interacts with a wide range of drugs to increase the risk of bleeding and/or peptic ulcers. Such drugs include aspirin and other NSAIDs, oral anticoagulants, and corticosteroids.
Ciprofloxacin The risk of seizures with this drug and related antibiotics may be increased by ibuprofen.
Antihypertensive drugs and diuretics The beneficial effects of these drugs may be reduced by ibuprofen.
Lithium, digoxin, and methotrexate Ibuprofen may increase the blood levels of these drugs to an undesirable extent.

SPECIAL PRECAUTIONS

Be sure to consult your doctor or pharmacist before taking this drug if:
◆ You have a long-term kidney problem.
◆ You have a long-term liver problem.

◆ You have high blood pressure.
◆ You have had a peptic ulcer, oesophagitis, or acid indigestion.
◆ You are allergic to aspirin.
◆ You have asthma.
◆ You are taking other medications.

Pregnancy Not usually prescribed. May affect the developing baby and may prolong labour. Discuss with your doctor.

Breast-feeding The drug passes into the breast milk, but at normal doses adverse effects on the baby are unlikely. Discuss with your doctor.

Infants and children Reduced dose necessary.

Over 60 Reduced dose may be necessary.

Driving and hazardous work No problems expected.

Alcohol Avoid. Alcohol may increase the risk of stomach disorders with ibuprofen.

Surgery and general anaesthetics Ibuprofen may prolong bleeding. Discuss the possibility of stopping treatment temporarily with your doctor or dentist.

PROLONGED USE

There is a small, but definite, increase in risk of bleeding from peptic ulcers and in the bowel with prolonged use of ibuprofen.

Imipramine

Brand name Tofranil
Used in the following combined preparations
None

QUICK REFERENCE

Drug group Tricyclic antidepressant (p.14) and drug for urinary disorders (p.112)
Overdose danger rating High
Dependence rating Low
Prescription needed Yes
Available as generic Yes

GENERAL INFORMATION

Imipramine belongs to the tricyclic class of antidepressant drugs. It is used mainly in the long-term treatment of depression to elevate mood, improve appetite, increase physical activity, and restore interest in everyday life. Because imipramine is less sedating than some other antidepressants, it is particularly useful when a depressed person is withdrawn or apathetic, although it can aggravate insomnia if it is taken in the evening. The drug is also prescribed to treat night-time enuresis (bedwetting) in children, although proof of its benefit is not conclusive.

Imipramine can cause a variety of side effects. In overdose, the drug may cause coma and dangerous heart rhythms.

INFORMATION FOR USERS

Your drug prescription is tailored for you. Do not alter dosage without checking with your doctor.

How taken Tablets, liquid.

Frequency and timing of doses 1–3 x daily.

Dosage range *Adults* Usually 75–200mg daily (up to a maximum of 300mg in hospital patients). *Children* Reduced dose according to age and weight.

Onset of effect Some benefits and effects may appear within hours, but full antidepressant effect may not be felt for 2–6 weeks.

Duration of action Following prolonged treatment, the antidepressant effect may persist for up to 6 weeks. Any adverse effects may wear off within days.

Diet advice None.

Storage Keep in a closed container in a cool, dry place out of reach of children.

Missed dose Take as soon as you remember. If your next dose is due within 3 hours, take a single dose now and skip the next.

Stopping the drug Unless giddy spells or palpitations occur, do not stop taking the drug without consulting your doctor, who will supervise gradual reduction in dosage. Stopping abruptly may cause withdrawal symptoms.

OVERDOSE ACTION

Seek immediate medical advice in all cases. Take emergency action if consciousness is lost.

POSSIBLE ADVERSE EFFECTS

Adverse effects are mainly due to the drug's anticholinergic (see Autonomic nervous system, p.8) action and its effect on heart rhythm. Sweating, flushing, dry mouth, constipation, difficulty in passing urine, blurred vision, and weight gain are common. Dizziness and drowsiness may also occur. If you develop a rash or palpitations, stop taking the drug and seek urgent medical advice.

INTERACTIONS

Sedatives Imipramine may increase the effects of sedative drugs.

MAOIs There is a possibility of a serious interaction. Such drugs are prescribed with imipramine only under strict supervision.

Antihypertensive drugs Imipramine may reduce the effectiveness of these drugs.

Phenytoin Imipramine may increase levels of phenytoin.

Terfenadine, amiodarone, and sotalol These drugs may increase the risk of abnormal heart rhythms.

SPECIAL PRECAUTIONS

Be sure to tell your doctor if:
◆ You have had heart problems.
◆ You have long-term liver or kidney problems.
◆ You have had epileptic fits.
◆ You have porphyria.
◆ You have had glaucoma.
◆ You have prostate trouble.
◆ You have had mania or a psychotic illness.
◆ You are taking other medications.

Pregnancy Safety in pregnancy not established. Discuss with your doctor.

Breast-feeding The drug passes into the breast milk, but at normal doses adverse effects on the baby are unlikely. Discuss with your doctor.

Infants and children Not recommended under 7 years. Reduced dose necessary in older children.

Over 60 Increased likelihood of adverse effects. Reduced dose may be necessary.

Driving and hazardous work Avoid such activities until you have learned how imipramine affects you because the drug can cause reduced alertness and blurred vision.

Alcohol Avoid. Alcohol may increase the sedative effect of imipramine.

Surgery and general anaesthetics Imipramine treatment may need to be stopped before you have a general anaesthetic. Discuss this with your doctor or dentist before having any operation.

PROLONGED USE

No problems expected with prolonged use of imipramine. The drug is not usually prescribed for children as a treatment for bedwetting for longer than three months.

Indapamide

Brand names Natrilix, Natrilix SR, Nindaxa
Used in the following combined preparations
Coversyl Plus

QUICK REFERENCE

Drug group Diuretic (p.32)
Overdose danger rating Low
Dependence rating Low
Prescription needed Yes
Available as generic Yes

GENERAL INFORMATION

Indapamide is related in its effects and uses to the thiazide diuretic group of drugs (see p.33) but is used to treat hypertension (high blood pressure). The drug prevents the hormone norepinephrine (noradrenaline) from constricting blood vessels, thereby allowing them to dilate. Indapamide is sometimes combined with other antihypertensive drugs but not with other diuretics.

The diuretic effects of this drug are slight at low doses, but susceptible people need to have blood levels of potassium and uric acid monitored. These include elderly people, those taking digitalis drugs, or those with gout or hyperaldosteronism (overproduction of the hormone aldosterone). Unlike thiazides, indapamide does not affect diabetic control.

INFORMATION FOR USERS

Your drug prescription is tailored for you. Do not alter dosage without checking with your doctor.

How taken Tablets, SR-tablets.
Frequency and timing of doses Once daily in the morning.
Adult dosage range 1.5–2.5mg.
Onset of effect 1–2 hours, but the full effect may not be felt for several months.
Duration of action 12–24 hours.
Diet advice None.
Storage Keep in a closed container in a cool, dry place out of reach of children.
Missed dose Take as soon as you remember. If your next dose is due within 4 hours, take a single dose now and skip the next.
Stopping the drug Do not stop taking the drug without consulting your doctor; high blood pressure may return.

Exceeding the dose An occasional unintentional extra dose is unlikely to cause problems. But if you notice any unusual symptoms, or if a large overdose has been taken, notify your doctor.

POSSIBLE ADVERSE EFFECTS

Headaches, fatigue, and muscle cramps are common adverse effects. Diarrhoea, constipation, and impotence are less common. If you experience dizziness, fainting, palpitations, tingling, or "pins and needles", consult your doctor. If you develop a sore throat, a rash, or jaundice, seek medical advice.

INTERACTIONS

Diuretics There is a risk of imbalance of salts in the blood if these drugs are taken with indapamide.

Digitalis drugs Loss of potassium may lead to toxicity of these drugs with indapamide.

Lithium Blood levels of lithium are increased when it is taken with indapamide.

Antiarrhythmics Potassium loss may make these drugs less effective if taken with indapamide.

SPECIAL PRECAUTIONS

Be sure to tell your doctor if:
◆ You have had a stroke.
◆ You have liver or kidney problems.
◆ You have gout.
◆ You have hyperaldosteronism or hyperparathyroidism.
◆ You are allergic to sulphonamide drugs.
◆ You are taking digitalis drugs.
◆ You are taking other medications.

Pregnancy Safety not established. Discuss with your doctor.

Breast-feeding Safety not established. Discuss with your doctor.

Infants and children Not prescribed.

Over 60 No special problems.

Driving and hazardous work No special problems.

Alcohol No special problems.

PROLONGED USE

Long-term use may lead to potassium loss in elderly people and certain other groups.

Monitoring Blood tests may be performed periodically to check kidney function and levels of potassium and other salts.

Indoramin

Brand names Baratol, Doralese
Used in the following combined preparations
None

QUICK REFERENCE

Drug group Antihypertensive drug (p.36) and drug for urinary retention (p.112)
Overdose danger rating Medium
Dependence rating Low
Prescription needed Yes
Available as generic No

GENERAL INFORMATION

Indoramin is a selective alpha blocker drug (see p.37) that is used to treat hypertension (high blood pressure). It works by relaxing the muscles in the blood vessel walls, dilating (widening) them and thereby easing the flow of blood. Indoramin may be combined with other antihypertensive drugs in order to achieve better control.

Indoramin is also used, in lower doses, to relieve urinary retention caused by an enlarged prostate gland. The drug works by relaxing the muscle of the prostate, enabling urine to be passed more easily.

Because indoramin can initially cause a rapid fall in blood pressure, the first dose is usually low, and should be taken lying down. The drug can also cause drowsiness at first and whenever dosage is increased. If unequal-sized daily doses are taken, the largest dose is usually prescribed for bedtime.

INFORMATION FOR USERS

Your drug prescription is tailored for you. Do not alter dosage without checking with your doctor.

How taken Tablets.

Frequency and timing of doses Hypertension 2–3 x daily. Urinary retention 1–2 x daily.

Adult dosage range Hypertension 25mg (starting dose), increased if necessary at 2-week intervals. Maximum daily dose 200mg. Urinary retention 20mg (starting dose), increased if necessary at 2-week intervals. Maximum daily dose 100mg.

Onset of effect 1 hour.

Duration of action 6–12 hours.

Diet advice None.

Storage Keep in a closed container in a cool, dry place out of reach of children.

Missed dose Take as soon as you remember. If your next dose is due within 2 hours, take a single dose now and skip the next.

Stopping the drug Do not stop taking the drug without consulting your doctor. Stopping the drug may lead to worsening of the underlying condition.

Exceeding the dose An occasional unintentional extra dose is unlikely to be a cause for concern. Large overdoses, however, may produce deep sedation and fits; notify your doctor immediately.

POSSIBLE ADVERSE EFFECTS
Drowsiness and dizziness are the most common adverse effects. Dry mouth, nasal congestion, fatigue, and headache may also occur but are often worse at the start of treatment or following an increase in dosage. If depression, tremor or abnormal movements, or ejaculation failure occur, consult your doctor.

INTERACTIONS
Antidepressants, beta-blockers, calcium channel blockers, diuretics, thymoxamine These drugs increase the blood-pressure-lowering effect of indoramin.

SPECIAL PRECAUTIONS
Be sure to tell your doctor if:
◆ You have liver or kidney problems.
◆ You have Parkinson's disease.
◆ You have epilepsy.
◆ You have heart failure.
◆ You have a history of depression.
◆ You are taking an MAOI drug.
◆ You are taking other medications.

Pregnancy Safety not established. Discuss with your doctor.

Breast-feeding Safety not established. Discuss with your doctor.

Infants and children Not recommended.

Over 60 Reduced dose may be necessary.

Driving and hazardous work Avoid such activities until you have learned how indoramin affects you because the drug can cause drowsiness and dizziness.

Alcohol Avoid. Alcohol increases the amount of indoramin absorbed, which increases its sedative effects.

Surgery and general anaesthetics Anaesthesia may increase the blood-pressure-lowering effect of indoramin. Discuss this with your doctor or dentist before having any surgery.

PROLONGED USE
No special problems.

Insulin

Brand names Humalog, Human Actrapid, Human Insulatard, Human Mixtard, Human Monotard, Human Ultratard, Human Velosulin, Humulin, Hypurin, Insuman, Lantus, NovoRapid, Pork Insulatard, Pork Mixtard, Pork Velosulin, and others

QUICK REFERENCE
Drug group Drug for diabetes (p.82)
Overdose danger rating High
Dependence rating Low
Prescription needed Yes
Available as generic No

GENERAL INFORMATION
Insulin is a hormone manufactured by the pancreas and is vital to the body's ability to use glucose. In people with diabetes mellitus, the body does not effectively make or respond to insulin, so the hormone is given by injection to supplement or replace natural levels. It is the only effective treatment in juvenile (insulin-dependent or Type 1) diabetes and may also be prescribed in the treatment of adult (maturity-onset or Type 2) diabetes. Insulin should be used in conjunction with a carefully controlled diet that is supervised by your practice nurse or a dietitian. Illness, vomiting, or alterations in diet or in exercise levels may require dosage adjustment.

Insulin is available in a wide variety of preparations, which can be short-, medium-, or long-acting. Combinations of these types are often given. People receiving insulin should carry a warning card or tag.

INFORMATION FOR USERS
Your drug prescription is tailored for you. Do not alter dosage without checking with your doctor.

How taken Injection, infusion pump, pen injection.

Frequency and timing of doses 1–4 x daily. Short-acting insulin usually 15–30 minutes before meals. Some newer forms can be given directly before or after eating. The exact time of injections and administration for longer-acting preparations will be tailored to your individual needs; follow the instructions you are given, and be sure to rotate injection sites.

Dosage range Dose (and type) is determined according to the needs of the individual.

Onset of effect 30–60 minutes (short-acting); 1–2 hours (medium- and long-acting).

Duration of action 6–8 hours (short-acting); 18–26 hours (medium-acting); 28–36 hours (long-acting).

Diet advice A low-carbohydrate diet is necessary. Follow your doctor's advice.

Storage Refrigerate (do not freeze), but once insulin is opened it may be stored at room temperature for 1 month. Follow the instructions on the container.

Missed dose Discuss with your doctor. Appropriate action depends on dose and type.

Stopping the drug Do not stop taking the drug without consulting your doctor; confusion and coma may occur.

OVERDOSE ACTION

Seek immediate medical advice. If you notice symptoms of low blood glucose, such as faintness, hunger, and trembling, eat or drink something sugary. Take emergency action if fits or loss of consciousness occur.

POSSIBLE ADVERSE EFFECTS

Symptoms such as dizziness, sweating, weakness, and confusion indicate low blood glucose. Serious allergic reactions such as rash, swelling, and shortness of breath are very rare and need urgent medical attention. If you have eyesight problems, or irritation or dimpling at the injection site, consult your doctor.

INTERACTIONS

General note 1 Many drugs, including some antibiotics, MAOIs, and oral antidiabetics, increase the risk of low blood glucose.

Corticosteroids and diuretics may oppose the effect of insulin.

General note 2 Check with your doctor or pharmacist before taking any medicines; some contain sugar and may upset diabetic control.

Beta blockers may affect insulin needs and could mask some signs of low blood glucose.

SPECIAL PRECAUTIONS

Be sure to tell your doctor if:
◆ You have had a previous allergic reaction to insulin.
◆ You are taking other medications, or your other drug treatment is changed.

Pregnancy No evidence of risk to the developing baby from insulin, but poor control of diabetes increases the risk of birth defects. Careful monitoring is required.

Breast-feeding No evidence of risk. Adjustment in dose may be necessary while breast-feeding.

Infants and children Reduced dose necessary.

Over 60 No special problems.

Driving and hazardous work Usually no problem, but strenuous exercise alters insulin and glucose requirements. Avoid these activities if you have warning signs of low blood glucose.

Alcohol Avoid. Alcohol upsets diabetic control.

Surgery and general anaesthetics Insulin requirements may increase during surgery, and blood glucose levels will need to be monitored during and after an operation. Notify your doctor or dentist that you are diabetic before having any surgery.

PROLONGED USE

No problems expected.

Monitoring Regular review by your doctor or diabetic clinic is essential to reduce the risk of your developing long-term complications of diabetes.

Interferon

Brand names Avonex, Betaferon, Immukin, IntronA, Pegasys, PegIntron, Rebif, Roferon-A, Viraferon, ViraferonPeg

Used in the following combined preparations
None

QUICK REFERENCE

Drug group Antiviral drug (p.69) and anticancer drug (p.96).

Overdose danger rating Medium

Dependence rating Low

Prescription needed Yes

Available as generic No

GENERAL INFORMATION

Interferons are a group of substances normally produced in human and animal cells in response to viruses or other substances. They are thought to promote resistance to several types of viral infection. Three main types of interferon (alfa, beta, and gamma) are used to treat a range of diseases. Interferon alfa is used for leukaemias, other cancers, and chronic active hepatitis B. Interferon beta may reduce the frequency and severity of relapses in some forms of multiple sclerosis. Interferon gamma is used in conjunction with antibiotics for patients with chronic granulomatous disease.

Interferons can cause severe adverse effects (see below).

INFORMATION FOR USERS

This drug is given only under medical supervision and is not for self-administration.

How taken Injection.

Frequency and timing of doses Once daily or once weekly depending on the product and the condition being treated.

Adult dosage range The dosage is calculated taking account of the body surface area of the patient and the condition being treated.

Onset of effect The drug is active inside the body within 1 hour, but its effects may not be noted for 1–2 months.

Duration of action Immediate effects last for about 12 hours.

Diet advice None.

Storage Store in a refrigerator at 2–8°C (36–46°F). Do not let it freeze, and protect from light. Keep out of reach of children.

Missed dose Not applicable. This drug is usually given only in hospital under close medical supervision.

Stopping the drug Discuss with your doctor.

Exceeding the dose Overdosage is unlikely since treatment is carefully monitored.

POSSIBLE ADVERSE EFFECTS

The most common problems are headache, lethargy, depression, dizziness, drowsiness, digestive disturbance, poor appetite, and weight loss. Discuss all unusual symptoms with your doctor without delay. Some of these symptoms may be dose-related, and a reduction in dosage may be necessary in order to eliminate them. If you develop a fever or experience muscle ache, or hair loss, consult your doctor.

INTERACTIONS

General note A number of drugs increase the risk of adverse effects on the blood, heart, or nervous system. This is taken into account whenever an interferon is prescribed with other drugs.

Vaccines Interferons may reduce the effectiveness of vaccines.

Theophylline/aminophylline The effects of this drug may be enhanced by interferons.

Sedatives All drugs that have a sedative effect on the central nervous system are likely to increase the sedative properties of interferons. Such drugs include opioid analgesics, anti-anxiety drugs, sleeping drugs, antihistamines, antidepressants, and antipsychotics.

SPECIAL PRECAUTIONS

Be sure to tell your doctor if:
◆ You have long-term liver or kidney problems.
◆ You have heart disease.
◆ You have had epileptic fits.
◆ You have previously suffered allergic reactions to any drugs.
◆ You have had asthma or eczema.
◆ You suffer from depression.
◆ You are taking other medications.

Pregnancy Not usually prescribed. Safety in pregnancy not established. Discuss with your doctor.

Breast-feeding It is not known whether the drug passes into the breast milk. Discuss with your doctor.

Infants and children Not usually used.

Over 60 Increased likelihood of adverse effects. Reduced dose may be necessary.

Driving and hazardous work Not applicable.

Alcohol Avoid. Alcohol may increase the sedative effects of this drug.

PROLONGED USE

Prolonged use increases the risk of liver damage. Blood cell production in the bone marrow may be reduced. Lethargy, fatigue, collapse, and coma may occur with repeated large doses.

Monitoring Frequent blood tests are required to monitor blood composition and liver function.

Ipratropium bromide

Brand names Atrovent, Rinatec, Respontin, Tropiovent
Used in the following combined preparations Combivent, Duovent

QUICK REFERENCE

Drug group Bronchodilator (p.23)
Overdose danger rating Low
Dependence rating Low
Prescription needed Yes
Available as generic Yes

GENERAL INFORMATION

Ipratropium bromide is a bronchodilator with an anticholinergic (see Autonomic nervous system, p.8) action that relaxes the muscles surrounding the bronchioles (airways in the lungs). It is used primarily in the maintenance treatment of reversible airway disorders (those in which the airways are temporarily swollen or obstructed), particularly chronic bronchitis. It is given by inhaler or via a nebulizer for these conditions.

Although its effect lasts longer, ipratropium bromide has a slower onset of action than the sympathomimetic bronchodilators (see p.24). For this reason, it is not as effective in treating acute attacks of wheezing, or in the emergency treatment of asthma, and it is usually used together with the faster-acting drugs. It is also prescribed as a nasal spray for the treatment of a continually runny nose resulting from allergy.

Unlike other anticholinergic drugs, ipratropium bromide rarely causes side effects and is unlikely to affect the heart, eyes, bowel, or bladder. It must be used with caution by people with glaucoma, but problems are unlikely to arise at normal doses and if any inhalers are used correctly.

INFORMATION FOR USERS

Your drug prescription is tailored for you. Do not alter dosage without checking with your doctor.
How taken Inhaler, nasal spray, liquid for nebulizer.
Frequency and timing of doses 3–4 x daily.
Adult dosage range 80–320mcg daily (inhaler); 400–2,000mcg daily (nebulizer); 1–2 puffs to the affected nostril 2–3 x daily (nasal spray).
Onset of effect 5–15 minutes.
Duration of action Up to 8 hours.
Diet advice None.
Storage Keep in a cool, dry place out of reach of children. Do not puncture or burn containers.
Missed dose Take as soon as you remember. If your next dose is due within 2 hours, take a single dose now and skip the next.
Stopping the drug Do not stop taking the drug without consulting your doctor; symptoms may recur.
Exceeding the dose An occasional unintentional extra dose is unlikely to be a cause for concern. But if you notice any unusual symptoms, or if a large overdose has been taken, notify your doctor.

POSSIBLE ADVERSE EFFECTS

Adverse effects from ipratropium bromide are rare; the most common is a dry mouth or throat. Constipation and difficulty in passing urine may occur with high doses. If you develop blurred vision or a headache, notify your doctor.

INTERACTIONS

None.

SPECIAL PRECAUTIONS

Be sure to tell your doctor if:
◆ You have glaucoma.
◆ You have prostate problems.
◆ You have difficulty in passing urine.
◆ You are taking other medications.
Pregnancy There is no evidence of risk to the developing baby, but discuss with your doctor before using the drug during the first 3 months of pregnancy.
Breast-feeding No evidence of risk to the baby if the drug is used while the patient is breast-feeding, but discuss with your doctor.
Infants and children Reduced dose necessary.
Over 60 No special problems.
Driving and hazardous work No special problems.
Alcohol No known problems.

PROLONGED USE

No special problems.

Irbesartan

Brand name Aprovel
Used in the following combined preparations
CoAprovel

QUICK REFERENCE

Drug group Vasodilator (p.31) and antihypertensive drug (p.36)
Overdose danger rating Medium
Dependence rating Low
Prescription needed Yes
Available as generic No

GENERAL INFORMATION

Irbesartan belongs to a group of vasodilator drugs called angiotensin-II blockers. Used to treat hypertension, the drug works by blocking the action of angiotensin-II (a naturally occurring substance that constricts blood vessels). This causes the blood vessel walls to relax, thereby lowering blood pressure.

Unlike ACE inhibitors, irbesartan does not cause a persistent dry cough. Along with other angiotensin-II blockers, it is being evaluated for the treatment of other conditions, such as heart failure, for which ACE inhibitors are used. Irbesartan is also available in combination with a diuretic.

Irbesartan is prescribed with caution to people with stenosis (narrowing) of the arteries to the kidneys because the drug may make kidney function worse in people with this problem. It is important to notify your doctor if you know that you have this condition.

INFORMATION FOR USERS

Your drug prescription is tailored for you. Do not alter dosage without checking with your doctor.

How taken Tablets.
Frequency and timing of doses Once daily.
Adult dosage range 150–300mg, but 75mg may be used in people over 75 years.
Onset of effect Within 1 hour. Blood pressure is lowered within 1–2 weeks, and maximum beneficial effect is felt 4–6 weeks from the start of treatment.
Duration of action 24 hours.
Diet advice None.
Storage Keep in a closed container in a cool, dry place out of reach of children.

Missed dose Take as soon as you remember. If your next dose is due within 8 hours, take a single dose now and skip the next.
Stopping the drug Unless wheezing, itching, or rash occur, do not stop taking the drug without consulting your doctor. Stopping the drug may lead to worsening control of high blood pressure.
Exceeding the dose An occasional unintentional extra dose is unlikely to be a cause for concern. Large overdoses may cause dizziness and fainting; notify your doctor.

POSSIBLE ADVERSE EFFECTS

Adverse effects are usually mild. Dizziness, fatigue, and flushing are common; headaches are less so. If you develop wheezing, a blotchy rash, or itching, stop taking the drug immediately and consult your doctor urgently.

INTERACTIONS

Diuretics There is a risk of a sudden fall in blood pressure if these drugs are being taken when irbesartan treatment is started.
Potassium supplements, potassium-sparing diuretics, and ciclosporin Irbesartan enhances the effect of these drugs, leading to raised levels of potassium in the blood.
Lithium Irbesartan increases the blood levels and toxicity of lithium.
NSAIDs Certain of these drugs may act to reduce the blood-pressure-lowering effects of irbesartan.

SPECIAL PRECAUTIONS

Be sure to tell your doctor if:
◆ You have kidney problems or renal artery stenosis.
◆ You have heart problems.
◆ You have congestive heart failure.
◆ You have primary aldosteronism.
◆ You are taking other medications.
Pregnancy Not prescribed.
Breast-feeding Safety not established. Discuss with your doctor.
Infants and children Not prescribed.
Over 60 Reduced dose may be necessary in people over 75 years.
Driving and hazardous work Avoid such activities until you have learned how irbesartan affects you because the drug can cause dizziness and fatigue.

Alcohol Avoid. Regular alcohol intake may raise blood pressure and reduce the effectiveness of irbesartan. It may also increase the likelihood of an excessive fall in blood pressure.

PROLONGED USE
No special problems.

Monitoring Blood pressure will be monitored during treatment with irbesartan, as with all antihypertensive drugs. Periodic kidney function tests and checks on blood potassium levels may be performed.

Isoniazid

Brand names None
Used in the following combined preparations
Rifater, Rifinah, Rimactazid

QUICK REFERENCE
Drug group Antituberculous drug (p.67)
Overdose danger rating High
Dependence rating Low
Prescription needed Yes
Available as generic Yes

GENERAL INFORMATION
In use for over 40 years, isoniazid (also called INAH and INH) remains an effective drug for tuberculosis. It is given alone for tuberculosis prevention and in combination with other drugs for treatment. Treatment usually lasts for six months, but courses of nine months or a year may sometimes be given.

One side effect of isoniazid is the increased loss of pyridoxine (vitamin B_6) from the body. This effect, which is more likely with high doses, is rare in children but common among people with poor nutrition. Because pyridoxine deficiency can lead to irreversible nerve damage, supplements are usually given.

INFORMATION FOR USERS
Your drug prescription is tailored for you. Do not alter dosage without checking with your doctor.

How taken Tablets, liquid, injection.
Frequency and timing of doses Normally once daily.
Dosage range *Adults* 300mg daily.
Children According to age and weight.

Onset of effect Over 2–3 days.
Duration of action Up to 24 hours.
Diet advice Isoniazid may deplete pyridoxine (vitamin B_6) levels in the body. Supplements may therefore be prescribed.
Storage Keep in a closed container in a cool, dry place out of reach of children. Protect from light.
Missed dose Take as soon as you remember. If your next dose is scheduled within 8 hours, take a single dose now and skip the next.
Stopping the drug Unless serious adverse effects occur (see below), take the full course. Even if you feel better, the infection may still be present and may recur if treatment is stopped too soon.

OVERDOSE ACTION
Seek immediate medical advice in all cases. Take emergency action if breathing difficulties, fits, or loss of consciousness occur.

POSSIBLE ADVERSE EFFECTS
Serious problems are uncommon, but all adverse effects should receive prompt medical attention due to the possibility of nerve or liver damage. These effects include nausea, vomiting, fatigue, weakness, numbness, tingling, mood changes, and a rash. If you develop blurred vision, jaundice, twitching, or muscle weakness, stop taking the drug and consult your doctor without delay.

INTERACTIONS
Alcohol and rifampicin Large quantities of alcohol may reduce the effectiveness of isoniazid. If the two are taken together, the likelihood of liver damage is increased; if rifampicin is also being taken, the likelihood is increased even further.
Anticonvulsant drugs The effects of these drugs may be increased with isoniazid.
Antacids These drugs may reduce the absorption of isoniazid.
Ketoconazole Isoniazid reduces the blood concentration of ketoconazole.

SPECIAL PRECAUTIONS
Be sure to tell your doctor if:
◆ You have long-term liver or kidney problems.
◆ You have had liver damage following isoniazid treatment in the past.

◆ You have problems with drug or alcohol abuse.

◆ You have diabetes.

◆ You have porphyria.

◆ You have HIV infection.

◆ You have had epileptic fits.

◆ You are taking other medications.

Pregnancy The drug is not known to be harmful to the developing baby, but discuss with your doctor.

Breast-feeding The drug passes into the breast milk and may affect the baby. The infant should be monitored for signs of toxic effects. Discuss with your doctor.

Infants and children Reduced dose necessary.

Over 60 Increased likelihood of adverse effects.

Driving and hazardous work No special problems.

Alcohol Avoid excessive amounts.

PROLONGED USE

Pyridoxine (vitamin B$_6$) deficiency may occur with prolonged use and lead to nerve damage. Supplements are usually prescribed. There is also a risk of serious liver damage.

Monitoring Periodic blood tests are usually performed to monitor liver function.

Isosorbide dinitrate/ mononitrate

Brand names [Dinitrate] Cedocard, Isocard, Isoket, Isordil; [Mononitrate] Elantan, Imdur, Ismo, Isotard, Isotrate, MCR-50, Modisal, Monit, Monomax
Used in the following combined preparation
Imazin XL

QUICK REFERENCE

Drug group Nitrate vasodilator (p.31) and anti-angina drug (p.35)
Overdose danger rating Medium
Dependence rating Low
Prescription needed No (some preparations); yes (other preparations and injection)
Available as generic Yes

GENERAL INFORMATION

Isosorbide dinitrate and mononitrate are vasodilator drugs similar to glyceryl trinitrate. They are usually used to treat angina as well as some cases of heart failure.

Unlike glyceryl trinitrate, isosorbide dinitrate and mononitrate are stable and can be stored for long periods without losing their effectiveness. They are often sold as slow-release (SR) preparations, which have a longer action.

Headache, flushing, and dizziness are common side effects during the early stages of treatment with isosorbide dinitrate and mononitrate; small initial doses of the drug minimize these symptoms. The effectiveness of both forms of the drug may be reduced after a few months; a change in the timing of doses, with a gap for some hours in the day, may prevent this.

INFORMATION FOR USERS

Your drug prescription is tailored for you. Do not alter dosage without checking with your doctor.

How taken *Dinitrate* Tablets (held under the tongue, chewed, or swallowed), SR-tablets, SR-capsules, injection, spray. *Mononitrate* Tablets, SR-tablets, SR-capsules.

Frequency and timing of doses *Relief of angina attacks* Tablets chewed or held under the tongue, or spray, as needed (certain preparations only). *Prevention of angina* 2–4 x daily, not to be taken after 6pm; 1–2 x daily, maximum, to avoid loss of effectiveness (SR-tablets, capsules).

Adult dosage range *Relief of angina attacks* 5–10mg per dose. *Prevention of angina* 30–120mg daily.

Onset of effect 2–3 minutes when chewed or held under the tongue or used as spray (certain preparations only); 30 minutes when swallowed.

Duration of action Up to 2 hours (chewed); up to 5 hours (swallowed); up to 10 hours (SR-capsules).

Diet advice None.

Storage Keep in a closed container in a cool, dry place out of reach of children. Protect from light.

Missed dose Take as soon as you remember. If your next dose is due within 2 hours, take a single dose now and skip the next.

Stopping the drug Do not stop taking the drug without consulting your doctor; stopping the drug may lead to worsening of the underlying condition.

Exceeding the dose An occasional unintentional extra dose is unlikely to cause problems. Large overdoses, however, may cause dizziness and headache; notify your doctor.

POSSIBLE ADVERSE EFFECTS

Flushing and headache are common. The most serious problem is excessively low blood pressure, which may show itself as dizziness, fainting, or weakness, and should be discussed with your doctor. Other adverse effects of both forms of isosorbide usually improve after regular use, and adjusting the dose may help.

INTERACTIONS

Sildenafil This drug significantly enhances the blood-pressure-lowering effect of nitrates; the two drugs should not be used together.

Antihypertensives A further lowering of blood pressure occurs when such drugs are taken with isosorbide dinitrate.

SPECIAL PRECAUTIONS

Be sure to tell your doctor if:
◆ You have long-term liver or kidney problems.
◆ You have any blood disorders or anaemia.
◆ You have had glaucoma.
◆ You have low blood pressure.
◆ You have ever had a heart attack.
◆ You have an underactive thyroid.
◆ You are taking other medications.

Pregnancy Safety in pregnancy not established. Discuss with your doctor.

Breast-feeding Safety not established. Discuss with your doctor.

Infants and children Not usually prescribed.

Over 60 No special problems.

Driving and hazardous work Avoid such activities until you have learned how isosorbide dinitrate or mononitrate affect you because these drugs can cause dizziness.

Alcohol Avoid excessive intake. Alcohol may further lower blood pressure, depressing the heart and causing dizziness and fainting.

PROLONGED USE

The initial adverse effects may disappear with prolonged use. The beneficial effects, however, become weaker as the body adapts. This may be prevented by changing the timing of doses to allow a daily "gap" period during which blood levels of the drug are low.

Isotretinoin

Brand names Isotrex Gel, Roaccutane
Used in the following combined preparation
Isotrexin

QUICK REFERENCE

Drug group Drug for acne (p.123)
Overdose danger rating Medium
Dependence rating Low
Prescription needed Yes
Available as generic Yes

GENERAL INFORMATION

Isotretinoin, a drug that is chemically related to vitamin A, is prescribed to treat acne that has failed to respond to other treatments. It may be applied topically in moderate cases or taken orally for severe cases.

The drug reduces production of the skin's natural oils (sebum) and of the horny protein (keratin) in the outer layers of the skin. This action makes it useful in conditions such as ichthyosis, in which the skin thickens abnormally, causing scaling.

A single 16-week course of treatment often clears the acne. The skin may be very dry, flaky, and itchy at first but usually improves as treatment continues. Serious adverse effects include liver damage and bowel inflammation. The drug should never be taken during pregnancy or by women planning pregnancy as it may harm a developing baby.

INFORMATION FOR USERS

Your drug prescription is tailored for you. Do not alter dosage without checking with your doctor.

How taken Capsules, gel.

Frequency and timing of doses 1–2 x daily. Take capsules with food or milk.

Adult dosage range Dosage is determined individually.

Onset of effect 2–4 weeks. Acne may worsen during the first few weeks in some people.

Duration of action Effects persist for several weeks after the drug has been stopped. Acne is usually completely cleared.

Diet advice None.

Storage Keep in a closed container in a cool, dry place out of reach of children. Protect from light.

Missed dose Take as soon as you remember. If your next dose is due within 4 hours, take a single dose now and skip the next.

Stopping the drug Can be safely stopped as soon as you no longer need it, but best results are achieved when the course of treatment is completed as prescribed.

Exceeding the dose An occasional unintentional extra dose is unlikely to cause problems. Large overdoses, however, may cause headaches, vomiting, abdominal pain, facial flushing, loss of coordination, and dizziness; notify your doctor.

POSSIBLE ADVERSE EFFECTS

The most serious adverse effects occur when isotretinoin is taken by mouth. Dryness of the nose, mouth, and eyes, inflammation of the lips, and flaking of the skin occur in most cases. Mood changes, muscle or joint pains, and temporary loss or increased growth of hair may also occur.

If you experience headache, accompanied by symptoms such as nausea and vomiting, abdominal pain with diarrhoea and/or blood in the faeces, or visual impairment, consult your doctor promptly.

INTERACTIONS

Tetracycline antibiotics These drugs may increase the risk of pressure changes in the fluid around the brain, leading to headaches, nausea, and vomiting.

Skin-drying preparations Medicated cosmetics, soaps, toiletries, and anti-acne preparations increase the likelihood of dryness and irritation of the skin with isotretinoin.

Vitamin A Supplements of this vitamin increase the risk of adverse effects from isotretinoin.

SPECIAL PRECAUTIONS

Do not donate blood during, or for at least a month after, taking oral isotretinoin. Be sure to tell your doctor if:
◆ You have long-term liver or kidney problems.
◆ You suffer from arthritis.
◆ You have diabetes.
◆ You have high levels of fat in the blood.
◆ You wear contact lenses.
◆ You suffer from gout.
◆ You are taking other medications.

Pregnancy Must not be prescribed. May cause abnormalities in the developing baby. Effective contraception must be used during treatment and for at least a month before and afterwards.

Breast-feeding The drug passes into the breast milk and may affect the baby. Discuss with your doctor.

Infants and children Not prescribed.

Over 60 Not usually prescribed.

Driving and hazardous work Avoid such activities until you have learned how the drug affects you because it can cause vision problems in dim light or darkness.

Alcohol Regular heavy intake of alcohol may raise blood fat levels with isotretinoin.

Sunlight Avoid exposure to the sun and do not use a sunlamp or sunbed.

PROLONGED USE

A course of treatment rarely exceeds 16 weeks. Prolonged use may raise fat levels in the blood, thereby increasing the risk of heart and blood vessel disease. Bone changes may also occur.

Monitoring Liver function tests and periodic checks on fat levels in the blood are usually performed.

Ketoconazole

Brand names Daktarin Gold, Nizoral
Used in the following combined preparations
None

QUICK REFERENCE

Drug group Antifungal drug (p.76)
Overdose danger rating Medium
Dependence rating Low
Prescription needed Yes (except for some shampoos)
Available as generic No

GENERAL INFORMATION

Ketoconazole is an antifungal drug prescribed, in the form of tablets, to treat severe, internal systemic fungal infections. The drug is also given to treat serious infections of the skin and mucous membranes caused by the candida yeast. People who have rare fungal diseases (for example, paracoccidioidomycosis, histoplasmosis, and coccidioidomycosis) may also be given ketoconazole.

The drug is also available as a cream to treat fungal skin infections, and as a shampoo for the treatment of scalp infections and seborrhoeic dermatitis.

The most common side effect of ketoconazole is nausea, but this can be reduced if the doses are taken at bedtime or with meals. Rarely, the drug may also cause liver damage.

INFORMATION FOR USERS

Your drug prescription is tailored for you. Do not alter dosage without checking with your doctor.
How taken Tablets, liquid, cream, shampoo.
Frequency and timing of doses Once daily with food (by mouth); 1–2 x daily (cream); 1–2 times weekly (shampoo used for seborrhoeic dermatitis).
Dosage range *Adults* 200–400mg daily (by mouth). *Children* Reduced dose according to age and weight.
Onset of effect Ketoconazole begins to work within a few hours; the full beneficial effect may take several days to develop.
Duration of action Up to 24 hours.
Diet advice None.
Storage Keep in a closed container in a cool, dry place out of reach of children.

Missed dose (oral) Take as soon as you remember. If your next dose is due within 6 hours, take a single dose now and skip the next.
Stopping the drug Unless severe adverse effects occur (see below), take the full course. Even if you feel better, the infection may still be present; symptoms may recur if treatment is stopped too soon.
Exceeding the dose An occasional unintentional extra dose is unlikely to be a cause for concern. Large overdoses, however, may cause gastric problems; notify your doctor.

POSSIBLE ADVERSE EFFECTS

Nausea and vomiting are the most common side effects of treatment with ketoconazole; abdominal pain and headache may also occur. If you develop itching or a rash, or if you are a man and develop painful breasts, stop taking the drug and consult your doctor. Liver damage is a rare but serious adverse effect of ketoconazole treatment; it causes jaundice (yellowing of the skin and the whites of the eyes) and may necessitate stopping the drug.

INTERACTIONS (ADMINISTRATION BY MOUTH ONLY)

Antacids, cimetidine, and ranitidine These drugs may reduce the effectiveness of ketoconazole if they are taken within 2 hours before or after ketoconazole is taken.
Rifampicin and phenytoin These drugs may reduce the effect of ketoconazole.
Sedatives, warfarin, ciclosporin, tacrolimus, sirolimus, theophylline, and sildenafil Ketoconazole increases the effects of these drugs.
Eletriptan Use of this drug with ketoconazole is not recommended.
Antiviral drugs Adjustments in the doses of these drugs may be necessary if they are used with ketoconazole.
Antimalarials The use of artemether with lumefantrine should be avoided when taking ketoconazole.
Terfenadine This drug increases the risk of adverse effects on the heart if it is taken with ketoconazole.
Simvastatin If this drug is taken with ketoconazole, there may be an increased risk of muscle damage.

SPECIAL PRECAUTIONS
Be sure to tell your doctor if:
◆ You have any long-term liver or kidney problems.
◆ You have porphyria.
◆ You have previously had an allergic reaction to antifungal drugs.
◆ You are taking other medications.
Pregnancy Not usually prescribed. May cause defects in the developing baby. Discuss with your doctor.
Breast-feeding The drug passes into the breast milk and may affect the baby. Discuss with your doctor.
Infants and children Reduced dose necessary.
Over 60 No special problems.
Driving and hazardous work No special problems.
Alcohol Avoid. Alcohol may interact with this drug to cause flushing and nausea.

PROLONGED USE
The risk of liver damage is increased with use of oral ketoconazole for more than 14 days.
Monitoring Periodic blood tests are usually performed to check the effect of the drug on the liver.

Ketoprofen

Brand names Ketocid, Ketovail, Ketozip, Larafen, Orudis, Oruvail, Powergel, and many others
Used in the following combined preparations
None

QUICK REFERENCE
Drug group Non-steroidal anti-inflammatory drug (p.50)
Overdose danger rating Medium
Dependence rating Low
Prescription needed No
Available as generic No

GENERAL INFORMATION
Ketoprofen is a member of the non-steroidal anti-inflammatory (NSAID) group of drugs. Like other NSAIDs, it relieves pain and reduces inflammation and stiffness in rheumatoid arthritis, osteoarthritis, and ankylosing spondylitis. It does not cure the underlying disease, however.

Ketoprofen is also given to relieve the mild to moderate pain of menstruation and soft tissue injuries, and the pain that occurs following operations.

The most common adverse reactions to ketoprofen, as with all NSAIDs, are gastrointestinal disturbances such as nausea and indigestion. If these unwanted effects are persistent or troublesome, your doctor may recommend that you change to using another NSAID.

INFORMATION FOR USERS
Follow instructions on the label. Call your doctor if symptoms worsen.
How taken Capsules, SR-capsules, injection, suppositories, gel.
Frequency and timing of doses 2–4 x daily with food (capsules); once daily (SR-capsules); 6 x daily for up to 3 days (injection); 2 x daily (suppositories).
Adult dosage range 100–200mg daily.
Onset of effect Pain relief may be felt in 30 minutes to 2 hours. Full anti-inflammatory effect may not be felt for up to 2 weeks.
Duration of action Up to 8–12 hours.
Diet advice None.
Storage Keep in a closed container in a cool, dry place out of reach of children.
Missed dose Take as soon as you remember. If your next dose is due within 4 hours, take a single dose now and skip the next.
Stopping the drug Unless severe adverse effects occur (see below), seek medical advice before stopping the drug.
Exceeding the dose An occasional unintentional extra dose is unlikely to be a cause for concern. However, large overdoses may cause vomiting, confusion, or irritability; notify your doctor.

POSSIBLE ADVERSE EFFECTS
Gastrointestinal disturbances, such as nausea, abdominal pain, indigestion, and heartburn commonly occur with ketoprofen when it is taken by mouth. Dizziness, drowsiness, and headache or fluid retention (resulting in swollen feet or legs and weight gain) may also occur. Suppositories may cause rectal irritation. Black or bloodstained faeces should be reported to your doctor promptly. If you develop a rash, itching,

wheezing, or breathlessness, stop taking the drug and consult your doctor urgently.

INTERACTIONS

General note Ketoprofen interacts with a wide range of drugs, such as other NSAIDs including aspirin, oral anticoagulants, and corticosteroids, to increase the risk of bleeding and/or stomach ulcers.

Lithium, digoxin, and methotrexate Ketoprofen may raise blood levels of these drugs to an undesirable extent.

Phenytoin Ketoprofen may enhance the effects of phenytoin.

Quinolone antibiotics Ketoprofen may increase the risk of seizures if it is taken with these drugs.

Antihypertensive drugs Ketoprofen may reduce the beneficial effects of these drugs.

SPECIAL PRECAUTIONS

Be sure to consult your doctor or pharmacist before taking this drug if:

◆ You have any long-term liver or kidney problems.

◆ You have heart problems.

◆ You have high blood pressure.

◆ You have asthma.

◆ You have had a peptic ulcer, oesophagitis, or acid indigestion.

◆ You have bleeding problems.

◆ You are allergic to aspirin or other NSAIDs.

◆ You are taking other medications.

Pregnancy Safety in pregnancy not established. Discuss with your doctor.

Breast-feeding The drug passes into the breast milk and may affect the baby. Discuss with your doctor.

Infants and children Not recommended under 12 years.

Over 60 Increased likelihood of adverse effects. Reduced dose may be necessary.

Driving and hazardous work Avoid such activities until you have learned how ketoprofen affects you because the drug can cause dizziness and drowsiness.

Alcohol Avoid. Alcohol may increase the risk of stomach disorders with ketoprofen.

Surgery and general anaesthetics Ketoprofen may prolong bleeding. Discuss this with your doctor or dentist before having any surgery.

PROLONGED USE

There is an increased risk of bleeding from peptic ulcers and in the bowel with prolonged use of ketoprofen.

Lactulose

Brand names Duphalac, Lactugal, Regulose
Used in the following combined preparations None

QUICK REFERENCE

Drug group Laxative (p.45)
Overdose danger rating Low
Dependence rating Low
Prescription needed No
Available as generic Yes

GENERAL INFORMATION

Lactulose is an effective laxative that softens faeces by increasing the amount of water in the large intestine. It is used for the relief of constipation and faecal impaction, especially in elderly people. It is less likely than some other laxatives to disrupt normal bowel action.

Lactulose is also used to treat and prevent hepatic encephalopathy, a form of brain disturbance associated with liver failure.

Because the drug acts locally in the large intestine and is not absorbed into the body, it is safer than many other laxatives, but it can cause stomach cramps and flatulence, especially at the start of treatment.

INFORMATION FOR USERS

Follow instructions on the label. Call your doctor if symptoms worsen.
How taken Liquid.
Frequency and timing of doses *Chronic constipation* 2 x daily. *Liver failure* 3–4 x daily.
Adult dosage range *Chronic constipation* 15–30ml daily. *Liver failure* 90–150ml daily.
Onset of effect 24–48 hours.
Duration of action 6–18 hours.
Diet advice You should maintain adequate intake of fluid (up to 8 glasses of water daily).
Storage Keep in a closed container in a cool, dry place out of reach of children. Do not store after diluting.
Missed dose Take as soon as you remember. If your next dose is due within 3 hours, take a single dose now and skip the next.
Stopping the drug In the treatment of constipation, lactulose can be safely stopped as soon as you no longer need it.
Exceeding the dose An occasional unintentional extra dose is unlikely to be a cause for concern. But if you notice any unusual symptoms, or if a large overdose has been taken, notify your doctor.

POSSIBLE ADVERSE EFFECTS

Adverse effects, including belching, flatulence, nausea, and abdominal cramps and distension, are rarely serious and often disappear as the body adjusts to the drug. Diarrhoea may indicate that the dosage is too high.

INTERACTIONS

Mesalazine Lactulose may reduce the release of mesalazine at the site of action.

SPECIAL PRECAUTIONS

Be sure to consult your doctor or pharmacist before taking this drug if:
◆ You have severe abdominal pain.
◆ You suffer from lactose intolerance or galactosaemia.
◆ You are taking other medications.
Pregnancy No evidence of risk. Discuss with your doctor.
Breast-feeding No evidence of risk.
Infants and children Reduced dose necessary.
Over 60 No special problems.
Driving and hazardous work No known problems.
Alcohol No known problems.

PROLONGED USE

In children, prolonged use may contribute to the development of dental caries.

Lamotrigine

Brand name Lamictal
Used in the following combined preparations None

QUICK REFERENCE

Drug group Anticonvulsant drug (p.16)
Overdose danger rating Medium
Dependence rating Low
Prescription needed Yes
Available as generic No

GENERAL INFORMATION

Lamotrigine, introduced in 1993, is an anticonvulsant drug prescribed, either alone or in combination with other anticonvulsants, in the treatment of epilepsy. It acts by restoring the balance between excitatory and inhibitory neurotransmitters in the brain. Lamotrigine may be less sedating than older anticonvulsants, and there is no need for tests to determine blood levels of the drug. Unlike many older anticonvulsants, lamotrigine does not interfere with the action of oral contraceptives.

INFORMATION FOR USERS

Your drug prescription is tailored for you. Do not alter dosage without checking with your doctor.

How taken Tablets, dispersible or chewable tablets.

Frequency and timing of doses 1–2 x daily.

Adult dosage range 100–500mg (100–200mg if given with sodium valproate) daily (maintenance dose). Smaller doses are used at the start of treatment. Dose may vary if other anticonvulsant drugs are being taken.

Onset of effect Approximately 5 days at a constant dose.

Duration of action Up to 24 hours.

Diet advice None.

Storage Keep in a closed container in a cool, dry place out of reach of children.

Missed dose Take as soon as you remember. If your next dose is due within 2 hours, take a single dose now and skip the next.

Stopping the drug Do not stop taking the drug without consulting your doctor, who will supervise a gradual reduction in dosage over a period of about 2 weeks. Abrupt cessation increases the risk of rebound fits.

Exceeding the dose An occasional unintentional extra dose is unlikely to be a cause for concern. Large overdoses, however, may cause sedation, double vision, loss of muscular coordination, nausea, and vomiting; contact your doctor immediately.

POSSIBLE ADVERSE EFFECTS

Serious effects are rare. Rash, nausea, headache, tiredness, insomnia, dizziness, agitation, confusion, and poor muscle coordination are common and respond to dosage reduction; a rash is less likely if treatment is started at a low dose (25mg), increasing gradually over about 4 weeks. If sore throat, facial swelling, flu-like symptoms, blurred or double vision, or persistent or unusual bruising occur, consult your doctor immediately.

INTERACTIONS

Sodium valproate This drug increases and prolongs the effectiveness of lamotrigine; a reduced dose of lamotrigine will be used.

Antidepressants, antipsychotics, mefloquine, and chloroquine These may counteract the anticonvulsant effect of lamotrigine.

Carbamazepine This drug may reduce lamotrigine blood levels, but lamotrigine may increase the side effects of carbamazepine.

Phenytoin and phenobarbital Both of these drugs may decrease blood levels of lamotrigine; a higher dose of lamotrigine may be needed.

SPECIAL PRECAUTIONS

Be sure to tell your doctor if:
◆ You have long-term liver or kidney problems.
◆ You suffer from thalassaemia.
◆ You have heart disease.
◆ You are taking other medications.

Pregnancy Safety in pregnancy not established. Discuss with your doctor.

Breast-feeding The drug passes into breast milk and may affect the baby. Discuss with your doctor.

Infants and children Not recommended under 2 years or as single therapy under 12 years. Doses may be relatively higher than adult doses due to increased metabolism.

Over 60s No special problems.

Driving and hazardous work Your underlying condition, as well as the possibility of sedation, dizziness, and visual disturbances while taking lamotrigine, may make such activities inadvisable. Discuss with your doctor.

Alcohol Alcohol may increase adverse effects.

PROLONGED USE

No special problems.

Lansoprazole

Brand name Zoton
Used in the following combined preparations None

QUICK REFERENCE

Drug group Anti-ulcer drug (p.43)
Overdose danger rating Low
Dependence rating Low
Prescription needed Yes
Available as generic No

GENERAL INFORMATION

Lansoprazole is a type of anti-ulcer drug called a proton pump inhibitor. It is used to treat peptic ulcers, gastro-oesophageal reflux (in which stomach acid enters and irritates the oesophagus), and Zollinger-Ellison syndrome (in which large quantities of stomach acid are produced, leading to ulceration).

Lansoprazole may be used alone or, for peptic ulcers, with two antibiotics, as part of a seven-day regimen to eradicate *Helicobacter pylori* bacteria, the main cause of such ulcers.

INFORMATION FOR USERS

Your drug prescription is tailored for you. Do not alter dosage without checking with your doctor.

How taken Capsules, oral suspension.

Frequency and timing of doses 1–2 x daily in the morning.

Dosage range *Benign gastric ulcer* 30mg daily. *NSAID-associated gastric ulcer* 15–30mg daily. *Duodenal ulcer* 30mg daily; 15mg daily in the morning (maintenance dose). *Helicobacter pylori-associated ulcer* 60mg daily, half of the dose in the morning and half in the evening.

Onset of effect 1–2 hours.

Duration of action 24 hours.

Diet advice Spicy foods and alcohol may exacerbate the condition.

Storage Keep in a closed container in a cool, dry place out of reach of children.

Missed dose Take as soon as you remember. If your next dose is due within 8 hours, take a single dose now and skip the next.

Stopping the drug Unless rash, itching, wheezing, or breathing difficulties occur (see below), do not stop taking the drug without consulting your doctor; symptoms may recur.

Exceeding the dose An occasional unintentional extra dose is unlikely to be a cause for concern. But if you notice any unusual symptoms, or if a large overdose has been taken, notify your doctor.

POSSIBLE ADVERSE EFFECTS

Common side effects include headache, fatigue or dizziness, indigestion, flatulence and abdominal pain, and diarrhoea or constipation. If you experience muscle or joint pain, excessive bruising, or swollen extremities, consult your doctor.

Sore throat and breathlessness are rare but should be reported to your doctor at once. If you develop a rash, itching, wheezing, or breathing difficulties, stop taking the drug and consult your doctor urgently.

INTERACTIONS

Oral contraceptives, phenytoin, carbamazepine, warfarin, and theophylline Lansoprazole may reduce the effect of these drugs.

Antacids and sucralfate These drugs should not be taken within an hour of lansoprazole; they may reduce its absorption into the body.

SPECIAL PRECAUTIONS

Be sure to tell your doctor if:
◆ You have liver problems.
◆ You are taking other medications.

Pregnancy Safety not established. Discuss with your doctor.

Breast-feeding Safety not established. Discuss with your doctor.

Infants and children Not recommended.

Over 60 No special problems.

Driving and hazardous work No special problems.

Alcohol Avoid. Alcohol may aggravate your condition and reduce the beneficial effects of lansoprazole.

PROLONGED USE

No problems expected.

Latanoprost

Brand name Xalatan
Used in the following combined preparation
Xalacom

QUICK REFERENCE

Drug group Drug for glaucoma (p.114)
Overdose danger rating Medium
Dependence rating Low
Prescription needed Yes
Available as generic No

GENERAL INFORMATION

Latanoprost is a synthetic derivative of the prostaglandin dinoprost, which constricts the smooth muscle in the blood vessels and bronchi (the main airways inside the lungs).

Latanoprost eye drops reduce pressure inside the eye in open-angle (chronic) glaucoma (see p.115) by constricting the pupils. The drug is used when patients have not responded to, or cannot tolerate, the first-choice drug – usually a beta blocker such as timolol (see p.406). Sometimes, latanoprost and timolol eye drops may be prescribed if timolol alone is not adequately controlling the pressure.

Latanoprost eye drops can gradually increase the amount of brown pigment (melanin) in the eye, thereby darkening the iris. This will be particularly noticeable if only one eye needs treatment. Irises of mixed coloration are especially susceptible; pure blue eyes do not seem to be affected. Latanoprost has also been reported to cause darkening, thickening, and lengthening of the eyelashes.

INFORMATION FOR USERS

Your drug prescription is tailored for you. Do not alter dosage without checking with your doctor.

How taken Eye drops.

Frequency and timing of doses 1x daily, in the evening.

Adult dosage range 1 drop per eye, daily.

Onset of effect 15–30 minutes.

Duration of action 24 hours.

Diet advice None.

Storage Keep the eye drops in the outer cardboard package to protect from light. Store in a refrigerator at 2–8°C (36–46°F), out of reach of children.

Missed dose Take the next dose as normal.

Stopping the drug Do not stop taking the drug without consulting your doctor; symptoms may recur.

Exceeding the dose An occasional unintentional extra application is unlikely to cause problems. Excessive use, however, may irritate the eye and produce adverse effects in other parts of the body; notify your doctor.

POSSIBLE ADVERSE EFFECTS

Darkening of the iris, eye irritation, and eyelash changes are common. Consult your doctor if these are severe, or if you have eye pain, bloodshot or swollen eyes, inflamed eyelids, or facial swelling. Stop taking the drug and seek medical advice if you develop chest pains, wheezing, or breathing difficulties.

INTERACTIONS

Thiomersal-containing eye drops These preparations should not be used within 5 minutes of using latanoprost. (Thiomersal is a preservative used in some eye drops.)

SPECIAL PRECAUTIONS

Be sure to tell your doctor if:
◆ You wear contact lenses.
◆ You are allergic to benzalkonium chloride or latanoprost.
◆ You have asthma.
◆ You are taking other medications.

Pregnancy Safety in pregnancy not established. Prostaglandins may affect the developing baby.

Breast-feeding The drug may pass into the breast milk and may affect the baby. Discuss with your doctor.

Infants and children Not recommended.

Over 60 No special problems.

Driving and hazardous work No known problems.

Alcohol No known problems.

PROLONGED USE

No known problems apart from changes to iris pigment and eyelash colour.

Monitoring No problems expected with long-term use of latanoprost, but your doctor will continue to monitor any eye pigmentation as well as control of the glaucoma.

Levodopa

Brand names None

Used in the following combined preparations
Half Sinemet CR, Madopar, Madopar CR, Sinemet, Sinemet CR

QUICK REFERENCE

Drug group Drug for parkinsonism (p.18)

Overdose danger rating Medium

Dependence rating Low

Prescription needed Yes

Available as generic Yes

GENERAL INFORMATION

The introduction of levodopa in the 1960s dramatically changed the treatment of Parkinson's disease. The body can transform levodopa into dopamine, the chemical messenger in the brain whose absence or shortage causes Parkinson's disease. Therefore, the use of this drug enabled rapid improvements in control to be obtained. These effects were a marked relief of symptoms but were not a cure for the disease.

However, while levodopa was effective, it produced severe side effects, such as nausea, dizziness, and palpitations. Even when treatment was initiated gradually, it was difficult to balance the benefits against these adverse reactions.

Today, the drug is combined with carbidopa or benserazide, which enhance its effects in the brain and help to reduce its side effects.

INFORMATION FOR USERS

Your drug prescription is tailored for you. Do not alter dosage without checking with your doctor.

How taken Tablets, dispersible tablets, capsules.

Frequency and timing of doses 3–6 x daily with food or milk.

Adult dosage range 125–500mg initially, increased until the benefits and the side effects are balanced.

Onset of effect Within 1 hour.

Duration of action 2–12 hours.

Diet advice None.

Storage Keep in a closed container in a cool, dry place out of reach of children. Protect from light.

Missed dose Take as soon as you remember. If your next dose is due within 2 hours, take a single dose now and skip the next.

Stopping the drug Unless palpitations occur, do not stop the drug without consulting your doctor. Stopping the drug may lead to severe worsening of the underlying condition.

Exceeding the dose An occasional unintentional extra dose is unlikely to cause problems. Larger overdoses may cause vomiting or drowsiness; notify your doctor.

POSSIBLE ADVERSE EFFECTS

Adverse effects are closely related to dosage levels. At the start of treatment, when the dosage is usually low, unwanted effects such as digestive disturbances, abnormal movement, and nervousness or agitation are usually mild. Dizziness, fainting, confusion, and vivid dreams may also occur and may worsen as the drug's dosage is increased to boost beneficial effects. Darkening of the urine can be ignored; all other adverse effects should be discussed with your doctor. If palpitations occur, stop taking the drug and seek urgent medical advice.

INTERACTIONS

Antidepressants Levodopa may interact with MAOIs, to cause a dangerous rise in blood pressure, and with tricyclic antidepressants.

Iron This may reduce absorption of levodopa.

Antipsychotic drugs Some of these drugs may reduce the effect of levodopa.

Pyridoxine (vitamin B_6) Excessive intake of this vitamin may reduce the effect of levodopa if levodopa is used on its own.

Bupropion The side effects of levodopa will be increased if used with this drug.

SPECIAL PRECAUTIONS

Be sure to tell your doctor if:

◆ You have heart problems.

◆ You have long-term liver or kidney problems.

◆ You have a lung disorder, such as asthma or bronchitis.

◆ You have an overactive thyroid gland.

◆ You have had glaucoma.

◆ You have a peptic ulcer.

◆ You have diabetes.

◆ You have any serious mental illness.

◆ You have ever had malignant melanoma.

◆ You are taking other medications.

Pregnancy Unlikely to be required.

Breast-feeding Unlikely to be required.

Infants and children Not normally used (and rarely given to patients under 25 years).

Over 60 No special problems.

Driving and hazardous work Your underlying condition, and the possibility of the drug causing fainting and dizziness, may make such activities inadvisable. Discuss with your doctor.

Alcohol No known problems.

PROLONGED USE

The effectiveness of levodopa usually declines in time, necessitating increased dosage or the addition of other drugs (see p.18). The adverse effects may become so severe that ultimately the drug has to be stopped.

Levofloxacin

Brand name Tavanic
Used in the following combined preparations None

QUICK REFERENCE

Drug group Antibacterial drug (p.66)
Overdose danger rating Medium
Dependence rating Low
Prescription needed Yes
Available as generic No

GENERAL INFORMATION

Levofloxacin is a quinolone antibacterial drug used for soft-tissue infections and respiratory and urinary tract infections that have not responded to other antibiotics.

The drug is usually prescribed as tablets, but it is administered by intravenous infusion to people with serious systemic infections or those who cannot take drugs by mouth.

Like other quinolones, levofloxacin may occasionally cause tendon inflammation and damage, especially in elderly people or those taking corticosteroids. If you have tendon pain or inflammation, therefore, you should stop taking it and consult your doctor immediately. You should also rest the affected limb or limbs until the symptoms have subsided.

INFORMATION FOR USERS

Your drug prescription is tailored for you. Do not alter dosage without checking with your doctor.

How taken Tablets, injection.
Frequency and timing of doses 1–2 x daily for 7–14 days, depending on infection (tablets).
Adult dosage range 250–1,000mg daily.
Onset of effect 1 hour.
Duration of action 12–24 hours.
Diet advice None.
Storage Keep in a closed container in a cool, dry place out of reach of children.
Missed dose Take as soon as you remember, then take your next dose when it is due.
Stopping the drug Unless severe adverse effects occur (see below), take the full course. Even if you feel better, the original infection may still be present, and symptoms may recur if treatment is stopped too soon.
Exceeding the dose An occasional unintentional extra dose is unlikely to cause problems.

Larger overdoses may cause mental disturbances and fits; notify your doctor.

POSSIBLE ADVERSE EFFECTS

Nausea and vomiting are the most common adverse effects of oral forms. Abdominal pain, diarrhoea, dizziness, headache, restlessness, drowsiness, itching, and rash may also occur. Injections of the drug may cause palpitations and giddiness due to a fall in blood pressure. If jaundice, confusion, hallucinations, fever, rash, painful or inflamed tendons, itching, wheezing, or breathlessness occur, stop taking the drug and consult your doctor urgently.

INTERACTIONS

NSAIDs and theophylline There is an increased risk of convulsions when these drugs are taken with levofloxacin.
Anticoagulants The effect of these drugs may be increased by levofloxacin.
Antacids, adsorbents, sucralfate, iron, and zinc These drugs may reduce the absorption of levofloxacin.
Ciclosporin Taken with levofloxacin, there is an increased risk of kidney damage.

SPECIAL PRECAUTIONS

Be sure to tell your doctor if:
◆ You have kidney problems.
◆ You suffer from epilepsy.
◆ You have glucose-6-phosphate dehydrogenase (G6PD) deficiency.
◆ You are taking aspirin or another NSAID.
◆ You have had a previous allergic reaction to a quinolone antibacterial.
◆ You have had a previous tendon problem with a quinolone.
◆ You are taking other medications.
Pregnancy Safety not established. Discuss with your doctor.
Breast-feeding Safety not established. Discuss with your doctor.
Infants and children Not recommended.
Over 60 No special problems, except that tendon damage is more likely over the age of 60.
Driving and hazardous work Avoid such activities until you have learned how levofloxacin affects you as it can cause dizziness, drowsiness, visual disturbances, and hallucinations.
Alcohol Avoid. Alcohol may increase the sedative effects of levofloxacin.

Sunlight Avoid exposing skin to strong sunlight or ultraviolet rays as photosensitization (abnormal sensitization to light) may occur.

PROLONGED USE
Not usually prescribed for long-term use.

Levonorgestrel

Brand names Levonelle-2, Microval, Norgeston
Used in the following combined preparations
Ciclo-progynova, Eugynon 30, Microgynon 30, Ovranette, and others

QUICK REFERENCE
Drug group Female sex hormone (p.88) and oral contraceptive (p.105)
Overdose danger rating Low
Dependence rating Low
Prescription needed Yes
Available as generic No

GENERAL INFORMATION
Levonorgestrel is a synthetic hormone similar to progesterone, a natural female sex hormone. The drug's primary use is as an ingredient in oral contraceptives. It performs this function by thickening the mucus at the neck of the uterus (cervix), thereby making it difficult for sperm to enter the uterus.

Levonorgestrel is available both in combined oral contraceptives with an oestrogen drug and in progestogen-only preparations. It is occasionally given alone or with an oestrogen for emergency post-coital contraception. It is also given in combination with an oestrogen drug in hormone replacement therapy (HRT) to treat menopausal symptoms.

Levonorgestrel rarely causes serious adverse effects. When it is used without an oestrogen, menstrual irregularities, especially mid-cycle, or "breakthrough", bleeding, are common.

INFORMATION FOR USERS
Your drug prescription is tailored for you. Do not alter dosage without checking with your doctor.
How taken Tablets, implant, intrauterine device (IUD).
Frequency and timing of doses Once daily, at the same time each day.

Adult dosage range *Progestogen-only contraceptive* 30mcg daily. *Postcoital contraceptive* 1.5mg (2 tablets) as a single dose as soon as possible, within 12 hours, but no later than after 72 hours.
Onset of effect The drug starts to act within 4 hours, but contraceptive protection may not be fully effective for 14 days, depending on which day of the cycle the tablets are started.
Duration of action 24 hours. Some effects, not including contraception, may persist for up to 3 months after levonorgestrel is stopped.
Diet advice None.
Storage Keep in a closed container in a cool, dry place out of reach of children.
Missed dose *Progestogen-only contraceptive* Take as soon as you remember, but if a pill is delayed by 3 hours or more, regard it as a missed dose. See What to do if you miss a pill (p.109). *Postcoital contraceptive* If vomiting occurs within 3 hours, take another 2 tablets immediately.
Stopping the drug Can be safely stopped as soon as contraception is no longer required. For treatment of menopausal symptoms, consult your doctor before stopping the drug.
Exceeding the dose An occasional unintentional extra dose is unlikely to be a cause for concern. But if you notice any unusual symptoms, or if a large overdose has been taken, notify your doctor.

POSSIBLE ADVERSE EFFECTS
Menstrual irregularities (blood spotting between periods or absence of menstruation) are the most common side effects of levonorgestrel used alone. Fluid retention, leading to swollen feet or ankles, and weight gain may also occur. Nausea, vomiting, and breast tenderness are less common effects. If headache or depression occur, consult your doctor.

INTERACTIONS
General note The beneficial effects of many drugs, including bromocriptine, oral anticoagulants, anticonvulsants, and antihypertensive and antidiabetic drugs, may be affected by levonorgestrel. Many other drugs may affect the action of oral contraceptives, reducing contraceptive protection; these drug types include anticonvulsants, antituberculous drugs, and antibiotics. Inform your doctor that you are taking levonorgestrel before taking additional prescribed medication.

SPECIAL PRECAUTIONS

Be sure to tell your doctor if:
◆ You have a liver problem.
◆ You have heart failure or hypertension (high blood pressure).
◆ You have diabetes.
◆ You have unexplained abnormal vaginal bleeding.
◆ You have had blood clots or a stroke.
◆ You have ever suffered from migraines or severe headaches.
◆ You are taking other medications.

Pregnancy Not prescribed. May cause abnormalities in the developing baby. Discuss with your doctor.

Breast-feeding The drug passes into the breast milk, but at normal doses adverse effects on the baby are unlikely. Discuss with your doctor.

Infants and children Not prescribed.

Over 60 Not prescribed.

Driving and hazardous work No known problems.

Alcohol No known problems.

PROLONGED USE

Problems are rare.

Levothyroxine

Brand name Eltroxin
Used in the following combined preparations
None

QUICK REFERENCE

Drug group Drug for thyroid disorders (p.84)
Overdose danger rating Medium
Dependence rating Low
Prescription needed Yes
Available as generic Yes

GENERAL INFORMATION

Thyroxine is the major hormone produced by the thyroid gland. A deficiency of the natural hormone causes hypothyroidism and may sometimes lead to myxoedema, characterized by slowing of body functions and facial puffiness. Levothyroxine, a synthetic form of the hormone, is used to correct this deficiency.

Levothyroxine reduces the excessive thyroid activity that causes certain types of goitre (enlarged thyroid gland), so it may be used to prevent goitre from developing during treatment with antithyroid drugs. It is also prescribed for some forms of thyroid cancer.

Adults with a severe thyroid deficiency are sensitive to thyroid hormones, so treatment is introduced gradually, and increased slowly, to prevent adverse effects. Particular care is taken for those with heart problems such as angina.

INFORMATION FOR USERS

Your drug prescription is tailored for you. Do not alter dosage without checking with your doctor.

How taken Tablets.

Frequency and timing of doses Once daily.

Dosage range Adults Doses of 50–100mcg daily, increased at 3–4-week intervals as required. The maximum dose is 200mcg daily.

Onset of effect Within 48 hours. Full beneficial effects may not be felt for several weeks.

Duration of action 1–3 weeks.

Diet advice None.

Storage Keep in a closed container in a cool, dry place out of reach of children. Protect from light.

Missed dose Take as soon as you remember. If your next dose is due within 8 hours, take a single dose now and skip the next.

Stopping the drug Do not stop without consulting your doctor; symptoms may recur.

Exceeding the dose An occasional unintentional extra dose is unlikely to cause problems. Large overdoses may cause palpitations during the next few days; notify your doctor.

POSSIBLE ADVERSE EFFECTS

Adverse effects are rare and are usually the result of overdosage causing thyroid overactivity. These effects diminish as the dose is lowered. Too low a dose of levothyroxine may cause signs of thyroid underactivity. The rarest adverse effects include anxiety, diarrhoea, sweating, muscle cramps and palpitations. If these occur, seek medical advice.

INTERACTIONS

Oral anticoagulants Levothyroxine may increase the effect of these drugs.

Antidiabetic agents The doses of these drugs may need to be increased once levothyroxine treatment has been started.

Colestyramine This drug may reduce the absorption of levothyroxine.

Amiodarone This drug may affect thyroid activity and levothyroxine dosage may need to be adjusted.

Anticonvulsant drugs These drugs may reduce the effect of levothyroxine.

Sucralfate Absorption of levothyroxine may be reduced by sucralfate.

SPECIAL PRECAUTIONS

Be sure to tell your doctor if:
◆ You have high blood pressure.
◆ You have heart problems.
◆ You have diabetes.
◆ You are taking other medications.

Pregnancy No evidence of risk, but dosage adjustment may be necessary.

Breast-feeding The drug passes into the breast milk, but at normal doses adverse effects on the baby are unlikely. Discuss with your doctor.

Infants and children Dosage depends on age and weight.

Over 60 Reduced dose usually necessary.

Driving and hazardous work No known problems.

Alcohol No known problems.

PROLONGED USE

No special problems.

Monitoring Periodic tests of thyroid function are usually required.

Lisinopril

Brand names Carace, Zestril
Used in the following combined preparations
Carace Plus, Zestoretic

QUICK REFERENCE

Drug group Vasodilator (p.31)
Overdose danger rating Medium
Dependence rating Low
Prescription needed Yes
Available as generic Yes

GENERAL INFORMATION

Lisinopril is an ACE (angiotensin-converting enzyme) inhibitor drug used to treat hypertension, or high blood pressure (see p.36), and heart failure (in which the heart is unable to deal with its workload). It works by relaxing the muscles in blood vessel walls, allowing the vessels to dilate (widen), which enables the blood to circulate more easily and helps to lower blood pressure.

Lisinopril may also be given to patients following a heart attack and is sometimes used to prevent or delay kidney damage (nephropathy) in patients with diabetes. In addition, it is often given with a diuretic to increase its effect on high blood pressure and heart failure.

The drug is long-acting and may be taken once daily. The first dose may cause a sudden drop in blood pressure, especially in patients taking a diuretic. For this reason, you should lie down for 2–3 hours afterwards.

Various minor side effects may occur with lisinopril. Many people develop a persistent dry cough; others experience taste disturbance, which can be minimized by dosage reduction.

INFORMATION FOR USERS

Your drug prescription is tailored for you. Do not alter dosage without checking with your doctor.

How taken Tablets.

Frequency and timing of doses Once daily.

Adult dosage range *Hypertension* 2.5mg (starting dose) up to 40mg. *Heart failure/diabetic nephropathy* 2.5mg (starting dose) up to 20mg. *Prevention of further heart attacks* 2.5–5mg (starting dose) up to 10mg.

Onset of effect 1–2 hours. Full beneficial effect may take several weeks.

Duration of action 12–24 hours.

Diet advice None.

Storage Keep in a closed container in a cool, dry place out of reach of children.

Missed dose Take as soon as you remember. If your next dose is due within 8 hours, take a single dose now and skip the next.

Stopping the drug Unless severe adverse effects occur (see below), do not stop taking the drug without consulting your doctor. Stopping the drug may lead to worsening of the underlying condition.

Exceeding the dose An occasional unintentional extra dose is unlikely to be a cause for concern. Larger overdoses, however, may cause dizziness or fainting; notify your doctor.

POSSIBLE ADVERSE EFFECTS

Dizziness on standing is likely to occur after the first dose of lisinopril. Nausea and headache are common but are usually mild and transient. A persistent dry cough is the most common effect but can be minimized by taking smaller, more frequent doses; some people may have to stop taking the drug. Rash or itching may occur. If dizziness or fainting, runny nose or sore throat, confusion or mood changes, and chest pain or palpitations occur, or if you develop jaundice, consult your doctor. If you develop facial swelling, stop taking the drug and seek urgent medical advice.

INTERACTIONS

Potassium supplements, potassium-sparing diuretics, and ciclosporin Taken with lisinopril, these increase the risk of high blood potassium.

NSAIDs Some of these drugs may reduce the effect of lisinopril, and the risk of kidney damage is increased.

Vasodilators, diuretics, and other drugs for hypertension These drugs may increase the effect of lisinopril.

Lithium Blood levels of lithium may be raised by lisinopril.

Insulin and antidiabetic drugs Lisinopril may increase the effect of these drugs.

SPECIAL PRECAUTIONS

Be sure to tell your doctor if:
◆ You have suffered from severe allergies.
◆ You have long-term kidney problems.
◆ You have coronary artery disease.
◆ You peripheral vascular disease.
◆ You are on a low-sodium diet.
◆ You are allergic to other ACE inhibitors.
◆ You are taking other medications.

Pregnancy Not prescribed. May cause defects in the developing baby.

Breast-feeding The drug passes into breast milk, but at normal doses adverse effects on the baby are unlikely. Discuss with your doctor.

Infants and children Not usually prescribed.

Over 60 Reduced dose may be necessary.

Driving and hazardous work Avoid such activities until you have learned how lisinopril affects you because the drug can cause dizziness and fainting.

Alcohol Avoid excessive amounts. Alcohol may increase the blood-pressure-lowering and adverse effects of this drug.

Surgery and general anaesthetics Notify your doctor or dentist that you are taking lisinopril.

PROLONGED USE

Rarely, prolonged use of lisinopril can lead to changes in blood count or kidney function.

Monitoring Periodic checks on blood potassium levels, white blood cell counts, and urine are usually performed.

Lithium

Brand names Camcolit, Li-liquid, Liskonum, Priadel
Used in the following combined preparations
None

QUICK REFERENCE

Drug group Antimanic drug (p.16)
Overdose danger rating High
Dependence rating Low
Prescription needed Yes
Available as generic No

GENERAL INFORMATION

Lithium, the lightest known metal, has been used since the 1940s to treat manic depression (or bipolar affective disorder). It decreases the intensity and frequency of the episodic mood swings from extreme excitement to deep depression that are characteristic of the disorder. It is sometimes used with an antidepressant for depression that has not responded to an antidepressant alone.

Lithium treatment may be started in hospital for more seriously ill people. Careful monitoring is required because high blood levels of lithium can cause serious adverse effects. Since it may take two to three weeks for any benefit to become apparent, an antipsychotic drug (see p.15) is often given as well until the lithium becomes effective. Lithium cards, with details of side effects and other information, are available from pharmacies.

INFORMATION FOR USERS

Your drug prescription is tailored for you. Do not alter dosage without checking with your doctor.

How taken Tablets, SR-tablets, liquid, ointment.

Frequency and timing of doses 1–2 x daily with meals. Always take the same brand of lithium to ensure a consistent effect; any change of brand must be closely supervised.

Adult dosage range 0.3–1.6g daily. Dosage may vary according to individual response.

Onset of effect Some effects may be noticed in 3–5 days, but full benefits may not be felt for 3 weeks.

Duration of action 18–36 hours. Some effects may last for several days.

Diet advice Blood levels of lithium are affected by the amount of sodium present in the body; do not suddenly increase or reduce the amount of salt in your diet. Be sure to drink adequate volumes of fluids, especially during hot weather.

Storage Keep in a closed container in a cool, dry place out of reach of children.

Missed dose Take as soon as you remember. If your next dose is due within 4 hours, take a single dose now and skip the next.

Stopping the drug Unless severe adverse effects occur (see below), do not stop taking the drug without consulting your doctor; symptoms may recur.

OVERDOSE ACTION

Seek immediate medical advice in all cases. Take emergency action if convulsions or loss of consciousness occur.

POSSIBLE ADVERSE EFFECTS

Many of the following adverse effects may be signs of high blood lithium levels: tremor, muscle weakness, thirst and increased urine production, weight gain, nausea, vomiting, diarrhoea, drowsiness, lethargy, and blurred vision. Stop taking the drug and seek medical advice promptly if any of these symptoms occur. Stop taking the drug and consult your doctor urgently if If you develop a rash.

INTERACTIONS

General note Many drugs interact with lithium. Do not take any over-the-counter or prescription drugs without consulting your doctor or pharmacist. Paracetamol should be used in preference to other analgesics for everyday pain relief.

SPECIAL PRECAUTIONS

Be sure to tell your doctor if:
◆ You have long-term liver or kidney problems.
◆ You have heart or circulation problems.
◆ You have an overactive thyroid gland.
◆ You have myasthenia gravis.
◆ You have Addison's disease.
◆ You are taking other medications.

Pregnancy Lithium is not usually prescribed. It may cause defects in the unborn baby. Discuss with your doctor.

Breast-feeding The drug passes into the breast milk and may affect the baby. Discuss with your doctor.

Infants and children Not recommended.

Over 60 Reduced dose may be necessary. Increased likelihood of adverse effects.

Driving and hazardous work Avoid such activities until you have learned how lithium affects you as it can cause reduced alertness.

Alcohol Avoid. Alcohol may increase the sedative effects of this drug.

PROLONGED USE

Prolonged use may lead to kidney problems. Treatment for periods of longer than 5 years is not normally advised unless the benefits are significant and tests show no sign of reduced kidney function.

Monitoring Once stabilized, lithium levels should be checked every 3 months, and thyroid function every 6–12 months. Kidney function should also be monitored regularly.

Lofepramine

Brand name Gamanil
Used in the following combined preparations
None

QUICK REFERENCE

Drug group Antidepressant drug (p.14)
Overdose danger rating Medium
Dependence rating Low
Prescription needed Yes
Available as generic Yes

GENERAL INFORMATION

Lofepramine is a tricyclic antidepressant drug used primarily in the long-term treatment of depression.The drug serves to elevate mood, improve appetite, increase physical activity, and restore interest in everyday activities.

Less sedating than some other tricyclics, it is particularly useful for depression accompanied by lethargy. It seems to have a weaker anticholinergic (see Autonomic nervous system p.8) action and milder side effects. In overdose, it is considered less harmful than older tricyclics.

INFORMATION FOR USERS

Your drug prescription is tailored for you. Do not alter dosage without checking with your doctor.

How taken Tablets, liquid.

Frequency and timing of doses 2–3 x daily.

Adult dosage range 140–210mg daily.

Onset of effect Can be felt within hours; full antidepressant effect may take 2–6 weeks.

Duration of action Antidepressant effect may last 6 weeks; adverse effects, only a few days.

Diet advice None.

Storage Keep in a closed container in a cool, dry place out of reach of children. Protect from light.

Missed dose Take as soon as you remember. If your next dose is due within 3 hours, take a single dose now and skip the next.

Stopping the drug Stopping abruptly can cause withdrawal symptoms and a recurrence of the original problem. Consult your doctor, who may supervise gradual dosage reduction.

Exceeding the dose An occasional unintentional extra dose is unlikely to cause problems. If you notice any unusual symptoms, or if a large overdose has been taken, notify your doctor.

POSSIBLE ADVERSE EFFECTS

Adverse effects such as sweating or flushing, drowsiness, dry mouth, or blurred vision are mainly due to the drug's mild anticholinergic action. Consult your doctor if constipation, dizziness, or difficulty in passing urine occur. If palpitations occur, stop taking the drug and seek prompt medical attention.

INTERACTIONS

Sedatives All drugs that have sedative effects may intensify those of lofepramine.

Smoking may reduce lofepramine's effects.

MAOIs Serious interactions are possible. These drugs are only prescribed together under close medical supervision.

Antihypertensive drugs Lofepramine may reduce the effectiveness of some of these drugs.

Warfarin Lofepramine may, rarely, increase the effects of warfarin.

Anti-arrhythmics and sotalol These drugs may increase the risk of abnormal heart rhythms.

Antihistamines Terfenadine intensifies some effects of lofepramine.

SPECIAL PRECAUTIONS

Be sure to tell your doctor if:
◆ You have heart problems.
◆ You have had epileptic fits.
◆ You have long-term liver or kidney problems.
◆ You have glaucoma.
◆ You have an overactive thyroid gland.
◆ You have prostate trouble.
◆ You have porphyria.
◆ You are taking other medications.

Pregnancy Safety in pregnancy not established. Discuss with your doctor.

Breast-feeding The drug passes into breast milk and may affect the baby. Consult your doctor.

Infants and children Not recommended.

Over 60 Reduced dose may be necessary.

Driving and hazardous work Avoid until you have learned how the drug affects you; it may cause blurred vision and reduced alertness.

Alcohol Avoid. Alcohol may increase the sedative effects of this drug.

Surgery and general anaesthetics Lofepramine may need to be stopped. Discuss this with your doctor or dentist before any surgery.

PROLONGED USE

No problems expected.

Loperamide

Brand names Arret, Boots Diareze, Diasorb, Diocalm Ultra, Diocaps, Imodium, LoperaGen, Norimode, Normaloe

Used in the following combined preparations
Diocalm Plus

QUICK REFERENCE

Drug group Antidiarrhoeal drug (p.44)

Overdose danger rating Medium

Dependence rating Low

Prescription needed No (most preparations)

Available as generic Yes

GENERAL INFORMATION

Loperamide is an antidiarrhoeal drug that slows bowel activity and reduces the loss of water and salts from the bowel, resulting in the passage of firmer bowel movements at less frequent intervals.

A fast-acting drug, loperamide is widely used for both sudden and recurrent bouts of diarrhoea. It is not generally recommended for diarrhoea due to infection, however, because it may delay the expulsion of harmful substances from the bowel. It is often prescribed following a colostomy or ileostomy, to reduce fluid loss from the stoma (outlet).

INFORMATION FOR USERS

Follow instructions on the label. Call your doctor if symptoms worsen.

How taken Tablets, capsules, liquid.

Frequency and timing of doses *Acute diarrhoea* A double starting dose, then a single dose after each loose bowel movement, up to maximum daily dose. *Chronic diarrhoea* 2 x daily.

Adult dosage range *Acute diarrhoea* 4mg (starting dose), then 2mg after each loose bowel movement (maximum 16mg daily); usual dose 6–8mg daily. Use for up to 5 days only (3 days only for children between 4 and 8 years), then consult your doctor. *Chronic diarrhoea* 4–8mg daily (up to 16mg daily).

Onset of effect Within 1–2 hours.

Duration of action 6–18 hours.

Diet advice Ensure adequate fluid, sugar, and salt intake during a diarrhoeal illness.

Storage Keep in a closed container in a cool, dry place out of reach of children.

Missed dose Do not take the missed dose. Take your next dose if needed.

Stopping the drug Can be safely stopped as soon as you no longer need it.

Exceeding the dose An occasional unintentional extra dose is unlikely to be a cause for concern. Large overdoses, however, may cause constipation, vomiting, or drowsiness, and affect breathing; notify your doctor.

POSSIBLE ADVERSE EFFECTS

Adverse effects are rare. Dry mouth, drowsiness, or dizziness may occur. Some effects are hard to distinguish from the effects of the diarrhoea that the drug is used to treat. If constipation occurs, stop taking the drug. If bloating, abdominal pain, or fever persist or worsen during treatment, consult your doctor. If itching occurs, unless it is only mild, stop taking the drug.

INTERACTIONS

None.

SPECIAL PRECAUTIONS

Be sure to consult your doctor or pharmacist before taking this drug if:
◆ You have long-term liver or kidney problems.
◆ You have had recent abdominal surgery.
◆ You have an infection or blockage in the intestine or ulcerative colitis.
◆ You are taking other medications.

Pregnancy Safety in pregnancy not established. Discuss with your doctor.

Breast-feeding The drug passes into the breast milk and may affect the baby. Discuss with your doctor.

Infants and children Not given under 4 years. Reduced dose necessary for older children. Children can be very sensitive to the drug's effect; the drug should be used with care.

Over 60 No special problems.

Driving and hazardous work No known problems.

Alcohol No known problems.

PROLONGED USE

Not usually taken for prolonged periods (except in medically diagnosed long-term gastrointestinal conditions), but special problems are not expected.

Lopinavir/Ritonavir

Brand name Kaletra
Used in the following combined preparations
(Lopinavir/Ritonavir is a combination of two drugs)

QUICK REFERENCE

Drug group Drug for HIV and AIDS (p.100)
Overdose danger rating Medium
Dependence rating Low
Prescription needed Yes
Available as generic No

GENERAL INFORMATION

Lopinavir and ritonavir are both antiretroviral drugs from the same class of drugs, known as protease inhibitors. Combined as a single drug, they are used in the treatment of HIV infection. The drugs work by interfering with an enzyme used by the virus to produce genetic material.

The combination drug is prescribed with other antiretroviral drugs, usually two reverse transcriptase inhibitors, which together slow down the production of HIV. The aim of this combination therapy is to reduce the damage that is done to the immune system by the virus.

Combination antiretroviral therapy is not a cure for HIV. Taken regularly on a long-term basis, it can reduce the level of the virus in the body and improve the outlook for the HIV patient. However, the patient will remain infectious, and will suffer a relapse if the treatment is stopped.

INFORMATION FOR USERS

Your drug prescription is tailored for you. Do not alter dosage without checking with your doctor.

How taken Capsules, liquid.

Frequency and timing of doses Every 12 hours, with food.

Adult dosage range 3 capsules or 5ml liquid.

Onset of effect Within 1 hour.

Duration of action 12 hours.

Diet advice None.

Storage Keep in the fridge in the original container, out of reach of children.

Missed dose Take as soon as you remember. If your next dose is due within 2 hours, take a single dose now and skip the next. It is very important not to miss doses on a regular basis because this could lead to the development of drug-resistant HIV.

Stopping the drug Do not stop taking the drug without consulting your doctor.

Exceeding the dose An occasional unintentional extra dose is unlikely to cause problems. But if you notice any unusual symptoms, or if a large overdose has been taken, notify your doctor.

POSSIBLE ADVERSE EFFECTS

Gastrointestinal upset, including nausea, vomiting, diarrhoea, and loss of appetite, and fatigue are the most common adverse effects, and medical consultation is needed only if the symptoms are severe. Other problems, which are more likely to occur with prolonged use, include changes in body shape; these problems should be discussed with your doctor.

If you develop severe abdominal pain, stop taking the drug and contact your doctor without delay.

INTERACTIONS

General note A wide range of drugs may interact with lopinavir and ritonavir, causing either an increase in adverse effects or a reduction in the effect of the antiretroviral drugs. Check with your doctor or pharmacist before taking any new drugs, including those from the dentist or the supermarket, and herbal medicines.

Ritonavir is known to interact with some recreational drugs, including ecstasy. It is essential, therefore, that you discuss the use of such drugs with your doctor or pharmacist.

SPECIAL PRECAUTIONS

Be sure to tell your doctor if:
◆ You have any long-term liver or kidney problems.
◆ You take recreational drugs.
◆ You are taking other medications.

Pregnancy Safety in pregnancy not established. Discuss with your doctor.

Breast-feeding Safety in breast-feeding not established. Breast-feeding is not recommended for HIV-positive mothers because the virus may be passed to the baby.

Infants and children Not recommended under 2 years. Reduced dose recommended for older children.

Over 60 Reduced dose may be necessary.

Driving and hazardous work No known problems.

Alcohol The liquid form of lopinavir and ritonavir contains a small amount of alcohol; care should be taken if alcoholic drinks are consumed as well.

PROLONGED USE

Changes in body shape may occur.

Monitoring Regular blood samples are taken to check the effect of the drugs on the virus. The blood will also be checked for changes in lipids, cholesterol, and glucose levels.

Loratadine/Desloratadine

Brand name Boots Hayfever and Allergy Relief All Day, Clarityn, Clarityn Allergy, NeoClarityn (desloratadine)
Used in the following combined preparations
None

QUICK REFERENCE

Drug group Antihistamine (p.58)
Overdose danger rating Low
Dependence rating Low
Prescription needed No (loratadine); yes (desloratadine)
Available as generic No

GENERAL INFORMATION

Loratadine, a long-acting antihistamine, relieves sneezing, runny nose, and itching and burning eyes in allergic rhinitis. It is also used to treat allergic skin conditions such as chronic urticaria. It has fewer sedative and anticholinergic (see Autonomic nervous system, p.8) effects than older antihistamines and is less likely to cause drowsiness. Desloratadine, an active breakdown product of loratadine, is available as a separate product.

The drug should be discontinued about four days prior to skin testing for allergy as it may decrease or prevent otherwise positive results.

INFORMATION FOR USERS

Follow instructions on the label. Call your doctor if symptoms worsen.
How taken Tablets, liquid.
Frequency and timing of doses Once daily.
Adult dosage range 10mg daily (loratadine); 5mg daily (desloratadine).
Onset of effect Usually within 1 hour.
Duration of action Up to 24 hours.
Diet advice None.
Storage Keep in a closed container in a cool, dry place out of reach of children.
Missed dose Take as soon as you remember. If your next dose is due within 6 hours, take a single dose now and skip the next.
Stopping the drug Can be safely stopped as soon as you no longer need it.
Exceeding the dose An occasional unintentional extra dose is unlikely to cause problems. But if you notice any unusual symptoms, or if a large overdose has been taken, notify your doctor.

POSSIBLE ADVERSE EFFECTS

Adverse effects are rare, but fatigue, nausea, and headache may occur. If fainting or palpitations occur, consult your doctor.

INTERACTIONS

Cimetidine, clarithromycin, erythromycin, ketoconazole, fluoxetine, fluconazole, and quinidine These drugs may increase the blood levels and effects of loratadine and desloratadine.

SPECIAL PRECAUTIONS

Be sure to consult your doctor or pharmacist before taking this drug if:
◆ You are taking other medications.
Pregnancy Safety in pregnancy not established. Discuss with your doctor.
Breast-feeding The drug passes into the breast milk. Discuss with your doctor.
Infants and children Not recommended under 2 years. Reduced dose necessary for older children.
Over 60 No problems expected.
Driving and hazardous work Problems are unlikely, but you need to be aware how loratadine may affect you before undertaking these activities.
Alcohol No known problems, but avoid excessive amounts.

PROLONGED USE

No problems expected.

Losartan

Brand name Cozaar
Used in the following combined preparation
Cozaar-Comp

QUICK REFERENCE

Drug group Vasodilator (p.31) and antihypertensive drug (p.36)
Overdose danger rating Medium
Dependence rating Low
Prescription needed Yes
Available as generic No

GENERAL INFORMATION

Losartan is an antihypertensive drug that acts by blocking the action of angiotensin-II, a naturally occurring substance that constricts blood vessels. This causes the blood vessel walls to relax, easing blood pressure.

Unlike ACE inhibitors, losartan does not cause a persistent dry cough, and its use is being evaluated in conditions such as heart failure, for which ACE inhibitors are used.

The drug is prescribed with caution to people who have stenosis (narrowing) of the arteries to the kidneys because it may make their kidney function worse. It is important to notify your doctor if you know you have this condition. In addition, the initial dose causes a sudden drop in blood pressure. Adverse effects, including diarrhoea, dizziness, and fatigue, are usually mild.

INFORMATION FOR USERS

Your drug prescription is tailored for you. Do not alter dosage without checking with your doctor.

How taken Tablets.

Frequency and timing of doses Once daily.

Adult dosage range 50–100mg. People over 75 years, and other groups especially sensitive to the drug's effects, may start on 25mg.

Onset of effect *Blood pressure* 1–2 weeks, with maximum effect in 3–6 weeks from start of treatment. *Other conditions* Within 1 hour.

Duration of action 12–24 hours.

Diet advice None.

Storage Keep in a closed container in a cool, dry place out of reach of children.

Missed dose Take as soon as you remember. If your next dose is due within 8 hours, take a single dose now and skip the next.

Stopping the drug Unless severe adverse effects occur (see below), do not stop taking the drug without consulting your doctor. Stopping the drug may lead to worsening of the underlying condition.

Exceeding the dose An occasional unintentional extra dose is unlikely to cause problems. Large overdoses, however, may cause dizziness and fainting; notify your doctor.

POSSIBLE ADVERSE EFFECTS

Dizziness and fatigue are common but are usually mild. Diarrhoea, migraine, taste disturbance, and rash or itching may also occur. Dizziness, lightheadedness, or feeling faint may be signs of an excessive fall in blood pressure;

consult your doctor. If wheezing occurs, or facial swelling develops, stop taking the drug and seek immediate medical advice.

INTERACTIONS

Diuretics There is a risk of a sudden fall in blood pressure when these drugs are taken with losartan for the first time.

Potassium supplements, potassium-sparing diuretics, and ciclosporin Losartan increases the effects of these drugs, leading to raised levels of potassium in the blood.

Lithium Losartan may increase the levels and toxicity of lithium.

NSAIDs Certain NSAIDs may reduce the blood-pressure-lowering effect of losartan.

SPECIAL PRECAUTIONS

Be sure to tell your doctor if:
◆ You have stenosis of the kidney arteries.
◆ You have liver or kidney problems.
◆ You have congestive heart failure.
◆ You have primary aldosteronism.
◆ You have experienced angioedema.
◆ You are taking other medications.

Pregnancy Not prescribed. May cause abnormalities in the developing baby.

Breast-feeding Not prescribed. Safety not established.

Infants and children Not prescribed. Safety not established.

Over 60 Reduced dose may be necessary for people over 75 years.

Driving and hazardous work Do not undertake such activities until you have learned how losartan affects you because the drug can cause dizziness and fatigue.

Alcohol Avoid excessive amounts. Alcohol may raise blood pressure, reducing the effectiveness of losartan. Alcohol also causes blood vessels to dilate, increasing the likelihood of an excessive fall in blood pressure.

PROLONGED USE

No special problems.

Monitoring Blood pressure will be monitored during treatment with losartan, as with all antihypertensive drugs. Periodic checks on blood potassium levels and kidney function may also be performed.

Magnesium hydroxide

Brand names Cream of Magnesia, Milk of Magnesia
Used in the following combined preparations
Carbellon, Maalox, Mucaine, Mucogel, and others

QUICK REFERENCE

Drug group Antacid (p.42) and laxative (p.45)
Overdose danger rating Low
Dependence rating Low
Prescription needed No
Available as generic Yes

GENERAL INFORMATION

Magnesium hydroxide, a fast-acting antacid given to neutralize stomach acid, is available in a number of over-the-counter preparations for indigestion and heartburn. It also relieves the pain of stomach and duodenal ulcers, gastritis, and reflux oesophagitis, but other drugs are normally used for these problems nowadays. In addition, it acts as a laxative by drawing water into the intestine from the surrounding blood vessels to soften the faeces.

Magnesium hydroxide is not often used alone as an antacid because of its laxative effect. However, this effect is countered when the drug is used in combination with aluminium hydroxide, which can cause constipation.

INFORMATION FOR USERS

Follow instructions on the label. Call your doctor if symptoms worsen.
How taken Tablets, liquid, powder.
Frequency and timing of doses 1–4 x daily as needed, with water, preferably an hour after food and at bedtime.
Adult dosage range *Antacid* 1–2g per dose (tablets); 5–20ml per dose (liquid).
Laxative 5–20ml per dose (liquid).
Onset of effect *Antacid* Within 15 minutes. *Laxative* 2–8 hours.
Duration of action *Antacid* 2–4 hours. *Laxative* 12–24 hours.
Diet advice None.
Storage Keep in a closed container in a cool (not cold), dry place, out of reach of children.
Missed dose Take as soon as you remember.
Stopping the drug When used as an antacid, can be safely stopped as soon as you no longer need it. When given as ulcer treatment, follow your doctor's advice.

Exceeding the dose An occasional unintentional extra dose is unlikely to be a cause for concern. But if you notice any unusual symptoms, or if a large overdose has been taken, notify your doctor.

POSSIBLE ADVERSE EFFECTS

Diarrhoea is the only common adverse effect. Dizziness and muscle weakness, due to absorption of excess magnesium in the body, may occur from prolonged heavy use of the drug in people with poor kidney function.

INTERACTIONS

General note Magnesium hydroxide interferes with the absorption of a wide range of drugs taken by mouth, including tetracycline antibiotics, iron supplements, diflunisal, phenytoin, and penicillamine.
Enteric-coated tablets As with other antacids, magnesium hydroxide may allow the break-up of the enteric coating of these tablets, sometimes leading to stomach irritation.

SPECIAL PRECAUTIONS

Be sure to consult your doctor or pharmacist before taking this drug if:
◆ You have a long-term kidney problem.
◆ You have a bowel disorder.
◆ You are taking other medications.
Pregnancy No evidence of risk, but discuss the most appropriate treatment with your doctor.
Breast-feeding No evidence of risk, but discuss the most appropriate treatment with your doctor.
Infants and children Not recommended for infants under 1 year except on the advice of a doctor. Reduced dose necessary for older children.
Over 60 No special problems.
Driving and hazardous work No known problems.
Alcohol Avoid excess alcohol; it irritates the stomach and may reduce the drug's benefits.

PROLONGED USE

You should not use magnesium hydroxide for prolonged periods without consulting your doctor. If you are over 40 years of age and are experiencing long-term indigestion or heartburn, your doctor will probably refer you to a specialist. Prolonged use of the drug in people with kidney damage may cause drowsiness, dizziness, and weakness due to the accumulation of magnesium in the body.

Malathion

Brand names Derbac M, Prioderm, Quellada M, Suleo-M
Used in the following combined preparations None

QUICK REFERENCE

Drug group Drug to treat skin parasites (p.122)
Overdose danger rating Low (medium if swallowed)
Dependence rating Low
Prescription needed No
Available as generic No

GENERAL INFORMATION

Malathion is an insecticide used in the treatment of lice and scabies mite infestations. It kills the parasites by interfering with their nervous system, causing paralysis and death.

Malathion is applied topically, either as shampoo or as lotion (which is more convenient to use, requiring only a single application, and more effective because shampoo is diluted in use). Lotions with a high alcohol content are unsuitable for small children or asthmatics, who may be affected by the solvent, or for treating crab lice in the genital area. However, the water-based liquid is suitable. Take care to avoid bringing the drug into contact with the eyes or broken skin.

If resistance occurs during treatment, your pharmacist will recommend an alternative.

INFORMATION FOR USERS

Follow instructions on the label. Call your doctor if symptoms worsen.
How taken Liquid, lotion, shampoo.
Frequency and timing of doses *Scabies* Once only (liquid or lotion). *Lice* 3 applications 3 days apart (shampoo); 2 doses, 7 days apart (liquid or lotion).
Adult dosage range As directed. Family members and close contacts should also be treated.
Onset of effect *Liquid or lotion* Leave on for 12 hours (lice), or 24 hours (scabies), before washing off. *Shampoo* Leave on for 5 minutes, rinse off, repeat, then use fine-toothed comb.

Duration of action Until washed off.
Diet advice None.
Storage Keep in a closed container in a cool, dry place out of reach of children. Protect from light.
Missed dose If a repeat application of the shampoo is missed, it should be carried out as soon as is practicable.
Stopping the drug Should be applied as a single application or short course of treatment.
Exceeding the dose An extra application of malathion is unlikely to cause problems. Take emergency action if the insecticide has been swallowed.

POSSIBLE ADVERSE EFFECTS

Used correctly, malathion preparations are unlikely to produce adverse effects, other than skin irritation, although the alcoholic fumes given off by some lotions may cause wheezing in asthmatics.

INTERACTIONS

None.

SPECIAL PRECAUTIONS

Be sure to consult your doctor or pharmacist before using this drug if:
◆ You have asthma.
Pregnancy No evidence of risk. It is unlikely that enough malathion would be absorbed after occasional application to affect the developing baby.
Breast-feeding No evidence of risk. It is unlikely that enough malathion would be absorbed after occasional application to affect the baby.
Infants and children No special problems, but seek medical advice for use on infants under 6 months.
Over 60 No special problems.
Driving and hazardous work No special problems.
Alcohol No special problems.

PROLONGED USE

Malathion is intended for intermittent use only. The lotions should not be used more than once a week for 3 weeks at a time. If there is a need to use malathion more frequently, it is possible that resistance has built up; seek your doctor's advice.

Mebeverine

Brand names Colofac, Colofac IBS, Colofac MR, Equilon
Used in the following combined preparation Fybogel-Mebeverine

QUICK REFERENCE

Drug group Drug for irritable bowel syndrome (p.45)
Overdose danger rating Low
Dependence rating Low
Prescription needed No (some preparations)
Available as generic Yes

GENERAL INFORMATION

Mebeverine is an antispasmodic drug used to relieve painful spasms of the intestine (colic), such as those that occur as a result of irritable bowel syndrome and other intestinal disorders such as diverticular disease. It has a direct relaxing effect on the muscle in the bowel wall and may also have an anticholinergic (see Autonomic nervous system, p.8) action, which reduces the transmission of nerve signals to the smooth muscle of the bowel wall, thereby preventing spasm. Mebeverine does not have serious side effects.

Mebeverine is also combined with ispaghula husk to provide roughage in an easily assimilable formulation. Both the drug itself and the combined form are commonly used to improve symptoms in the control of irritable bowel syndrome.

INFORMATION FOR USERS

Follow instructions on the label. Call your doctor if symptoms worsen.
How taken Tablets, SR-capsules, liquid, granules.
Frequency and timing of doses 2–3 x daily, 20 minutes before meals.
Adult dosage range 300–450mg daily.
Onset of effect 30–60 minutes.
Duration of action 6–8 hours.
Diet advice None.
Storage Keep in a closed container in a dry place at room temperature, out of reach of children. Protect from light.
Missed dose Take as soon as you remember, then return to your normal dosing schedule.
Stopping the drug The drug can be safely stopped as soon as you no longer need it.

Exceeding the dose An occasional unintentional extra dose is unlikely to be a cause for concern. Larger overdoses will probably cause constipation, and may cause central nervous system excitability.

POSSIBLE ADVERSE EFFECTS

Constipation is common. If, rarely, confusion and agitation occur, stop taking the drug and consult your doctor immediately

INTERACTIONS

None.

SPECIAL PRECAUTIONS

Be sure to consult your doctor or pharmacist before taking this drug if:
◆ You have cystic fibrosis.
◆ You have porphyria.
Pregnancy Safety in pregnancy not established. Discuss with your doctor.
Breast-feeding Safety in breast-feeding not established. Discuss with your doctor.
Infants and children Not used in infants and children under 10 years.
Over 60 No special problems.
Driving and hazardous work No special problems.
Alcohol No special problems.

PROLONGED USE

No problems expected.

Medroxyprogesterone

Brand names Adgyn-Medro, Depo-Provera, Farlutal, Provera
Used in the following combined preparations Indivina, Premique, Tridestra

QUICK REFERENCE

Drug group Female sex hormone (p.88)
Overdose danger rating Low
Dependence rating Low
Prescription needed Yes
Available as generic No

GENERAL INFORMATION

Medroxyprogesterone is a progestogen, a synthetic female sex hormone similar to the natural hormone progesterone. It is used to treat a range of menstrual disorders such as mid-cycle bleeding and amenorrhoea (absent periods).

The drug is also often used to treat endometriosis, in which there is abnormal growth of uterine-lining tissue in the pelvic cavity.

Depot injections of the drug are used as a contraceptive. However, since they may cause serious side effects, such as persistent bleeding from the uterus, amenorrhoea, and delayed return of fertility, their use remains controversial, and they are recommended only under special circumstances in the UK.

In addition, medroxyprogesterone may be used to treat some types of cancer, such as cancer of the breast, uterus, or prostate.

INFORMATION FOR USERS

Your drug prescription is tailored for you. Do not alter dosage without checking with your doctor.

How taken Tablets, depot injection.

Frequency and timing of doses 1–3 x daily with plenty of water (by mouth); tablets may need to be taken at certain times during your cycle; follow the instructions you have been given. Every 3 months (depot injection).

Adult dosage range *Menstrual disorders* 2.5–10mg daily. *Endometriosis* 30mg daily. *Cancer* 100–1,500mg daily. *Contraception* 150mg.

Onset of effect *Cancer* 1–2 months. *Other conditions* 1–2 weeks.

Duration of action 1–2 days (by mouth); up to a few months (depot injection).

Diet advice None.

Storage Keep in a closed container in a cool, dry place out of reach of children.

Missed dose Take as soon as you remember. If your next dose is due within 3 hours, take a single dose now and skip the next.

Stopping the drug Unless itching, rash, or acne occur, do not stop taking the drug without consulting your doctor; symptoms may recur.

Exceeding the dose An occasional unintentional extra dose is unlikely to be a cause for concern. But if you notice any unusual symptoms, or if a large overdose has been taken, notify your doctor.

POSSIBLE ADVERSE EFFECTS

Adverse effects are rare. Fluid retention may cause weight gain, swollen feet or ankles, and breast tenderness. Nausea, fatigue, depression, and irregular menstruation may also occur. If you develop itching, a rash, or acne, stop taking the drug and consult your doctor.

INTERACTIONS

Ciclosporin The effects of this drug may be increased by medroxyprogesterone.

SPECIAL PRECAUTIONS

Be sure to tell your doctor if:
◆ You have high blood pressure.
◆ You have diabetes.
◆ You have had blood clots or a stroke.
◆ You have long-term liver or kidney problems.
◆ You are taking other medications.

Pregnancy Not prescribed. May cause abnormalities in the developing baby. Discuss with your doctor.

Breast-feeding The drug passes into the breast milk, but at normal doses adverse effects on the baby are unlikely. Discuss with your doctor.

Infants and children Not usually prescribed.

Over 60 No special problems.

Driving and hazardous work No known problems.

Alcohol No known problems.

PROLONGED USE

Long-term use of this drug may slightly increase the risk of blood clots in the leg veins. Irregular menstrual bleeding or spotting between periods may also occur during long-term use.

Monitoring Periodic checks on blood pressure and annual cervical smear tests are usually required.

Mefenamic acid

Brand names Dysman, Ponstan
Used in the following combined preparations
None

QUICK REFERENCE

Drug group Non-steroidal anti-inflammatory drug (p.50)

Overdose danger rating Medium

Dependence rating Low

Prescription needed Yes

Available as generic Yes

GENERAL INFORMATION

Introduced in 1963, mefenamic acid is a non-steroidal anti-inflammatory drug (NSAID). Like other NSAIDs, it relieves pain and inflammation. The drug is an effective analgesic, and is used to treat headache, toothache, and menstrual pains (dysmenorrhoea), as well as to reduce excessive menstrual bleeding (menorrhagia). Mefenamic acid is also prescribed for long-term relief of pain and stiffness in rheumatoid arthritis and osteoarthritis.

The most common side effects of mefenamic acid are gastrointestinal: abdominal pain, nausea and vomiting, and indigestion. Other, more serious effects include kidney problems, blood disorders, and peptic ulcers (which may occasionally bleed).

INFORMATION FOR USERS

Your drug prescription is tailored for you. Do not alter dosage without checking with your doctor.

How taken Tablets, capsules, liquid.
Frequency and timing of doses 3 x daily with food.
Adult dosage range 1,500mg daily.
Onset of effect 1–2 hours.
Duration of action Up to 8 hours.
Diet advice None.
Storage Keep in a closed container in a cool, dry place out of reach of children.
Missed dose Take as soon as you remember. If your next dose is due within 2 hours, take a single dose now and skip the next.
Stopping the drug Can be safely stopped as soon as you no longer need it.
Exceeding the dose An occasional unintentional extra dose is unlikely to be a cause for concern. Large overdoses, however, may cause poor coordination, muscle twitching, or fits; notify your doctor.

POSSIBLE ADVERSE EFFECTS

Gastrointestinal disturbances such as indigestion and nausea are the most common side effects. Drowsiness and dizziness may also occur. The drug should be stopped if diarrhoea or rash occur, and not be used thereafter. If you have bloodstained or black faeces, wheezing or breathlessness, stop taking the drug and consult your doctor immediately.

INTERACTIONS

General note Mefenamic acid interacts with a wide range of drugs to increase the risk of bleeding and/or peptic ulcers. These drugs include other NSAIDs such as aspirin, oral anticoagulant drugs, and corticosteroids.
Antihypertensive drugs and diuretics The beneficial effects of these drugs may be reduced by mefenamic acid.
Lithium, digoxin, and methotrexate Mefenamic acid may raise blood levels of these drugs to an undesirable extent.
Oral antidiabetic drugs Mefenamic acid may increase the blood-glucose-lowering effect of these drugs.
Ciprofloxacin The risk of seizures with this drug and related antibiotics may be increased by mefenamic acid.

SPECIAL PRECAUTIONS

Be sure to tell your doctor if:
◆ You have liver or kidney problems.
◆ You have had a peptic ulcer, oesophagitis, or acid indigestion.
◆ You have inflammatory bowel disease.
◆ You have asthma.
◆ You have high blood pressure.
◆ You are allergic to aspirin.
◆ You have porphyria.
◆ You are taking other medications.

Pregnancy Not usually prescribed. May cause defects in the unborn baby and, taken in late pregnancy, may affect the baby's cardiovascular system. Discuss with your doctor.
Breast-feeding The drug passes into the breast milk, but at normal doses adverse effects on the baby are unlikely. Discuss with your doctor.
Infants and children Reduced dose necessary.
Over 60 Increased likelihood of adverse effects. Reduced dose necessary.
Driving and hazardous work Avoid such activities until you have learned how mefenamic acid affects you because the drug can cause drowsiness and dizziness.
Alcohol Avoid excessive intake. Alcohol may increase the risk of stomach irritation with mefenamic acid.
Surgery and general anaesthetics Mefenamic acid may prolong bleeding. Discuss the possibility of stopping treatment with your doctor or dentist before any surgery.

PROLONGED USE

Prolonged use increases the risk of bleeding from peptic ulcers and in the bowel. Rarely, the drug may affect the liver and blood. Blood tests may be carried out.

Mefloquine

Brand name Lariam
Used in the following combined preparations
None

QUICK REFERENCE

Drug group Antimalarial drug (p.75)
Overdose danger rating High
Dependence rating Low
Prescription needed Yes
Available as generic No

GENERAL INFORMATION

Mefloquine is used for the prevention and treatment of malaria. It is recommended for use in areas where malaria is resistant to other drugs (such as China, Southeast Asia, South America, and Central and Southern Africa).

However, the drug's use is limited by the fact that in some patients it can cause serious side effects including depression, suicidal tendencies, anxiety, panic, confusion, hallucinations, paranoid delusions, and convulsions.

For most people, the benefits of the use of mefloquine outweigh the risks, although this should be discussed with your doctor.

INFORMATION FOR USERS

Your drug prescription is tailored for you. Do not alter dosage without checking with your doctor.
How taken Tablets.
Frequency and timing of doses *Prevention* Once weekly. *Treatment* Up to 3 x daily, every 6–8 hours.
Adult dosage range *Prevention* 1 tablet once weekly starting 1–3 weeks before departure and continuing until 4 weeks after leaving the malarial area. *Treatment* 20–25mg/kg bodyweight up to a maximum dose of 1.5g.
Onset of effect 2–3 days.
Duration of action Over 1 week. Low levels of the drug may persist for several months.
Diet advice None.

Storage Keep in a cool, dry place out of reach of children.
Missed dose Take as soon as you remember. If your next dose is due within 48 hours (if taken once weekly for prevention), take a single dose now and skip the next.
Stopping the drug If you feel you need to stop taking the drug, consult your doctor about alternatives before the next dose is due.

OVERDOSE ACTION

Seek immediate medical advice in all cases. Take emergency action if dizziness, palpitations, collapse, or loss of consciousness occur.

POSSIBLE ADVERSE EFFECTS

Dizziness, vertigo, nausea, vomiting, abdominal pain, and headache are common. Rarely, serious adverse effects on the nervous system can occur, including anxiety or panic attacks, depression, hallucinations, and paranoid delusions. If these symptoms, hearing problems, or palpitations occur, stop taking the drug and consult your doctor immediately.

INTERACTIONS

General note Mefloquine may increase the effects on the heart of drugs such as beta blockers, calcium channel blockers, and digitalis drugs.
Anticonvulsants Mefloquine may decrease the effect of these drugs.
Other antimalarials Mefloquine may increase the risk of adverse effects with these drugs.

SPECIAL PRECAUTIONS

Be sure to tell your doctor if:
◆ You have long-term liver or kidney problems.
◆ You have had epileptic fits.
◆ You have had depression or other psychiatric illness.
◆ You have had a previous allergic reaction to mefloquine or quinine.
◆ You have heart problems.
◆ You are taking other medications.
Pregnancy Not usually prescribed. If unavoidable, the drug is given only after the first trimester. Pregnancy must be avoided during mefloquine use and for 3 months afterwards.
Breast-feeding Not prescribed. The drug passes into the breast milk.

Infants and children Not used in infants under 3 months old. Reduced dose necessary in older children.

Over 60 Careful monitoring is necessary if liver or kidney problems or heart disease are present.

Driving and hazardous work Avoid such activities when taking mefloquine for prevention until you know how the drug affects you. Also avoid during treatment and for 3 weeks afterwards as the drug can cause dizziness or disturb balance.

Alcohol Keep consumption low.

PROLONGED USE

May be taken for prevention for up to 1 year.

Megestrol

Brand name Megace
Used in the following combined preparations
None

QUICK REFERENCE

Drug group Female sex hormone (p.88 and anticancer drug (p.96)
Overdose danger rating Low
Dependence rating Low
Prescription needed Yes
Available as generic No

GENERAL INFORMATION

Megestrol is a progestogen (a synthetic female sex hormone similar to the natural hormone progesterone). It is used in the treatment of certain types of advanced cancer affecting the breast and uterus that are sensitive to hormone treatment. Megestrol is often prescribed when the tumour cannot be removed by surgery, when the disease has recurred after surgery, or when treatment with other anticancer drugs or radiotherapy has failed.

Successful treatment with the drug reduces the size of the tumour and may also cause secondary growths to disappear. Improvement usually occurs within two months of starting treatment. Because megestrol does not eradicate the cancer completely, the drug may need to be continued indefinitely.

Megestrol may also be used to prevent weight loss in other types of cancer.

INFORMATION FOR USERS

Your drug prescription is tailored for you. Do not alter dosage without checking with your doctor.
How taken Tablets.
Frequency and timing of doses 1–4 x daily.
Adult dosage range *Breast cancer* 160mg daily. *Cancer of the uterus* 40–320mg daily.
Onset of effect Within 2 months.
Duration of action 1–2 days.
Diet advice None.
Storage Keep in a closed container in a cool, dry place out of reach of children.
Missed dose Take as soon as you remember.
Stopping the drug Unless a rash occurs, do not stop taking the drug without consulting your doctor. Stopping the drug may lead to worsening of your underlying condition.
Exceeding the dose An occasional unintentional extra dose is unlikely to be a cause for concern. But if you notice any unusual symptoms, or if a large overdose has been taken, notify your doctor.

POSSIBLE ADVERSE EFFECTS

Adverse effects are rare with megestrol, but it may cause weight gain due to fluid retention (leading to swollen feet or ankles) or increased appetite and food intake. Other effects include nausea, headache, and hair loss. If you develop a rash, stop taking the drug and consult your doctor immediately.

INTERACTIONS

Ciclosporin The effects of this drug may be increased by megestrol.

SPECIAL PRECAUTIONS

Be sure to tell your doctor if:
◆ You have long-term liver or kidney problems.
◆ You have had thrombosis.
◆ You have high blood pressure.
◆ You have heart problems.
◆ You are taking other medications.
Pregnancy Not usually prescribed.
Breast-feeding Breast-feeding is usually discontinued. Discuss with your doctor.
Infants and children Not usually required.
Over 60 No special problems.
Driving and hazardous work No known problems.
Alcohol No known problems.

PROLONGED USE

Long-term use of this drug may increase the risk of blood clots in the leg veins.

Monitoring Periodic checks on blood pressure may be performed.

Meloxicam

Brand name Mobic
Used in the following combined preparations
None

QUICK REFERENCE

Drug group Non-steroidal anti-inflammatory drug (p.50)
Overdose danger rating Medium
Dependence rating Low
Prescription needed Yes
Available as generic No

GENERAL INFORMATION

Meloxicam is a member of the non-steroidal anti-inflammatory (NSAID) group of drugs. It reduces pain, stiffness, and inflammation and is used to relieve the symptoms of rheumatoid arthritis, ankylosing spondylitis, and acute episodes of osteoarthritis. It does not cure the underlying condition, however.

Meloxicam does not affect the stomach as severely as some NSAIDs and is therefore less likely to cause gastrointestinal bleeding, ulceration, and perforation. Elderly people, however, are more sensitive than others to the effects of the drug; for this reason, they are usually prescribed only half the normal adult dose.

INFORMATION FOR USERS

Your drug prescription is tailored for you. Do not alter dosage without checking with your doctor.

How taken Tablets, suppositories.
Frequency and timing of doses Once daily.
Adult dosage range 7.5–15mg.
Onset of effect 1 hour. However, the full anti-inflammatory effect may not be felt for up to 2 weeks.
Duration of action 24 hours.
Diet advice None.
Storage Keep in a closed container in a cool, dry place out of reach of children.

Missed dose Take as soon as you remember. If your next dose is due within 8 hours, take a single dose now and skip the next.

Stopping the drug In short-term use, the drug can be safely stopped as soon as you no longer need it. In long-term use, unless severe adverse effects occur (see below), do not stop taking it without consulting your doctor.

Exceeding the dose An occasional unintentional extra dose is unlikely to cause problems. Large overdoses can cause stomach and intestinal pain and damage; notify your doctor.

POSSIBLE ADVERSE EFFECTS

Gastrointestinal disturbances, which may include abdominal pain, indigestion, diarrhoea, or constipation, are common adverse effects. Headache, lightheadedness or drowsiness, rash, or itching may also occur. If you experience palpitations, vertigo, ringing in the ears, or a persistent sore throat, consult your doctor. If black or bloodstained faeces or wheezing occur, stop taking the drug and consult your doctor immediately.

INTERACTIONS

General note Meloxicam interacts with a wide range of drugs to increase the risk of bleeding and/or peptic ulcers. Such drugs include NSAIDs, aspirin, and also oral anticoagulants, and corticosteroids.

Ciclosporin There is an increased risk of kidney damage when meloxicam is taken with ciclosporin.

Lithium, digoxin, and methotrexate Meloxicam may increase the blood levels of these drugs to an undesirable extent.

Antibacterials Meloxicam may increase the risk of convulsions with ciprofloxacin and similar drugs.

SPECIAL PRECAUTIONS

Be sure to tell your doctor if:
◆ You have asthma.
◆ You are allergic to aspirin or other NSAIDs.
◆ You have had a peptic ulcer, oesophagitis, or acid indigestion.
◆ You have liver or kidney problems.
◆ You have a bleeding disorder, proctitis, or haemorrhoids.
◆ You are taking other medications.

Pregnancy Safety not established. The drug may affect the developing baby. Discuss with your doctor.

Breast-feeding Safety not established. Discuss with your doctor.

Infants and children Not recommended.

Over 60 Reduced doses necessary. Increased likelihood of adverse effects.

Driving and hazardous work Avoid such activities until you have learned how meloxicam affects you because the drug can cause vertigo and drowsiness.

Alcohol Keep consumption low. Alcohol may increase the risk of stomach irritation with meloxicam.

Surgery and general anaesthetics Meloxicam may prolong bleeding. Discuss the possibility of stopping treatment temporarily with your doctor or dentist.

PROLONGED USE
No special problems.

Monitoring Periodic tests on kidney function may be performed.

Mercaptopurine

Brand name Puri-Nethol
Used in the following combined preparations
None

QUICK REFERENCE
Drug group Anticancer drug (p.96)
Overdose danger rating Medium
Dependence rating Low
Prescription needed Yes
Available as generic No

GENERAL INFORMATION
Mercaptopurine is an anticancer drug that is widely used in the treatment of certain forms of leukaemia. It is usually given in combination with other anticancer drugs.

Nausea and vomiting, mouth ulcers, and loss of appetite are the drug's most common side effects. Such symptoms tend to be milder than those of other cytotoxic drugs, and often disappear as the body adjusts to the drug. More seriously, mercaptopurine can interfere with blood cell production, resulting in blood clotting disorders and anaemia, and can cause liver damage. The likelihood of infections is also increased.

INFORMATION FOR USERS
Your drug prescription is tailored for you. Do not alter dosage without checking with your doctor.

How taken Tablets.

Frequency and timing of doses Once daily.

Dosage range Dosage is determined individually according to bodyweight and response.

Onset of effect 1–2 weeks.

Duration of action Side effects may persist for several weeks after stopping treatment.

Diet advice None.

Storage Keep in a closed container in a cool, dry place out of reach of children. Protect from light.

Missed dose If your next dose is due within 6 hours, take a single dose now and skip the next. Tell your doctor that you missed a dose.

Stopping the drug Do not stop taking the drug without consulting your doctor. Stopping the drug may lead to worsening of your underlying condition.

Exceeding the dose An occasional unintentional extra dose is unlikely to cause problems. Large overdoses may cause nausea and vomiting; notify your doctor.

POSSIBLE ADVERSE EFFECTS
The most common adverse effects are nausea and vomiting and loss of appetite. Any other problems should be reported to your doctor urgently. Some people develop mouth ulcers, and infections are more likely. Jaundice may also occur but is reversible on stopping the drug. Because mercaptopurine interferes with the production of blood cells, it may cause anaemia and blood clotting disorders, and black faeces and bloodstained vomit may therefire occur due to bleeding in the intestine.

INTERACTIONS
Allopurinol This drug increases blood levels of mercaptopurine.

Warfarin The effects of warfarin may be decreased by mercaptopurine.

Co-trimoxazole and trimethoprim These drugs increase the risk of blood problems with mercaptopurine.

SPECIAL PRECAUTIONS
Be sure to tell your doctor if:
◆ You have long-term liver or kidney problems.
◆ You suffer from gout.
◆ You have recently had any infection.
◆ You have porphyria.
◆ You are taking other medications.

Pregnancy Not usually prescribed. Discuss with your doctor.

Breast-feeding Not advised. The drug passes into the breast milk and may affect the baby adversely. Discuss with your doctor.

Infants and children Reduced dose necessary.

Over 60 Reduced dose may be necessary. Increased risk of adverse effects.

Driving and hazardous work No known problems.

Alcohol Avoid. Alcohol may increase the adverse effects of this drug.

PROLONGED USE
Prolonged use of this drug may reduce bone marrow activity, leading to a reduction of all types of blood cells.

Monitoring Regular blood checks and tests on liver function are required.

Mesalazine

Brand names Asacol, Pentasa, Salofalk
Used in the following combined preparations
None

QUICK REFERENCE
Drug group Drug for inflammatory bowel disease (p.46)
Overdose danger rating Low
Dependence rating Low
Prescription needed Yes
Available as generic Yes

GENERAL INFORMATION
Mesalazine is prescribed for patients who have ulcerative colitis. It is also sometimes used in the treatment of Crohn's disease, which affects the large intestine. The drug is given to relieve symptoms in an acute attack and is also taken as a preventative measure. When mesalazine is used to treat severe cases, it is often taken with other drugs, such as corticosteroids.

When the drug is taken as tablets, its active component is released in the large intestine, where it acts locally to relieve the inflamed mucous membrane. Enemas and suppositories are also available and are particularly useful for disease in the rectum and lower colon.

This drug produces fewer side effects than some older treatments, such as sulfasalazine. People who cannot tolerate sulfasalazine may be able to take mesalazine without problems. However, it should not be used if people are hypersensitive to salicylates such as aspirin.

INFORMATION FOR USERS
Your drug prescription is tailored for you. Do not alter dosage without checking with your doctor.

How taken Tablets, SR-tablets, granules, suppositories, enema (foam or liquid).

Frequency and timing of doses 3 x daily, swallowed whole, not chewed (tablets); 3 x daily (suppositories); once daily at bedtime (enema).

Adult dosage range 1.5–2.4g daily (acute attack); 750mg–2.4g daily (maintenance dose).

Onset of effect Adverse effects may be noticed within a few days, but full beneficial effects may not be felt for a couple of weeks.

Duration of action Up to 12 hours.

Diet advice Your doctor may advise you, taking account of the condition affecting you.

Storage Keep in a closed container in a cool, dry place out of reach of children. Protect from light. Keep aerosol out of direct sunlight.

Missed dose Take as soon as you remember. If your next dose is due within 2 hours, take a single dose now and skip the next.

Stopping the drug Unless severe adverse effects occur (see below), do not stop taking the drug without consulting your doctor; symptoms may recur.

Exceeding the dose An occasional unintentional extra dose is unlikely to be a cause for concern. But if you notice any unusual symptoms, or if a large overdose has been taken, notify your doctor.

POSSIBLE ADVERSE EFFECTS
The common side effects of mesalazine involve the gastrointestinal tract; nausea, abdominal pain, or diarrhoea may occur. Other problems are uncommon. If unexplained

bleeding and bruising, sore throat, fever, wheezing, or malaise occur, stop taking the drug and contact your doctor immediately. If worsening of colitis or a rash occur, report them to your doctor without delay.

INTERACTIONS
Lactulose The release of mesalazine at its site of action may be reduced by lactulose.
Warfarin Mesalazine may reduce the effect of warfarin.

SPECIAL PRECAUTIONS
Be sure to tell your doctor if:
◆ You have long-term liver or kidney problems.
◆ You are allergic to aspirin.
◆ You are taking other medications.
Pregnancy Negligible amounts of the drug cross the placenta, but safety in pregnancy not established. Discuss with your doctor.
Breast-feeding Negligible amounts of the drug pass into the breast milk, but safety not established. Discuss with your doctor.
Infants and children Not recommended under 15 years.
Over 60 Dosage reduction not normally necessary unless there is kidney impairment.
Driving and hazardous work No special problems.
Alcohol No special problems.

PROLONGED USE
No problems expected.

Metformin

Brand names Duformin, Glucophage, Orabet
Used in the following combined preparations
None

QUICK REFERENCE
Drug group Drug used in diabetes (p.82)
Overdose danger rating High
Dependence rating Low
Prescription needed Yes
Available as generic Yes

GENERAL INFORMATION
Metformin is an antidiabetic drug used to treat adult (maturity-onset or Type 2) diabetes in which some insulin-secreting cells are still active in the pancreas. It is usually prescribed for patients who are overweight.

Metformin lowers blood glucose by reducing the absorption of glucose from the digestive tract into the bloodstream, by reducing the glucose production by cells in the liver and kidneys, and by increasing the sensitivity of cells to insulin so that they take up glucose more effectively from the blood.

The drug is given in conjunction with a special diabetic diet that limits sugar and fat intake. It is often given with another antidiabetic drug that stimulates insulin secretion by the pancreas, or with insulin (see p.271) for treatment of maturity-onset diabetes, especially to overweight patients.

INFORMATION FOR USERS
Your drug prescription is tailored for you. Do not alter dosage without checking with your doctor.
How taken Tablets.
Frequency and timing of doses 2–3 x daily with food.
Adult dosage range 1.5–3g daily, with a low dose at the start of the treatment.
Onset of effect Within 2 hours. It may take 2 weeks to achieve control of diabetes.
Duration of action 8–12 hours.
Diet advice For the drug to be fully effective, an individualized low-fat, low-sugar diet must be maintained. Follow your doctor's advice.
Storage Keep in a closed container in a cool, dry place out of reach of children.
Missed dose Take as soon as you remember. If your next dose is due within 2 hours, take a single dose now and skip the next.
Stopping the drug Do not stop taking the drug without consulting your doctor. Stopping the drug may lead to worsening of the underlying condition.

OVERDOSE ACTION
Seek immediate medical advice in all cases. Take emergency action if fits or loss of consciousness occur.

POSSIBLE ADVERSE EFFECTS
Minor gastrointestinal symptoms such as nausea, vomiting, appetite loss, and a metallic taste in the mouth may occur but are often helped by taking the drug with food.

Diarrhoea may also occur but usually settles after a few days of continued treatment. Dizziness, confusion, weakness, sweating, or rash are uncommon and should be discussed with your doctor.

INTERACTIONS

General note A number of drugs, including corticosteroids, oestrogens, and diuretics, reduce the effects of metformin. Others, notably MAOIs and beta blockers, increase its effects.

Warfarin Metformin may increase the effect of this anticoagulant. The dosage of warfarin may need to be adjusted accordingly.

SPECIAL PRECAUTIONS

Be sure to tell your doctor if:
◆ You have long-term liver or kidney problems.
◆ You have heart failure.
◆ You are a heavy drinker.
◆ You are taking other medications.

Pregnancy Not usually prescribed. Insulin is usually substituted because it provides better diabetic control during pregnancy. Discuss with your doctor.

Breast-feeding Safety not established. Discuss with your doctor.

Infants and children Not recommended.

Over 60 Reduced dose may be necessary. Increased likelihood of adverse effects.

Driving and hazardous work Usually no problems. Avoid such activities if you have warning signs of low blood glucose.

Alcohol Avoid excessive amounts. Alcohol increases the risk of low blood glucose and can cause coma by increasing the blood's acidity.

Surgery and general anaesthetics The response to this drug may be reduced. Notify your doctor that you are diabetic before any surgery; insulin treatment may need to be substituted. Tell your doctor if you are to have a contrast X-ray; metformin should be stopped before the procedure.

PROLONGED USE

Prolonged treatment with metformin can deplete reserves of vitamin B_{12}, and this may, rarely, cause anaemia.

Monitoring Regular checks on kidney function and on levels of sugar in the urine and/or blood are usually required. Vitamin B_{12} levels may also be checked annually.

Methadone

Brand names Methadose, Metharose, Physeptone, Synastone
Used in the following combined preparations
None

QUICK REFERENCE

Drug group Opioid analgesic (p.9)
Overdose danger rating High
Dependence rating High
Prescription needed Yes
Available as generic Yes

GENERAL INFORMATION

Methadone is a synthetic drug belonging to the opioid analgesic group. It is used in the control of severe pain, but it is more widely used to replace morphine or heroin in the treatment of dependence. In this situation, methadone can be given once daily to prevent withdrawal symptoms. In some cases, dosage can be reduced until the drug is no longer needed.

Tolerance to methadone is marked. Although the initial dose for a person not used to taking opioids is very low, the dose needed by someone who regularly takes them could be fatal for a non-user.

INFORMATION FOR USERS

Your drug prescription is tailored for you. Do not alter dosage without checking with your doctor.

How taken Tablets, liquid, injection.

Frequency and timing of doses *Pain* 3–4 x daily; 2 x daily (prolonged use). *Opioid addiction* 1 x daily.

Adult dosage range *Pain* 5–10mg per dose initially, adjusted according to response. *Opioid addiction* 10–20mg (starting dose); 40–60mg daily (maintenance dose).

Onset of effect 15–60 minutes.

Duration of action 36–48 hours.

Diet advice None.

Storage Keep in a closed container in a cool, dry place out of reach of children. Protect injections and liquids from light.

Missed dose Take the missed dose as soon as you remember and return to your normal dosing schedule as soon as possible. If you missed the dose because it caused you to vomit, or if you cannot swallow anything, consult your doctor.

Stopping the drug If the reason for taking the drug no longer exists, it can be safely stopped. Discuss with your doctor.

OVERDOSE ACTION

Seek immediate medical advice in all cases. Take emergency action if symptoms such as slow or irregular breathing, severe drowsiness, or loss of consciousness occur.

POSSIBLE ADVERSE EFFECTS

Drowsiness and nausea are the most common side effects, but these diminish as the body adapts. Constipation is also common and may be longer-lasting. Other adverse effects include dizziness and confusion. If you experience loss of consciousness or slow, difficult breathing, stop taking the drug and seek immediate medical attention.

INTERACTIONS

Phenytoin, carbamazepine, rifampicin, and ritonavir These drugs may reduce the effects of methadone.

MAOIs and selegiline Taken with methadone, these drugs may produce a dangerous rise or fall in blood pressure.

Sedatives The effects of all drugs that have a sedative effect on the central nervous system are likely to be increased by methadone.

SPECIAL PRECAUTIONS

Be sure to tell your doctor if:
◆ You have heart or circulatory problems.
◆ You have liver or kidney problems.
◆ You have lung problems such as asthma or bronchitis.
◆ You have thyroid disease.
◆ You have a history of epileptic fits.
◆ You are an alcoholic.
◆ You are taking other medications.

Pregnancy Methadone is not prescribed in late pregnancy if possible. It may cause breathing difficulties in the newborn baby. Discuss with your doctor.

Breast-feeding Safety not established. The drug passes into breast milk and may affect the baby adversely. Discuss with your doctor.

Infants and children Not recommended.

Over 60 Not recommended.

Driving and hazardous work Your underlying condition may make such activities inadvisable. Discuss with your doctor.

Alcohol Avoid. Alcohol increases the sedative effects of the drug and may depress breathing.

PROLONGED USE

Treatment is always closely monitored. In long-term treatment, the dose must be carefully reduced before the drug is stopped.

Methotrexate

Brand name Maxtrex
Used in the following combined preparations
None

QUICK REFERENCE

Drug group Anticancer drug (p.96), antirheumatic drug (p.52), and drug for psoriasis (p.124)
Overdose danger rating Medium
Dependence rating Low
Prescription needed Yes
Available as generic Yes

GENERAL INFORMATION

Methotrexate is an anticancer drug used, together with other anticancer drugs, in treating leukaemia, lymphomas, and solid cancers such as those of the breast, bone, lung, bladder, head, and neck. It is also used for severe psoriasis until less potent drugs can be reintroduced. In addition, it is given to people with severe acute rheumatoid arthritis that has not responded to other treatment. Once the condition is under control, the dose is reduced.

As with most anticancer drugs, methotrexate affects both healthy and cancerous cells, so that its usefulness is limited by its adverse effects and toxicity. When given in high doses, it is usually given with folinic acid to prevent the destruction of bone marrow cells that occurs when high doses are used.

Methotrexate has been reported to reduce the IQ of children. It may also reduce fertility by depressing sperm and egg development.

INFORMATION FOR USERS

Your drug prescription is tailored for you. Do not alter dosage without checking with your doctor.

How taken Tablets, injection.

Frequency and timing of doses *Cancer* Single dose once weekly or every 3 weeks. *Other conditions* Usually, single dose once weekly.

Adult dosage range *Cancer* Determined individually according to nature of condition, bodyweight, and response. *Rheumatoid arthritis* 7.5–20mg weekly. *Psoriasis* 10–25mg weekly.

Onset of effect 30–60 minutes.

Duration of action 10–15 hours (short term).

Diet advice None.

Storage Keep in a closed container in a cool, dry place out of reach of children. Wash your hands after handling the tablets.

Missed dose Take as soon as you remember and consult your doctor.

Stopping the drug Unless sore throat, fever, or a rash occur, do not stop taking the drug without consulting your doctor. Stopping the drug may lead to worsening of the underlying condition.

Exceeding the dose Tell your doctor if you accidentally take an extra tablet. Large overdoses damage the bone marrow and cause nausea and abdominal pain; notify your doctor immediately.

POSSIBLE ADVERSE EFFECTS

Nausea and vomiting may occur within a few hours. Diarrhoea and mouth ulcers, which are also common, may occur a few days after treatment starts. If these, or jaundice, mood changes, or confusion occur, notify your doctor. Dry cough or chest pain may also occur. If you develop a sore throat, fever, or a rash, stop taking the drug and consult your doctor immediately.

INTERACTIONS

General Note Many drugs, including NSAIDs, diuretics, ciclosporin, phenytoin, and probenecid, may increase the blood levels and toxicity of methotrexate.

Co-trimoxazole, trimethoprim, and certain antimalarial drugs These drugs may enhance the effects of methotrexate.

SPECIAL PRECAUTIONS

Be sure to tell your doctor if:
◆ You have liver or kidney problems.
◆ You have porphyria.
◆ You have a problem with alcohol abuse.

◆ You have a peptic or other digestive-tract ulcer.
◆ You are taking other medications.

Pregnancy Not prescribed. Methotrexate may cause birth defects in the unborn baby.

Breast-feeding Not advised. The drug passes into the breast milk and may affect the baby adversely.

Infants and children For cancer treatment only. Reduced dose necessary.

Over 60 Reduced dose necessary. Increased likelihood of adverse effects.

Driving and hazardous work No special problems.

Alcohol Avoid. Alcohol may increase the adverse effects of methotrexate.

PROLONGED USE

Long-term treatment may be needed for rheumatoid arthritis. Once the condition is controlled, the drug is reduced as much as possible to the lowest effective dose.

Monitoring Full blood counts and kidney and liver function tests will be performed before treatment starts and at intervals during treatment. Blood concentrations of methotrexate may also be measured periodically.

Methylcellulose

Brand name Celevac
Used in the following combined preparations
None

QUICK REFERENCE

Drug group Laxative (p.45) and antidiarrhoeal drug (p.44)
Overdose danger rating Low
Dependence rating Low
Prescription needed No
Available as generic Yes

GENERAL INFORMATION

Methylcellulose is a laxative used in treating constipation, diverticular disease, and irritable bowel syndrome. Taken by mouth, it is not absorbed into the bloodstream but remains in the intestine, absorbing up to 25 times its volume of water, and thereby softening faeces and increasing their volume. It is also used to reduce the frequency and increase the firmness of faeces in chronic diarrhoea, and to control the consistency of faeces after colostomies and ileostomies.

The drug is used with appropriate dieting in some cases of obesity. The bulking agent swells to give a feeling of fullness, encouraging adherence to a reducing diet.

INFORMATION FOR USERS

Follow instructions on the label. Call your doctor if symptoms worsen.

How taken Tablets.

Frequency and timing of doses 1–2 x daily. If being used as a laxative, and unless otherwise instructed, take with a full glass of water.

Adult dosage range 1.5–6g daily.

Onset of effect Within 24 hours.

Duration of action Up to 3 days.

Diet advice If taken as a laxative, drink plenty of fluids, at least 6–8 glasses daily.

Storage Keep in a closed container in a cool, dry place out of reach of children.

Missed dose Take as soon as you remember. Take the next dose as scheduled.

Stopping the drug Can be safely stopped as soon as you no longer need it.

Exceeding the dose An occasional unintentional extra dose is unlikely to be a cause for concern. But if you notice any unusual symptoms, or if a large overdose has been taken, notify your doctor.

POSSIBLE ADVERSE EFFECTS

Taken by mouth, the drug may cause bloating and excess wind. Insufficient fluid intake may cause blockage of the oesophagus (gullet) or intestine. Consult your doctor if severe abdominal pain occurs or if no bowel movement occurs for 2 days after taking the drug.

INTERACTIONS

None.

SPECIAL PRECAUTIONS

Be sure to consult your doctor or pharmacist before taking this drug if:
◆ You have severe constipation and/or abdominal pain.
◆ You have unexplained rectal bleeding.
◆ You have difficulty in swallowing.
◆ You vomit readily.
◆ You are taking other medications.

Pregnancy No evidence of risk to the developing baby, but discuss with your doctor.

Breast-feeding No evidence of risk.

Infants and children Reduced dose necessary.

Over 60 No special problems.

Driving and hazardous work No known problems.

Alcohol No known problems.

PROLONGED USE

No problems expected.

Methyldopa

Brand name Aldomet
Used in the following combined preparations
None

QUICK REFERENCE

Drug group Antihypertensive drug (p.36)
Overdose danger rating Medium
Dependence rating Low
Prescription needed Yes
Available as generic Yes

GENERAL INFORMATION

Introduced in the 1960s, methyldopa was, for many years, one of the most widely prescribed drugs for the treatment of high blood pressure. In recent years, its use has declined as newer antihypertensives with fewer side effects have been introduced. It is effective when other, newer drugs are ineffective and for patients who have taken it for many years without experiencing any of the side effects.

Because it does not reduce blood flow to the kidneys, methyldopa is sometimes used for patients with kidney disorders. In addition, methyldopa is often prescribed to women who experience high blood pressure during late pregnancy because it does not affect the developing baby.

INFORMATION FOR USERS

Your drug prescription is tailored for you. Do not alter dosage without checking with your doctor.

How taken Tablets.

Frequency and timing of doses 2–3 x daily.

Dosage range *Adults* 500mg–3g daily.

Children Reduced dose necessary.

Onset of effect 3–6 hours. Full effect begins in 2–3 days.

Duration of action 6–12 hours. Some effect may last for 1–2 days after stopping the drug.

Diet advice None.

Storage Keep in a closed container in a cool, dry place out of reach of children. Protect from light.

Missed dose Take as soon as you remember. If your next dose is due within 2 hours, take a single dose now and skip the next.

Stopping the drug Unless jaundice or a rash occur, do not stop taking the drug without consulting your doctor, who will gradually reduce your dose. Stopping suddenly may lead to an increase in blood pressure.

Exceeding the dose An occasional unintentional extra dose is unlikely to cause problems. Large overdoses may cause excessive drowsiness or palpitations; notify your doctor.

POSSIBLE ADVERSE EFFECTS

Most adverse effects diminish in time. The fluid retention that occurs during treatment is counteracted by taking a diuretic. Drowsiness and impotence are common. If depression, nightmares, headaches, or decreased libido occur, consult your doctor. Fever, stuffy nose, dizziness, and nausea are uncommon and require medical attention. If you develop a rash or jaundice, stop taking the drug and consult your doctor immediately.

INTERACTIONS

Antidepressants Tricyclic antidepressants may increase the effects of methyldopa.

MAOIs These should not be taken at the same time as methyldopa because they may cause a dangerous drop in blood pressure.

Lithium Methyldopa may raise blood lithium levels, causing lithium toxicity.

Levodopa The effects of methyldopa may be enhanced by levodopa.

SPECIAL PRECAUTIONS

Be sure to tell your doctor if:
◆ You have long-term liver or kidney problems.
◆ You have anaemia.
◆ You have angina.
◆ You have porphyria.
◆ You suffer from depression.
◆ You are taking other medications.

Pregnancy No evidence of risk.

Breast-feeding The drug passes into the breast milk, but at normal doses adverse effects on the baby are unlikely. Discuss with your doctor.

Infants and children Reduced dose necessary.

Over 60 Reduced dose necessary.

Driving and hazardous work Avoid such activities until you have learned how methyldopa affects you; the drug can cause drowsiness.

Alcohol Avoid. Alcohol may increase the hypotensive and sedative effects of this drug.

Surgery and general anaesthetics Discuss with your doctor or dentist before any surgery.

PROLONGED USE

Liver and blood problems may occur rarely.

Monitoring Periodic checks on blood and urine are usually required.

Metoclopramide

Brand names Gastrobid Continus, Maxolon, Maxolon SR, Primperan
Used in the following combined preparations MigraMax, Paramax

QUICK REFERENCE

Drug group Gastrointestinal motility regulator and anti-emetic drug (p.21)
Overdose danger rating Medium
Dependence rating Low
Prescription needed Yes
Available as generic Yes

GENERAL INFORMATION

Metoclopramide is a drug that encourages the normal propulsion of food through the stomach and intestine by direct action on the gastrointestinal tract. The drug has powerful anti-emetic properties and is most commonly used in the prevention and treatment of nausea and vomiting, particularly the nausea that sometimes accompanies migraine and the nausea caused by treatment with anticancer drugs. It is also given to alleviate symptoms of hiatus hernia resulting from stomach acid reflux into the oesophagus.

One side effect of the drug is muscle spasm of the face and neck, which is more likely in children and young adults under 20 years. Other side effects are not usually troublesome.

INFORMATION FOR USERS

Your drug prescription is tailored for you. Do not alter dosage without checking with your doctor.

How taken Tablets, SR-tablets/capsules, liquid, powder, injection.

Frequency and timing of doses Usually 3 x daily; 1–2 x daily (SR-preparations).

Adult dosage range Usually 15–30mg daily; may be higher for nausea due to anticancer drugs.

Onset of effect Within 1 hour.

Duration of action 6–8 hours.

Diet advice Fatty and spicy foods and alcohol are best avoided if nausea is a problem.

Storage Keep in a closed container in a cool, dry place out of reach of children.

Missed dose Take as soon as you remember. If your next dose is due within 3 hours, take a single dose now and skip the next.

Stopping the drug Can be safely stopped as soon as you no longer need it.

Exceeding the dose An occasional unintentional extra dose is unlikely to be a cause for concern. Large overdoses may cause drowsiness and muscle spasms; notify your doctor.

POSSIBLE ADVERSE EFFECTS

Adverse effects are rare; drowsiness or restlessness may occur. If uncontrolled muscle spasm occurs, stop taking the drug and consult your doctor immediately.

INTERACTIONS

Sedatives The sedative properties of metoclopramide are increased by all drugs that have a sedative effect on the central nervous system. Such drugs include anti-anxiety and sleeping drugs, antihistamines, antidepressants, opioid analgesics, and antipsychotics.

Ciclosporin Metoclopramide may increase the blood levels of this drug.

Phenothiazine antipsychotics Metoclopramide increases the likelihood of adverse effects from these drugs.

Lithium Metoclopramide increases the risk of central nervous system side effects.

SPECIAL PRECAUTIONS

Be sure to tell your doctor if:
◆ You have long-term liver or kidney problems.
◆ You have epilepsy.
◆ You have Parkinson's disease.

◆ You have acute porphyria.
◆ You have a history of depression.
◆ You are taking other medications.

Pregnancy Safety in pregnancy not established. Discuss with your doctor.

Breast-feeding The drug passes into the breast milk, but at normal doses adverse effects on the baby are unlikely. Discuss with your doctor.

Infants and children Restricted use for those under 20 years. Reduced dose necessary.

Over 60 Reduced dose may be necessary.

Driving and hazardous work Avoid such activities until you have learned how metoclopramide affects you because the drug can cause drowsiness.

Alcohol Avoid. Alcohol may oppose the drug's beneficial effects and increase sedative effect.

PROLONGED USE

Not normally used in the long term, except under specialist supervision for certain gastrointestinal disorders.

Metoprolol

Brand names Betaloc, Betaloc SA, Lopresor, Lopresor SR
Used in the following combined preparations Co-Betaloc, Co-Betaloc SA

QUICK REFERENCE

Drug group Beta blocker (p.30)
Overdose danger rating High
Dependence rating Low
Prescription needed Yes
Available as generic Yes

GENERAL INFORMATION

Metoprolol belongs to the beta blocker group of drugs. It is used to prevent the heart from beating too fast in conditions such as angina, hypertension (high blood pressure), arrhythmias (abnormal heart rhythms), heart failure, and hyperthyroidism (overactive thyroid gland). Metoprolol is also used to prevent migraine attacks, and to protect the heart from further damage following a heart attack.

Because metoprolol is cardioselective, it is less likely to provoke breathing difficulties than other, non-cardioselective beta blockers. It should not be used by people with asthma, however, but can be used, with caution, by people with bronchitis.

INFORMATION FOR USERS

Your drug prescription is tailored for you. Do not alter dosage without checking with your doctor.

How taken Tablets, SR-tablets, injection.

Frequency and timing of doses *Hypertension* 1–2 x daily. *Angina/arrhythmias* 2–3 x daily. *Heart attack prevention* 4 x daily for 2 days, then 2 x daily. *Migraine prevention* 2 x daily. *Hyperthyroidism* 4 x daily.

Adult dosage range 100–300mg daily.

Onset of effect 1–2 hours.

Duration of action 3–7 hours.

Diet advice None.

Storage Keep in a closed container in a cool, dry place out of reach of children.

Missed dose Take as soon as you remember. If your next dose is due within 2 hours, take a single dose now and skip the next.

Stopping the drug Do not stop taking the drug without consulting your doctor. Stopping suddenly may lead to worsening of the underlying condition.

OVERDOSE ACTION

Seek immediate medical advice in all cases. Take emergency action if breathing difficulties, collapse, or loss of consciousness occur.

POSSIBLE ADVERSE EFFECTS

Like all beta blockers, metoprolol is associated with nightmares and cold fingers and toes. Fatigue, dizziness, headache, nausea, vomiting, and abdominal pain may also occur. Other common adverse effects, which should be reported to your doctor immediately, include breathing difficulties and slow heart beat, which may lead to fainting.

INTERACTIONS

Verapamil should not be taken with metoprolol because it may seriously slow or stop the heart beat and lower the blood pressure.

Decongestants Taken with metoprolol, these drugs may increase the blood pressure and heart rate.

Ergotamine This drug increases constriction of blood vessels in the extremities with metoprolol.

NSAIDs These drugs may oppose the blood-pressure-lowering effects of metoprolol.

SPECIAL PRECAUTIONS

Be sure to tell your doctor if:
◆ You have liver or kidney problems.
◆ You have asthma, bronchitis, or emphysema.
◆ You have heart failure.
◆ You have diabetes.
◆ You have hyperthyroidism.
◆ You have phaeochromocytoma.
◆ You have psoriasis.
◆ You have poor circulation in the legs.
◆ You are taking other medications.

Pregnancy Not usually prescribed; may affect the baby, but may be given under close supervision. Discuss with your doctor.

Breast-feeding The drug passes into the breast milk, but at normal doses adverse effects on the baby are unlikely. Discuss with your doctor.

Infants and children Not recommended.

Over 60 Increased risk of adverse effects.

Driving and hazardous work Avoid such activities until you have learned how metoprolol affects you because the drug can cause fatigue, dizziness, and drowsiness.

Alcohol No special problems.

PROLONGED USE

No special problems.

Metronidazole

Brand names Anabact, Elyzol, Flagyl, Metrogel, Metrolyl, Metrotop, Metrozol, Noritate, Rozex, Vaginyl, Zidoval, Zyomet
Used in the following combined preparations
None

QUICK REFERENCE

Drug group Antibacterial drug (p.66) and antiprotozoal drug (p.73)
Overdose danger rating Low
Dependence rating Low
Prescription needed Yes
Available as generic Yes

GENERAL INFORMATION

Metronidazole is prescribed to fight both protozoal infections and a variety of bacterial infections. It is widely used in the treatment of vaginal trichomonas infection; because the organism responsible is sexually transmitted and may not cause symptoms, a simultaneous course of treatment is usually advised for the sexual partner.

Certain infections of the abdomen, pelvis, and gums respond well to metronidazole. The drug is also used to treat *Helicobacter pylori* infection of the stomach, as well as septicaemia and infected leg ulcers and pressure sores. It may be given to prevent or treat infections after surgery; and because, in high doses, it can penetrate the brain, it is prescribed to treat abscesses occurring there.

Metronidazole is also prescribed for the treatment of amoebic dysentery and for giardiasis, a rare protozoal infection.

Metronidazole may be applied topically in the form of a gel to treat some forms of acne, rosacea, infected tumours, and gum disease.

INFORMATION FOR USERS
Your drug prescription is tailored for you. Do not alter dosage without checking with your doctor.

How taken Tablets, liquid, injection, suppositories, gel, cream.

Frequency and timing of doses 3 x daily for 5–10 days, depending on the condition being treated. Sometimes a single large dose is prescribed. Tablets should be taken after meals and swallowed whole with plenty of water.

Adult dosage range 600–1,200mg daily (by mouth); 3g daily (suppositories); 1.5g daily (injection).

Onset of effect Within an hour or so, but beneficial effects may not be felt for 1–2 days.

Duration of action 6–12 hours.

Diet advice None.

Storage Keep in a closed container in a cool, dry place out of reach of children. Protect from light.

Missed dose Take as soon as you remember. If your next dose is due within 2 hours, take a single dose now and skip the next.

Stopping the drug Take the full course. Even if you feel better, the infection may still be present and symptoms may recur if treatment is stopped too soon.

Exceeding the dose An occasional unintentional extra dose is unlikely to cause problems. But if you notice unusual symptoms,

especially numbness or tingling, or if a large overdose has been taken, notify your doctor.

POSSIBLE ADVERSE EFFECTS
Minor gastrointestinal problems, such as dry mouth, metallic taste, nausea, and appetite loss, are common but tend to diminish with time. Headache, dizziness, and darkening of the urine (which is of no concern) may occur. More serious effects on the nervous system, causing numbness or tingling, are very rare.

INTERACTIONS
Oral anticoagulants Metronidazole may increase the effect of oral anticoagulants.

Lithium Metronidazole increases the risk of adverse effects on the kidneys.

Phenytoin Metronidazole may increase the effects of phenytoin.

Cimetidine This drug may increase the levels of metronidazole in the body.

Phenobarbital This drug may reduce the effects of metronidazole.

SPECIAL PRECAUTIONS
Be sure to tell your doctor if:
◆ You have long-term liver problems.
◆ You have a blood disorder.
◆ You have a disorder of the central nervous system, such as epilepsy.
◆ You are taking other medications.

Pregnancy Safety in pregnancy not established. Discuss with your doctor

Breast-feeding The drug passes into the breast milk, but at normal doses adverse effects on the baby are unlikely; may give the milk a bitter taste. Discuss with your doctor.

Infants and children Reduced dose necessary.

Over 60 No special problems.

Driving and hazardous work Avoid such activities until you have learned how metronidazole affects you because the drug can cause dizziness and drowsiness.

Alcohol Avoid. Taken with metronidazole, alcohol may cause flushing, nausea, vomiting, abdominal pain, and headache.

PROLONGED USE
Not usually prescribed for longer than 10 days because loss of sensation in the hands and feet (usually temporary) may occur, and white blood cell production may be reduced.

Miconazole

Brand names Daktarin, Gyno-Daktarin
Used in the following combined preparation
Daktacort

QUICK REFERENCE
Drug group Antifungal drug (p.76)
Overdose danger rating Low
Dependence rating Low
Prescription needed No
Available as generic No

GENERAL INFORMATION

Miconazole is an antifungal drug used to treat candida (yeast) infections of the mouth, candida and bacterial infections of the vagina, and a range of other fungal skin infections. It is available as a gel for oral infections or a special gel for use on dentures. Cream, powder, or ointment are used for skin infections, and several vaginal preparations are available.

Side effects usually only occur with oral forms. Vaginal pessaries, capsules, and cream may damage latex condoms and diaphragms.

INFORMATION FOR USERS

Follow instructions on the label. Call your doctor if symptoms worsen.
How taken Pessaries, vaginal cream/capsules, cream, ointment, gel, dusting powder.
Frequency and timing of doses 4 x daily after food (gel); .1 x weekly for 3 weeks (dental gel); 1–2 x daily (vaginal/skin preparations).
Adult dosage range *Vaginal infections* 1 x 5g applicatorful (cream); 1 x 100mg pessary; 1 x 1.2g capsule. *Oral and skin infections* As directed.
Onset of effect 2–3 days.
Duration of action Up to 12 hours.
Diet advice None.
Storage Keep in a closed container in a cool, dry place out of reach of children.
Missed dose No cause for concern, but apply the missed dose as soon as you remember.
Stopping the drug Unless wheezing or rash occur, apply the full course. Even if you feel better, the infection may still be present and may recur if treatment is stopped too soon.
Exceeding the dose An occasional unintentional extra dose is unlikely to cause problems. However, if you notice any unusual symptoms, or if you have swallowed a large amount, notify your doctor.

POSSIBLE ADVERSE EFFECTS

Apart from local irritation, adverse effects are rare and usually only occur with oral use. Nausea and vomiting may occur. If you have wheezing or a blotchy rash, stop taking the drug and seek urgent medical attention.

INTERACTIONS

Oral anticoagulants, ciclosporin, phenytoin, anti-diabetics, terfenadine, quinidine, and pimozide Miconazole oral gel may increase the effects and toxicity of these drugs.

SPECIAL PRECAUTIONS

Be sure to consult your doctor or pharmacist before taking this drug if:
◆ You have porphyria.
◆ You have liver problems.
◆ You are taking other medications.
Pregnancy Safety not established. Discuss with your doctor.
Breast-feeding Safety not established. Discuss with your doctor.
Infants and children Reduced dose necessary (oral gel).
Over 60 No special problems.
Driving and hazardous work No special problems.
Alcohol No special problems.

PROLONGED USE

No problems expected. Miconazole is not usually prescribed long term, but oral gel may cause diarrhoea if used for a long time.

Minocycline

Brand names Aknemin, Blemix, Dentomycin, Minocin, Minocin MR
Used in the following combined preparations
None

QUICK REFERENCE
Drug group Antibiotic (p.62)
Overdose danger rating Low
Dependence rating Low
Prescription needed Yes
Available as generic Yes

GENERAL INFORMATION

Minocycline is a tetracycline antibiotic but has a substantially longer duration of action than tetracycline itself. The drug is most commonly used to treat acne.

Minocycline may be given to treat pneumonia or to prevent infection in people with chronic bronchitis. It is also used for the treatment of gonorrhea and non-gonococcal urethritis and may be used to treat other sexually transmitted diseases. In addition, it is used to treat chronic gum disease in adults.

The most frequent side effects of minocycline are nausea, vomiting, and diarrhoea. The drug also interferes with the functioning of the balance mechanism in the inner ear, with resultant nausea, dizziness, and unsteadiness, but these symptoms generally disappear after the drug is stopped. Minocycline is not prescribed for people with poor kidney function.

INFORMATION FOR USERS

Your drug prescription is tailored for you. Do not alter dosage without checking with your doctor.

How taken Tablets, capsules, gel.

Frequency and timing of doses 1–2 x daily.

Dosage range *Adults* 100–200mg daily. *Children* Reduced dose according to age and weight.

Onset of effect 4–12 hours.

Duration of action Up to 24 hours.

Diet advice Milk products may impair absorption of minocycline; avoid from 1 hour before, to 2 hours after, dosage.

Storage Keep in a closed container in a cool, dry, well-secured place out of reach of children.

Missed dose Take as soon as you remember. If your next dose is due within 4 hours, take a single dose now and skip the next.

Stopping the drug Unless you experience severe adverse effects (see below), use the full course. Even if you feel better, the original infection may still be present and symptoms may recur if treatment is stopped too soon.

Exceeding the dose An occasional unintentional extra dose is unlikely to be a cause for concern. But if you notice any unusual symptoms, or if a large overdose has been taken, notify your doctor.

POSSIBLE ADVERSE EFFECTS

Nausea, vomiting, or diarrhoea may occasionally occur and, less commonly, rash and increased sensitivity of the skin to sunlight. If dizziness, loss of balance (vertigo), headache, or blurred vision occur, stop taking the drug and consult your doctor immediately.

INTERACTIONS

Oral anticoagulants Minocycline may increase the anticoagulant action of these drugs.

Retinoids Taken with minocycline, these drugs may increase the risk of benign intracranial hypertension (high pressure in the skull), leading to headaches, nausea, and vomiting.

Penicillin antibiotics Minocycline interferes with the antibacterial action of these drugs.

Oral contraceptive drugs Minocycline can reduce the effectiveness of these drugs.

Iron This may interfere with absorption of minocycline and may reduce its effectiveness.

Antacids and milk These interfere with the absorption of minocycline and may reduce its effectiveness. Doses should be separated by 1–2 hours.

SPECIAL PRECAUTIONS

Be sure to tell your doctor if:

◆ You have liver or kidney problems.

◆ You have previously suffered an allergic reaction to a tetracycline antibiotic.

◆ You are taking other medications.

Pregnancy Not prescribed. May damage the developing baby's teeth and bones as well as the mother's liver. Discuss with your doctor.

Breast-feeding The drug passes into the breast milk and may lead to discoloration of the baby's teeth. Discuss with your doctor.

Infants and children Not recommended under 13 years. Reduced dose necessary in older children.

Over 60 No special problems.

Driving and hazardous work Avoid such activities until you have learned how minocycline affects you; the drug can cause dizziness.

Alcohol No known problems.

How to take your tablets To prevent the medication from sticking in your throat, take a few sips of water before, and a full glass after, each dose; swallow the dose while you are sitting or standing; and do not lie down immediately afterwards.

PROLONGED USE

Skin darkening and discoloration of the teeth may occasionally occur with prolonged use.

Monitoring Regular blood tests should be carried out to assess liver function.

Minoxidil

Brand names Loniten, Regaine
Used in the following combined preparations
None

QUICK REFERENCE

Drug group Antihypertensive drug (p.36) and drug for hair loss (p.127)

Overdose danger rating Medium (oral forms); low (topical solution)

Dependence rating Low

Prescription needed Yes (except for scalp lotions)

Available as generic No

GENERAL INFORMATION

Minoxidil is a vasodilator drug (see p.31) that works by relaxing the muscles of artery walls and dilating blood vessels. It is effective in controlling dangerously high, rapidly rising blood pressure. Because the drug is stronger than many other antihypertensives, it is particularly useful for people whose blood pressure is not controlled by other treatment.

Because the drug can cause fluid retention and an increased heart rate, it is usually prescribed with a diuretic (see p.32) and a beta blocker (see p.30) to increase effectiveness and counteract its side effects. Unlike many other antihypertensives, minoxidil rarely causes dizziness and fainting. Its major drawback is that, if taken for more than two months, it increases hair growth, especially on the face. The abnormal growth can be controlled by shaving or depilatories, but can be distressing. This effect is put to use, however, to treat baldness in men and women; for this purpose minoxidil is applied locally as a solution.

INFORMATION FOR USERS

Your drug prescription is tailored for you. Do not alter dosage without checking with your doctor.

How taken Tablets, topical solution.
Frequency and timing of doses 1 x 2 times daily.

Adult dosage range 5mg daily initially, increasing gradually to maximum 50mg daily.

Onset of effect *Blood pressure* Within 1 hour (tablets). *Hair growth* Up to 1 year (solution).

Duration of action Up to 24 hours. Some effect may last for 2–5 days after drug is stopped.

Diet advice None.

Storage Keep in a closed container in a cool, dry place out of reach of children.

Missed dose Take as soon as you remember (tablets). If your next dose is due within 5 hours, take one dose now and skip the next.

Stopping the drug Unless palpitations occur, do not stop taking the drug without consulting your doctor. Stopping the drug may lead to worsening of the underlying condition.

Exceeding the dose An occasional unintentional extra dose is unlikely to cause problems. Large overdoses, however, may cause nausea, vomiting, palpitations, or dizziness; notify your doctor.

POSSIBLE ADVERSE EFFECTS

Side effects are very rare with the lotion. Fluid retention is common with the tablets and may lead to increased bodyweight; diuretics are often given to control this. Allergic and irritant dermatitis may occur with the lotion. Increased body hair growth may occur. Nausea, breast tenderness, dizziness or lightheadedness, and rash are also recognized side effects. If palpitations develop, stop taking the drug and call your doctor without delay.

INTERACTIONS

Antidepressant drugs The hypotensive effects of minoxidil may be enhanced by these drugs.

Other antihypertensives These drugs may increase the effects of minoxidil.

Oestrogens and progestogens These drugs (including those in some contraceptive pills) may reduce the effects of minoxidil.

SPECIAL PRECAUTIONS

Be sure to tell your doctor if:
◆ You have a long-term kidney problem.
◆ You have heart problems.
◆ You retain fluid.
◆ You are taking other medications.

Pregnancy Safety in pregnancy not established. Discuss with your doctor.

Breast-feeding The drug passes into the breast milk, but at normal doses adverse effects on the baby are unlikely. Discuss with your doctor.

Infants and children Reduced dose necessary.

Over 60 Reduced dose may be necessary.

Driving and hazardous work Avoid such activities until you have learned how minoxidil affects you because the drug can cause dizziness and lightheadedness.

Alcohol Avoid. Alcohol may further reduce blood pressure.

Surgery and general anaesthetics Minoxidil may need to be stopped before you have a general anaesthetic. Discuss this with your doctor or dentist before any surgery.

PROLONGED USE

Prolonged use of this drug may lead to swelling of the ankles and increased hair growth.

Misoprostol

Brand name Cytotec
Used in the following combined preparations
Arthrotec, Napratec

QUICK REFERENCE

Drug group Anti-ulcer drug (p.43)
Overdose danger rating Low
Dependence rating Low
Prescription needed Yes
Available as generic No

GENERAL INFORMATION

Misoprostol is related to naturally occurring chemicals called prostaglandins. The drug reduces the amount of acid secreted in the stomach and promotes the healing of gastric and duodenal ulcers. These ulcers may be caused by aspirin (see p.146) and NSAIDs (see p.50) that block certain prostaglandins; the drug can be used to prevent or cure them, and they usually heal after a few weeks of misoprostol treatment. In some cases, misoprostol is given during treatment with these drugs as a preventative; and combined preparations are available that reduce the likelihood of ulcers occurring.

The most likely adverse effects are diarrhoea and abdominal pain, which, if severe, may necessitate stopping treatment. Diarrhoea can be made worse by antacids containing magnesium; these should therefore be avoided.

INFORMATION FOR USERS

Your drug prescription is tailored for you. Do not alter dosage without checking with your doctor.

How taken Tablets.

Frequency and timing of doses 2–4 x daily with or after food.

Adult dosage range 400–800mcg daily.

Onset of effect Within 24 hours.

Duration of action Up to 24 hours; some effects may be longer lasting.

Diet advice None.

Storage Keep in a closed container in a cool, dry place out of reach of children.

Missed dose Take as soon as you remember. If your next dose is due within 3 hours, take a single dose now and skip the next.

Stopping the drug Unless a rash occurs, do not stop taking the drug without consulting your doctor; symptoms may recur.

Exceeding the dose An occasional unintentional extra dose is unlikely to be a cause for concern. But if you notice any unusual symptoms, or if a large overdose has been taken, notify your doctor.

POSSIBLE ADVERSE EFFECTS

Diarrhoea and nausea or vomiting may occur but can be reduced by spreading the doses out during the day. Taking the drug with food may be recommended. Bleeding between periods and abdominal pain may occur. If a rash develops, stop taking the drug and consult your doctor immediately.

INTERACTIONS

Magnesium-containing antacids These may increase the severity of any diarrhoea caused by misoprostol.

SPECIAL PRECAUTIONS

Be sure to tell your doctor if:
◆ You are, or intend to become, pregnant.
◆ You have had a stroke.
◆ You have heart or circulation problems.
◆ You have high blood pressure.
◆ You have bowel problems.
◆ You are taking other medications.

Pregnancy Not prescribed. The drug can cause the uterus to contract before the baby is due.
Breast-feeding Safety not established. Discuss with your doctor.
Infants and children Not recommended.
Over 60 No special problems.
Driving and hazardous work No problems expected.
Alcohol No problems expected, but excessive amounts may impair the drug's desired effect.

PROLONGED USE
No problems expected.

Mometasone

Brand names Elocon, Nasonex
Used in the following combined preparations
None

QUICK REFERENCE
Drug group Corticosteroid (p.78)
Overdose danger rating Low
Dependence rating Low
Prescription needed Yes
Available as generic No

GENERAL INFORMATION
Mometasone is a corticosteroid drug used as a nasal spray to relieve the symptoms of allergic rhinitis. It is also used topically for the treatment of severe inflammatory skin disorders, and in conditions such as eczema that have not responded to other corticosteroids (see Topical corticosteroids, p.120).

Serious adverse effects are rare if the drug is used for short periods or in small amounts. Prolonged or excessive topical use may cause local side effects, such as thin skin with enlarged capillaries, and systemic effects such as weak bones, muscle weakness, and peptic ulcers. Corticosteroids can affect growth, so children using the nasal spray long term may need to have their growth (height) monitored.

INFORMATION FOR USERS
Your drug prescription is tailored for you. Do not alter dosage without checking with your doctor.
How taken Cream, ointment, scalp lotion, nasal spray.

Frequency and timing of doses Once daily.
Dosage range *Nasal spray* 100mcg (2 puffs) into each nostril. *Topical preparations* As directed, applied thinly.
Onset of effect 12 hours. Full beneficial effect develops after 48 hours.
Duration of action 24 hours.
Diet advice None.
Storage Keep in a cool, dry place out of reach of children.
Missed dose Take as soon as you remember. If your next dose/application is due within 8 hours, take a single dose or apply the usual amount now and skip the next.
Stopping the drug Do not stop taking the drug without consulting your doctor; symptoms may recur.
Exceeding the dose An occasional unintentional extra dose or application may not be a cause for concern, but if you notice unusual symptoms, notify your doctor.

POSSIBLE ADVERSE EFFECTS
Irritation of, and sometimes bleeding from, the nose are the most common side effects of mometasone. In the skin, loss of colour, thinning, and increases in the size of capillaries may occur. Acne or dermatitis may develop around the mouth. Sore throat, weight gain, and mood changes are also recognized adverse effects. Discuss all unwanted effects with your doctor.

INTERACTIONS
None.

SPECIAL PRECAUTIONS
Be sure to tell your doctor if:
◆ You have a cold sore, measles, or chickenpox.
◆ You have any other nasal or skin infection.
◆ You have rosacea or acne.
Avoid exposure to chickenpox, measles, or shingles while using mometasone.
Pregnancy Safety not established. Discuss with your doctor.
Breast-feeding No evidence of risk. Discuss with your doctor.
Infants and children Only used for very short courses in children.
Over 60 No special problems.
Driving and hazardous work No special problems.
Alcohol No special problems.

PROLONGED USE

Not advisable. Prolonged use of topical preparations can cause permanent skin changes and should be avoided whenever possible.

Montelukast

Brand name Singulair
Used in the following combined preparations
None

QUICK REFERENCE

Drug group Anti-allergy drug (p.24)
Overdose danger rating Low
Dependence rating Low
Prescription needed Yes
Available as generic No

GENERAL INFORMATION

Montelukast belongs to the leukotriene receptor antagonist group of anti-allergy drugs and is used in the prevention of asthma attacks. It is thought that chemicals called leukotrienes released in the lungs play a part in causing asthma; montelukast works by blocking the receptors for these leukotrienes.

The drug is given as additional medication when combined treatment with corticosteroids and bronchodilators does not give adequate control. It is not a bronchodilator, and cannot be used to treat an acute asthma attack.

INFORMATION FOR USERS

Your drug prescription is tailored for you. Do not alter dosage without checking with your doctor.
How taken Tablets, chewable tablets.
Frequency and timing of doses Once daily, at bedtime, on an empty stomach.
Adult dosage range 10mg.
Onset of effect 2 hours.
Duration of action 24 hours.
Diet advice None.
Storage Keep in a closed container in a cool, dry place out of the reach of children. Protect from light.
Missed dose Take as soon as you remember. If your next dose is due within 8 hours, take a single dose now and skip the next.
Stopping the drug Do not stop the drug without consulting your doctor; symptoms may recur.

Exceeding the dose An occasional unintentional extra dose is unlikely to cause problems. But if you notice unusual symptoms, or if a large overdose has been taken, notify your doctor.

POSSIBLE ADVERSE EFFECTS

Severe adverse effects are rare. There seems to be an increase in incidence of chest infections in people taking this drug. If fever, cough, rash, numbness or tingling, or worsening chest symptoms occur, seek medical advice.

INTERACTIONS

None.

SPECIAL PRECAUTIONS

Be sure to tell your doctor if:
◆ You have phenylketonuria.
◆ You are taking other medications.
Pregnancy Safety not established. Discuss with your doctor.
Breast-feeding Safety not established. Discuss with your doctor.
Infants and children Reduced dose necessary.
Over 60 No special problems.
Driving and hazardous work Avoid such activities until you have learned how montelukast affects you; the drug can cause dizziness.
Alcohol No special problems.

PROLONGED USE

No special problems.

Morphine/Diamorphine

Brand names Morcap SR, MST Continus, MXL, Oramorph, Oramorph SR, Sevredol, Zomorph
Used in the following combined preparations
Cyclimorph

QUICK REFERENCE

Drug group Opioid analgesic (p.9)
Overdose danger rating High
Dependence rating High
Prescription needed Yes
Available as generic Yes

GENERAL INFORMATION

Morphine and diamorphine are opioid analgesic drugs (see p.11). The drugs are derived from opium, obtained from the unripe seed capsules of the opium poppy.

Morphine and diamorphine are used to relieve the severe pain of heart attacks, injury, surgery, or chronic diseases such as cancer. They are also sometimes given as premedication before surgery.

The painkilling effect of the drugs wears off quickly, in contrast to some other opioid analgesics, and morphine may be given in a special slow-release (long-acting) form to relieve continuous severe pain.

These drugs are habit-forming, and, unless they are taken for pain relief over brief periods of time, dependence and addiction can occur. Long-term use for painful conditions does not lead to dependence, but constipation can be a problem.

INFORMATION FOR USERS

Your drug prescription is tailored for you. Do not alter your dosage without checking with your doctor.

How taken Tablets, SR-tablets, capsules, SR-capsules, liquid, SR-granules, injection, suppositories, SR-suppositories.

Frequency and timing of doses Every 4 hours. *SR-preparations* Every 12–24 hours.

Adult dosage range 5–25mg per dose, although some people may need 75mg or more per dose.

Onset of effect Within 1 hour. *SR-preparations* Within 4 hours.

Duration of action 4 hours. *SR-preparations* Up to 24 hours.

Diet advice None.

Storage Keep in a closed container in a cool, dry place out of reach of children.

Missed dose Take as soon as you remember. Return to your normal dosing schedule as soon as possible.

Stopping the drug If the reason for taking morphine or diamorphine no longer exists, you may stop taking the drugs and notify your doctor.

OVERDOSE ACTION

Seek immediate medical advice in all cases. Take emergency action if symptoms such as slow or irregular breathing, severe drowsiness, or loss of consciousness develop.

POSSIBLE ADVERSE EFFECTS

Nausea, vomiting, and constipation are common, especially with high doses, and anti-nausea drugs or laxatives may be needed. Drowsiness, dizziness, and confusion may occur. Slow or irregular breathing may be a sign of overdosage; stop taking the drugs and seek urgent medical attention.

INTERACTIONS

Sedatives Morphine and diamorphine increase the sedative effects of other sedating drugs including antidepressants, antipsychotics, sleeping drugs, and antihistamines.

MAOIs These drugs may produce a severe rise in blood pressure when taken with morphine or diamorphine.

Esmolol The effects of this beta blocker may be increased by morphine or diamorphine.

SPECIAL PRECAUTIONS

Be sure to tell your doctor if:
◆ You have long-term liver or kidney problems.
◆ You have heart or circulatory problems.
◆ You have a lung disorder such as asthma or bronchitis.
◆ You have thyroid disease.
◆ You have a history of epileptic fits.
◆ You are taking other medications.

Pregnancy Not usually prescribed. May cause breathing difficulties in the newborn baby. Discuss with your doctor.

Breast-feeding The drugs pass into the breast milk, but at low doses adverse effects on the baby are unlikely. Discuss with your doctor.

Infants and children Reduced dose necessary.

Over 60 Increased likelihood of adverse effects. Reduced dose may be necessary.

Driving and hazardous work People having morphine treatment are unlikely to be well enough to undertake such activities.

Alcohol Avoid. Alcohol may increase the sedative effects of these drugs.

PROLONGED USE

The effects of these drugs usually become weaker during prolonged use as the body adapts. Dependence may occur if the drugs are taken for extended periods, although this is unusual in patients who are taking the correct dose for pain relief.

Moxonidine

Brand name Physiotens
Used in the following combined preparations
None

QUICK REFERENCE

Drug group Antihypertensive drug (p.36)
Overdose danger rating Medium
Dependence rating Low
Prescription needed Yes
Available as generic No

GENERAL INFORMATION

Moxonidine is an antihypertensive drug that is related to the drug clonidine but is more selective and may therefore have fewer side effects. It works by stimulating receptors within the central nervous system, reducing the signals that constrict the blood vessels. Moxonidine reduces resistance to blood flow in the peripheral blood vessels. It also seems to have actions on the kidneys that result in more sodium and water being excreted.

The drug is less likely than clonidine to cause a dry mouth, and, unlike clonidine, has no effect on blood fat levels or glucose.

INFORMATION FOR USERS

Your drug prescription is tailored for you. Do not alter dosage without checking with your doctor.
How taken Tablets.
Frequency and timing of doses
Once daily in the morning (initially); 1–2 x daily.
Adult dosage range 200mcg daily, increasing after 3 weeks to 400mcg daily (if needed) and again after a further 3 weeks to a maximum of 600mcg daily in 2 divided doses if necessary.
Onset of effect 30–180 minutes.
Duration of action 12 hours.
Diet advice None.
Storage Keep in a closed container in a cool, dry place out of reach of children.
Missed dose Take as soon as you remember. If your next dose is due within 4 hours, take a single dose now and skip the next.
Stopping the drug Do not stop taking the drug without consulting your doctor, who will supervise a gradual reduction in dosage over a period of 2 weeks.

Exceeding the dose An occasional unintentional extra dose is unlikely to cause problems. Large overdoses may cause drowsiness and a fall in blood pressure.

POSSIBLE ADVERSE EFFECTS

Side effects that appear at the start of treatment with moxonidine often decrease in frequency and intensity during the course of treatment. The most common of these are a dry mouth, headache, and weakness or fatigue. Dizziness, drowsiness, nausea, rash, and sleep disturbance are less common.

INTERACTIONS

Other antihypertensives, thymoxamine, and muscle relaxants These may increase the blood-pressure-lowering effect of moxonidine.
Sedatives and hypnotics The effect of these drugs may be increased by moxonidine.

SPECIAL PRECAUTIONS

Be sure to tell your doctor if:
◆ You have liver or kidney problems.
◆ You have heart problems.
◆ You have a history of angioedema.
◆ You have Raynaud's syndrome.
◆ You have epilepsy.
◆ You suffer from depression.
◆ You have Parkinson's disease.
◆ You have glaucoma.
◆ You are taking other medications.
Pregnancy Safety not established. Discuss with your doctor.
Breast-feeding Safety in breast-feeding not established. Discuss with your doctor.
Infants and children Not recommended.
Over 60 No special problems.
Driving and hazardous work Avoid such activities until you have learned how moxonidine affects you because the drug can cause drowsiness and dizziness.
Alcohol Avoid excessive amounts. Alcohol may increase the sedative effects of this drug.

PROLONGED USE

No special problems.

Naftidrofuryl

Brand name Praxilene
Used in the following combined preparations
None

QUICK REFERENCE

Drug group Vasodilator (p.31)
Overdose danger rating Medium
Dependence rating Low
Prescription needed Yes
Available as generic Yes

GENERAL INFORMATION

Naftidrofuryl is a vasodilator drug used in the treatment of peripheral circulatory disorders such as Raynaud's syndrome or intermittent claudication (cramplike pain). Most of these conditions are caused by the blockage of blood vessels due to spasms or sclerosis (hardening) of the vessel walls.

The drug may improve symptoms and mobility, but it is not known if it has any influence on the progress of these disorders. Lifestyle changes such as giving up smoking and taking exercise (and keeping warm in the case of Raynaud's) are often helpful.

Naftidrofuryl has also been tried for treating night cramps and to treat circulatory disorders in the brain.

INFORMATION FOR USERS

Your drug prescription is tailored for you. Do not alter dosage without checking with your doctor.
How taken Capsules.
Frequency and timing of doses 3 x daily.
Adult dosage range 300–600mg daily.
Onset of effect 1 hour.
Duration of action 8 hours.
Diet advice None.
Storage Keep in a closed container in a cool, dry place out of reach of children.
Missed dose Take when you remember. If your next dose is due within 2 hours, take a single dose now and skip the next.
Stopping the drug Unless you experience severe adverse effects, do not stop taking the drug without consulting your doctor; symptoms may recur.
Exceeding the dose An occasional unintentional extra dose is unlikely to cause problems. But large overdoses may cause heart problems and convulsions; notify your doctor immediately.

POSSIBLE ADVERSE EFFECTS

The drug is generally well tolerated, but nausea is common. If, rarely, a rash, chest pain, jaundice, or convulsions occur, stop taking the drug and consult your doctor immediately.

INTERACTIONS

None.

SPECIAL PRECAUTIONS

Be sure to tell your doctor if:
◆ You have liver or kidney problems.
◆ You are taking other medications.
Pregnancy Safety not established. Discuss with your doctor.
Breast-feeding Safety not established. Discuss with your doctor.
Infants and children Not recommended.
Over 60 No special problems.
Driving and hazardous work No special problems.
Alcohol No special problems.

PROLONGED USE

Treatment should be reviewed after 3 months to see if the condition is improving, or if the drug should be stopped.

Naproxen

Brand names Arthrosin, Arthroxen, Naprosyn, Nycopren, Synflex, Timpron, and others
Used in the following combined preparations
Napratec

QUICK REFERENCE

Drug group Non-steroidal anti-inflammatory drug (p50) and drug for gout (p.53)
Overdose danger rating Medium
Dependence rating Low
Prescription needed Yes
Available as generic Yes

GENERAL INFORMATION

Naproxen, one of the non-steroidal anti-inflammatory drugs (NSAIDs), is used to reduce pain, stiffness, and inflammation. The drug relieves the symptoms of adult and juvenile rheumatoid arthritis, ankylosing spondylitis, and osteoarthritis, although it does not cure the underlying disease.

Naproxen is also used to treat acute attacks of gout, and may sometimes be prescribed for the relief of migraine and pain following orthopaedic surgery, dental treatment, strains, and sprains. In addition, it is effective for treating painful menstrual cramps.

Gastrointestinal side effects are fairly common, and there is an increased risk of bleeding. However, naproxen may be safer than aspirin, and in long-term use it needs to be taken only twice daily.

INFORMATION FOR USERS

Your drug prescription is tailored for you. Do not alter dosage without checking with your doctor.

How taken Tablets, liquid, granules, suppositories.

Frequency and timing of doses *General pain relief* Every 6–8 hours as required. *Muscular pain and arthritis* 1–2 x daily. *Gout* Every 8 hours. All doses should be taken with food.

Adult dosage range *Mild to moderate pain, menstrual cramps* 500mg (starting dose), then 250mg every 6–8 hours as required. *Muscular pain and arthritis* 500–1,250mg daily. *Gout* 750mg (starting dose), then 250mg every 8 hours until attack has subsided.

Onset of effect Pain relief begins within 1 hour. Full anti-inflammatory effect may take 2 weeks to develop.

Duration of action Up to 12 hours.

Diet advice None.

Storage Keep in a closed container in a cool, dry place out of reach of children. Protect from light.

Missed dose Take as soon as you remember. If your next dose is due within 4 hours, take a single dose now and skip the next.

Stopping the drug When taken for short-term pain relief, naproxen can be safely stopped as soon as you no longer need it. Seek medical advice before stopping long-term treatment unless serious adverse effects occur (see below).

Exceeding the dose An occasional unintentional extra dose is unlikely to be a cause for concern. But if you notice any unusual symptoms, or if a large overdose has been taken, notify your doctor.

POSSIBLE ADVERSE EFFECTS

Most adverse effects of naproxen are not serious and may diminish with time. Stomach irritation is common and may lead to dyspepsia or abdominal pain. If you have a headache, inability to concentrate, ringing in the ears, or swollen feet or ankles, discuss with your doctor. Stop taking the drug and notify your doctor immediately if rash or itching, wheezing or breathlessness, or black or bloodstained bowel movements occur.

INTERACTIONS

General note Naproxen interacts with a wide range of drugs to increase the risk of bleeding and/or peptic ulcers. It may also increase the blood levels of lithium, methotrexate, and digoxin to an undesirable extent.

Antihypertensive drugs and diuretics The beneficial effects of these drugs may be reduced by naproxen.

SPECIAL PRECAUTIONS

Be sure to tell your doctor if:
♦ You have any long-term liver or kidney problems.
♦ You have heart problems.
♦ You have a bleeding disorder.
♦ You have high blood pressure.
♦ You have had a peptic ulcer, oesophagitis, or acid indigestion.
♦ You are allergic to aspirin.
♦ You suffer from asthma.
♦ You are taking other medications.

Pregnancy Not usually prescribed. When taken in the last 3 months of pregnancy, the drug may increase the risk of adverse effects on the baby's heart and may prolong labour. Discuss with your doctor.

Breast-feeding The drug passes into the breast milk, but at normal doses adverse effects on the baby are unlikely. Discuss with your doctor.

Infants and children Prescribed only to treat juvenile arthritis. Reduced dose necessary.

Over 60 Reduced dose may be necessary. Increased likelihood of adverse effects.

Driving and hazardous work Avoid such activities until you have learned how naproxen affects you because the drug may reduce your ability to concentrate.

Alcohol Keep consumption low. Alcohol may increase the risk of stomach irritation with naproxen.

Surgery and general anaesthetics Naproxen may prolong bleeding. Discuss with your doctor or dentist before surgery.

PROLONGED USE

There is an increased risk of bleeding from peptic ulcers and in the bowel when naproxen is used long term.

Nicorandil

Brand name Ikorel
Used in the following combined preparations
None

QUICK REFERENCE

Drug group Anti-angina drug (p.35
Overdose danger rating Medium
Dependence rating Low
Prescription needed Yes
Available as generic No

GENERAL INFORMATION

Nicorandil is the only generally available member of a group of drugs known as potassium channel openers. It is used to treat angina pectoris.

The chest pain of angina results from the failure of narrowed coronary blood vessels to deliver sufficient oxygen to the heart. Nicorandil acts by widening blood vessels by a different mechanism to other anti-angina drugs, and is notable because it widens both veins and arteries. As a result of this action, more oxygen-carrying blood reaches the heart muscle. In addition, the heart's work load is reduced, since the resistance against which it has to pump is decreased.

Nicorandil is as effective as other drugs used to treat angina, and when used in combination with others may add to their effects.

INFORMATION FOR USERS

Your drug prescription is tailored for you. Do not alter dosage without checking with your doctor.

How taken Tablets.
Frequency and timing of doses 2 x daily.
Adult dosage range 10–60mg daily.
Onset of effect Within 1 hour.
Duration of action Approximately 12 hours.
Diet advice None.
Storage Keep in a closed container in a cool, dry place out of reach of children.
Missed dose Take as soon as you remember. If your next dose is due within 4 hours, take a single dose now and skip the next.
Stopping the drug Unless you experience palpitations, do not stop the drug without consulting your doctor. Stopping the drug may lead to worsening of the underlying condition.
Exceeding the dose An occasional unintentional extra dose is unlikely to cause problems. Large overdoses, however, may cause unusual dizziness and dangerously low blood pressure; notify your doctor.

POSSIBLE ADVERSE EFFECTS

Adverse effects, such as headache, flushing, and nausea and vomiting, are usually minor and usually wear off with continued treatment, but they may necessitate a dose reduction in some cases. Stop taking the drug and consult your doctor immediately if you experience palpitations or develop jaundice.

INTERACTIONS

Tricyclic antidepressant drugs These may increase the effects of nicorandil on blood pressure, resulting in dizziness.
Antihypertensive drugs Nicorandil may increase the effects of these drugs.
Sildenafil This drug greatly increases the effects of nicorandil on blood pressure.

SPECIAL PRECAUTIONS

Be sure to tell your doctor if:
◆ You are taking other medications.
◆ You have low blood pressure.
◆ You have other heart problems.
Pregnancy Safety in pregnancy not established. Discuss with your doctor.
Breast-feeding Safety not established. Discuss with your doctor.
Infants and children Not recommended.
Over 60 No special problems.
Driving and hazardous work Avoid such activities until you have learned how nicorandil

affects you because the drug can cause dizziness as a result of lowered blood pressure.

Alcohol Avoid until you are accustomed to the effect of nicorandil. Alcohol may further reduce blood pressure, causing dizziness or other symptoms.

PROLONGED USE

No problems expected.

Nicotine

Brand names Boots Nicotine Gum, Boots Nicotine Inhalator, Boots NRT Patch, Nicorette, Nicotinell, NiQuitin CQ
Used in the following combined preparations
None

QUICK REFERENCE

Drug group Tobacco-smoking deterrent
Overdose danger rating Medium
Dependence rating Low
Prescription needed No
Available as generic No

GENERAL INFORMATION

Smoking is a difficult habit to stop due to the addiction to nicotine and the psychological attachment to cigarettes or other forms of tobacco. Taking nicotine in a different form can help a smoker deal with the two aspects of the habit separately. Nicotine is available as chewing gum, nasal spray, sublingual tablets, skin patches, lozenges, and an inhalator for the relief of withdrawal symptoms.

The patches should be applied every 24 hours to unbroken, dry, and non-hairy skin on the trunk or the upper arm. Replacement patches should be placed on a different area, and the same area of application avoided for several days. The strength of the patch is gradually reduced, and abstinence is generally achieved within 3 months.

The chewing gum or nasal spray are used when the urge to smoke occurs. The gum is chewed slowly for up to 30 minutes, by which time all available nicotine has been released.

INFORMATION FOR USERS

Follow instructions on the label. Call your doctor if symptoms worsen.

How taken Sublingual tablets, lozenges, skin patch, nasal spray, inhalator, chewing gum.
Frequency and timing of doses Hourly (tablets and lozenges); every 24 hours, removing the patch after 16 hours (patches); when the urge to smoke is felt (gum, inhalator).
Adult dosage range Depends on previous smoking habits. 7–22mg per day (patches); 1 x 2mg piece to 15 x 4mg pieces per day (gum); up to 64 x 0.5mg puffs (spray).
Onset of effect A few hours (patches); within minutes (other forms).
Duration of action Up to 24 hours (patches); 30 minutes (other forms).
Diet advice None.
Storage Keep in a cool, dry place out of reach of children.
Missed dose Change your patch as soon as you remember, and keep the new patch on for the required amount of time before removing it.
Stopping the drug The dose of nicotine is normally reduced gradually.
Exceeding the dose Application of several nicotine patches at the same time could result in serious overdosage. Seek immediate medical help. Overdosage with the tablets, lozenges, gum, or spray can occur only if tablets or lozenges are taken more often than every hour, if many pieces of gum are chewed at once, or if the spray is used more than 4 times an hour. Seek immediate medical help.

POSSIBLE ADVERSE EFFECTS

Any skin reaction to nicotine patches will usually disappear in a couple of days. The chewing gum and nasal spray may cause local irritation of the throat or nose and increased salivation. Other recognized side effects of the drug include headache, dizziness, nausea, flu-like symptoms, indigestion, and insomnia.

INTERACTIONS

General note Nicotine patches, chewing gum, and nasal spray should not be used with other nicotine-containing products, including cigarettes. Stopping smoking may increase the blood levels of some drugs (such as warfarin and theophylline/aminophylline). Discuss with your doctor or pharmacist.

SPECIAL PRECAUTIONS

Be sure to consult your doctor or pharmacist before taking this drug if:

◆ You have long-term liver or kidney problems.

◆ You have diabetes mellitus.

◆ You have thyroid disease.

◆ You have circulation problems.

◆ You have heart problems.

◆ You have a peptic ulcer.

◆ You have phaeochromocytoma.

◆ You have any skin disorders.

◆ You are taking other medications.

Pregnancy Nicotine should not be used (in any form) during pregnancy.

Breast-feeding Nicotine should not be used (in any form) while breast-feeding.

Infants and children Nicotine products should not be administered to children.

Over 60 No special problems.

Driving and hazardous work Usually no problems.

Alcohol No special problems.

PROLONGED USE

Nicotine replacement therapy should not normally be used for more than 3 months.

Nifedipine

Brand names Adalat, Adipine MR, Angiopine, Cardilate MR, Coracten, Coroday MR, Fortipine LA, Tensipine MR, and others
Used in the following combined preparations
Beta-Adalat, Tenif

QUICK REFERENCE

Drug group Anti-angina drug (p.35) and antihypertensive drug (p.36)
Overdose danger rating Medium
Dependence rating Low
Prescription needed Yes
Available as generic Yes

GENERAL INFORMATION

Nifedipine belongs to a group of drugs called calcium channel blockers, which interfere with conduction of signals in the muscles of the heart and blood vessels.

Nifedipine is given for the treatment of angina, as a regular medication to help prevent attacks. Unlike some other anti-angina drugs, such as beta blockers, the drug can be used safely by people with asthma.

Nifedipine is also widely used to reduce high blood pressure and is often helpful in improving circulation to the limbs in disorders such as Raynaud's disease.

In common with other drugs of its class, nifedipine may cause blood pressure to fall too low, and may occasionally cause disturbances of heart rhythm. In rare cases, angina worsens as a result of taking nifedipine, and another drug must be substituted.

INFORMATION FOR USERS

Your drug prescription is tailored for you. Do not alter dosage without checking with your doctor.

How taken Tablets, capsules, SR-tablets, SR-capsules.

Frequency and timing of doses 3 x daily; 1–2 x daily (SR-preparations). For angina attacks, a capsule may be bitten and the liquid kept in the mouth or swallowed.

Adult dosage range 15–90mg daily.

Onset of effect 30–60 minutes. When capsules are bitten, the effects may be felt within minutes.

Duration of action 6–24 hours.

Diet advice Nifedipine should not be taken together with grapefruit juice (see Interactions, below).

Storage Keep in a closed container in a cool, dry place out of reach of children. Protect from light.

Missed dose Take as soon as you remember, or when needed. If your next dose is due within 3 hours, take a single dose now and skip the next.

Stopping the drug Do not stop taking the drug without consulting your doctor; sudden withdrawal may make angina worse.

Exceeding the dose An occasional unintentional extra dose is unlikely to cause problems. Large overdoses may cause dizziness; notify your doctor.

POSSIBLE ADVERSE EFFECTS

Nifedipine can cause various minor adverse effects such as headache, flushing, ankle swelling, dizziness, and fatigue. Rarer effects include rash, palpitations, and frequency in passing urine. If any of these symptoms are severe, contact your doctor. Patients with angina may notice an increase in the severity or frequency of attacks after starting treatment. If this occurs, stop taking the drug and consult your doctor immediately. Sometimes dosage adjustment or a change of drug may be necessary.

INTERACTIONS

Antihypertensive and anti-angina drugs Nifedipine may increase the effects of these drugs.

Phenytoin Nifedipine may increase the effects of phenytoin.

Digoxin Nifedipine may increase the effects and toxicity of digoxin.

Rifampicin This drug may decrease the effects of nifedipine.

Grapefruit juice This may block the breakdown of nifedipine, increasing its effects.

SPECIAL PRECAUTIONS

Be sure to tell your doctor if:
◆ You have liver or kidney problems.
◆ You have heart failure.
◆ You have had a recent heart attack.
◆ You have aortic stenosis.
◆ You have diabetes.
◆ You are taking other medications.

Pregnancy Not usually prescribed. The drug may cause abnormalities in the developing baby and delay labour. Discuss with your doctor.

Breast-feeding The drug passes into the breast milk and may affect the baby. Discuss with your doctor.

Infants and children Not recommended.

Over 60 Reduced dose may be necessary. Increased likelihood of adverse effects.

Driving and hazardous work Avoid such activities until you have learned how nifedipine affects you because the drug can cause dizziness as a result of lowered blood pressure.

Alcohol Keep consumption low. Alcohol may further reduce blood pressure, causing dizziness or other symptoms.

Surgery and general anaesthetics Nifedipine may interact with some general anaesthetics, causing a fall in blood pressure. Discuss this with your doctor or dentist before any surgery.

PROLONGED USE

No problems expected.

Nitrazepam

Brand names Mogadon, Remnos, Somnite
Used in the following combined preparations
None

QUICK REFERENCE

Drug group Sleeping drug (p.11)
Overdose danger rating Medium
Dependence rating High
Prescription needed Yes
Available as generic Yes

GENERAL INFORMATION

Nitrazepam is a long-acting benzodiazepine drug that is used as a sleeping drug. Benzodiazepine drugs relieve tension and nervousness, relax muscles, and encourage sleep. When nitrazepam is taken at night, it has effects that are still present the next day. When nitrazepam is taken every night, its effects gradually accumulate. Therefore, the drug is usually only prescribed in short courses of one or two weeks. Long-term use of nitrazepam leads to daytime sedation, tolerance, and dependence.

Stopping treatment with nitrazepam after prolonged use results in rebound insomnia, anxiety, and a withdrawal syndrome that may include confusion, toxic psychosis, and convulsions. In such cases, a tapering-off period will be necessary. The actual time that is needed for withdrawal can vary from a few weeks to many months.

The use of benzodiazepine drugs to treat insomnia is recommended only for people in whom the problem is severe, disabling, or very distressing.

INFORMATION FOR USERS

Your drug prescription is tailored for you. Do not alter dosage without checking with your doctor.

How taken Tablets, liquid.
Frequency and timing of doses Once daily, at bedtime.
Adult dosage range 5–10mg daily.
Onset of effect 30–60 minutes.
Duration of action 24 hours or more.
Diet advice None.
Storage Keep in a closed container in a cool, dry place out of reach of children.

Missed dose If you fall asleep without having taken a dose and wake some hours later, do not take the missed dose. If necessary, return to your normal dosing schedule the following night.

Stopping the drug If you have been taking the drug for 2 weeks or less, it can be safely stopped. If you have been taking the drug for longer, consult your doctor, who may supervise a gradual reduction in dosage. Stopping abruptly may lead to withdrawal symptoms.

Exceeding the dose An occasional unintentional extra dose is unlikely to be a cause for concern. Large overdoses may cause unusual drowsiness; notify your doctor.

POSSIBLE ADVERSE EFFECTS

The main adverse effects are related primarily to the sedative and tranquillizing properties of nitrazepam; they include drowsiness (the next day), confusion and forgetfulness, dizziness or double vision, and uncoordinated walking. Consult your doctor if any of these effects are severe. Headache, vertigo, and rash may also occur but are less common. If you suffer from any mood changes or restlessness, consult your doctor.

INTERACTIONS

Sedatives All drugs that have a sedative effect on the central nervous system are likely to increase the sedative properties of nitrazepam. Such drug include other sleeping drugs, anti-anxiety drugs, antihistamines, opioid analgesics, antidepressants, and antipsychotics.

Rifampicin This drug reduces the effect of nitrazepam.

Antiepileptic drugs The side effects and toxicity of these drugs may be increased by nitrazepam.

Macrolide antibacterials and imidazole and triazole antifungals These drugs increase the levels and toxicity of nitrazepam.

SPECIAL PRECAUTIONS

Be sure to tell your doctor if:
◆ You have severe respiratory disease.
◆ You have porphyria.
◆ You have kidney or liver problems.
◆ You suffer from depression.
◆ You have myasthenia gravis.
◆ You suffer from sleep apnoea.

◆ You have had problems with alcohol or drug abuse.
◆ You are taking other medications.

Pregnancy Safety not established. The drug affects the developing baby, who may be born with dependence and suffer withdrawal symptoms. Discuss with your doctor.

Breast-feeding Avoid. Nitrazepam passes into the breast milk and may affect the baby.

Infants and children Not recommended.

Over 60 Reduced dose necessary.

Driving and hazardous work Do not undertake such activities. Nitrazepam will still affect you the day after taking a dose. The drug reduces alertness, slows reactions, impairs concentration, and causes drowsiness.

Alcohol Avoid. Alcohol enhances the sedative effects of nitrazepam.

PROLONGED USE

Not recommended. Nitrazepam produces tolerance and dependence.

Norethisterone

Brand names Micronor, Noriday, Noristerat, Primolut N, Utovlan
Used in the following combined preparations Brevinor, Climagest, Loestrin, Norinyl, Synphase, TriNovum, and others

QUICK REFERENCE

Drug group Female sex hormone (p.88)
Overdose danger rating Low
Dependence rating Low
Prescription needed Yes
Available as generic Yes

GENERAL INFORMATION

Norethisterone is a progestogen: a synthetic hormone similar to a natural female sex hormone, progesterone. It has a wide variety of uses including the postponement of menstruation and the treatment of menstrual disorders such as endometriosis (see p.105). In these cases, it is only taken on certain days during the menstrual cycle. It is also used in hormone replacement therapy (HRT) and in treating certain types of breast cancer.

One of the major uses of norethisterone is as an oral contraceptive, either on its own or together with an oestrogen. Norethisterone is also available, in special circumstances, in an injectable contraceptive preparation.

Adverse effects from the drug are rare, but contraceptive preparations containing it may cause "breakthrough" bleeding (see p.107).

INFORMATION FOR USERS

Your drug prescription is tailored for you. Do not alter dosage without checking with your doctor.

How taken Tablets, injection, skin patches.

Frequency and timing of doses 1–3 x daily (tablets); once every 8 weeks (injection); 2 x weekly (skin patches).

Adult dosage range *Menstrual disorders* 10–15mg daily. *Postponement of menstruation* 15mg daily. *Progestogen-only contraceptives* 350mcg daily. *HRT* 700mcg–1mg daily. *Cancer* 30–60mg daily.

Onset of effect The drug starts to act within a few hours.

Duration of action 24 hours.

Diet advice None.

Storage Keep in a closed container in a cool, dry place out of reach of children. Protect from light.

Missed dose Take as soon as you remember. If you are taking the drug for contraception, see What to do if you miss a pill (p.109).

Stopping the drug The drug can be safely stopped as soon as contraceptive protection is no longer required. If it is prescribed for an underlying disorder, do not stop taking it without consulting your doctor.

Exceeding the dose An occasional unintentional extra dose is unlikely to be a cause for concern. But if you notice any unusual symptoms, or if a large overdose has been taken, notify your doctor.

POSSIBLE ADVERSE EFFECTS

Adverse effects are rare. They include breakthrough bleeding, swollen feet or ankles, weight gain, headache, and depression. Prolonged treatment may cause jaundice due to liver damage. If this develops, stop taking the drug and notify your doctor immediately.

INTERACTIONS

General note Norethisterone may interfere with the beneficial effects of many drugs, including oral anticoagulants, anticonvulsants, antihypertensives, and antidiabetic drugs. Many other drugs, including anticonvulsants, antituberculous drugs, and antibiotics, may reduce the contraceptive effect of pills containing norethisterone. Always inform your doctor that you are taking norethisterone before taking additional prescribed medication.

Ciclosporin Levels of ciclosporin may be raised by norethisterone.

SPECIAL PRECAUTIONS

Be sure to tell your doctor if:
◆ You have liver or kidney problems.
◆ You have diabetes.
◆ You have had epileptic fits.
◆ You suffer from migraines.
◆ You have acute porphyria.
◆ You have heart or circulatory problems.
◆ You are taking other medications.

Pregnancy Not usually prescribed. May cause defects in the unborn baby. Discuss with your doctor.

Breast-feeding The drug passes into the breast milk, but at normal doses adverse effects on the baby are unlikely. Discuss with your doctor.

Infants and children Not prescribed.

Over 60 Not usually prescribed.

Driving and hazardous work No special problems.

Alcohol No special problems.

PROLONGED USE

Prolonged use may in rare cases cause liver damage.

Monitoring Blood tests to check liver function may be carried out.

Nystatin

Brand names Nystamont, Nystan
Used in the following combined preparations
Dermovate-NN, Nystaform, Timodine, Tinaderm-M, and others

QUICK REFERENCE

Drug group Antifungal drug (p.76)
Overdose danger rating Low
Dependence rating Low
Prescription needed Yes
Available as generic Yes

GENERAL INFORMATION

Nystatin is an antifungal drug named after the New York State Institute of Health, where it was developed in the early 1950s.

Nystatin has been used effectively against candidiasis (thrush), an infection caused by the *Candida* yeast. Available in a variety of dosage forms, it is used for infections of the skin, mouth, throat, intestinal tract, oesophagus, and vagina. It is of little use against systemic infections, however, because it is poorly absorbed into the bloodstream from the digestive tract. Nystatin is not given by injection.

Nystatin rarely causes adverse effects and can be used during pregnancy to treat vaginal candidiasis.

INFORMATION FOR USERS

Your drug prescription is tailored for you. Do not alter dosage without checking with your doctor.

How taken Tablets, pastilles, liquid, pessaries, cream, ointment.

Frequency and timing of doses *Mouth or throat infections* 4 x daily; liquid should be held in the mouth for several minutes before being swallowed. *Intestinal infections* 4 x daily. *Skin infections* 2–4 x daily. *Vaginal infections* Once daily for 2 weeks.

Adult dosage range 2–4 million units daily (by mouth); 100,000–200,000 units at night (pessaries); 1–2 applicatorfuls (vaginal cream); as directed (skin preparations).

Onset of effect The full beneficial effect may not be felt for 7–14 days.

Duration of action Up to 6 hours.

Diet advice None.

Storage Keep in a closed container in a cool, dry place out of reach of children. Protect from light.

Missed dose Take as soon as you remember. Take your next dose as usual.

Stopping the drug Take the full course. Even if the affected area seems to be cured, the original infection may still be present, and symptoms may recur if treatment is stopped too soon.

Exceeding the dose An occasional unintentional extra dose is unlikely to be a cause for concern. But if you notice any unusual symptoms, or if a large overdose has been taken, notify your doctor.

POSSIBLE ADVERSE EFFECTS

Adverse effects are uncommon and are usually mild and transient. Nausea and vomiting may occur when high doses of the drug are taken by mouth. If you develop diarrhoea or a rash, consult your doctor.

INTERACTIONS

None.

SPECIAL PRECAUTIONS

Be sure to tell your doctor if:
◆ You are taking other medications.

Pregnancy No evidence of risk to the developing baby.

Breast-feeding No evidence of risk.

Infants and children Reduced dose necessary.

Over 60 No special problems.

Driving and hazardous work No known problems.

Alcohol No known problems.

PROLONGED USE

No problems expected. Nystatin is usually given as a course of treatment until the infection is cured.

Olanzapine

Brand name Zyprexa
Used in the following combined preparations
None

QUICK REFERENCE

Drug group Antipsychotic drug (p.15)
Overdose danger rating Medium
Dependence rating Low
Prescription needed Yes
Available as generic No

GENERAL INFORMATION

Olanzapine is an atypical antipsychotic drug
that is prescribed for the treatment of
schizophrenia and mania. The drug works by
blocking several different receptors in the
brain, including dopamine, histamine, and
serotonin receptors.

In schizophrenia, the drug can be used to
treat both "positive" symptoms (delusions,
hallucinations, and thought disorders) and
"negative" symptoms (blunted affect and
emotional and social withdrawal). In mania,
olanzapine can be used alone or in combination with other drugs.

The drug stays in the body longer in
women, non-smokers, and elderly people.
Lower starting and maintenance doses may
be used in these groups.

INFORMATION FOR USERS

Your drug prescription is tailored for you.
Do not alter dosage without checking with
your doctor.
How taken Tablets, dispersible tablets.
Frequency and timing of doses Once daily.
Adult dosage range *Schizophrenia* 10mg (starting dose). *Mania* 15mg if used alone or 10mg
if used in combination with other drugs
(starting dose). For both conditions, the
dose can be adjusted to between 5mg
and 20mg daily.
Onset of effect 4–8 hours.
Duration of action 30–38 hours, but longer
in women than in men, and longer in elderly
people.
Diet advice None.
Storage Keep in a closed container in a cool,
dry place out of reach of children. Protect
from light.

Missed dose Take as soon as you remember. If
your next dose is due within 8 hours, take a
single dose now and skip the next.
Stopping the drug Do not stop taking the
drug without consulting your doctor; symptoms may recur.
Exceeding the dose An occasional unintentional extra dose is unlikely to cause problems. Large overdoses, however, may cause
unusual drowsiness, depressed breathing,
and low blood pressure; notify your doctor.

POSSIBLE ADVERSE EFFECTS

Unusual drowsiness and weight gain are common. Consult your doctor if fainting or dizziness, tremor, or a persistent sore throat occur.
Rarely, the drug may cause parkinsonism.

INTERACTIONS

Sedatives All drugs that have a sedative effect
on the central nervous system may increase
the sedative effects of olanzapine.
Anticonvulsants Olanzapine opposes the effects of these drugs. Carbamazepine decreases the effects of olanzapine.
Anti-arrhythmics There is an increased risk of
arrhythmias when certain of these drugs are
used with olanzapine.

SPECIAL PRECAUTIONS

Be sure to tell your doctor if:
◆ You have an enlarged prostate.
◆ You have kidney or liver problems.
◆ You have diabetes.
◆ You have glaucoma.
◆ You have epilepsy.
◆ You are taking other medications.
Pregnancy Safety not established. Discuss
with your doctor.
Breast-feeding Safety not established. Discuss
with your doctor.
Infants and children Not recommended.
Over 60 Reduced dose necessary.
Driving and hazardous work Avoid. Olanza-
pine can cause unusual drowsiness.
Alcohol Avoid. Alcohol increases the sedative
effects of olanzapine.

PROLONGED USE

Prolonged use may, in rare cases, cause tardive dyskinesia, in which there are involuntary movements of the tongue and face.

Omeprazole

Brand name Losec
Used in the following combined preparations
None

QUICK REFERENCE

Drug group Anti-ulcer drug (p.43)
Overdose danger rating Low
Dependence rating Low
Prescription needed Yes
Available as generic Yes

GENERAL INFORMATION

Omeprazole, an anti-ulcer drug, was introduced in 1989 and is used to treat stomach and duodenal ulcers as well as reflux oesophagitis, a condition in which acid from the stomach rises into the oesophagus. It reduces (by about 70 per cent) the amount of acid produced by the stomach and works in a different way to some of the other anti-ulcer drugs that reduce acid secretion.

The drug is usually given for four to eight weeks, depending on the condition that is being treated. Omeprazole may also be given with antibiotics to eradicate *Helicobacter pylori* bacteria, which cause many gastric ulcers. Reflux oesophagitis may be treated for four to 12 weeks.

Omeprazole causes few serious side effects. However, because the drug may affect the actions of enzymes in the liver, where many drugs are broken down, it may increase the effects of ciclosporin, warfarin, and phenytoin, and these drugs require more careful monitoring when they are being used with omeprazole.

INFORMATION FOR USERS

Your drug prescription is tailored for you. Do not alter dosage without checking with your doctor.
How taken Tablets, capsules, injection, intravenous infusion.
Frequency and timing of doses 1–2 x daily.
Adult dosage range 10–40mg daily and sometimes up to 120mg daily.
Onset of effect 2–5 hours.
Duration of action 24 hours.
Diet advice None, but spicy foods and alcohol may exacerbate the underlying condition.

Storage Keep in a closed container in a cool, dry place out of reach of children. Omeprazole is very sensitive to moisture. It must not be transferred to another container and must be used within 3 months of opening.
Missed dose Take as soon as you remember. If your next dose is due within 8 hours, take a single dose now and skip the next.
Stopping the drug Unless a rash occurs, do not stop taking the drug without consulting your doctor; symptoms may recur.
Exceeding the dose An occasional unintentional extra dose is unlikely to be a cause for concern. But if you notice any unusual symptoms, or if a large overdose has been taken, notify your doctor.

POSSIBLE ADVERSE EFFECTS

Adverse effects such as headache and diarrhoea are usually mild, and often diminish with continued use of the drug. Less commonly, rash, nausea and constipation may occur. If you develop a rash, stop taking the drug and notify your doctor.

INTERACTIONS

Warfarin The effects of warfarin may be increased by omeprazole.
Phenytoin The effects of phenytoin may be increased by omeprazole.
Ciclosporin Blood levels of ciclosporin are raised by omeprazole.

SPECIAL PRECAUTIONS

Be sure to tell your doctor if:
◆ You have a long-term liver problem.
◆ You are taking other medications.
Pregnancy Safety in pregnancy not established. Discuss with your doctor.
Breast-feeding The drug may pass into the breast milk. Safety in breast-feeding not established. Discuss with your doctor.
Infants and children Not recommended.
Over 60 No special problems.
Driving and hazardous work No special problems.
Alcohol Avoid. Alcohol may aggravate your underlying condition and reduce the beneficial effects of this drug.

PROLONGED USE

No problems expected.

Ondansetron

Brand name Zofran
Used in the following combined preparations
None

QUICK REFERENCE

Drug group Anti-emetic (p.21
Overdose danger rating Low
Dependence rating Low
Prescription needed Yes
Available as generic No

GENERAL INFORMATION

Ondansetron, an anti-emetic, is used especially for treating the nausea and vomiting associated with radiotherapy and anticancer drugs such as cisplatin. It may also be given for nausea and vomiting following surgery.

The dose and frequency of ondansetron treatment depend on the anticancer drug. In most cases, you will receive a dose, either by mouth or injection, before infusion of the anticancer agent, then tablets for up to 5 days after the treatment has finished. Ondansetron is less effective against the delayed nausea and vomiting that occur several days after chemotherapy than it is against the symptoms that occur soon after anticancer treatment.

To enhance its effectiveness, the drug is usually taken with others, such as dexamethasone (see p.210). Serious adverse effects are unlikely.

INFORMATION FOR USERS

Your drug prescription is tailored for you. Do not alter dosage without checking with your doctor.
How taken Tablets, sublingual tablets, liquid, injection, suppositories.
Frequency and timing of doses Normally 2 x daily; frequency depends on reason for use.
Adult dosage range 4–32mg daily depending on the reason for which it is being used.
Onset of effect Within 1 hour.
Duration of action Approximately 12 hours.
Diet advice None.
Storage Keep in a closed container in a cool, dry place out of reach of children. Protect from light.
Missed dose Take as soon as you remember. If your next dose is due within 2 hours, take a single dose now and skip the next.

Stopping the drug Can be safely stopped as soon as you no longer need it.
Exceeding the dose An occasional unintentional extra dose is unlikely to be a problem. If you notice unusual symptoms, or if a large overdose has been taken, notify your doctor.

POSSIBLE ADVERSE EFFECTS

Unlike some other anti-emetics, the drug does not cause sedation and movement disorders. You may have a headache and constipation, or (less commonly) a warm feeling in the head or stomach. If palpitations or fits occur, consult your doctor.

INTERACTIONS

None.

SPECIAL PRECAUTIONS

Be sure to tell your doctor if:
◆ You have a long-term liver problem.
◆ You are taking other medications.
Pregnancy Safety in pregnancy not established. Discuss with your doctor.
Breast-feeding The drug passes into the breast milk. Discuss with your doctor.
Infants and children Reduced dose necessary.
Over 60 No special problems.
Driving and hazardous work No problems expected.
Alcohol No known problems.

PROLONGED USE

Not generally prescribed long term.

Orlistat

Brand name Xenical
Used in the following combined preparations
None

QUICK REFERENCE

Drug group Anti-obesity drug
Overdose danger rating Low
Dependence rating Low
Prescription needed Yes
Available as generic No

GENERAL INFORMATION

Orlistat blocks the action of stomach and pancreatic enzymes (lipases) that digest fats, so that the fats are not absorbed into the body but pass through to be excreted in the faeces. As a result, the body must burn stored fat to provide energy, which gradually reduces fat stores and produces weight loss. The drug's effectiveness varies from person to person.

Because orlistat works by making the faeces oily, flatulence can occur. Its effectiveness may be partly due to people reducing their fat intake to avoid the unpleasant side effects.

As fat absorption is greatly reduced, there is a danger that fat-soluble vitamins (A, D, E, and K) might be lost to the body. Vitamin supplements may be prescribed to compensate. The vitamins should be taken at a different time from the orlistat; bedtime might be best, or at least 2 hours apart from an orlistat dose.

INFORMATION FOR USERS

Your drug prescription is tailored for you. Do not alter dosage without checking with your doctor.

How taken Capsules.

Frequency and timing of doses Just before, during, or up to 1 hour after each main meal (up to 3 x daily). If a meal is omitted or contains no fat, do not take the dose of orlistat.

Adult dosage range 120–360mg daily.

Onset of effect 30 minutes; excretion of excess faecal fat begins about 24–48 hours after the first dose.

Duration of action The drug is not absorbed from the gut and can continue to work as it passes through the intestines. Faeces return to normal 48–72 hours after treatment is stopped.

Diet advice Eat a balanced diet that does not contain quite enough calories, and that provides about 30 per cent of the calories as fat. Eat lots of fruit and vegetables. The intake of fat, carbohydrate, and protein should be distributed over the three main meals.

Storage Keep in a closed container in a cool, dry place. Keep out of reach of children.

Missed dose No cause for concern. Take the next dose with the next meal.

Stopping the drug The drug can be safely stopped as soon as it is no longer needed, but notify your doctor.

POSSIBLE ADVERSE EFFECTS

Most side effects depend on the dose and on how much fat is eaten. Side effects include liquid, oily stools, faecal urgency, abdominal or rectal pain, headache, nausea, flatulence, menstrual irregularities, anxiety, and fatigue.

INTERACTIONS

Acarbose, metformin, and fibrates increase the effects of orlistat.

SPECIAL PRECAUTIONS

Be sure to tell your doctor if:
◆ You have diabetes.
◆ You have chronic malabsorption syndrome.
◆ You have gallbladder or liver problems.
◆ You take lipid-lowering drugs (see p.37).
◆ You are taking other medications.

Pregnancy Safety not established. Discuss with your doctor.

Breast-feeding Safety not established. Discuss with your doctor.

Infants and children Not prescribed.

Over 60 No known problems.

Driving and hazardous work No special problems.

Alcohol No special problems.

PROLONGED USE

Treatment should be stopped after 12 weeks if you have not lost 5 per cent of your bodyweight since starting treatment. If you have, the drug may be continued for a maximum of 2 years until target weight is approached.

When orlistat treatment is stopped, there may be gradual weight gain.

Orphenadrine

Brand names Biorphen, Disipal
Used in the following combined preparations None

QUICK REFERENCE

Drug group Muscle relaxant (p.54) and drug for parkinsonism (p.18)
Overdose danger rating High
Dependence rating Low
Prescription needed Yes
Available as generic Yes

GENERAL INFORMATION

Orphenadrine is an anticholinergic (see Autonomic nervous system, p8) drug prescribed to treat all forms of Parkinson's disease. It is less effective than other drugs for this disorder but is often preferred because its adverse effects tend to be less severe. It is particularly valuable for relieving the muscle rigidity that often occurs with Parkinson's disease, but it is less helpful for improving the slowing of movement that also commonly occurs.

Orphenadrine has significant muscle-relaxant properties. It produces this effect by blocking nerve pathways responsible for muscle rigidity and spasm. Consequently, the drug is prescribed for the relief of muscle spasm caused by muscle injury, prolapsed ("slipped") disc, and whiplash injuries.

INFORMATION FOR USERS

Your drug prescription is tailored for you. Do not alter dosage without checking with your doctor.

How taken Tablets, liquid.
Frequency and timing of doses 2–3 x daily.
Adult dosage range 150–400mg daily.
Onset of effect Within 60 minutes.
Duration of action 8–12 hours.
Diet advice None.
Storage Keep in a closed container in a cool, dry place out of reach of children. Protect from light.
Missed dose Take as soon as you remember. If your next dose is due within 2 hours, take a single dose now and skip the next.
Stopping the drug Unless a rash, itching, or palpitations occur, do not stop taking the drug without consulting your doctor; symptoms may recur.

OVERDOSE ACTION

Seek immediate medical advice in all cases. Take emergency action if palpitations, fits, or loss of consciousness occur.

POSSIBLE ADVERSE EFFECTS

The drug's adverse effects are similar to those of other anticholinergic drugs. The more common symptoms, such as dry mouth and blurred vision, can often be overcome by an adjustment in dosage. Other anticholinergic symptoms include difficulty in passing urine, constipation, dizziness, and confusion or agitation. If any of these symptoms, a rash, itching, or palpitations occur, stop taking the drug and consult your doctor immediately.

INTERACTIONS

Anticholinergics These drugs are likely to increase orphenadrine's anticholinergic effects.
Dextropropoxyphene/co-proxamol Confusion, anxiety, and tremors may occur if these drugs are taken with orphenadrine.
Metoclopramide and domperidone Orphenadrine opposes the effect of these on the gut.

SPECIAL PRECAUTIONS

Be sure to tell your doctor if:
◆ You have long-term liver or kidney problems.
◆ You have heart problems.
◆ You have had glaucoma.
◆ You have difficulty in passing urine and have an enlarged prostate.
◆ You have myasthenia gravis.
◆ You are taking other medications.
Pregnancy Safety in pregnancy not established. Discuss with your doctor.
Breast-feeding The drug passes into the breast milk, but at normal doses adverse effects on the baby are unlikely. Discuss with your doctor.
Infants and children Not usually prescribed.
Over 60 Increased likelihood of adverse effects. Reduced dose may be necessary.
Driving and hazardous work Avoid until you have learned how orphenadrine affects you because the drug can cause dizziness, lightheadedness, and blurred vision.
Alcohol Avoid until you have learned how orphenadrine affects you because alcohol may worsen the adverse effects of the drug.

PROLONGED USE

No problems expected. The effectiveness of orphenadrine in treating Parkinson's disease may diminish with time.

Oxybutynin

Brand names Contimin, Cystrin, Ditropan XL
Used in the following combined preparations None

QUICK REFERENCE

Drug group Drug for urinary disorders (p.112)
Overdose danger rating Medium
Dependence rating Low
Prescription needed Yes
Available as generic Yes

GENERAL INFORMATION

Oxybutynin is an anticholinergic (see Autonomic nervous system, p.8) and antispasmodic drug that is used to treat urinary incontinence and urinary frequency in adults and bedwetting in children. The drug acts by reducing bladder contraction, allowing the bladder to hold more urine. It stops bladder spasms and delays the desire to empty the bladder. It also has some local anaesthetic effect.

The drug's usefulness is, to some extent, limited by its side effects, especially in children and elderly people. It can aggravate conditions such as an enlarged prostate or coronary heart disease in elderly people. Children are more susceptible to effects on the central nervous system (CNS), such as restlessness, disorientation, hallucinations, and convulsions.

INFORMATION FOR USERS

Your drug prescription is tailored for you. Do not alter dosage without checking with your doctor.

How taken Tablets, liquid.

Frequency and timing of doses 2–4 x daily.

Adult dosage range 10–20mg daily.

Onset of effect 1 hour.

Duration of action Up to 10 hours.

Diet advice None.

Storage Keep in a closed container in a cool, dry place out of reach of children. Protect liquid from light.

Missed dose Take as soon as you remember. If your next dose is due within 2 hours, take a single dose now and skip the next.

Stopping the drug Do not stop taking the drug without consulting your doctor; symptoms may recur.

Exceeding the dose An occasional unintentional extra dose is unlikely to cause problems. Larger overdoses may cause restlessness or psychotic behaviour, a fall in blood pressure, breathing difficulties, paralysis, or coma; notify your doctor immediately.

POSSIBLE ADVERSE EFFECTS

Dosage adjustment is necessary in children and elderly people to minimize adverse effects. The drug can precipitate glaucoma. Dry mouth, constipation, nausea, facial flushing, dry skin, and difficulty in passing urine may occur. Consult your doctor if headache, confusion, rash, eye pain, or blurred vision occur.

INTERACTIONS

General note If oxybutynin is taken with other drugs that have anticholinergic effects, the risk of accumulated side effects is increased.

SPECIAL PRECAUTIONS

Be sure to tell your doctor if:
◆ You have liver or kidney problems.
◆ You have hyperthyroidism.
◆ You have heart problems.
◆ You have an enlarged prostate.
◆ You have hiatus hernia.
◆ You have ulcerative colitis.
◆ You have glaucoma.
◆ You have myasthenia gravis.
◆ You are taking other medications.

Pregnancy Safety not established. The drug may harm the developing baby. Discuss with your doctor.

Breast-feeding Safety not established. Discuss with your doctor.

Infants and children Not recommended under 5 years. Reduced dose necessary in older children.

Over 60 Reduced dose necessary.

Driving and hazardous work Avoid such activities until you have learned how oxybutynin affects you because the drug can cause drowsiness, disorientation, and blurred vision.

Alcohol Avoid excessive amounts. Alcohol increases the sedative effects of oxybutynin.

PROLONGED USE

No special problems. The need for continued treatment may be reviewed after 6 months.

Paracetamol

Brand names Alvedon, Calpol, Disprol, Hedex, Panadol, Panaleve, and many others
Used in the following combined preparations
Anadin Extra, Migraleve, Panadeine, Paradote, Tylex, and others

QUICK REFERENCE

Drug group Non-opioid analgesic (p.9)
Overdose danger rating High
Dependence rating Low
Prescription needed No
Available as generic Yes

GENERAL INFORMATION

Although paracetamol has been known since the early 1900s, it was not widely used as an analgesic until the 1950s. One of a group of drugs known as the non-opioid analgesics, it is kept in the home to relieve occasional bouts of mild pain and to reduce fever. It is suitable for children as well as adults.

One of the primary advantages of paracetamol is that it does not cause stomach upset or bleeding problems. This makes it particularly useful for people who suffer from peptic ulcers or those who cannot tolerate aspirin. It is also safe for occasional use by those being treated with anticoagulants.

Although safe when used as directed, paracetamol is dangerous when taken in overdose, and it is capable of causing serious damage to the liver and kidneys. Large doses may also be toxic if you regularly drink even moderate amounts of alcohol.

INFORMATION FOR USERS

Follow instructions on the label. Call your doctor if symptoms worsen.
How taken Tablets, capsules, liquid, suppositories.
Frequency and timing of doses Every 4–6 hours as necessary, but not more than 4 doses per 24 hours in children.
Dosage range *Adults* 500mg–1g per dose up to 4g daily. *Children* 60–120mg per dose (3 months–1 year); 120–250mg per dose (1–5 years); 250–500mg per dose (6–12 years).
Onset of effect Within 15–60 minutes.
Duration of action Up to 6 hours.
Diet advice None.

Storage Keep in a closed container in a cool, dry place out of reach of children.
Missed dose Take as soon as you remember if required to relieve pain. Otherwise do not take the missed dose, and take a further dose only when you are in pain.
Stopping the drug Can be safely stopped as soon as you no longer need it.

OVERDOSE ACTION

Seek immediate medical advice in all cases. Take emergency action if nausea, vomiting, or stomach pain occur.

POSSIBLE ADVERSE EFFECTS

Paracetamol has rarely been found to produce any side effects when taken as recommended, although nausea may occur. If you develop a rash, stop taking the drug and notify your doctor.

INTERACTIONS

Anticoagulants such as warfarin may need dosage adjustment if paracetamol is taken regularly in high doses.
Cholestyramine reduces the absorption of paracetamol and may reduce its effectiveness.

SPECIAL PRECAUTIONS

Be sure to consult your doctor or pharmacist before using this drug if:
◆ You have long-term liver or kidney problems.
◆ You are taking other medications.
Pregnancy No evidence of risk with occasional use.
Breast-feeding No evidence of risk.
Infants and children Not to be given to infants under 3 months, except on a doctor's advice or to treat fever following immunization. Reduced dose necessary up to 12 years.
Over 60 No special problems.
Driving and hazardous work No special problems.
Alcohol Prolonged heavy intake in combination with excess paracetamol may substantially increase the risk of injury to the liver.

PROLONGED USE

You should not normally take this drug for longer than 48 hours except on the advice of your doctor. However, there is no evidence of harm from long-term use.

Paroxetine

Brand name Seroxat
Used in the following combined preparations
None

QUICK REFERENCE

Drug group Antidepressant drug (p.14)
Overdose danger rating Medium
Dependence rating Low
Prescription needed Yes
Available as generic No

GENERAL INFORMATION

Paroxetine belongs to the group of antidepressant drugs known as selective serotonin re-uptake inhibitors (SSRIs). It is used to treat mild to moderate depression and helps to control the anxiety that often accompanies depression. It is also used to treat generalized anxiety disorder, social phobia, panic disorder, and obsessive-compulsive disorders.

Unlike tricyclics, paroxetine and other SSRIs are less likely to cause anticholinergic (see Autonomic nervous system, p.8) side effects such as dry mouth, blurred vision, and difficulty in passing urine. They are also much less dangerous if taken in overdose.

Common adverse effects include nausea, diarrhoea, drowsiness, sweating, tremor, weakness, insomnia, and sexual dysfunction (lack of orgasm/male ejaculation problems).

INFORMATION FOR USERS

Your drug prescription is tailored for you. Do not alter dosage without checking with your doctor.

How taken Tablets, liquid.
Frequency and timing of doses Once daily, in the morning.
Dosage range 20–60mg daily.
Onset of effect The onset of therapeutic response usually occurs within 7–14 days of starting treatment, but the full antidepressant effect may not be felt for 3–4 weeks.
Duration of action Up to 24 hours.
Diet advice None.
Storage Keep in a closed container in a cool, dry place out of reach of children.
Missed dose Take as soon as you remember.
Stopping the drug Unless rash or joint pains occur, do not stop taking the drug without consulting your doctor. Stopping abruptly can cause withdrawal symptoms.
Exceeding the dose An occasional unintentional extra dose is unlikely to be a cause for concern. Large doses may cause unusual drowsiness; notify your doctor immediately.

POSSIBLE ADVERSE EFFECTS

The most common adverse effects are nausea, drowsiness, sweating, tremor, weakness, insomnia, and sexual dysfunction. Less commonly, nervousness, anxiety, agitation, worsening appetite, and weight loss may occur. Convulsions are a rare complication. If you develop a blotchy or irritating rash or joint pains, stop taking the drug and consult your doctor immediately.

INTERACTIONS

General note Any drug that affects the breakdown of others in the liver may alter blood levels of paroxetine or vice versa.
Anticoagulants Paroxetine may increase the effects of these drugs.
Sedatives All sedatives are likely to increase the sedative effects of paroxetine.
Tricyclic antidepressants Paroxetine may increase the toxicity of these drugs.
MAOIs Paroxetine should not be taken during or within 14 days of MAOI treatment because serious reactions may occur.

SPECIAL PRECAUTIONS

Be sure to tell your doctor if:
◆ You have long-term liver or kidney problems.
◆ You have a heart problem.
◆ You have a history, or family history, of fits.
◆ You are taking other medications.
Pregnancy Safety in pregnancy not established. Discuss with your doctor.
Breast-feeding The drug passes into the breast milk. Discuss with your doctor.
Infants and children Not recommended under 18 years.
Over 60 Increased likelihood of adverse effects. Reduced dose may be necessary.
Driving and hazardous work Avoid such activities until you have learned how paroxetine affects you because the drug can cause drowsiness.
Alcohol Avoid. Alcohol may increase the sedative effects of this drug.

PROLONGED USE

Withdrawal symptoms may occur if the drug is not stopped gradually. Such symptoms include dizziness, electric shock sensations, anxiety, nausea, and insomnia. These rarely last for more than 1–2 weeks.

Perindopril

Brand name Coversyl
Used in the following combined preparations
Coversyl Plus

QUICK REFERENCE

Drug group Vasodilator (p.31)
Overdose danger rating Medium
Dependence rating Low
Prescription needed Yes
Available as generic No

GENERAL INFORMATION

Perindopril is an ACE inhibitor, a group of drugs used to treat high blood pressure and heart failure. The drug relaxes the muscles around the blood vessels, allowing them to dilate and thereby easing blood flow. Perindopril lowers blood pressure promptly but may need to be taken for several weeks to achieve maximum effect. When used to treat heart failure, it is usually combined with a diuretic. This can produce dramatic improvement, relaxing the muscle in blood vessel walls and reducing the heart's workload.

At the start of treatment, ACE inhibitors can cause a very rapid fall in blood pressure. Therefore, the first dose is usually low and is taken at bedtime to enable the patient to remain lying down.

The most characteristic adverse effect is a persistent dry cough. This may occur in up to 20 per cent of patients. The throat may become irritated, and the voice husky or hoarse.

INFORMATION FOR USERS

Your drug prescription is tailored for you. Do not alter dosage without checking with your doctor.
How taken Tablets.
Frequency and timing of doses Once daily, 30 minutes before food. Taken in the morning for the treatment of heart failure.

Adult dosage range 2mg initially, then 4–8mg daily.
Onset of effect 30–60 minutes.
Duration of action 24 hours.
Diet advice None.
Storage Keep in a closed container in a cool, dry place out of the reach of children.
Missed dose Take as soon as you remember. If your next dose is due within the next 8 hours, take a single dose now, and skip the next.
Stopping the drug Do not stop taking the drug without consulting your doctor; stopping the drug may lead to worsening of the underlying condition.
Exceeding the dose An occasional unintentional extra dose is unlikely to cause problems. Large overdoses, however, may cause dizziness or fainting; notify your doctor.

POSSIBLE ADVERSE EFFECTS

Perindopril may cause kidney impairment and large falls in blood pressure. Loss of taste, nausea and abdominal pain, rash, and a persistent dry cough are common adverse effects. If you develop a sore throat and fever, or suffer from dizziness or fainting, seek medical advice. Perindopril may also cause fatigue.

INTERACTIONS

Lithium Blood levels and toxicity of this drug may be raised by perindopril.
Diuretics These drugs cause a very rapid fall in blood pressure when taken with perindopril.
Ciclosporin, potassium salts, and potassium-sparing diuretics These drugs increase the risk of high potassium blood levels when taken with perindopril.
NSAIDs These drugs may reduce the effects of perindopril. There is also a risk of kidney damage when they are taken together.
Vasodilators (such as nitrates) Taken with perindopril, these may reduce blood pressure even further.

SPECIAL PRECAUTIONS

Be sure to tell your doctor if:
◆ You have long-term liver or kidney problems.
◆ You have a history of allergy to any ACE inhibitor.

◆ You are on a low-sodium diet.
◆ You are taking other medications.

Pregnancy Safety in pregnancy not established. Discuss with your doctor.

Breast-feeding Safety in breast-feeding not established. Discuss with your doctor.

Infants and children Not recommended.

Over 60 Elderly people may be more sensitive to the drug. Reduced dose necessary.

Driving and hazardous work Avoid such activities until you have learned how perindopril affects you. The drug can cause dizziness and fainting.

Alcohol Avoid. Alcohol may increase the blood-pressure-lowering and adverse effects of the drug.

Surgery and general anaesthetics Perindopril may need to be stopped before you have a general anaesthetic. Discuss with your doctor or dentist before any operation.

PROLONGED USE

Rarely, long-term use can lead to changes in the blood count or kidney function.

Monitoring Periodic checks on potassium levels, white blood cell count, kidney function, and urine are usually performed.

Permethrin

Brand name Lyclear
Used in the following combined preparations
None

QUICK REFERENCE

Drug group Drug to treat skin parasites (p.122)
Overdose danger rating Low
Dependence rating Low
Prescription needed No
Available as generic No

GENERAL INFORMATION

Permethrin is an insecticide used to treat head lice and scabies infestations. It works by interfering with the nervous system function of the parasites, causing paralysis and death. The drug has the advantage of being less toxic than some other types of insecticide.

Permethrin is used topically as a liquid for head lice and a cream for scabies infestation. In children and elderly people, the entire body surface, including the face, scalp, neck, and ears, may have to be covered; adults are treated from the neck downwards. For pubic lice, the entire body should be treated and the permethrin left on overnight. A second treatment seven days later is needed.

For both head lice and scabies, all family members should be treated at the same time, to prevent recontamination, and the process repeated after a week.

There are signs that the parasites are developing resistance to permethrin. If it does not work for you, your pharmacist should be able to suggest an alternative treatment.

INFORMATION FOR USERS

Follow instructions on the label. Call your doctor if symptoms worsen.

How taken Cream, topical liquid.

Frequency and timing of doses Once only, repeating after 7 days. Avoid contact with eyes and broken or infected skin.

Adult dosage range As directed.

Onset of effect Liquid should be rinsed off after 10 minutes (head lice) or 12 hours (pubic lice); cream should be washed off after 8–12 hours (scabies).

Duration of action Until washed off.

Diet advice None.

Storage Keep in a closed container in a cool, dry place out of reach of children. Protect from light.

Missed dose Timing of second application is not rigid; use as soon as you remember.

Stopping the drug Not applicable.

Exceeding the dose An occasional extra application is unlikely to cause problems. If accidentally swallowed, take emergency action.

POSSIBLE ADVERSE EFFECTS

In general, permethrin is well tolerated on the skin, although mild skin irritation is common. The skin may be reddened or stinging, and occasionally a rash may occur.

INTERACTIONS

None.

SPECIAL PRECAUTIONS

Be sure to consult your doctor or pharmacist before taking this drug if:
◆ You are taking other medications.

Pregnancy Safety not established. Discuss with your doctor.
Breast-feeding Safety not established. Discuss with your doctor.
Infants and children No special problems.
Over 60 No special problems.
Driving and hazardous work No special problems.
Alcohol No special problems.

PROLONGED USE

Permethrin is intended for intermittent use only; it should not be used for the long term.

Phenobarbital

Brand name Gardenal
Used in the following combined preparations
None

QUICK REFERENCE

Drug group Anticonvulsant drug (p.16)
Overdose danger rating High
Dependence rating High
Prescription needed Yes
Available as generic Yes

GENERAL INFORMATION

Introduced more than 70 years ago, phenobarbital belongs to the group of drugs known as barbiturates. It is used mainly in the treatment of epilepsy but is now being superseded by newer drugs. It was also used as a sleeping drug and sedative before the development of safer drugs.

In the treatment of epilepsy, the drug is usually given together with another anticonvulsant drug, such as phenytoin (see p.348).

The main disadvantage of the drug is that it often causes unwanted sedation. However, tolerance develops within a week or two, and most patients have no problem in long-term use. In children and elderly people, it may occasionally cause excessive excitement.

Phenobarbital and other barbiturates are sometimes abused for their sedative effects.

INFORMATION FOR USERS

Your drug prescription is tailored for you. Do not alter dosage without checking with your doctor.

How taken Tablets, liquid, injection.
Frequency and timing of doses Once daily, usually at night.
Dosage range Adults 60–180mg daily.
Onset of effect 30–60 minutes (by mouth).
Duration of action 24–48 hours (some effect may persist for up to 6 days).
Diet advice None.
Storage Keep in a closed container in a cool, dry place out of reach of children.
Missed dose Take as soon as you remember. If you take once daily and the next dose is due within 10 hours, take a single dose now and skip the next. If you take 2–3 times daily and the next dose is due within 2 hours, take a single dose now and skip the next.
Stopping the drug Unless rash or swelling occur, do not stop taking the drug without consulting your doctor. He or she may supervise a gradual reduction in dosage because abrupt cessation may cause fits or lead to restlessness, trembling, and insomnia.

OVERDOSE ACTION

Seek immediate medical advice in all cases. Take emergency action if unsteadiness, severe weakness, confusion, or loss of consciousness occur.

POSSIBLE ADVERSE EFFECTS

Most adverse effects of phenobarbital are the result of its sedative effect. These include drowsiness, clumsiness or unsteadiness, dizziness, fainting, and confusion, which can sometimes be minimized by a medically supervised reduction of dosage. If a rash or localized swellings occur, stop taking the drug and call your doctor urgently.

INTERACTIONS

Antipsychotics, antidepressants, St John's wort, mefloquine, and chloroquine These may reduce the anticonvulsant effect of phenobarbital.
Anticoagulants, corticosteroids, oral contraceptives, and protease inhibitors Phenobarbital may decrease the effect of these drugs.
Sedatives All drugs that have a sedative effect on the central nervous system are likely to increase the sedative properties of phenobarbital. Such drugs include sleeping drugs, antihistamines, opioid analgesics, antidepressants, and antipsychotics.

PHENOXYMETHYLPENICILLIN

SPECIAL PRECAUTIONS

Be sure to tell your doctor if:

◆ You have long-term liver or kidney problems.
◆ You have heart problems.
◆ You have poor circulation.
◆ You have porphyria.
◆ You have breathing problems.
◆ You are taking other medications.

Pregnancy The drug may affect the developing baby and increase the tendency of bleeding in newborn babies. Discuss with your doctor.

Breast-feeding The drug passes into the breast milk and can make the baby drowsy. Discuss with your doctor.

Infants and children Reduced dose necessary.

Over 60 Increased likelihood of confusion. Reduced dose may therefore be necessary.

Driving and hazardous work Your underlying condition, and the possibility of reduced alertness while taking the drug, may make such activities inadvisable. Discuss with your doctor.

Alcohol Never drink while under treatment with phenobarbital. Alcohol may interact dangerously with this drug.

PROLONGED USE

After starting the drug, its sedative effect can build up, causing excessive drowsiness and lethargy. However, tolerance may develop, reducing these effects. Dependence may also result. Withdrawal symptoms may occur if the drug is stopped suddenly.

Monitoring Blood samples may be taken periodically to test blood levels of the drug.

Phenoxymethylpenicillin

Brand names Apsin, Tenkicin
Used in the following combined preparations
None

QUICK REFERENCE

Drug group Antibiotic (p.62)
Overdose danger rating Low
Dependence rating Low
Prescription needed Yes
Available as generic Yes

GENERAL INFORMATION

Phenoxymethylpenicillin, also known as penicillin V, is a synthetic penicillin-type antibiotic prescribed for a wide range of infections. A variety of commonly occurring respiratory tract infections, such as some types of tonsillitis and pharyngitis, as well as ear infections, often respond well to this drug. Phenoxymethylpenicillin is also effective in treating the gum disease Vincent's gingivitis.

Phenoxymethylpenicillin is used to treat less common infections caused by the Streptococcus bacterium, such as scarlet fever and erysipelas (a skin infection). It is also used for the long term to prevent recurrence of rheumatic fever, a rare but potentially serious condition. In addition, it is prescribed long-term to prevent infections following removal of the spleen or in sickle cell disease.

As with other penicillins, the most serious adverse effect that may rarely occur is an allergic reaction that may cause collapse, wheezing, and a rash in susceptible people.

INFORMATION FOR USERS

Your drug prescription is tailored for you. Do not alter dosage without checking with your doctor.

How taken Tablets, liquid.
Frequency and timing of doses 4 x daily, at least 30 minutes before food.
Dosage range *Adults* 2–4g daily. *Children* Reduced dose according to age.
Onset of effect 1–2 days.
Duration of action Up to 12 hours.
Diet advice None.
Storage Keep in a closed container in a cool, dry place out of reach of children.
Missed dose Take as soon as you remember. If your next dose is due within 2 hours, take a single dose now and skip the next.
Stopping the drug Take the full course. Only stop if rash, itching, wheezing, or breathing difficulties occur. Even if you feel better, the original infection may still be present and may recur if treatment is stopped too soon.
Exceeding the dose An occasional unintentional extra dose is unlikely to be a cause for concern. But if you notice any unusual symptoms, or if a large overdose has been taken, notify your doctor.

POSSIBLE ADVERSE EFFECTS

Most people have no serious adverse effects. However, nausea, vomiting, and diarrhoea may occur. The drug may also provoke an allergic reaction in susceptible people. Stop taking the drug and call your doctor urgently if you experience rash, itching, wheezing, or breathing difficulties.

INTERACTIONS
Oral contraceptives Phenoxymethylpenicillin may reduce the contraceptive effect of these drugs. Discuss with your doctor.
Probenecid This drug increases the level of phenoxymethylpenicillin in the blood.
Methotrexate Excretion of this drug may be greatly reduced by phenoxymethylpenicillin, leading to toxicity.

SPECIAL PRECAUTIONS
Be sure to tell your doctor if:
◆ You have a long-term kidney problem.
◆ You have had a previous allergic reaction to a penicillin or cephalosporin antibiotic.
◆ You have an allergic disorder such as asthma or urticaria.
◆ You are taking other medications.
Pregnancy No evidence of risk.
Breast-feeding The drug passes into the breast milk, but at normal doses adverse effects on the baby are unlikely. Discuss with your doctor.
Infants and children Reduced dose necessary.
Over 60 No special problems.
Driving and hazardous work No known problems.
Alcohol No known problems.

PROLONGED USE
Prolonged use may slightly increase the risk of *Candida* infections and diarrhoea.

Phenylpropanolamine

Brand names None
Used in the following combined preparations
Contac 400, Day Nurse Capsules, Dimotapp, Eskornade, Mucron, Sinutab

QUICK REFERENCE
Drug group Decongestant (p.26)
Overdose danger rating High
Dependence rating Low
Prescription needed No
Available as generic No

GENERAL INFORMATION
Phenylpropanolamine is used as a decongestant in many over-the-counter cold relief preparations. By reducing inflammation and swelling of blood vessels in the lining of the nose, it relieves nasal congestion in head colds, hay fever, and sinusitis.

Phenylpropanolamine mimics some of the actions of the sympathetic nervous system (see Autonomic nervous system, p.8), and as a consequence it can produce undesirable stimulant side effects. It may raise the heart rate and severely elevate blood pressure and can also cause palpitations and wakefulness.

INFORMATION FOR USERS
Follow instructions on the label. Call your doctor if symptoms worsen.
How taken Tablets, SR-tablets, capsules, liquid.
Frequency and timing of doses 3–4 x daily; 2 x daily (SR-tablets).
Dosage range 75–100mg daily.
Onset of effect Within 30 minutes.
Duration of action 4–6 hours. Up to 12 hours (SR-tablets).
Diet advice None.
Storage Keep in a closed container in a cool, dry place out of reach of children. Protect from light.
Missed dose Take as soon as you remember if needed. If you take the medication twice daily and your next dose is due within 12 hours, take a single dose now and skip the next. If you take it 3–4 times daily and your next dose is due within 2 hours, take a single dose now and skip the next.
Stopping the drug Can be safely stopped as soon as you no longer need it.

OVERDOSE ACTION
Seek immediate medical advice in all cases. Take emergency action if shortness of breath, delirium, convulsions, or loss of consciousness occur.

POSSIBLE ADVERSE EFFECTS
High doses may be associated with anxiety, nausea, dizziness, and, rarely, with a marked rise in blood pressure, causing palpitations, headache, and breathlessness. If these signs or a rash or headache occur, stop taking the drug and call your doctor urgently.

INTERACTIONS

Other sympathomimetics These increase the risk of adverse effects with the drug.

Beta blockers A severe rise in blood pressure can occur if beta blockers are taken with phenylpropanolamine.

Tricyclic antidepressants and digoxin There is an increased risk of abnormal heart rhythms if these drugs are taken with phenylpropanolamine.

MAOIs These dangerously increase the risk of high blood pressure with phenylpropanolamine. It should not be taken during or within 14 days of MAOI treatment.

Antihypertensive drugs The blood-pressure-lowering effects of these drugs are reduced by phenylpropanolamine.

SPECIAL PRECAUTIONS

Be sure to consult your doctor or pharmacist before taking this drug if:
◆ You have high blood pressure.
◆ You have heart problems.
◆ You have had glaucoma.
◆ You have an overactive thyroid gland.
◆ You have diabetes.
◆ You have urinary difficulties.
◆ You are taking other medications.

Pregnancy Safety in pregnancy not established. Discuss with your doctor.

Breast-feeding The drug passes into the breast milk and may affect the baby. Discuss with your doctor.

Infants and children Not recommended under 8 years.

Over 60 Increased likelihood of adverse effects. Reduced dose may be necessary.

Driving and hazardous work Do not undertake such activities until you know how phenylpropanolamine affects you because the drug can cause dizziness.

Alcohol No known problems, but phenylpropanolamine is only available combined with other drugs that might interact with alcohol.

PROLONGED USE

The drug should not be taken long term without medical supervision because it may raise the blood pressure, straining the heart. Phenylpropanolamine may also lose its effectiveness over time as the body becomes tolerant of its actions.

Phenytoin/fosphenytoin

Brand names Epanutin, Pro-Epanutin (fosphenytoin)
Used in the following combined preparations
None

QUICK REFERENCE

Drug group Anticonvulsant drug (p.16)
Overdose danger rating Medium
Dependence rating Low
Prescription needed Yes
Available as generic Yes

GENERAL INFORMATION

Phenytoin decreases the likelihood of convulsions by reducing abnormal electrical discharges within the brain. Introduced in the 1930s, it is prescribed for the treatment of epilepsy, including grand mal and temporal lobe epilepsy. Fosphenytoin is a new type of phenytoin given by injection for severe fits.

The drug has also been given for migraine, trigeminal neuralgia, and the correction of certain abnormal heart rhythms.

Some adverse effects (such as overgrowth of the gums) are more pronounced in children, so the drug is prescribed for children only when other drugs are unsuitable.

It is recommended that patients remain on the same brand of phenytoin.

INFORMATION FOR USERS

Your drug prescription is tailored for you. Do not alter dosage without checking with your doctor.

How taken Tablets, chewable tablets, capsules, liquid, injection.

Frequency and timing of doses 1–3 x daily with food or plenty of water.

Dosage range *Adults* 200–500mg daily (usually as a single dose). *Children* According to age and weight.

Onset of effect The full anticonvulsant effect may not be felt for 7–10 days.

Duration of action 24 hours.

Diet advice Folic acid and vitamin D deficiency may occasionally occur while taking this drug. Make sure you eat a balanced diet containing fresh green vegetables.

Storage Keep in a tightly closed container in a cool, dry place out of reach of children.

Missed dose Take as soon as you remember.

Stopping the drug Do not stop taking the drug without consulting your doctor; symptoms may recur.

Exceeding the dose An occasional, unintentional extra dose is unlikely to cause problems. But if excessive drowsiness, confusion, or slurred speech occur, notify your doctor.

POSSIBLE ADVERSE EFFECTS

There are a number of adverse effects, many of which appear only after prolonged use. Dizziness or headache, confusion, nausea, and insomnia are common. If they become severe, your doctor may prescribe a different anticonvulsant. Long-term effects include increased body hair and overgrowth of gums. Consult your doctor immediately if a rash, fever, sore throat, or mouth ulcers develop.

INTERACTIONS

General note Many drugs may interact with phenytoin, causing either an increase or a reduction in the phenytoin blood level. The dosage of phenytoin may need to be adjusted. Consult your doctor.

Ciclosporin Blood levels of ciclosporin may be reduced with phenytoin.

Antidepressants/antipsychotics, mefloquine, chloroquine, and St John's wort These may reduce the effect of phenytoin.

Warfarin The anticoagulant effect of this drug may be altered. An adjustment in its dosage may be necessary.

Oral contraceptives Phenytoin may reduce their effectiveness.

SPECIAL PRECAUTIONS

Be sure to tell your doctor if:
◆ You have long-term liver or kidney problems.
◆ You have diabetes.
◆ You have porphyria.
◆ You are taking other medications.

Pregnancy May be associated with malformation and a tendency to bleeding in newborn babies. Folic acid supplements should be taken by the mother. Discuss with your doctor.

Breast-feeding The drug passes into the breast milk, but at normal doses adverse effects on the baby are unlikely. Discuss with your doctor.

Infants and children Reduced dose necessary. Increased likelihood of overgrowth of the gums and excessive growth of body hair.

Over 60 Reduced dose may be necessary.

Driving and hazardous work Your underlying condition, as well as the effects of phenytoin, may make such activities inadvisable. Discuss with your doctor.

Alcohol Avoid. Alcohol increases the sedative effects of this drug.

PROLONGED USE

There is a slight risk that blood abnormalities may occur. Prolonged use may also lead to adverse effects on skin, gums, and bones. It may also disrupt control of diabetes.

Monitoring Periodic blood tests may be performed to monitor levels of the drug in the body and composition of the blood cells and blood chemistry.

Pilocarpine

Brand names Minims Pilocarpine, Pilogel, Salagen
Used in the following combined preparation
None

QUICK REFERENCE

Drug group Drug for glaucoma (p.114)
Overdose danger rating Medium
Dependence rating Low
Prescription needed Yes
Available as generic Yes

GENERAL INFORMATION

Pilocarpine is a miotic drug used to treat chronic glaucoma and severe glaucoma prior to surgery. It is also used, in the form of tablets, to treat dry mouth following radiotherapy to the head and neck.

The eye drops are quick-acting but have to be re-applied every four to eight hours. Eye gel is longer acting and needs to be applied only once a day. Pilocarpine frequently causes blurred vision; and excessive spasm of the eye muscles may cause headaches, particularly at the start of treatment. However, serious adverse effects are rare.

INFORMATION FOR USERS

Your drug prescription is tailored for you. Do not alter dosage without checking with your doctor.

How taken Tablets, eye drops, eye gel.

Frequency and timing of doses *Eye drops* 3–6 x daily (chronic glaucoma); 5-minute intervals until the condition is controlled (acute glaucoma).
Eye gel Once daily. *Tablets* 3 x daily after food with plenty of water .

Dosage range According to formulation and condition. In general, 1–2 eye drops are used per application; 15–30 mg daily (tablets).

Onset of effect 15–30 minutes.

Duration of action 4–8 weeks for maximum effect (tablets); 3–8 hours (eye drops); up to 24 hours (eye gel).

Diet advice None.

Storage Keep tablets or eye drops in a closed container in a cool, dry place out of reach of children. Discard eye drops 1 month after opening them.

Missed dose Use as soon as you remember. If you have not remembered until 2 hours before your next dose, skip the missed dose and take the next dose now.

Stopping the drug Do not stop taking the drug without consulting your doctor; symptoms may recur.

Exceeding the dose An occasional unintentional extra application is unlikely to cause problems. Excessive use may cause facial flushing, an increase in the flow of saliva, and sweating. If the drug is accidentally swallowed, seek medical attention immediately.

POSSIBLE ADVERSE EFFECTS

Eye drops, eye gel Alterations in vision, such as blurred vision or poor night vision, are common. Headache, brow ache, eye pain or irritation, and sweating are also common at the start of treatment, but usually wear off after a few days. If they do not, or the symptoms are severe, consult your doctor. Twitching eyelids and red, watery eyes may also occur in rare cases. If there is eye pain or irritation, stop using the drug and contact your doctor.
Tablets Nausea, diarrhoea, dizziness, and urinary frequency are common. If the symptoms are severe, seek medical advice.

INTERACTIONS

General note Many drugs, including aminoglycoside antibiotics, clindamycin, colistin, chloroquine, quinine, quinidine, lithium, and procainamide, may block pilocarpine's effects.

Beta blockers These drugs may reduce the effects of pilocarpine.

Calcium channel blockers These drugs may increase pilocarpine's systemic effects.

SPECIAL PRECAUTIONS

Be sure to tell your doctor if:
◆ You have asthma.
◆ You have inflamed eyes.
◆ You wear contact lenses.
◆ You have heart, liver, or gastrointestinal problems.
◆ You are taking other medications.

Pregnancy No evidence of risk at the doses used for chronic glaucoma.

Breast-feeding The drug passes into the breast milk, but at normal doses adverse effects on the baby are unlikely. Discuss with your doctor.

Infants and children Not usually prescribed.

Over 60 Reduced night vision is particularly noticeable.

Driving and hazardous work Avoid such activities, especially in poor light, until you have learned how pilocarpine affects you; the drug may cause short sight and poor night vision.

Alcohol No known problems.

PROLONGED USE

The effect of the drug may occasionally wear off with prolonged use as the body adapts, but may be restored by changing temporarily to another antiglaucoma drug.

Piroxicam

Brand names Brexidol, Feldene, Pirozip
Used in the following combined preparations
None

QUICK REFERENCE

Drug group Non-steroidal anti-inflammatory drug (p.50) and drug for gout (p.53)
Overdose danger rating Medium
Dependence rating Low
Prescription needed Yes
Available as generic Yes

GENERAL INFORMATION

Piroxicam, introduced in 1980, is a non-steroidal anti-inflammatory drug (NSAID). Like other drugs in this group, it reduces pain, stiffness, and inflammation. Blood levels of the drug remain high for many hours after a dose; therefore, it needs to be taken only once daily.

Piroxicam is used to treat osteoarthritis, rheumatoid arthritis, acute attacks of gout, and ankylosing spondylitis. The drug relieves the symptoms of arthritis but does not cure the disease. It is sometimes prescribed in conjunction with slow-acting drugs in the treatment of rheumatoid arthritis to relieve pain and inflammation while the slow-acting drugs take effect. Piroxicam may also be given for pain relief after sports injuries, to treat conditions such as tendinitis and bursitis, and following minor surgery.

As with all NSAIDs, there is a risk of stomach ulcers occurring.

INFORMATION FOR USERS

Your drug prescription is tailored for you. Do not alter dosage without checking with your doctor.

How taken Tablets, dispersible tablets, capsules, injection, suppositories, gel.

Frequency and timing of doses 1–3 x daily with food or plenty of water.

Adult dosage range 10–40mg daily.

Onset of effect Pain relief begins in 3–4 hours. Used for arthritis, the full anti-inflammatory effect develops over 2–4 weeks. Used for gout, this effect develops over 4–5 days.

Duration of action Up to 2 days. Some effect may last for 7–10 days after treatment has been stopped.

Diet advice None.

Storage Keep in a closed container in a cool, dry place out of reach of children. Protect from light.

Missed dose Take as soon as you remember. If your next dose is due within 4 hours, take a single dose now and skip the next.

Stopping the drug When taken for short-term pain relief, the drug can be safely stopped as soon as you no longer need it. Unless serious adverse effects occur (see below), seek medical advice before stopping long-term treatment of arthritis.

Exceeding the dose An occasional unintentional extra dose is unlikely to be a cause for concern. Large overdoses may cause nausea and vomiting; notify your doctor.

POSSIBLE ADVERSE EFFECTS

Dizziness, headache and gastrointestinal effects, such as nausea and indigestion, may occur but are not usually serious. If you have symptoms such as abdominal pain and swollen feet or ankles, discuss with your doctor. If a rash develops, or if wheezing, breathlessness, bruising or bleeding, or black bowel movements occur, stop taking the drug and call your doctor immediately.

INTERACTIONS

General note Piroxicam interacts with many drugs, including other NSAIDs, corticosteroids, and oral anticoagulant drugs, to increase the risk of bleeding and/or peptic ulcers.

Lithium, digoxin, and methotrexate Piroxicam may raise blood levels of these drugs to an undesirable extent.

Antihypertensive drugs and diuretics The beneficial effects of these drugs may be reduced by piroxicam.

Ciprofloxacin, norfloxacin, and ofloxacin Piroxicam may increase the risk of convulsions when taken with these drugs.

SPECIAL PRECAUTIONS

Be sure to tell your doctor if:
◆ You have liver or kidney problems.
◆ You have heart problems or hypertension (high blood pressure).
◆ You have had a peptic ulcer, oesophagitis, or acid indigestion.
◆ You have porphyria.
◆ You have asthma.
◆ You are allergic to aspirin.
◆ You are taking other medications.

Pregnancy Not usually prescribed. When taken in the last 3 months of pregnancy, the drug increases the risk of adverse effects on the baby's heart and may prolong labour. Discuss with your doctor.

Breast-feeding The drug passes into the breast milk but at normal doses adverse effects are unlikely. Discuss with your doctor.

Infants and children Not recommended under 6 years. Reduced dose necessary.

Over 60 Reduced dose may be necessary. Increased likelihood of adverse effects.

Driving and hazardous work Avoid such activities until you have learned how piroxicam affects you; the drug can cause dizziness.

Alcohol Avoid. Alcohol may increase the risk of stomach disorders with piroxicam.

Surgery and general anaesthetics Piroxicam may prolong bleeding. Discuss with your doctor or dentist before any surgery.

PROLONGED USE

There is an increased risk of bleeding from peptic ulcers and in the bowel.

Monitoring Periodic blood counts and liver function tests may be performed.

Pizotifen

Brand name Sanomigran
Used in the following combined preparations
None

QUICK REFERENCE

Drug group Drug used for migraine (p.20)
Overdose danger rating Medium
Dependence rating Low
Prescription needed Yes
Available as generic Yes

GENERAL INFORMATION

Pizotifen is an antihistamine drug with a chemical structure similar to that of the tricyclic antidepressants (see p.14); it also has similar anticholinergic (see Autnomic nervous system, p.8) effects. It is prescribed for the prevention of migraine headaches in people who suffer from frequent, disabling attacks. The drug is thought to work by blocking the chemicals (histamine and serotonin) that act on blood vessels in the brain.

Pizotifen has also been prescribed to relieve the symptoms of carcinoid syndrome, a disorder in which excess production of serotonin by the body causes attacks of flushing and diarrhoea.

The main disadvantage of prolonged use of pizotifen is that it stimulates the appetite and, as a result, often causes weight gain. It is usually prescribed only for people in whom other measures for migraine prevention – for example, avoidance of stress and foods that trigger attacks – have failed.

The sweetener used in the liquid medication is hydrogenated glucose syrup, and this may affect levels of blood glucose.

INFORMATION FOR USERS

Your drug prescription is tailored for you. Do not alter dosage without checking with your doctor.

How taken Tablets, liquid.

Frequency and timing of doses Once a day (at night) or 3 x daily.

Adult dosage range 1.5–4.5mg daily. Maximum single dose 3mg.

Onset of effect Full beneficial effects may not be felt for several days.

Duration of action The effects of this drug may last for several weeks.

Diet advice Migraine sufferers may be advised to avoid foods that trigger headaches in their case.

Storage Keep in a closed container in a cool, dry place out of reach of children. Protect from light.

Missed dose Take as soon as you remember. If your next dose is due within 4 hours, take a single dose now and skip the next.

Stopping the drug Do not stop taking the drug without consulting your doctor; symptoms may recur.

Exceeding the dose An occasional unintentional extra dose is unlikely to be a cause for concern. Large overdoses, however, may cause drowsiness, nausea, palpitations, and fits; notify your doctor.

POSSIBLE ADVERSE EFFECTS

Drowsiness is a common adverse effect of pizotifen treatment; it can often be minimized by starting treatment with a low dose that is gradually increased. Increased appetite may lead to weight gain. Other adverse effects include nausea, a dry mouth, dizziness, blurred vision, and muscle pains. If you begin to become depressed, be sure to consult your doctor.

INTERACTIONS

Anticholinergic drugs The weak anticholinergic effects of pizotifen may be increased by other anticholinergic drugs, including tricyclic antidepressants.

Sedatives All drugs that have a sedative effect on the central nervous system are likely to increase pizotifen's sedative properties. These include sleeping drugs, anti-anxiety drugs, opioid analgesic drugs, and antihistamines.

SPECIAL PRECAUTIONS

Be sure to tell your doctor if:
◆ You have a long-term kidney problem.
◆ You have glaucoma.
◆ You have urinary retention.
◆ You have prostate trouble.
◆ You are taking other medications.

Pregnancy Safety in pregnancy not established. Discuss with your doctor.

Breast-feeding The drug passes into the breast milk, but at normal doses adverse effects on the baby are unlikely. Discuss with your doctor.

Infants and children Reduced dose usually necessary.

Over 60 No special problems.

Driving and hazardous work Avoid such activities until you have learned how pizotifen affects you because the drug can cause drowsiness and blurred vision.

Alcohol Avoid. Alcohol may increase the sedative effects of this drug.

PROLONGED USE

Pizotifen often causes weight gain during long-term use. Treatment is usually reviewed every 6 months.

Pravastatin

Brand name Lipostat
Used in the following combined preparations
None

QUICK REFERENCE

Drug group Lipid-lowering drug (p.37)
Overdose danger rating Medium
Dependence rating Low
Prescription needed Yes
Available as generic No

GENERAL INFORMATION

Pravastatin belongs to the statin group of lipid-lowering drugs. It is prescribed for people with hypercholesterolaemia (high levels of cholesterol in the blood) who have not responded to other treatments, such as a special diet, and who are at risk of developing heart disease. The drug works by blocking the action of an enzyme that is needed for the manufacture of cholesterol, mainly in the liver. As a result, blood levels of cholesterol are lowered, which can help to prevent heart disease.

Rarely, statins can cause muscle pain, inflammation, and damage. This seems to be more likely if another kind of lipid-lowering drug called a fibrate is given with the statin.

INFORMATION FOR USERS

Your drug prescription is tailored for you. Do not alter dosage without checking with your doctor.

How taken Tablets.

Frequency and timing of doses Once daily at night.

Adult dosage range 10–40mg daily, changed after intervals of at least 4 weeks.

Onset of effect Within 2 weeks. Full beneficial effect may be felt within 4 weeks.

Duration of action 24 hours.

Diet advice A low-fat diet is usually recommended for people taking pravastatin.

Storage Keep in a closed container in a cool, dry place out of the reach of children. Protect from light.

Missed dose Take as soon as you remember. If your next dose is due within 8 hours, do not take the missed dose, but take the next dose as usual.

Stopping the drug Do not stop taking the drug without consulting your doctor. Stopping the drug may lead to worsening of the underlying condition.

Exceeding the dose An occasional unintentional extra dose is unlikely to cause problems. Large overdoses, however, may cause liver problems; notify your doctor.

POSSIBLE ADVERSE EFFECTS

Most adverse effects, such as headache, nausea, and fatigue, are mild and usually disappear with time. If you have symptoms such as jaundice, abdominal pain, rash, or muscle pain or weakness, notify your doctor urgently.

INTERACTIONS

Anticoagulants Pravastatin may increase the effect of these drugs.

Antifungal drugs Taken with pravastatin, itraconazole, ketoconazole, and possibly other antifungal drugs may increase the risk of muscle damage.

Orlistat This drug increases the blood levels and toxicity of pravastatin.

Other lipid-lowering drugs (fibrates) Taken with pravastatin, these drugs may increase the risk of muscle damage.

Ciclosporin and other immunosuppressant drugs There is an increased risk of muscle damage if these drug are taken with pravastatin. For this reason, they are not usually prescribed together with pravastatin.

SPECIAL PRECAUTIONS

Be sure to tell your doctor if:
◆ You have had liver problems.
◆ You are taking other medications.

Pregnancy Not usually prescribed. Safety not established. Consult your doctor.

Breast-feeding Safety not established. Discuss with your doctor.

Infants and children Not recommended.

Over 60 No special problems.

Driving and hazardous work No special problems.

Alcohol Avoid excessive amounts. Alcohol may increase the risk of developing liver problems with this drug.

PROLONGED USE

Long-term use of pravastatin can affect liver function.

Monitoring Regular blood tests to check liver and muscle function are usually required.

Prednisolone

Brand names Deltacortril, Deltastab, Minims prednisolone, Predenema, Predfoam, Pred Forte, Predsol, and others
Used in the following combined preparations Predsol-N, Scheriproct

QUICK REFERENCE

Drug group Corticosteroid (p.80)
Overdose danger rating Low
Dependence rating Low
Prescription needed Yes
Available as generic Yes

GENERAL INFORMATION

Prednisolone, a powerful corticosteroid drug, is used for a wide range of conditions, including some skin diseases, rheumatic disorders, allergic states, and certain blood disorders. It is used in the form of eye drops to reduce inflammation in conjunctivitis or iritis and may be given as an enema to treat inflammatory bowel disease. The drug can also be injected into joints to relieve rheumatoid and other forms of arthritis. In addition, prednisolone is prescribed with fludrocortisone for pituitary or adrenal gland disorders.

Low doses taken for the short term orally or topically rarely cause serious side effects. However, long-term treatment with large doses can cause fluid retention, indigestion, diabetes, hypertension, and acne. Enteric-coated tablets reduce the drug's local effects on the stomach but not the systemic effects.

INFORMATION FOR USERS

Your drug prescription is tailored for you. Do not alter dosage without checking with your doctor.

How taken Tablets, injection, suppositories, enema, foam, eye and ear drops.

Frequency and timing of doses 1–2 x daily or on alternate days with food (tablets/injection); 2–4 x daily, more frequently initially (eye/ear drops).

Adult dosage range Considerable variation. Follow your doctor's instructions.

Onset of effect 2–4 days.

Duration of action 12–72 hours.

Diet advice A low-sodium/high-potassium diet is recommended when the oral or injected form of prednisolone is prescribed for extended periods. Follow your doctor's advice.

Storage Keep in a closed container in a cool, dry place out of reach of children. Protect from light.

Missed dose Take as soon as you remember. If your next dose is due within 6 hours, take a single dose now and skip the next.

Stopping the drug Do not stop taking the drug without consulting your doctor. Abrupt cessation of long-term treatment by mouth or injection may be dangerous.

Exceeding the dose An occasional unintentional extra dose is unlikely to be a cause for concern. But if you notice any unusual symptoms, or if a large overdose has been taken, notify your doctor.

POSSIBLE ADVERSE EFFECTS

Indigestion, acne, weight gain, muscle weakness, and mood changes or depression are among the wide range of adverse effects of prednisolone taken by mouth and should be reported to your doctor.

If you have black or bloodstained bowel movements, call your doctor urgently. This adverse effect only occurs when high doses of prednisolone are taken by mouth or injection or for long periods.

If you are taking prednisolone by mouth, avoid close personal contact with chickenpox or herpes zoster (shingles), and seek urgent medical attention if exposed.

INTERACTIONS

Anticonvulsant drugs Carbamazepine, phenytoin, and phenobarbital can reduce the effects of prednisolone.

Anticoagulant drugs Prednisolone may affect the response to these drugs.

Diuretics Prednisolone may increase the adverse effects of these drugs.

Antihypertensive, and antidiabetic drugs and insulin Prednisolone may reduce the effects of these drugs.

Vaccines Serious reactions can occur when vaccinations are given with this drug. Discuss with your doctor.

Ciclosporin This drug increases the effects of prednisolone.

SPECIAL PRECAUTIONS

Be sure to tell your doctor if:
◆ You have had a peptic ulcer.
◆ You have glaucoma.
◆ You have had tuberculosis.
◆ You suffer from depression.
◆ You have any infection.
◆ You have diabetes.
◆ You have osteoporosis.
◆ You are taking other medications.

Pregnancy No evidence of risk with drops or joint injections. If prednisolone is taken as tablets in low doses, harm to the developing baby is unlikely. Discuss with your doctor.

Breast-feeding No evidence of risk with drops or injections. Taken by mouth, it passes into the breast milk, but at low doses adverse effects on the baby are unlikely. Discuss with your doctor.

Infants and children Not prescribed unless essential. Reduced dose may be necessary.

Over 60 Increased likelihood of adverse effects. Reduced dose may be necessary.

Driving and hazardous work No known problems.

Alcohol Keep consumption low. Alcohol may increase the risk of peptic ulcers with prednisolone taken by mouth or injection.

PROLONGED USE

Prolonged systemic use can lead to adverse effects such as diabetes, glaucoma, cataracts, and osteoporosis, and may retard growth in children. Dosages are usually tailored to minimize these problems. People who are on long-term treatment are advised to carry a "steroid treatment" card.

Prochlorperazine

Brand names Buccastem, Prozière, Stemetil
Used in the following combined preparations
None

QUICK REFERENCE

Drug group Antipsychotic drug (p.15) and antiemetic (p.21)
Overdose danger rating Medium
Dependence rating Low
Prescription needed Yes
Available as generic Yes

GENERAL INFORMATION

Introduced in the late 1950s, prochlorperazine belongs to a group of drugs known as the phenothiazines, which act on the central nervous system.

In small doses, prochlorperazine controls nausea and vomiting, especially when they occur as side effects of medical treatment by drugs or radiation, or of anaesthesia. It is also used to treat the nausea that occurs with inner-ear disorders such as vertigo. In large doses, the drug is used as an antipsychotic to tranquillize, reduce aggressiveness, and suppress abnormal behaviour. It therefore minimizes and controls the abnormal behaviour of schizophrenia, mania, and other mental disorders. It does not cure any of these diseases but helps to relieve symptoms.

INFORMATION FOR USERS

Your drug prescription is tailored for you. Do not alter the dosage without checking with your doctor.

How taken Tablets, buccal tablets, liquid, powder, injection, suppositories.

Frequency and timing of doses 2–3 x daily (tablets); 2–3 x daily (suppositories); 2–3 x daily (injection).

Adult dosage range *Nausea and vomiting* 20mg initially; then 5–10mg per dose (tablets); 5–25mg per dose (suppositories). *Mental illness* 15–40mg daily. Larger doses may be given.

Onset of effect Within 60 minutes (by mouth or suppository); 10–20 minutes (injection).

Duration of action 3–6 hours.

Diet advice None.

Storage Keep in a closed container in a cool, dry place out of reach of children. Protect from light.

Missed dose Take as soon as you remember. If your next dose is due within 2 hours, take a single dose now and skip the next.

Stopping the drug Can be safely stopped as soon as it is no longer needed for nausea or vomiting. When used for mental illness, do not stop taking the drug without consulting your doctor; symptoms may recur.

Exceeding the dose An occasional unintentional extra dose is unlikely to be a cause for concern. Large overdoses, however, may cause unusual drowsiness and may affect the heart; notify your doctor.

POSSIBLE ADVERSE EFFECTS

Prochlorperazine has a strong anticholinergic (see Autonomic nervous system, p.8) effect, which can cause drowsiness, lethargy, dry mouth, and dizziness, that often diminish with time. The main adverse effect with high doses is parkinsonism due to changes in the balance of brain chemicals. If this or rash, jaundice, fever, and a stiff neck, tongue, or jaws occur, discuss urgently with your doctor.

INTERACTIONS

Sedatives All drugs with a sedative effect are likely to increase prochlorperazine's effects.

Drugs for parkinsonism Prochlorperazine may block the beneficial effect of these drugs.

Terfenadine Taken with prochlorperazine, this increases the risk of abnormal heart rhythms.

Anticholinergic drugs Prochlorperazine may increase the side effects of these drugs.

SPECIAL PRECAUTIONS

Be sure to tell your doctor if:
◆ You have heart problems.
◆ You have liver or kidney problems.
◆ You have had epileptic fits.
◆ You have Parkinson's disease.
◆ You have an underactive thyroid gland.
◆ You have prostate problems.
◆ You have glaucoma.
◆ You are taking other medications.

Pregnancy Safety in pregnancy not established. Discuss with your doctor.

Breast-feeding The drug passes into breast milk and may affect the baby. Discuss with your doctor.

Infants and children Not recommended for infants or young children weighing less than 10kg (22lb). Reduced dose necessary for older children due to increased risk of adverse effects.

Over 60 Reduced dose may be necessary. Increased likelihood of adverse effects.

Driving and hazardous work Avoid such activities until you have learned how prochlorperazine affects you because the drug can cause drowsiness and reduced alertness.

Alcohol Avoid. Alcohol may increase and prolong the sedative effects of this drug.

PROLONGED USE

Use for more than a few months may lead to tardive dyskinesia (involuntary, potentially irreversible eye, mouth, and tongue movements). Occasionally, jaundice may occur.

Monitoring Periodic blood tests may be performed.

Procyclidine

Brand names Arpicolin, Kemadrin
Used in the following combined preparations None

QUICK REFERENCE

Drug group Drug for parkinsonism (p.18)
Overdose danger rating High
Dependence rating Low
Prescription needed Yes
Available as generic Yes

GENERAL INFORMATION

Introduced in the 1950s, procyclidine is an anticholinergic (see Autonomic nervous system, p.8) drug that is used to treat Parkinson's disease. It is especially helpful in the early stages of the disorder for treating muscle rigidity, and it helps to reduce muscle tremor and excessive salivation. However, the drug has less effect on the shuffling gait and slowness of muscular movement that characterize Parkinson's disease.

Procyclidine is also often used to treat parkinsonism resulting from treatment with antipsychotic drugs.

The drug may produce various minor adverse effects (see below), but these effects are rarely serious enough to warrant stopping treatment.

INFORMATION FOR USERS

Your drug prescription is tailored for you. Do not alter dosage without checking with your doctor.

How taken Tablets, liquid.

Frequency and timing of doses 2–3 x daily.

Adult dosage range 7.5–30mg daily; in exceptional cases, up to 60mg daily. The dosage is determined individually in order to find the best balance between the effective relief of symptoms and the occurrence of adverse effects.

Onset of effect Within 30 minutes.

Duration of action 8–12 hours.

Diet advice None.

Storage Keep in a closed container in a cool, dry place out of reach of children.

Missed dose Take the missed dose as soon as you remember. If your next dose is due within 2 hours, take a single dose now and skip the next one.

Stopping the drug Do not stop taking the drug without consulting your doctor; symptoms may recur.

OVERDOSE ACTION

Seek immediate medical advice in all cases. Take emergency action if palpitations, fits, or unconsciousness occur.

POSSIBLE ADVERSE EFFECTS

The possible adverse effects of procyclidine are mainly the result of its anticholinergic action. Some of the more common symptoms include a dry mouth, constipation, and blurred vision; these effects may be overcome by an adjustment in dosage. Nausea and vomiting, nervousness, confusion, drowsiness, and rash have also occasionally been reported. If you experience difficulty in passing urine, notify your doctor. If palpitations occur, seek immediate medical attention.

INTERACTIONS

Anticholinergics and antihistamines These drugs may increase the adverse effects of procyclidine.

Antidepressants These drugs may increase the adverse effects of procyclidine.

Glyceryl trinitrate This drug, when taken with procyclidine, may be less effective than normal in the relief of angina (heart pain) because a dry mouth may prevent it from dissolving under the tongue.

SPECIAL PRECAUTIONS

Be sure to tell your doctor if:

◆ You have any long-term liver or kidney problems.

◆ You suffer from, or have a family history of, glaucoma.

◆ You have high blood pressure.

◆ You suffer from constipation.

◆ You have prostate trouble.

◆ You are taking other medications.

Pregnancy Safety in pregnancy not established. Discuss with your doctor.

Breast-feeding The drug passes into the breast milk and may affect the baby. Discuss with your doctor.

Infants and children Not recommended.

Over 60 Reduced dose may be necessary.

Driving and hazardous work Avoid these activities until you have learned how procyclidine affects you because the drug can cause drowsiness, blurred vision, and mild confusion.

Alcohol Avoid. Alcohol may increase the sedative effect of this drug.

PROLONGED USE

Prolonged use of this drug may provoke the onset of glaucoma.

Monitoring Periodic eye examinations are usually advised.

Proguanil with atovaquone

Brand name Malarone
Used in the following combined preparations
None

QUICK REFERENCE
Drug group Antimalarial drug (p.75)
Overdose danger rating Medium
Dependence rating Low
Prescription needed Yes
Available as generic No

GENERAL INFORMATION
Proguanil is an antimalarial drug given to prevent the development of malaria. Microbial resistance to its effects can occur, and this has led to it being used in combination with other drugs.

Atovaquone is an antiprotozoal drug that is also active against the fungus Pneumocystis carinii (a cause of pneumonia in people with poor immunity). Atovaquone is less useful on its own for malaria, but when it is combined with proguanil it rapidly treats the infection. The combination is also used for prevention of malaria, especially in areas where resistance to other drugs is present.

When using proguanil for prevention, you should start taking it with atovaquone a day or two before travelling. Continue taking the tablets during your stay, and for 7 days after your return. It is important to take other precautions, such as using an insect repellent at all times and a mosquito net at night. If you develop an illness after your return from a malarial zone, and especially in the first 3 months, go to your doctor immediately and tell him or her where you have been.

INFORMATION FOR USERS
Follow instructions on the label.
How taken Tablets.
Frequency and timing of doses *Prevention* Once daily with food or a milky drink, at the same time each day. Start 1–2 days before travel, and continue for 7 days after return. *Treatment* Once daily for 3 days, with food or a milky drink.
Adult dosage range *Prevention* 1 tablet. *Treatment* 4 tablets.

Onset of effect After 24 hours.
Duration of action 24–48 hours.
Diet advice None.
Storage Keep in a closed container in a cool, dry place out of reach of children.
Missed dose Take as soon as you remember. If your next dose is due at this time, take both doses together.
Stopping the drug Do not stop taking the drug for 4 weeks after leaving a malaria-infected area, otherwise there is a risk that you may develop the disease.
Exceeding the dose An occasional unintentional extra dose is unlikely to cause problems. Large overdoses may cause abdominal pain and vomiting; notify your doctor.

POSSIBLE ADVERSE EFFECTS
Adverse effects are generally fairly mild. The most frequent is diarrhoea. Other effects include headache, nausea, vomiting, indigestion, and abdominal pain, but these usually settle as the treatment continues. Mouth ulcers and hair loss are also recognized adverse effects. If you develop a rash or jaundice, or suffer hair loss, consult your doctor. If a sore throat or fever occurs, consult your doctor immediately.

INTERACTIONS
Warfarin The effects of warfarin may be enhanced by proguanil.
Antacids The absorption of proguanil may be reduced by antacids.
Rifampicin, metoclopramide, and tetracycline antibiotics These drugs reduce the effect of proguanil with atovaquone.

SPECIAL PRECAUTIONS
Be sure to tell your doctor if:
◆ You have a long-term kidney problem.
◆ You have a liver problem.
◆ You are suffering from diarrhoea and vomiting.
◆ You are taking other medications.
Pregnancy Safety in pregnancy not established, but benefits are generally considered to outweigh risks. Folic acid supplements must be taken. Discuss with your doctor.
Breast-feeding The drug passes into the breast milk, but at normal doses adverse effects on the baby are unlikely. Breast-

feeding while taking proguanil will not protect the baby from malaria. Discuss with your doctor.

Infants and children Reduced dose necessary.

Over 60 No known problems.

Driving and hazardous work Avoid such activities until you have learned how the drug affects you because it can cause dizziness.

Alcohol No special problems.

PROLONGED USE
No known problems.

Promazine

Brand name Sparine
Used in the following combined preparations
None

QUICK REFERENCE
Drug group Anti-anxiety drug (p.13)
Overdose danger rating Medium
Dependence rating Low
Prescription needed Yes
Available as generic Yes

GENERAL INFORMATION
Promazine, introduced in the late 1950s, is one of a class of drugs called phenothiazines, which act on the brain to regulate abnormal behaviour (see Antipsychotic drugs, p.15).

The main use of promazine is to calm agitated and restless behaviour. The drug is also given as a sedative for the short-term treatment of severe anxiety, especially in elderly people and during terminal illness. In addition, promazine may be given for the control of nausea and vomiting, and to help stop persistent hiccups.

In theory, promazine may cause unpleasant side effects, in particular parkinsonism (abnormal movements and shaking of the arms and legs). In practice, however, the drug is rarely used for long enough to produce these problems.

INFORMATION FOR USERS
Your drug prescription is tailored for you. Do not alter dosage without checking with your doctor.

How taken Tablets, liquid, injection.

Frequency and timing of doses 4 x daily.

Adult dosage range 100–800mg daily (tablets).

Onset of effect 30 minutes–1 hour.

Duration of action 4–6 hours.

Diet advice None.

Storage Keep in a closed container in a cool, dry place out of reach of children. Protect from light.

Missed dose Take as soon as you remember. If your next dose is due within 2 hours, take a single dose now and skip the next.

Stopping the drug Do not stop taking the drug without consulting your doctor; symptoms may recur.

Exceeding the dose An occasional unintentional extra dose is unlikely to be a cause for concern. Large overdoses, however, may cause drowsiness, dizziness, unsteadiness, fits, and coma; notify your doctor.

POSSIBLE ADVERSE EFFECTS
The more common adverse effects of promazine, such as drowsiness, dry mouth, constipation, and blurred vision, may be helped by adjustment of dosage. Promazine may affect the body's ability to regulate its own temperature (especially in elderly people). The most significant adverse effect with high doses is parkinsonism, caused by changes in the balance of brain chemicals. Discuss this with your doctor.

INTERACTIONS
Sedatives All drugs that have a sedative effect are likely to increase the sedative properties of promazine.

Anticonvulsants Promazine may reduce the effectiveness of anticonvulsants by lowering the seizure threshold.

Drugs for parkinsonism The effectiveness of these drugs may be reduced by promazine.

Anti-emetics There is an increased risk of parkinsonism if antiemetic drugs such as metoclopramide are taken with promazine.

Antihistamines There may be an increased risk of abnormal heart rhythms occurring with terfenadine.

SPECIAL PRECAUTIONS
Be sure to tell your doctor if:
◆ You have heart problems.
◆ You have long-term liver or kidney problems.

◆ You have myasthenia gravis or phaeochromocytoma.

◆ You have had epileptic fits.

◆ You have breathing problems.

◆ You have prostate problems.

◆ You have glaucoma.

◆ You have Parkinson's disease.

◆ You are diabetic.

◆ You are taking other medications.

Pregnancy Safety in early pregnancy not established. The drug is sometimes injected during labour. Consult your doctor.

Breast-feeding The drug passes into the breast milk, but at normal doses adverse effects on the baby are unlikely. Discuss with your doctor.

Infants and children Not recommended.

Over 60 Increased likelihood of adverse effects. Reduced dose may be necessary.

Driving and hazardous work Avoid such activities until you have learned how promazine affects you because the drug can cause drowsiness and reduced alertness.

Alcohol Avoid. Alcohol may increase the sedative effect of this drug.

PROLONGED USE

Use of this drug for more than a few months may be associated with jaundice and abnormal movements. Sometimes a reduction in dose may be recommended.

Monitoring Periodic blood tests and eye examinations may be performed.

Promethazine

Brand names Avomine, Phenergan, Sominex
Used in the following combined preparations
Medised, Night Nurse, Pamergan P100, Tixylix Night-time

QUICK REFERENCE

Drug group Antihistamine (p.58) and anti-emetic (p.21)
Overdose danger rating Medium
Dependence rating Low
Prescription needed No
Available as generic No

GENERAL INFORMATION

Promethazine is one of a class of drugs called phenothiazines, developed in the 1950s for their beneficial effect on abnormal behaviour arising from mental illnesses (see Antipsychotic drugs, p.15). Promethazine was found, however, to have effects more like the antihistamines used to treat allergies (see p.58) and some types of nausea and vomiting (see Anti-emetics, p.21). The drug is widely used to reduce itching in a variety of skin conditions including urticaria (hives), chickenpox, and eczema. It can also relieve the nausea and vomiting caused by inner ear disturbances such as Ménière's disease and motion sickness. Due to its sedative effect, promethazine is sometimes used for short periods as a sleeping medicine, and is also given as premedication before surgery.

Promethazine is used in combined preparations together with opioid cough suppressants for the relief of coughs and nasal congestion, and it is given at night for its sedative effect.

INFORMATION FOR USERS

Follow instructions on the label. Call your doctor if symptoms worsen.

How taken Tablets, liquid, injection.

Frequency and timing of doses *Allergic symptoms* 1–3 x daily or as a single dose at night. *Motion sickness* Bedtime on night before travelling, repeating following morning if necessary, then every 6–8 hours as necessary. *Nausea and vomiting* Every 4–6 hours as necessary.

Dosage range (promethazine hydrochloride) *Adults* 20–75mg per dose.
Children Reduced dose according to age.

Onset of effect Within 1 hour. If a dose is taken after nausea has started, the onset of the effect is delayed.

Duration of action 8–16 hours.

Diet advice None.

Storage Keep in a closed container in a cool, dry place out of reach of children. Protect from light.

Missed dose No cause for concern, but take as soon as you remember. Adjust the timing of your next dose accordingly.

Stopping the drug Can be safely stopped as soon as symptoms disappear.

Exceeding the dose An occasional unintentional extra dose is unlikely to cause problems. Large overdoses, however, may cause drowsiness or agitation, fits, unsteadiness, and coma; notify your doctor.

POSSIBLE ADVERSE EFFECTS

Promethazine usually causes only minor anticholinergic effects, including drowsiness and lethargy, a dry mouth, and blurred vision. Consult your doctor if urinary retention or palpitations occur. If a rash develops on areas of skin exposed to light, stop taking the drug and consult your doctor immediately.

INTERACTIONS

MAOIs These drugs may cause a severe reaction if taken with promethazine. Avoid taking promethazine if MAOIs have been taken in the last 14 days.

Sedatives All drugs that have a sedative effect, such as other antihistamines, sleeping drugs, and antipsychotics, are likely to increase the sedative properties of promethazine.

SPECIAL PRECAUTIONS

Be sure to consult your doctor or pharmacist before taking this drug if:
◆ You have liver or kidney problems.
◆ You have had epileptic fits.
◆ You have heart disease.
◆ You have glaucoma.
◆ You suffer from asthma or bronchitis.
◆ You have Parkinson's disease.
◆ You have urinary retention or prostate problems.
◆ You are taking other medications.

Pregnancy Safety in pregnancy not established. Discuss with your doctor.

Breast-feeding The drug passes into the breast milk, but at normal doses adverse effects on the baby are unlikely. Discuss with your doctor.

Infants and children Not recommended under 2 years. Reduced dose necessary for older children.

Over 60 Adverse effects may be more likely.

Driving and hazardous work Avoid such activities until you have learned how promethazine affects you because the drug can cause drowsiness.

Alcohol Avoid. Alcohol may increase the sedative effects of this drug.

Sunlight Avoid exposure to strong sunlight.

PROLONGED USE

Prolonged use is rarely necessary. The drug may sometimes cause abnormal movements of the face and limbs (parkinsonism), but this normally disappears on stopping the drug.

Propranolol

Brand names Angilol, Apsolol, Bedranol SR, Beta-Prograne, Cardinol, Inderal, Inderal-LA, Propanix, Syprol, and others

Used in the following combined preparations Inderetic, Inderex

QUICK REFERENCE

Drug group Beta blocker (p.30) and anti-anxiety drug (p.13)
Overdose danger rating High
Dependence rating Low
Prescription needed Yes
Available as generic Yes

GENERAL INFORMATION

Introduced in 1965, propranolol was the first widely available beta blocker in the UK. It is most often used to treat hypertension, angina, and abnormal heart rhythms, but it is also helpful in controlling the fast heart rate and other symptoms of an overactive thyroid gland (hyperthyroidism). In addition, propranolol helps to reduce the palpitations, sweating, and tremor of severe anxiety and is used to prevent migraine headaches.

Propranolol is not prescribed to people with asthma because it can cause breathing difficulties. It can be useful for diabetics who are at high risk of heart disease, but, like all beta blockers, it may affect the body's response to low blood glucose.

INFORMATION FOR USERS

Your drug prescription is tailored for you. Do not alter dosage without checking with your doctor.

How taken Tablets, SR-capsules, liquid, injection.

Frequency and timing of doses 2–4 x daily. Once daily (SR-capsules).

Adult dosage range *Abnormal heart rhythms* 30–160mg daily. *Angina* 80–240mg daily. *Hypertension* 160–320mg daily. *Migraine prevention and anxiety* 40–160mg daily.

Onset of effect 1–2 hours (tablets); after 4 hours (SR-capsules). In hypertension and migraine, it may be several weeks before the full benefits of this drug are felt.

Duration of action 6–12 hours (tablets); 24–30 hours (SR-capsules).

Diet advice None.

Storage Keep in a closed container in a cool, dry place out of reach of children. Protect from light.

Missed dose Take as soon as you remember. If your next dose is due within 2 hours (tablets) or 12 hours (SR-capsules), take a single dose now and skip the next.

Stopping the drug Do not stop taking the drug without consulting your doctor. Abrupt cessation may lead to worsening of the underlying condition.

OVERDOSE ACTION

Seek immediate medical advice in all cases. Take emergency action if breathing difficulties, collapse, or loss of consciousness occur.

POSSIBLE ADVERSE EFFECTS

Cold hands and feet, dry eyes, aching muscles, and nightmares or vivid dreams are adverse effects that are common to most beta blockers. Symptoms such as fatigue and nausea are usually temporary and diminish with long-term use. Fainting may be a sign that the drug has slowed the heart beat excessively and should be reported to your doctor promptly. You should also report any shortness of breath or wheezing.

INTERACTIONS

Antihypertensives Propranolol may enhance the blood-pressure-lowering effect.

Diltiazem and verapamil Combining either of these drugs with propranolol may have adverse effects on heart function.

Cimetidine and hydralazine These drugs may increase the effects of propranolol.

NSAIDs (such as indometacin) These may reduce the antihypertensive effect of propranolol.

SPECIAL PRECAUTIONS

Be sure to tell your doctor if:
◆ You have long-term liver or kidney problems.
◆ You have a breathing disorder such as asthma, bronchitis, or emphysema.
◆ You have heart failure.
◆ You have diabetes.

◆ You have poor circulation in the legs.
◆ You are taking other medications.

Pregnancy The drug may affect the baby. Discuss with your doctor.

Breast-feeding The drug passes into the breast milk but at normal doses adverse effects on the baby are unlikely. Discuss with your doctor.

Infants and children Reduced dose necessary.

Over 60 Increased risk of adverse effects.

Driving and hazardous work No special problems.

Alcohol No special problems.

Surgery and general anaesthetics Propranolol may need to be stopped before you have a general anaesthetic. Discuss this with your doctor or dentist before any surgery.

PROLONGED USE

No problems expected.

Propylthiouracil

Brand names None
Used in the following combined preparations
None

QUICK REFERENCE

Drug group Antithyroid drug (p.84)
Overdose danger rating Medium
Dependence rating Low
Prescription needed Yes
Available as generic Yes

GENERAL INFORMATION

Propylthiouracil is an antithyroid drug used to manage an overactive thyroid gland (hyperthyroidism). In some people, particularly those with Graves' disease (the most common form of the disorder), drug treatment alone may bring on a remission. The drug may also be prescribed for the long term to people who may be at special risk from surgery, such as children and pregnant women.

The drug is used to restore the normal functioning of the thyroid gland before its partial removal by surgery, and it is sometimes given with thyroxine to prevent the development of hypothyroidism (low thyroid hormone levels). Propylthiouracil is preferred to other antithyroid drugs when treatment is essential during pregnancy.

The most important adverse effect that sometimes occurs is a reduction in white blood cells, leading to the risk of infection. If you develop a sore throat or mouth ulceration, see your doctor immediately; this might be a sign that your blood is being affected.

INFORMATION FOR USERS

Your drug prescription is tailored for you. Do not alter dosage without consulting your doctor.

How taken Tablets.
Frequency and timing of doses 1–3 x daily.
Dosage range Initially 300–600mg daily. Dose can usually be reduced to 50–150mg daily.
Onset of effect 10–20 days. Full beneficial effects may not be felt for 6–10 weeks.
Duration of action 24–36 hours.
Diet advice Your doctor may advise you to avoid foods that are high in iodine.
Storage Keep in a closed container in a cool, dry place out of reach of children. Protect from light.
Missed dose Take as soon as you remember. If your next dose is due within 3 hours, take a single dose now and skip the next.
Stopping the drug Do not stop taking the drug without consulting your doctor. Stopping the drug may lead to a recurrence of the hyperthyroidism.
Exceeding the dose An occasional unintentional extra dose is unlikely to cause problems. Large overdoses may cause nausea, vomiting, and headache; notify your doctor.

POSSIBLE ADVERSE EFFECTS

Serious side effects are rare with propylthiouracil. A rash and itching are fairly common. Nausea, vomiting, headache, and joint pain may also occur. A sore throat or fever may indicate adverse effects on the blood. If these problems or jaundice occur, consult your doctor immediately.

INTERACTIONS

None.

SPECIAL PRECAUTIONS

Be sure to tell your doctor if:
◆ You have long-term liver or kidney problems.
◆ You are pregnant.
◆ You are taking other medications.

Pregnancy Prescribed with caution. There is a risk of goitre and hypothyroidism in the newborn baby if the dose is too high. Discuss with your doctor.
Breast-feeding The drug passes into the breast milk and may affect the baby. Discuss with your doctor.
Infants and children Reduced dose necessary.
Over 60 No special problems.
Driving and hazardous work No problems expected.
Alcohol No known problems.

PROLONGED USE

High doses over a prolonged period may reduce the number of white blood cells.
Monitoring Periodic tests of thyroid function are usually required, and blood cell counts may also be carried out.

Pyridostigmine

Brand name Mestinon
Used in the following combined preparations None

QUICK REFERENCE

Drug group Drug for myasthenia gravis (p.55)
Overdose danger rating High
Dependence rating Low
Prescription needed Yes
Available as generic No

GENERAL INFORMATION

Pyridostigmine is used to treat a rare auto-immune condition called myasthenia gravis, which involves faulty transmission of nerve impulses to the muscles. The drug improves muscle strength by prolonging nerve signals but does not cure the disease. In severe cases, it may be given with corticosteroids or other drugs. Pyridostigmine may also be given to reverse temporary paralysis of the bowel and urinary retention following operations.

Side effects, including abdominal cramps, nausea, and diarrhoea, may occur but usually disappear when the dosage is reduced.

INFORMATION FOR USERS

Your drug prescription is tailored for you. Do not alter dosage without checking with your doctor.

How taken Tablets.

Frequency and timing of doses Every 3–4 hours initially. Thereafter, according to the needs of the individual.

Dosage range *Adults* 150mg–1.2g daily (by mouth) according to response and side effects. *Children* Reduced dose necessary according to age and weight.

Onset of effect 30–60 minutes.

Duration of action 3–6 hours.

Diet advice None.

Storage Keep in a closed container in a cool, dry place out of reach of children. Protect from light.

Missed dose Take as soon as you remember. If your next dose is due within 2 hours, take a single dose now and skip the next.

Stopping the drug Do not stop the drug without consulting your doctor; symptoms may recur.

OVERDOSE ACTION

Seek immediate medical advice in all cases. You may experience severe abdominal cramps, vomiting, weakness, and tremor. Take emergency action if wheezing, unusually slow heart beat, fits, or loss of consciousness occur.

POSSIBLE ADVERSE EFFECTS

Adverse effects are usually dose-related and can be avoided by adjusting the dose. These effects include nausea, vomiting, increased salivation, abdominal cramps, diarrhoea, watering eyes, small pupils, sweating, and headache. In rare cases hypersensitivity may occur, leading to an allergic rash.

INTERACTIONS

General note Drugs that suppress the transmission of nerve signals may oppose the effect of pyridostigmine; they include aminoglycoside antibiotics, digoxin, procainamide, quinidine, lithium, and chloroquine.

Propranolol This beta blocker antagonizes the effect of pyridostigmine.

SPECIAL PRECAUTIONS

Be sure to tell your doctor if:
◆ You have a long-term kidney problem.
◆ You have heart problems.
◆ You have had epileptic fits.
◆ You have asthma.
◆ You have difficulty in passing urine.
◆ You have a peptic ulcer.
◆ You have Parkinson's disease.
◆ You are taking other medications.

Pregnancy No evidence of risk to the developing baby in the first 6 months. Large doses near the time of delivery may cause premature labour and temporary muscle weakness in the baby. Discuss with your doctor.

Breast-feeding No evidence of risk, but the baby should be monitored for signs of muscle weakness.

Infants and children Reduced dose necessary, calculated according to age and weight.

Over 60 Increased likelihood of adverse effects. Reduced dose may be necessary.

Driving and hazardous work Your underlying condition may make such activities inadvisable. Discuss with your doctor.

Alcohol No special problems.

Surgery and general anaesthetics Pyridostigmine interacts with some anaesthetic agents. Discuss your treatment with your doctor, dentist, and anaesthetist before any surgery.

PROLONGED USE

No problems expected.

Pyrimethamine

Brand name Daraprim
Used in the following combined preparations
Fansidar

QUICK REFERENCE

Drug group Antimalarial drug (p.75)
Overdose danger rating Medium
Dependence rating Low
Prescription needed Yes
Available as generic No

GENERAL INFORMATION

Pyrimethamine is an antimalarial drug. Because malaria parasites can readily develop resistance to pyrimethamine, the drug is now always given combined with the antibacterial drug sulfadoxine (as Fansidar) in the treatment of malaria. The activity of the combination greatly exceeds that of either drug alone. Fansidar is also used with quinine in the treatment of malaria. Pyrimethamine is not used for the prevention of malaria.

Pyrimethamine and sulfadiazine are given together to treat toxoplasmosis in immuno-compromised patients.

Because blood disorders can arise during prolonged use, blood counts are monitored regularly and vitamin supplements are given.

INFORMATION FOR USERS

Your drug prescription is tailored for you. Do not alter dosage without checking with your doctor.

How taken Tablets.

Frequency and timing of doses Taken once only.

Dosage range *Adults* 3 tablets. *Children* Reduced dose necessary according to age.

Onset of effect 24 hours.

Duration of action Up to 1 week.

Diet advice None.

Storage Keep in a closed container in a cool, dry place out of reach of children. Protect from light.

Missed dose If you are being treated for toxoplasmosis, take as soon as you remember. If your next dose is due within 24 hours, take a single dose now and alter the dosing day so that your next dose is one week later.

Stopping the drug Do not stop taking the drug without consulting your doctor.

Exceeding the dose An occasional unintentional extra dose is unlikely to cause problems. Large overdoses, however, may cause trembling, breathing difficulty, fits, and blood disorders; notify your doctor.

POSSIBLE ADVERSE EFFECTS

Side effects of pyrimethamine, such as indigestion and insomnia, occur only rarely with the low doses that are given for the treatment of malaria. Unusual tiredness, weakness, bleeding, bruising, and sore throat may be signs of a blood disorder. Notify your doctor promptly if these occur. Breathing difficulties, rash, or signs of chest infection should also be reported to your doctor.

INTERACTIONS

General note Drugs that suppress the bone marrow or cause folic acid deficiency may increase the risk of serious blood disorders when taken with pyrimethamine. These drug types include anticancer and antirheumatic drugs, phenylbutazone, sulfasalazine, co-trimoxazole, trimethoprim, and phenytoin.

SPECIAL PRECAUTIONS

Be sure to tell your doctor if:
◆ You have any long-term liver or kidney problems.
◆ You have had epileptic fits.
◆ You have anaemia.
◆ You are allergic to sulphonamides.
◆ You have glucose-6-phosphate dehydrogenase (G6PD) deficiency.
◆ You are taking other medications.

Pregnancy Pyrimethamine may cause folic acid deficiency in the developing baby. Pregnant women receiving this drug should also take a folic acid supplement. Discuss with your doctor.

Breast-feeding The drug passes into the breast milk, but at normal doses adverse effects on the baby are unlikely. Discuss with your doctor.

Infants and children Reduced dose necessary.

Over 60 No special problems.

Driving and hazardous work No special problems.

Alcohol No known problems.

PROLONGED USE

Prolonged use of this drug may cause folic acid deficiency, leading to serious blood disorders. Supplements of folic acid may be recommended (in the form of folinic acid).

Monitoring Regular blood cell counts are required during high-dose or long-term treatment.

Quetiapine

Brand name Seroquel
Used in the following combined preparations
None

QUICK REFERENCE

Drug group Antipsychotic drug (p.15)
Overdose danger rating Medium
Dependence rating Low
Prescription needed Yes
Available as generic No

GENERAL INFORMATION

Quetiapine is an antipsychotic drug that is prescribed for the treatment of schizophrenia. It can be used to treat "positive" symptoms (thought disorders, delusions, and hallucinations) and "negative" symptoms (blunted affect and emotional and social withdrawal). Quetiapine may be more effective when it is used to treat positive symptoms, however.

Elderly people excrete the drug up to 50 per cent more slowly than the usual adult rate. Therefore, in order for adverse effects to be avoided, it is necessary for elderly people to be prescribed much lower doses.

INFORMATION FOR USERS

Your drug prescription is tailored for you. Do not alter dosage without checking with your doctor.
How taken Tablets.
Frequency and timing of doses 2 x daily.
Adult dosage range 50mg daily (day 1), 100mg daily (day 2), 200mg daily (day 3), 300mg daily (day 4), then changing according to individual response. Usual dosage range is 300–450mg daily, with a maximum of 750mg daily.
Onset of effect 1 hour.
Duration of action Up to 12 hours.
Diet advice None.
Storage Keep in a closed container in a cool, dry place out of reach of children.
Missed dose Take as soon as you remember. If your next dose is due within 4 hours, take a single dose now and skip the next.
Stopping the drug Do not stop taking the drug without consulting your doctor; symptoms may recur.

Exceeding the dose

An occasional unintentional extra dose is unlikely to cause problems. Large overdoses may cause unusual drowsiness, palpitations, and low blood pressure; notify your doctor.

POSSIBLE ADVERSE EFFECTS

Unusual drowsiness and weight gain are common adverse effects. Digestive upset and parkinsonism are less common. If persistent sore throat, dizziness or fainting, or palpitations occur, consult your doctor immediately.

INTERACTIONS

Anticonvulsant drugs Quetiapine opposes the effect of these drugs. However, phenytoin decreases the effect of quetiapine; it increases the levels of certain liver enzymes that break down drugs, thus making quetiapine ineffective. Other anticonvulsant drugs with a similar action, such as carbamazepine and barbiturates, may have a similar effect.

Sedatives All drugs with a sedative effect on the central nervous system are likely to increase the sedative properties of quetiapine.

SPECIAL PRECAUTIONS

Be sure to tell your doctor if:
◆ You have epilepsy.
◆ You have Parkinson's disease.
◆ You have liver or kidney problems.
◆ You have heart problems.
◆ You have blood problems.
◆ You are taking other medications.
Pregnancy Safety not established. Discuss with your doctor.
Breast-feeding Safety not established. Discuss with your doctor.
Infants and children Not recommended.
Over 60 Reduced doses necessary. Elderly people eliminate quetiapine much more slowly than younger adults.
Driving and hazardous work Avoid. Quetiapine can cause drowsiness.
Alcohol Avoid. Alcohol increases the sedative effects of this drug.

PROLONGED USE

Prolonged use of quetiapine has been reported to produce tardive dyskinesia (in which there are involuntary movements of the tongue and face).

Quinine

Brand names None
Used in the following combined preparations
None

QUICK REFERENCE

Drug group Antimalarial drug (p.75) and muscle
relaxant (p.54)
Overdose danger rating High
Dependence rating Low
Prescription needed Yes
Available as generic Yes

GENERAL INFORMATION

Quinine, which is obtained from the bark of
the cinchona tree, is the earliest antimalarial
drug. The drug often causes side effects, but
it is still given for malaria that is resistant to
safer treatments. Because the malaria parasite has become resistant to chloroquine and
some of the more modern antimalarials, quinine remains the mainstay of treatment. It is
not, however, used as a preventative.

At the high doses used to treat malaria,
quinine may cause a group of symptoms
known as cinchonism. These include ringing
in the ears, headaches, nausea, hearing loss,
and blurred vision. In rare cases, quinine
may cause bleeding into the skin due to
reduced blood platelets.

In many countries quinine is often used,
in small doses, to prevent painful night-time
leg cramps.

INFORMATION FOR USERS

Your drug prescription is tailored for you.
Do not alter dosage without checking with
your doctor.
How taken Tablets, injection.
Frequency and timing of doses *Malaria*
Every 8 hours. *Muscle cramps* Once daily at
bedtime.
Adult dosage range *Malaria* 1.8g daily. *Cramps*
200–300mg daily.
Onset of effect *Malaria* 1–2 days. *Cramps* Up to
4 weeks.
Duration of action Up to 24 hours.
Diet advice None.
Storage Keep in a closed container in a cool,
dry place out of the reach of children. Pro-
tect from light.

Missed dose Take as soon as you remember. If
your next dose is due within 4 hours, skip the
missed one and return to your normal dosing schedule thereafter.
Stopping the drug If prescribed for malaria,
take the full course. Even if you feel better,
the original infection may still be present
and may recur if treatment is stopped too
soon. If taken for muscle cramps, the drug
can safely be stopped as soon as you no
longer need it.

OVERDOSE ACTION

Seek immediate medical advice in all cases.
Take emergency action if breathing problems, fits, or loss of consciousness occur.

POSSIBLE ADVERSE EFFECTS

Adverse effects are unlikely with quinine at
low doses. At antimalarial doses, however,
headache and blurred vision are more common; and dizziness, ringing in the ears, and
temporary deafness may occur. Quinine
may also cause nausea and diarrhoea. If any
rash, loss of hearing, and blurred vision occurs, stop taking the drug and consult your
doctor immediately.

INTERACTIONS

Antihistamines There is an increased risk of
adverse effects on the heart if quinine is
taken together with antihistamines such as
terfenadine.
Cimetidine This drug increases the blood
levels of quinine.
Digoxin Quinine increases the blood levels of
digoxin, the dose of digoxin should therefore
be reduced. Discuss with your doctor.

SPECIAL PRECAUTIONS

Be sure to consult your doctor if:
♦ You have a long-term kidney problem.
♦ You have tinnitus (ringing in the ears).
♦ You have optic neuritis.
♦ You have myasthenia gravis.
♦ You have glucose-6-phosphate dehydro-
genase (G6PD) deficiency.
♦ You have heart problems.
♦ You are taking other medications.
Pregnancy Not usually prescribed. May cause
defects in the developing baby. Discuss with
your doctor.

Breast-feeding The drug passes into the breast milk, but at normal doses adverse effects on the baby are unlikely. Discuss with your doctor.

Infants and children Reduced dose necessary.

Over 60 No special problems.

Driving and hazardous work Avoid these activities until you know how quinine affects you because the drug's side effects may distract you.

Alcohol No known problems.

PROLONGED USE

No problems expected with low doses used to control night-time leg cramps. Treatment may be stopped after 3 months to assess the need to continue.

Raloxifene

Brand name Evista
Used in the following combined preparations
None

QUICK REFERENCE

Drug group Drug for bone disorders (p.56)
Overdose danger rating Low
Dependence rating Low
Prescription needed Yes
Available as generic No

GENERAL INFORMATION

Raloxifene is a non-steroidal drug that is related to clomifene (see p.192) and tamoxifen (see p.395). It is prescribed to prevent vertebral fractures in postmenopausal women, who are at increased risk of osteoporosis. It works by mimicking the effects of oestrogen, a naturally occurring female sex hormone (see p.88), in protecting bones. There is some evidence that the drug would also be useful for preventing fractures of the hip, but its use in the prevention of other bone fractures is uncertain.

Raloxifene has no beneficial effect on other menopausal problems, such as hot flushes. The drug is not prescribed to women who might become pregnant because it may harm the developing baby, and it is not prescribed to men.

There is an increased risk of deep vein thrombosis (a blood clot developing in a vein in the leg), but the risk is similar to that due to HRT (see p.89). However, because of this risk, raloxifene is usually stopped if the woman becomes immobile or bedbound, when clots are more likely to form. Treatment is restarted when full activity is resumed.

INFORMATION FOR USERS

Your drug prescription is tailored for you. Do not alter dosage without checking with your doctor.
How taken Tablets.
Frequency and timing of doses Once daily.
Adult dosage range 60mg daily.
Onset of effect 1–4 hours.
Duration of action 24–48 hours.

Diet advice Calcium supplements are recommended if dietary calcium is low.
Storage Keep in a closed container in a cool, dry place out of reach of children. Protect from light.
Missed dose Take as soon as you remember. If your next dose is due within 8 hours, take a single dose now and skip the next.
Stopping the drug Do not stop taking the drug without consulting your doctor except under specified conditions, such as immobility (which increases the risk of deep vein thrombosis).
Exceeding the dose An occasional unintentional extra dose is unlikely to be a cause for concern. But if you notice any unusual symptoms, or if a large overdose has been taken, notify your doctor.

POSSIBLE ADVERSE EFFECTS

Hot flushes, leg cramps, and swollen feet or ankles are common. If headaches and rash occur, consult your doctor. Pain, tenderness, or swelling in one leg, and discoloration or ulceration, indicate the possibility of a deep vein thrombosis. If any of these adverse effects occur, stop taking the drug and contact your doctor immediately.

INTERACTIONS

Anticoagulants Raloxifene reduces the effect of warfarin and acenocoumarol.
Colestyramine This drug reduces the absorption of raloxifene by the body.

SPECIAL PRECAUTIONS

Be sure to tell your doctor if:
◆ You have had a blood clot in a vein.
◆ You have uterine bleeding.
◆ You have liver or kidney problems.
◆ You are taking other medications.
Pregnancy Not prescribed to premenopausal women.
Breast-feeding Not prescribed to premenopausal women.
Infants and children Not prescribed.
Over 60 No special problems.
Driving and hazardous work No special problems.
Alcohol No special problems.

PROLONGED USE

No special problems. Raloxifene is normally used long term.

Ramipril

Brand name Tritace
Used in the following combined preparations
Triapin, Triapin mite

QUICK REFERENCE

Drug group Vasodilator (p.31) and antihypertensive drug (p.36)
Overdose danger rating Medium
Dependence rating Low
Prescription needed Yes
Available as generic No

GENERAL INFORMATION

Ramipril is an ACE (angiotensin-converting enzyme) inhibitor drug used to treat high blood pressure (see p.31) and heart failure (in which the heart cannot deal with its workload). It acts by relaxing the muscles in blood vessel walls, allowing the vessels to dilate (widen), which enables the blood to circulate more easily and helps to lower blood pressure.

The drug may also be given to patients following a heart attack, and is sometimes used to prevent or delay kidney damage in patients with diabetes. In addition, it is often given with a diuretic to increase its effect on high blood pressure and heart failure. The drug is long-acting and is taken once or twice daily. The first dose may cause a sudden drop in blood pressure, especially in patients taking a diuretic. For this reason, you should lie down for 2–3 hours afterwards.

A variety of minor side effects may occur with ramipril; many people develop a persistent dry cough, while others experience taste disturbance, which a reduction in dose may help to minimize.

INFORMATION FOR USERS

Your drug prescription is tailored for you. Do not alter dosage without checking with your doctor.
How taken Tablets, capsules.

Frequency and timing of doses With water, with or after food. *High blood pressure* Usually once daily. *Heart failure* After a heart attack, 2 x daily.
Adult dosage range *High blood pressure* 1.25–10mg daily. *Heart failure* After a heart attack, 5–10mg daily.
Onset of effect Within 2 hours.
Duration of action Up to 24 hours.
Diet advice You may be advised to lower your salt intake to help control your blood pressure.
Storage Keep in a closed container in a cool, dry place out of reach of children.
Missed dose Take as soon as you remember. If your next dose is due within 6 hours, take a single dose now and skip the next. Subsequently, continue with your usual routine.
Stopping the drug Unless severe adverse effects occur (see below), do not stop taking the drug without consulting your doctor. Treatment of hypertension and heart failure is normally lifelong, so if you need to stop it may be necessary to substitute alternative therapy.
Exceeding the dose If you notice any unusual symptoms or if a large overdose has been taken, notify your doctor.

POSSIBLE ADVERSE EFFECTS

Dizziness on standing is likely to occur after the first dose. Nausea and headache are common, but are usually mild and transient. A persistent dry cough is the most common adverse effect, but this can be minimized by taking smaller, more frequent, doses; some people may have to stop taking the drug. If jaundice and rash or itching occur, consult your doctor. If chest pain, swelling of the face or mouth, breathing difficulties, or unconsciousness occur, stop taking the drug and contact your doctor immediately.

INTERACTIONS

NSAIDs (such as ibuprofen) These may reduce the antihypertensive effect of ramipril and increase the risk of kidney damage.
Ciclosporin This drug increases the risk of high potassium levels.
Potassium supplements and potassium-sparing diuretics These may cause excess levels of potassium in the body.

Lithium Like all ACE inhibitors, ramipril may cause raised blood lithium levels and toxicity.

SPECIAL PRECAUTIONS

◆ You have long-term liver or kidney problems.
◆ You have ever suffered from severe allergies.
◆ You have had heart-valve problems.
◆ You have peripheral vascular disease or atherosclerosis.
◆ You suffer from systemic lupus erythematosus or scleroderma.
◆ You are taking other medications.

Pregnancy Not prescribed. May cause defects in the developing baby. Discuss with your doctor.

Breast-feeding The drug passes into the breast milk, but at normal doses adverse effects on the baby are unlikely. Discuss with your doctor.

Infants and children Not usually prescribed.

Over 60 Reduced dose may be necessary.

Driving and hazardous work Avoid such activities until you have learned how ramipril affects you; it can cause dizziness and fainting.

Alcohol Avoid excessive amounts. Alcohol may increase the blood-pressure-lowering and adverse effects of this drug.

Surgery and general anaesthetics Notify your doctor or dentist that you are taking ramipril because anaesthetics can increase its effects.

PROLONGED USE

No problems expected.

Monitoring If you have other medical conditions, blood counts and kidney function tests may be performed at intervals.

Ranitidine

Brand name Ranitic, Rantec, Zaedoc, Zantac
Used in the following combined preparations None

QUICK REFERENCE

Drug group Anti-ulcer drug (p.43)
Overdose danger rating Low
Dependence rating Low
Prescription needed No (tablets in limited quantities); Yes (other preparations)
Available as generic Yes

GENERAL INFORMATION

Ranitidine is prescribed in the treatment of stomach and duodenal ulcers. In combination with antibiotics, it is used for ulcers caused by *Helicobacter pylori* infection. It is also used to protect against duodenal (but not stomach) ulcers in people taking NSAIDs (see p.50), who may be prone to ulcers. In addition, this drug reduces the discomfort and ulceration of reflux oesophagitis and may prevent stress ulceration and gastric bleeding in severely ill patients. Ranitidine reduces the amount of stomach acid produced, allowing ulcers to heal. It is usually given in courses of four to eight weeks, with further courses if symptoms recur.

Ranitidine does not affect the actions of enzymes in the liver, where many drugs are broken down. Consequently, unlike the similar drug cimetidine, it does not increase blood levels of other drugs such as anticoagulants and anticonvulsants, which might reduce their effectiveness.

Most people experience no serious adverse effects. However, as it promotes healing of the stomach lining, there is a risk of it masking stomach cancer, delaying diagnosis. Therefore, it is usually given only when the possibility of stomach cancer has been ruled out.

INFORMATION FOR USERS

Your drug prescription is tailored for you. Do not alter dosage without checking with your doctor.

How taken Tablets, oral liquid, injection.

Frequency and timing of doses Once daily at bedtime or 2–3 x daily.

Adult dosage range 150mg–6g daily, depending on the condition being treated. Usual dose is 150mg twice daily.

Onset of effect Within 1 hour.

Duration of action 12 hours.

Diet advice None.

Storage Keep in a closed container in a cool, dry place out of reach of children. Protect from light.

Missed dose Take as soon as you remember. If your next dose is due within 3 hours, take a single dose now and skip the next.

Stopping the drug Do not stop taking the

drug without consulting your doctor; symptoms may recur.

Exceeding the dose An occasional unintentional extra dose is unlikely to be a cause for concern. But if you notice any unusual symptoms, or if a large overdose has been taken, notify your doctor.

POSSIBLE ADVERSE EFFECTS

Headache and dizziness are common. Other adverse effects, including, nausea, vomiting, constipation, and diarrhoea, are uncommon but are usually related to dosage levels and almost always disappear when treatment ends. If jaundice or confusion, depression, or hallucinations occur, consult your doctor. If you develop a sore throat or fever, contact your doctor immediately.

INTERACTIONS

Ketoconazole Ranitidine may reduce the absorption of ketoconazole. Ranitidine should be taken at least 2 hours after ketoconazole.

Sucralfate High doses (2g) of sucralfate may reduce the absorption of ranitidine. Sucralfate should be taken at least 2 hours after ranitidine.

SPECIAL PRECAUTIONS

Be sure to tell your doctor if:
♦ You have long-term liver or kidney problems.
♦ You have porphyria.
♦ You are taking other medications.
Pregnancy Safety in pregnancy not established. Discuss with your doctor.
Breast-feeding The drug passes into the breast milk and may affect the baby. Discuss with your doctor.
Infants and children Reduced dose necessary.
Over 60 No special problems.
Driving and hazardous work No known problems. Dizziness can occur in a very small proportion of patients.
Alcohol Avoid. Alcohol may aggravate your underlying condition and reduce the beneficial effects of this drug.

PROLONGED USE

No problems expected.

Repaglinide

Brand name NovoNorm
Used in the following combined preparations
None

QUICK REFERENCE

Drug group Drug used in diabetes (p.82)
Overdose danger rating Medium
Dependence rating Low
Prescription needed Yes
Available as generic No

GENERAL INFORMATION

Repaglinide is used to treat non-insulin-dependent diabetes (see p.82) that cannot be adequately controlled by diet and exercise alone. Like sulphonylurea drugs, it acts by stimulating release of insulin from the pancreas. Therefore, for it to be effective, some pancreatic cells need to be functioning.

The drug is fast-acting, but its effects last for only about four hours. It is sometimes given with metformin if that drug is not providing adequate diabetic control.

Repaglinide is best taken just before a meal in order for the insulin released to be able to cope with the food. If a meal is likely to be missed, the dose of repaglinide should not be taken. If a tablet has been taken and a meal is not forthcoming, some carbohydrate (as specified by your doctor or dietitian) should be eaten as soon as possible.

INFORMATION FOR USERS

Your drug prescription is tailored for you. Do not alter dosage without checking with your doctor.
How taken Tablets.
Frequency and timing of doses 1–4 x daily (up to 30 minutes before a meal, and up to 4 meals a day). If you are going to miss a meal, do not take the tablet.
Adult dosage range 500mcg (starting dose), increased at intervals of 1–2 weeks according to response; 4–16mg daily (maintenance dose).
Onset of effect 30 minutes.
Duration of action 4 hours.

Diet advice Follow the diet advised by your doctor or dietitian.

Storage Keep in a closed container in a cool, dry place out of reach of children.

Missed dose Do not take tablets between meals. Discuss with your doctor.

Stopping the drug Do not stop taking the drug without consulting your doctor.

Exceeding the dose An overdose of repaglinide will cause hypoglycaemia, with dizziness, sweating, trembling, confusion, and headache; notify your doctor.

POSSIBLE ADVERSE EFFECTS

Intestinal problems such as nausea, vomiting, abdominal pain, and diarrhoea or constipation are common at the start of treatment but tend to become less troublesome as treatment continues. If rash or itching occur, consult your doctor.

INTERACTIONS

MAOIs, beta-blockers, ACE inhibitors, and NSAIDs These drugs may increase the effect of repaglinide.

Oral contraceptives, thiazide diuretics, corticosteroids, danazol, thyroid hormones, and sympathomimetics These drugs may decrease the effect of repaglinide.

SPECIAL PRECAUTIONS

Be sure to tell your doctor if:
◆ You have liver or kidney problems.
◆ You are taking other medications.
Pregnancy Safety not established. Discuss with your doctor.
Breast-feeding Safety not established. Discuss with your doctor.
Infants and children Not recommended.
Over 60 No special problems, but safety not established for people over 75 years.
Driving and hazardous work Avoid if low blood glucose without warning signs is likely.
Alcohol Avoid. Alcohol may upset diabetic control and may increase and prolong the effects of repaglinide.

PROLONGED USE

No special problems. Repaglinide is usually prescribed indefinitely.

Rifampicin

Brand names Rifadin, Rimactane
Used in the following combined preparations
Rifater, Rifinah, Rimactazid

QUICK REFERENCE

Drug group Antituberculous drug (p.67)
Overdose danger rating Medium
Dependence rating Low
Prescription needed Yes
Available as generic Yes

GENERAL INFORMATION

Rifampicin is an antibacterial drug that is highly effective in the treatment of tuberculosis. Taken by mouth, the drug is well absorbed in the intestine and widely distributed throughout the body, including the brain. As a result, rifampicin is particularly useful in the treatment of tuberculous meningitis. To prevent recurrent disease in later life, a course of treatment may last up to a year.

Rifampicin is also used to treat leprosy and other serious infections, including Legionnaires' disease and infections of the bone (osteomyelitis). Additionally, it is given to anyone in close contact with meningococcal meningitis in order to prevent infection. Rifampicin is always prescribed with other antibiotics or antituberculous drugs because some bacteria rapidly develop resistance to it.

The drug may cause urine, saliva, and tears to take on a harmless red-orange colour; soft contact lenses may be permanently stained.

INFORMATION FOR USERS

Your drug prescription is tailored for you. Do not alter dosage without checking with your doctor.

How taken Tablets, capsules, liquid, injection.
Frequency and timing of doses *Tuberculosis* 1 x daily, 30 minutes before breakfast. *Leprosy* Once a month (as part of a combined treatment that is given daily). *Prevention of meningococcal meningitis* 2 x daily. *Other serious infections* 2–4 x daily, 30 minutes before or 2 hours after meals.
Adult dosage range *Tuberculosis* According to

bodyweight; usually 450–600mg daily. *Leprosy* 600mg once a month. *Meningococcal meningitis* 1.2g daily for 2 days. *Other serious infections* 600mg–1.2g daily.

Onset of effect Over several days.

Duration of action Up to 24 hours.

Diet advice None.

Storage Keep in a closed container in a cool, dry place out of reach of children. Protect from light.

Missed dose Take as soon as you remember. If your next dose is due within 6 hours, take a single dose now, then return to normal dosing schedule.

Stopping the drug Take the full course. Even if you feel better, the original infection may still be present and symptoms may recur if treatment is stopped too soon. In rare cases stopping the drug suddenly after high-dose treatment can lead to a severe flu-like illness.

Exceeding the dose An occasional unintentional extra dose is unlikely to cause problems. Large overdoses may cause liver damage, nausea, vomiting, and lethargy. Notify your doctor immediately.

POSSIBLE ADVERSE EFFECTS

A harmless red-orange coloration of body fluids normally occurs. Serious adverse effects are rare, but may include nausea, vomiting, diarrhoea, muscle cramps or aches, and jaundice, which usually improves during treatment. If you develop a rash or itching or jaundice, consult your doctor. Headache and breathing difficulties may occur after stopping high-dose treatment. If a flu-like illness occurs, stop taking the drug and contact your doctor immediately.

INTERACTIONS

General note Rifampicin may reduce the effectiveness of a wide variety of drugs, such as oral contraceptives (in which case alternative contraceptive methods may be necessary), phenytoin, corticosteroids, oral antidiabetics, disopyramide, and oral anticoagulants. Dosage adjustment of these drugs may be necessary at the start or end of treatment with rifampicin. Consult your doctor or pharmacist for advice.

SPECIAL PRECAUTIONS

Be sure to tell your doctor if:

◆ You have any long-term liver or kidney problems.

◆ You wear contact lenses.

◆ You have porphyria.

◆ You are taking other medications.

Pregnancy Safety in pregnancy not established. Discuss with your doctor.

Breast-feeding The drug passes into the breast milk, but at normal doses adverse effects on the baby are unlikely. Discuss with your doctor.

Infants and children Reduced dose necessary.

Over 60 Reduced dose may be necessary. Increased risk of adverse effects.

Driving and hazardous work No problems expected.

Alcohol Avoid excessive amounts. Heavy alcohol consumption may increase the risk of liver damage.

PROLONGED USE

Prolonged use of rifampicin may cause liver damage.

Monitoring Periodic blood tests may be performed to monitor liver function.

Risperidone

Brand names Risperdal
Used in the following combined preparations
None

QUICK REFERENCE

Drug group Antipsychotic drug (p.15)
Overdose danger rating Medium
Dependence rating Low
Prescription needed Yes
Available as generic No

GENERAL INFORMATION

Risperidone is used to treat acute psychiatric disorders and long-term psychotic illness such as schizophrenia. Although it does not cure the underlying disorder, it helps to alleviate the distressing symptoms. It is effective for relieving both "positive" symptoms (for example, hallucinations, thought disturbances, and hostility) and "negative" symptoms (such as emotional and social withdrawal). The drug may also help with various other symptoms often associated with schizophrenia, such as depression and anxiety. Risperidone has less of a sedative effect, and is also less likely to cause movement disorders as a side effect, than some other antipsychotics.

INFORMATION FOR USERS

Your drug prescription is tailored for you. Do not alter dosage without checking with your doctor.

How taken Tablets, liquid, injection.

Frequency and timing of doses 1–2 x daily (tablets, liquid).

Adult dosage range *Tablets* 2mg daily (starting dose) increasing to 4–6mg daily (usual maintenance dose); maximum 16mg daily. *Liquid* 2ml daily (starting dose) increasing to 4–6ml daily (usual maintenance dose); maximum 16 ml daily. *Injection* 25mg every 2 weeks (starting dose) increasing to 50mg every 2 weeks (maximum maintenance dose).

Onset of effect *Tablets/liquid* Within 2–3 days; maximum effect may take up to 4 weeks. *Injection* Up to 3 weeks.

Duration of action Approximately 2 days.

Diet advice None.

Storage Keep in a closed container in a cool, dry place out of reach of children. Protect from light.

Missed dose Take as soon as you remember. If your next dose is due within 3 hours, take a single dose now and skip the next.

Stopping the drug Unless severe adverse effects occur (see below), do not stop without consulting your doctor; symptoms may recur.

Exceeding the dose An occasional unintentional extra dose is unlikely to cause problems. If larger doses have been taken, notify your doctor.

POSSIBLE ADVERSE EFFECTS

Risperidone is generally well tolerated and movement disorders are rare. It is less sedating than some other antipsychotics, but adverse effects include insomnia, anxiety, agitation, headache, drowsiness, difficulty in concentrating, and dizziness. Weight gain, shakiness and tremor, rash and excessive thirst may also occur; consult your doctor. If you develop a high fever or rigid muscles, stop taking the drug and contact your doctor urgently.

INTERACTIONS

Drugs for parkinsonism Risperidone may reduce the effect of these drugs.

Carbamazepine This drug increases the levels of certain liver enzymes that break down drugs, thus making risperidone ineffective. Other drugs with a similar action, such as phenytoin, may have the same effect.

Sedatives All drugs that have a sedative effect on the central nervous system are likely to increase any sedative effect of risperidone.

Fluoxetine This drug increases the blood levels of risperidone and the risk of side effects.

SPECIAL PRECAUTIONS

Be sure to tell your doctor if:

◆ You have liver or kidney problems.

◆ You have heart or circulation problems.

◆ You have had epileptic fits.

◆ You have Parkinson's disease.

◆ You are taking other medications.

Pregnancy Safety in pregnancy not established. Discuss with your doctor.

Breast-feeding The drug probably passes into breast milk. Discuss with your doctor.

Infants and children Not recommended under 15 years.

Over 60 Reduced dose necessary.

Driving and hazardous work Avoid such activities until you have learned how risperidone affects you because the drug may cause difficulty in concentration and slowed reactions.

Alcohol Avoid excessive amounts. Alcohol may increase the sedative effects of this drug.

Surgery and general anaesthetics Risperidone treatment may need to be stopped before you have a general anaesthetic. Discuss this with your doctor or dentist before any operation.

PROLONGED USE

Permanent movement disorders (tardive dyskinesia) may occur but are less likely than with many other antipsychotics.

Rivastigmine

Brand names Exelon
Used in the following combined preparations
None

QUICK REFERENCE

Drug group Drug for dementia (p.19)
Overdose danger rating Medium
Dependence rating Low
Prescription needed Yes
Available as generic No

GENERAL INFORMATION

Rivastigmine is an inhibitor of the enzyme acetylcholinesterase. The enzyme breaks down the naturally occurring neurotransmitter acetylcholine to limit its effects. Blocking the enzyme raises the levels of acetylcholine in the brain, which increases alertness.

It has been found that rivastigmine can improve mild to moderate dementia in Alzheimer's disease, and the drug is used to slow the rate of deterioration in that disease. Rivastigmine is not, however, currently recommended for dementia due to other causes. It is usual for anyone treated with rivastigmine to be assessed after about three months to decide whether it is helping and whether it is worth continuing treatment. As the disease progresses, the beneficial effect may diminish.

Side effects may include agitation, confusion and depression (which could be thought due to Alzheimer's disease). Weight should be monitored in case of weight loss.

INFORMATION FOR USERS

Your drug prescription is tailored for you. Do not alter dosage without checking with your doctor.
How taken Capsules, liquid.
Frequency and timing of doses 2 x daily.
Adult dosage range 3mg daily (starting dose); 6–12mg daily (maintenance dose).
Onset of effect 30–60 minutes.
Duration of action 9–12 hours.
Diet advice None.
Storage Keep in a closed container in a cool, dry place out of reach of children.

Missed dose Take as soon as you remember. If your next dose is due within 4 hours, take a single dose now and skip the next. A carer should be overseeing the taking of tablets.
Stopping the drug Do not stop the drug without consulting your doctor; symptoms may recur.
Exceeding the dose An occasional unintentional extra dose is unlikely to be a problem. Large overdoses, however, may cause nausea, vomiting and diarrhoea; notify your doctor.

POSSIBLE ADVERSE EFFECTS

Common, usually mild problems include agitation, confusion and depression, drowsiness and dizziness, and intestinal problems such as reduced appetite, nausea, abdominal pain, and weight loss. Women may be more susceptible to nausea, vomiting, and weight loss. Weakness, trembling, sweating, malaise, headache, and insomnia may also occur. If convulsions occur, seek medical attention.

INTERACTIONS

General note Rivastigmine is a relatively new drug, and interactions with other drugs are not fully established. If you notice changes in the effect of the drug after taking or stopping other medications, consult your doctor.
Muscle relaxants used in surgery Rivastigmine may increase the effects of some muscle relaxants and may block the effects of others.

SPECIAL PRECAUTIONS

Be sure to tell your doctor if:
◆ You have a heart problem.
◆ You have liver or kidney problems.
◆ You have asthma or respiratory problems.
◆ You have had a gastric or duodenal ulcer.
◆ You are taking other medications.
Pregnancy Safety not established.
Breast-feeding Not recommended.
Infants and children Not recommended.
Over 60 No special problems.
Driving and hazardous work Your underlying condition may make such activities inadvisable. Discuss with your doctor.
Alcohol Avoid. Alcohol increases the sedative effects of rivastigmine.
Surgery and general anaesthetics Treatment may need to be stopped before you have a

general anaesthetic. Discuss this with your doctor or dentist before any operation.

PROLONGED USE

May be continued for as long as there is benefit. Stopping the drug leads to a gradual loss of the improvements.
Monitoring Periodic checks may be carried out to test whether the drug is still providing some benefit.

Rosiglitazone

Brand name Avandia
Used in the following combined preparation
None

QUICK REFERENCE

Drug group Drug used in diabetes (p.82)
Overdose danger rating High
Dependence rating Low
Prescription needed Yes
Available as generic No

GENERAL INFORMATION

Rosiglitazone is used to treat non-insulin-dependent diabetes mellitus (NIDDM; Type 2 diabetes). It works by reducing insulin resistance in fatty tissue, skeletal muscle, and the liver, which leads to a reduction of blood glucose levels. The effects appear gradually and reach their full extent in about 8 weeks.

The drug is not used on its own, but is usually prescribed with metformin (see p.309) or a sulphonylurea (see p.83) if metformin is contraindicated. The combined treatment can produce a significant improvement in diabetic control. Rosiglitazone works better in obese people, although it often causes weight gain. Anaemia is another adverse effect.

Rosiglitazone is not used with insulin.

INFORMATION FOR USERS

Your drug prescription is tailored for you. Do not alter dosage without checking with your doctor.
How taken Tablets.
Frequency and timing of doses 1–2 x daily.

Adult dosage range 4–8mg daily.
Onset of effect 60 minutes; full beneficial effects may not be felt for up to 8 weeks.
Duration of action 12–24 hours.
Diet advice An individualized low-fat, low-sugar diet must be maintained in order for the drug to be fully effective. Follow your doctor's advice.
Storage Keep in a closed container in a cool dry place out of the reach of children.
Missed dose Take as soon as you remember. If your next dose is due within 2 hours, take a single dose now and skip the next.
Stopping the drug Do not stop taking the drug without consulting your doctor; stopping it may lead to worsening of the underlying condition.

OVERDOSE ACTION

Seek immediate medical advice in all cases. Take emergency action if loss of consciousness occurs.

POSSIBLE ADVERSE EFFECTS

Fatigue and weakness (as a result of anaemia) and weight gain (even in those on a strict diabetic diet) are two of the more common side effects of rosiglitazone. Nausea and abdominal disturbances are also common. Fatigue or weakness, headache, or weight gain may occur. Less common effects include dark urine, dizziness, pins and needles, sleepiness, swollen ankles, and painful breathing or a night-time cough. If any of these occur, consult your doctor.

INTERACTIONS

Paclitaxel may reduce the metabolism and increase the effects of rosiglitazone.
ACE inhibitors may increase the effects of rosiglitazone.
Diazoxide reduces the effects of rosiglitazone.

SPECIAL PRECAUTIONS

Be sure to tell your doctor if:
◆ You have liver problems.
◆ You are anaemic.
◆ You have heart failure.
◆ You have severe kidney failure.
◆ You are taking other medications.

Pregnancy Safety not established. Discuss with your doctor.

Breast-feeding Safety not established. Discuss with your doctor.

Infants and children Not recommended.

Over 60 No special problems.

Driving and hazardous work No known problems.

Alcohol No known problems.

PROLONGED USE

Rosiglitazone, like other antidiabetic drugs, is used indefinitely.

Monitoring Periodic blood tests of liver function and haemoglobin levels will be performed. The heart's performance will be monitored regularly. Weight will be measured at intervals.

Salbutamol

Brand name Aerolin, Airomir, Asmasal, Maxivent, Salamol, Salbulin, Ventmax, Ventodisks, Ventolin, Volmax, and others
Used in the following combined preparations Aerocrom, Combivent, Ventide

QUICK REFERENCE
Drug group Bronchodilator (p.23) and drug used in premature labour (p.110)
Overdose danger rating Low
Dependence rating Low
Prescription needed Yes
Available as generic Yes

GENERAL INFORMATION
Salbutamol is a sympathomimetic bronchodilator that relaxes the muscle surrounding the bronchioles (airways in the lungs).

It is used to relieve symptoms of asthma, and may help some people with chronic bronchitis or emphysema. Although it can be taken by mouth, inhalation is considered more effective because the drug is delivered directly to the bronchioles, thus giving rapid relief, allowing smaller doses, and causing fewer side effects. Inhaled corticosteroids are commonly also given with salbutamol.

Compared with some similar drugs, salbutamol has little stimulant effect on the heart rate and blood pressure, making it safer for people with heart problems or high blood pressure. Because it relaxes the muscles of the uterus, it is also used to prevent premature labour.

The most common side effect of salbutamol is fine tremor of the hands, which may interfere with precise manual work. Anxiety, tension, and restlessness may also occur.

INFORMATION FOR USERS
Your drug prescription is tailored for you. Do not alter dosage without checking with your doctor.
How taken Tablets, SR-tablets, capsules, liquid, injection, inhaler, powder for inhalation.
Frequency and timing of doses 1–2 inhalations 3–4 x daily (inhaler); 3–4 x daily (tablets/liquid); 2 x daily (SR-tablets).
Dosage range 400–800mcg daily (inhaler); 8–32mg daily (by mouth).

Onset of effect Within 5–15 minutes (inhaler); within 30–60 minutes (by mouth).
Duration of action Up to 6 hours (inhaler); up to 8 hours (by mouth).
Diet advice None.
Storage Keep in a closed container in a cool, dry place out of reach of children. Protect from light. Do not puncture or burn inhalers.
Missed dose Take as soon as you remember if needed. If your next dose is due within 2 hours, take a single dose now and skip the next.
Stopping the drug Do not stop taking the drug without consulting your doctor; symptoms may recur.
Exceeding the dose An occasional unintentional extra dose is unlikely to be a cause for concern. But if you notice any unusual symptoms, or if a large overdose has been taken, notify your doctor.

POSSIBLE ADVERSE EFFECTS
Muscle tremor (which particularly affects the hands), anxiety, and restlessness are the most common adverse effects. Seek medical advice if the symptoms are severe. Muscle cramps and headache may also occur. If you suffer from palpitations, stop taking the drug and consult your doctor.

INTERACTIONS
Theophylline There is a risk that blood potassium levels may become too low if this drug is taken with salbutamol.
MAOIs These drugs can interact with salbutamol to produce a dangerous rise in blood pressure.
Other sympathomimetics These drugs may increase the effects of salbutamol, thereby also increasing the risk of adverse effects.
Beta blockers These drugs may oppose the action of salbutamol and should not be taken with it; but salbutamol may be given to relieve the airways when beta blockers cause wheezing.

SPECIAL PRECAUTIONS
Be sure to tell your doctor if:
◆ You have heart problems.
◆ You have high blood pressure.
◆ You have an overactive thyroid gland.
◆ You have diabetes.
◆ You are taking other medications.

Pregnancy No evidence of risk when used to treat asthma, or to treat or prevent premature labour. Discuss with your doctor.

Breast-feeding The drug passes into the breast milk, but at normal doses adverse effects on the baby are unlikely. Discuss with your doctor.

Infants and children Reduced dose necessary.

Over 60 Reduced dose may be necessary. Increased likelihood of adverse effects.

Driving and hazardous work Avoid such activities until you have learned how salbutamol affects you because the drug can cause tremors.

Alcohol No known problems.

PROLONGED USE

No problems expected, but contact your doctor if you need to use your inhaler more often than usual because this may be a result of worsening asthma that requires urgent medical attention.

Monitoring Periodic blood tests for potassium may be needed in people on high-dose treatment with salbutamol combined with other asthma drugs.

Salmeterol

Brand name Serevent
Used in the following combined preparation
Seretide

QUICK REFERENCE

Drug group Bronchodilator (p.23)
Overdose danger rating Low
Dependence rating Low
Prescription needed Yes
Available as generic No

GENERAL INFORMATION

Salmeterol is a sympathomimetic bronchodilator used to treat conditions, such as asthma and bronchospasm, in which the airways become constricted. Its advantage over salbutamol (see p.379) is that it is longer-acting.

Salmeterol relaxes the muscle surrounding the airways in the lungs. Because the effect develops slowly, it is not used to relieve the immediate symptoms of asthma. It is prescribed to prevent attacks, however, and can be helpful in controlling night-time asthma.

Inhalers deliver salmeterol directly to the airways. This allows smaller doses to be taken and reduces the risk of adverse effects.

INFORMATION FOR USERS

Your drug prescription is tailored for you. Do not alter dosage without checking with your doctor.

How taken Inhaler, powder for inhalation.
Frequency and timing of doses 2 x daily.
Adult dosage range 100–200mcg daily.
Onset of effect 10–20 minutes.
Duration of action 12 hours.
Diet advice None.
Storage Keep in a cool, dry place out of reach of children.
Missed dose Take as soon as you remember. If your next dose is due within 4 hours, take a single dose now and skip the next.
Stopping the drug Unless wheezing and breathlessness occur, do not stop taking the drug without consulting your doctor; symptoms may recur.
Exceeding the dose An occasional unintentional extra dose is unlikely to be a cause for concern. But if you notice any unusual symptoms, or if a large overdose has been taken, notify your doctor.

POSSIBLE ADVERSE EFFECTS

Side effects are usually mild. The most common is tremor. If headache and palpitations occur, consult your doctor. If wheezing and breathlessness (paradoxical bronchospasm) occur, stop taking the drug and contact your doctor immediately.

INTERACTIONS

Corticosteroids, theophylline, and diuretics These increase the risk of low blood potassium levels with high doses of salmeterol.

SPECIAL PRECAUTIONS

Be sure to tell your doctor if:
◆ You have heart problems.
◆ You have high blood pressure.
◆ You have an overactive thyroid.
◆ You have diabetes.
◆ You are taking other medications.
Pregnancy No evidence of risk when used to treat asthma. Discuss with your doctor.
Breast-feeding No known problems.

Infants and children Reduced dose necessary. Not recommended under 4 years.
Over 60 No special problems.
Driving and hazardous work No special problems.
Alcohol No known problems.

PROLONGED USE

Salmeterol is intended to be used long term. The main problem comes from using combinations of anti-asthma drugs, leading to low blood potassium levels.

Sertraline

Brand name Lustral
Used in the following combined preparations None

QUICK REFERENCE

Drug group Antidepressant (p.14)
Overdose danger rating Medium
Dependence rating Low
Prescription needed Yes
Available as generic No

GENERAL INFORMATION

Sertraline belongs to a group of antidepressants called selective serotonin re-uptake inhibitors (SSRIs). These drugs tend to cause less sedation and have different side effects from older types of antidepressants. Sertraline elevates mood, increases physical activity, and restores interest in everyday activities. It is used to treat depression, including accompanying anxiety, and for obsessive-compulsive disorder. Sertraline is also prescribed for post-traumatic stress disorder in women; it has not been shown to work in men with this condition.

The drug is usually stopped gradually, because symptoms such as headache, nausea, and dizziness may occur if sertraline is withdrawn suddenly.

INFORMATION FOR USERS

Your drug prescription is tailored for you. Do not alter dosage without checking with your doctor.
How taken Tablets.
Frequency and timing of doses Once daily.
Adult dosage range 50–200mg daily.
Onset of effect Some benefits may appear within 14 days, but full beneficial effects may take a further 2 weeks.
Duration of action 24 hours.
Diet advice None.
Storage Keep in a closed container in a cool, dry place out of reach of children.
Missed dose Take as soon as you remember. If your next dose is due within 8 hours, take a single dose now and skip the next.
Stopping the drug Do not stop taking the drug without consulting your doctor, who may supervise a gradual reduction in dosage.
Exceeding the dose An occasional unintentional extra dose is unlikely to cause problems. Large overdoses, however, may cause adverse effects; notify your doctor.

POSSIBLE ADVERSE EFFECTS

Restlessness, insomnia, and gastrointestinal problems such as diarrhoea, loose stools, loss of appetite and indigestion are common. If dizziness, tremor, confusion, palpitations, fainting, and impotence occur, consult your doctor. If a rash develops, or there is itching or skin eruptions, stop taking the drug and contact your doctor immediately.

INTERACTIONS

St John's wort There is a danger of greatly increasing the effects of both substances.
MAOIs Sertraline's effects and toxicity are greatly increased by MAOIs.
Terfenadine There is an increased risk of heart arrhythmias if this is taken with sertraline.
Artemether with lumefantrine This drug should not be taken with sertraline.
Antiepileptics Sertraline opposes the effects of these drugs and increases the risk of seizures.
Tramadol There is an increased risk of toxicity if tramadol is taken with sertraline.
Clozapine, haloperidol, and zotepine Sertraline increases the levels and effects of these drugs.

SPECIAL PRECAUTIONS

Be sure to tell your doctor if:
◆ You have long-term liver or kidney problems.
◆ You have had epileptic fits.
◆ You have heart problems.
◆ You have a history of bleeding disorders.
◆ You have diabetes.

◆ You have glaucoma.
◆ You have had a previous allergic reaction to an SSRI.
◆ You have a history of mania.
◆ You are taking other medications.

Pregnancy Safety not established. Discuss with your doctor.

Breast-feeding Safety not established. Discuss with your doctor.

Infants and children Not recommended under 6 years. Reduced dose necessary for children over 6 years with obsessive-compulsive disorder.

Over 60 No special problems.

Driving and hazardous work Avoid such activities until you have learned how sertraline affects you because the drug can cause drowsiness, dizziness, visual disturbances, and hallucinations.

Alcohol Avoid. SSRIs may increase the sedative effects of alcohol.

PROLONGED USE

No known problems.

Sibutramine

Brand name Reductil
Used in the following combined preparations
None

QUICK REFERENCE

Drug group Appetite suppressant (see Nervous system stimulants, p.19)
Overdose danger rating Medium
Dependence rating Low
Prescription needed Yes
Available as generic No

GENERAL INFORMATION

Sibutramine acts on brain neurotransmitters. The drug is used to suppress appetite in people who are obese (having a Body Mass Index, or BMI, of $30kg/m^2$ or more) or overweight (having a BMI of $27kg/m^2$ or more) and who have a condition such as Type 2 diabetes (see p.82) or high blood lipid levels (see p.37). Losing weight reduces the risk of stroke, improves the control of diabetes and gallstones, and reduces the load on joints in conditions such as osteoarthritis.

Drug treatment must be accompanied by a suitable diet. Sibutramine is prescribed when diet alone has failed. Lifestyle changes are also necessary to avoid weight being regained when the drug is withdrawn. Psychological help from a support group is beneficial for some people.

INFORMATION FOR USERS

Your drug prescription is tailored for you. Do not alter dosage without checking with your doctor.

How taken Capsules.

Frequency and timing of doses Once daily, in the morning.

Adult dosage range 10–15mg daily.

Onset of effect 30–60 minutes.

Duration of action 24 hours.

Diet advice Follow a low-fat, low-calorie diet.

Storage Keep in a closed container (the original pack) in a cool, dry place out of the reach of children.

Missed dose Take as soon as you remember. If your next dose is due within 12 hours, wait until you are due to take the next dose.

Stopping the drug Do not stop the drug without consulting your doctor. Stopping it can result in weight being regained.

Exceeding the dose An occasional unintentional extra dose is unlikely to cause problems. Large overdoses, however, may cause adverse effects; notify your doctor.

POSSIBLE ADVERSE EFFECTS

The most common side effects involve the cardiovascular system, and include palpitations and a rapid heart beat. Constipation and haemorrhoids, a dry mouth, nausea, insomnia, anxiety, lightheadedness, headache, hot flushes, and sweating may also occur.

INTERACTIONS

Erythromycin, clarithromycin, ciclosporin, ketoconazole, and itraconazole All of these drugs increase the blood levels and the effects of sibutramine.

Cough and cold remedies These may add to sibutramine's blood-pressure-raising effect.

Dihydroergotamine, sumatriptan, SSRIs, St John's wort, and some opioid analgesics All of these drugs inhibit serotonin re-uptake and can increase the effects of sibutramine.

SPECIAL PRECAUTIONS

Be sure to tell your doctor if:

◆ You have high blood pressure.

◆ You have a psychiatric illness.

◆ You have heart problems.

◆ You have an overactive thyroid.

◆ You have prostate problems.

◆ You have phaeochromocytoma.

◆ You have glaucoma.

◆ You have a history of drug abuse.

◆ You are taking other medications.

Pregnancy Safety not established. Weight-reducing drugs should not be used during pregnancy.

Breast-feeding It is not known whether sibutramine is secreted in breast milk; do not use throughout the breast-feeding period.

Infants and children Not recommended under 18 years.

Over 60 Not recommended over 65 years.

Driving and hazardous work Avoid until you have learned how sibutramine affects you; the drug can cause lightheadedness, blurred vision, seizures, and impaired thinking.

Alcohol Alcohol contains calories and should not be part of a diet supported by sibutramine.

PROLONGED USE

Sibutramine must be stopped after a year. Appetite often increases on withdrawal.

Monitoring Pulse rate, blood pressure, and bodyweight are checked regularly. If weight loss is less than 5 per cent of starting weight, the drug will be stopped.

Sildenafil

Brand name Viagra
Used in the following combined preparations None

QUICK REFERENCE

Drug group Drug for impotence (p.110)
Overdose danger rating Medium
Dependence rating Low
Prescription needed Yes
Available as generic No

GENERAL INFORMATION

Sildenafil is a new type of drug used to treat impotence. It does not cause an erection directly, but it produces a chemical change that prevents the muscle walls of the blood-filled chambers in the penis from relaxing.

Sildenafil does not need to be taken regularly; it is only used to produce an erection and only needs to be taken before sexual activity is initiated.

Because it is a vasodilator, sildenafil can cause a small drop in blood pressure while it is active, and it may increase the effect of antihypertensive drugs (see p.36). The drug is not usually prescribed with nitrates (see p.32) because it greatly increases their effects.

INFORMATION FOR USERS

Your drug prescription is tailored for you. Do not alter dosage without checking with your doctor.

How taken Tablets.

Frequency and timing of doses Once daily (maximum dose), 1 hour before sexual activity.

Adult dosage range 25–100mg.

Onset of effect 30 minutes.

Duration of action 4 hours.

Diet advice None, but sildenafil takes longer to work after food, especially a high-fat meal. It is absorbed faster on an empty stomach.

Storage Keep in a closed container in a cool, dry place out of reach of children.

Missed dose Take the next dose when you need to use it. Do not use more than one dose in a 24-hour period.

Stopping the drug Sildenafil can be safely stopped as soon as you no longer need it.

Exceeding the dose An occasional unintentional extra dose is unlikely to cause problems. Large overdoses, however, may cause headache, dizziness, flushing, altered vision, and nasal congestion; notify your doctor.

POSSIBLE ADVERSE EFFECTS

Most adverse effects of sildenafil are common and short-lived. These include headache, flushing, dizziness, indigestion, nasal congestion, and a bluish colour to vision. If priapism (a prolonged, painful erection) or chest pain occur, stop taking the drug and contact your doctor immediately. Sildenafil has been reported to cause muscle aches when taken more frequently than recommended. It is not certain, however, that this effect is due to the drug.

INTERACTIONS

Nitrates The effects of these drugs are greatly increased by sildenafil, and they are therefore not prescribed with it.

Cimetidine, erythromycin, nicorandil, ketoconazole (oral), and antiviral drugs These drugs increase both the blood levels and the toxicity of sildenafil.

Antihypertensives Sildenafil may enhance the blood-pressure-lowering effect of these drugs.

Other drugs for impotence Safety not established. Use of these drugs with sildenafil is not recommended.

SPECIAL PRECAUTIONS

Be sure to tell your doctor if:
◆ You have heart problems.
◆ You have had a stroke or heart attack.
◆ You have sickle cell anaemia.
◆ You have multiple myeloma.
◆ You have leukaemia.
◆ You have liver or kidney problems.
◆ You have an inherited eye problem.
◆ You have an abnormality of the penis.
◆ You are taking a nitrate drug.
◆ You are taking other medications.

Pregnancy Not prescribed.

Breast-feeding Not prescribed.

Infants and children Not prescribed for anyone under 18 years.

Over 60 Reduced dose may be necessary.

Driving and hazardous work Avoid such activities until you have learned how sildenafil affects you because it can cause dizziness.

Alcohol No special problems.

PROLONGED USE

No problems expected.

Simvastatin

Brand name Zocor
Used in the following combined preparations
None

QUICK REFERENCE

Drug group Lipid-lowering drug (p.37)
Overdose danger rating Medium
Dependence rating Low
Prescription needed Yes
Available as generic No

GENERAL INFORMATION

Simvastatin is a lipid-lowering drug introduced in 1989. It works by blocking the action of an enzyme that enables cholesterol to be manufactured in the liver; as a result, it lowers blood levels of cholesterol. The drug is prescribed for people with hypercholesterolaemia (high blood levels of cholesterol) who have not responded to other treatments, such as a special diet, and who are at risk of developing heart disease. It is also sometimes prescribed for people who have had a heart attack, to reduce the risk of a further attack. Studies are currently being carried out on simvastatin because it may have a beneficial effect on bone strength and mental function.

Side effects are usually mild and often wear off with time. In the body, simvastatin is found mainly in the liver, and it may raise the levels of various liver enzymes. This effect does not usually indicate serious liver damage.

INFORMATION FOR USERS

Your drug prescription is tailored for you. Do not alter dosage without checking with your doctor.

How taken Tablets.

Frequency and timing of doses Once daily at night.

Adult dosage range 10–80mg daily.

Onset of effect Within 2 weeks; full beneficial effects may not be felt for 4–6 weeks.

Duration of action Up to 24 hours.

Diet advice A low-fat diet is usually recommended for people taking simvastatin.

Storage Keep in a closed container in a cool, dry place out of reach of children. Protect from light.

Missed dose Take as soon as you remember. If your next dose is due within 8 hours, do not take the missed dose, but take the next dose on schedule.

Stopping the drug Unless a rash occurs, do not stop taking the drug without consulting your doctor. Stopping the drug has no effect in the short term but may eventually lead to worsening of the underlying condition.

Exceeding the dose An occasional unintentional extra dose is unlikely to cause problems. Large overdoses, however, may cause liver problems; notify your doctor.

POSSIBLE ADVERSE EFFECTS

Adverse effects with simvastatin are usually mild and do not last long. The most common effects are those that affect the gastrointestinal system, such as nausea, flatulence, abdominal pain, and constipation or diarrhoea. Headaches may also occur. If you develop a rash, muscle pain, or weakness, stop taking the drug and contact your doctor immediately.

INTERACTIONS

Anticoagulants Simvastatin may increase the effect of anticoagulants. The dose may need to be adjusted, and prothrombin time (a measure of the speed of blood clotting) should be monitored regularly.

Ciclosporin and other immunosuppressant drugs, and antiviral drugs Simvastatin and these drugs are not usually prescribed together because of the risk of muscle toxicity.

Other lipid-lowering drugs Taken with simvastatin, these drugs may increase the risk of muscle toxicity.

Itraconazole, ketoconazole, telithromycin, and erythromycin When taken with simvastatin, any of these drugs may increase the risk of muscle toxicity.

SPECIAL PRECAUTIONS

Be sure to tell your doctor if:
◆ You have liver or kidney problems.
◆ You have eye or vision problems.
◆ You have muscle weakness.
◆ You have a thyroid disorder.
◆ You have had problems with alcohol abuse.
◆ You have porphyria.
◆ You have angina.
◆ You have high blood pressure.
◆ You are taking other medications.

Pregnancy Not usually prescribed. Safety in pregnancy not established. Discuss with your doctor.

Breast-feeding Safety not established. Discuss with your doctor.

Infants and children Not recommended.

Over 60 No special problems.

Driving and hazardous work No special problems.

Alcohol Avoid excessive amounts. Alcohol may increase your risk of developing liver problems with this drug.

PROLONGED USE

Prolonged treatment can adversely affect liver function.

Monitoring Regular blood tests to assess liver function and muscle strength are recommended for people taking simvastatin.

Sodium bicarbonate

Used in the following combined preparations
Alka-Seltzer, Bismag, Bisodol, Carbalax, Dioralyte, Gastrocote, Gaviscon, Mictral, Roter, and many others

QUICK REFERENCE

Drug group Antacid (p.42)
Overdose danger rating Medium
Dependence rating Low
Prescription needed No
Available as generic Yes

GENERAL INFORMATION

Sodium bicarbonate is available without prescription for the relief of occasional episodes of indigestion and heartburn, either alone or in multi-ingredient preparations. The drug may also relieve the discomfort caused by peptic ulcers. However, sodium bicarbonate is now seldom recommended by doctors because other drugs are safer and more effective.

Because sodium bicarbonate also reduces the acidity of the urine, relieving painful urination, it is sometimes recommended for cystitis. It should be avoided by people with heart failure and a history of kidney disease, however. It is sometimes given by injection to reduce the acidity of the blood and body tissues in metabolic acidosis, a potentially fatal condition that may occur in life-threatening illnesses or following cardiac arrest. Ear drops containing sodium bicarbonate are sometimes used for softening ear wax prior to removing it.

INFORMATION FOR USERS

Follow instructions on the label. Call your doctor if symptoms worsen.

How taken Tablets, capsules, liquid, powder (dissolved in water), injection, ear drops.

Frequency and timing of doses *Indigestion* As required (by mouth).

Adult dosage range Dependent on the condition being treated. As an antacid: 1–5g per dose.

Onset of effect Within 15 minutes as an antacid.

Duration of action 30–60 minutes as an antacid.

Diet advice None.

Storage Keep in a closed container in a cool, dry place out of reach of children.

Missed dose No cause for concern.

Stopping the drug When taken for indigestion, sodium bicarbonate can be safely stopped. If it is being used to treat other disorders, consult your doctor.

Exceeding the dose An occasional unintentional extra dose is unlikely to cause problems. Large overdoses, however, may cause unusual weakness, dizziness, or headache; notify your doctor.

POSSIBLE ADVERSE EFFECTS

Belching and stomach pain may arise from the carbon dioxide that is produced as sodium bicarbonate neutralizes stomach acid, and can be caused by a single dose. Other effects, such as muscle cramps, weakness, vomiting, shortness of breath, and swollen ankles, result from the long-term, regular use of sodium bicarbonate.

INTERACTIONS

General note Sodium bicarbonate interferes with the absorption or excretion of a wide range of drugs taken by mouth. Consult your doctor if you are taking oral anticoagulants, tetracycline antibiotics, phenothiazine antipsychotics, oral iron preparations, or lithium and you wish to take more than an occasional dose of sodium bicarbonate.

Diuretics The beneficial effects of these drugs may be reduced by sodium bicarbonate.

Corticosteroids Large doses of sodium bicarbonate may hasten potassium loss and increase fluid retention and high blood pressure with these drugs.

SPECIAL PRECAUTIONS

Be sure to consult your doctor or pharmacist before taking this drug if:

◆ You have long-term liver or kidney problems.

◆ You have heart problems.

◆ You have high blood pressure.

◆ You have severe abdominal pain or vomiting.

◆ You are on a low-sodium diet.

◆ You are taking other medications.

Pregnancy No evidence of risk, but it is not likely to help morning sickness, and can encourage fluid retention.

Breast-feeding No evidence of risk.

Infants and children Not recommended under 6 years except on the advice of a doctor. Reduced dose necessary.

Over 60 Reduced dose may be necessary.

Driving and hazardous work No special problems.

Alcohol Avoid excessive amounts. Alcohol irritates the stomach and may counter the beneficial effects of this drug.

PROLONGED USE

Severe weakness, fatigue, and muscle cramps may occur when this drug is taken regularly for extended periods. You should not use it daily for longer than 2 weeks without consulting your doctor.

Monitoring Blood and urine tests may be performed during prolonged use.

Sodium cromoglicate

Brand names Cromogen, Hay-Crom, Intal, Nalcrom, Opticrom, Rynacrom, Vividrin

Used in the following combined preparations Aerocrom, Rynacrom Compound

QUICK REFERENCE

Drug group Anti-allergy drug (p.24)

Overdose danger rating Low

Dependence rating Low

Prescription needed No (some preparations)

Available as generic Yes

GENERAL INFORMATION

Sodium cromoglicate, introduced in the 1970s, is used primarily to prevent asthma and allergic conditions.

When taken by inhaler as a powder (Spinhaler) or spray, it is commonly used to reduce the frequency and severity of asthma attacks, and is also effective in helping to prevent attacks induced by exercise or cold air. The drug has a slow onset of action, and it may take up to 6 weeks to produce its full anti-asthmatic effect. It is not effective for the relief of an asthma attack. Taken as a nasal spray, the drug is used to prevent allergic rhinitis (hay fever). It is also given as capsules for food allergy, and given as eye drops to prevent allergic conjunctivitis.

Adverse effects from sodium cromoglicate are mild. If you suffer from coughing and wheezing when inhaling the drug, the problem may be prevented by using a sympathomimetic bronchodilator (see p.23) first. Hoarseness and throat irritation can be avoided by rinsing the mouth with water after inhalation.

INFORMATION FOR USERS

Follow instructions on the label. Call your doctor if symptoms worsen.

How taken Capsules, inhaler (various types), eye drops, nasal spray.

Frequency and timing of doses
4 x daily before meals, swallowed whole or dissolved in water (capsules); 4–6 x daily (inhaler/nasal preparations); 4 x daily (eye drops); 2–3 x daily (eye ointment).

Dosage range 800mg daily (capsules); as directed (inhaler); apply to each nostril as directed (nasal preparations); 1–2 drops in each eye per dose (eye drops).

Onset of effect Varies with dosage, form, and condition treated. Eye conditions and allergic rhinitis may respond after a few days' treatment with drops, while asthma and chronic allergic rhinitis may take take 2–6 weeks to show improvement.

Duration of action 4–6 hours. Some effect will persist for several days after treatment has been stopped.

Diet advice If you are taking capsules for food allergy, you may need to avoid foods that trigger symptoms. Follow your doctor's advice.

Storage Keep in a closed container in a cool, dry place out of reach of children. Protect from light.

Missed dose Take as soon as you remember. If your next dose is due within 2 hours, take a single dose now and skip the next.

Stopping the drug Do not stop taking the drug without consulting your doctor; symptoms may recur.

Exceeding the dose An occasional unintentional extra dose is unlikely to be a cause for concern. But if you notice any unusual symptoms, or if a large overdose has been taken, notify your doctor.

POSSIBLE ADVERSE EFFECTS

Coughing and hoarseness, and local irritation, are common with inhalation of sodium cromoglicate. Nasal spray may cause sneezing. These symptoms usually diminish with continued use. If they continue or are severe, consult your doctor. Capsules may cause nausea and vomiting, joint pain, wheezing, and breathlessness. If these occur, seek medical advice. If you develop a rash, stop taking the drug immediately.

INTERACTIONS

None.

SPECIAL PRECAUTIONS

Be sure to consult your doctor or pharmacist before taking this drug if:
◆ You are taking other medications.
Pregnancy No evidence of risk.
Breast-feeding No evidence of risk.
Infants and children Reduced dose necessary.
Over 60 No special problems.
Driving and hazardous work No known problems.
Alcohol No known problems.

PROLONGED USE

No problems expected.

Sodium valproate (Valproate)

Brand names Convulex (valproic acid), Epilim, Epilim Chrono, Orlept
Used in the following combined preparations None

QUICK REFERENCE

Drug group Anticonvulsant drug (p.16)
Overdose danger rating Medium
Dependency rating Low
Prescription needed Yes
Available as generic Yes

GENERAL INFORMATION

Sodium valproate is an anticonvulsant drug that is often used for the treatment of various types of epilepsy. Its action is similar to that of other anticonvulsants; it reduces electrical discharges in the brain, thereby preventing the excessive build-up that can lead to epileptic fits.

The drug is beneficial in long-term treatment and has no sedative effect. This makes it particularly suitable for children who suffer from either atonic epilepsy (the sudden relaxing of the muscles throughout the body) or absence seizures (during which the person appears to be daydreaming).

Care should be taken if you are changing from sodium valproate to valproic acid (Convulex).

INFORMATION FOR USERS

Your drug prescription is tailored for you. Do not alter dosage without checking with your doctor.

How taken Tablets, capsules, liquid, injection.

Frequency and timing of doses 1–2 x daily, after food.

Dosage range 600mg–2.5g daily, adjusted as necessary.

Onset of effect Within 60 minutes.

Duration of action 12 hours or more.

Diet advice None.

Storage Keep in a tightly closed container in a cool, dry place out of reach of children. Protect from light.

Missed dose Take as soon as you remember. If your next dose is due within 2 hours, take a single dose now and skip the next.

Stopping the drug Do not stop taking the drug without consulting your doctor; symptoms may recur.

Exceeding the dose An occasional unintentional extra dose is unlikely to cause problems. Large overdoses, however, may lead to coma; notify your doctor.

POSSIBLE ADVERSE EFFECTS

The common adverse effects of sodium valproate include temporary hair loss and weight gain. However, most of the adverse effects are uncommon. The most serious, though rare, effects include liver failure or platelet and bleeding abnormalities. If you experience nausea, vomiting, jaundice, or drowsiness, consult your doctor urgently. Menstrual periods may become irregular or cease altogether.

INTERACTIONS

Other anticonvulsant drugs These drugs may reduce blood levels of sodium valproate.

Aspirin This drug may increase the effects of sodium valproate.

Antidepressants, antipsychotics, mefloquine, and chloroquine These drugs may reduce sodium valproate's effectiveness.

Colestyramine This drug may reduce the absorption of oral sodium valproate.

Cimetidine and erythromycin These drugs may increase the effects of sodium valproate.

Zidovudine When zidovudine and sodium valproate are taken together, the blood levels of zidovudine may increase, leading to stronger adverse effects.

SPECIAL PRECAUTIONS

Be sure to tell your doctor if:
◆ You have any long-term liver or kidney problems.
◆ You are taking other medications.
◆ You have porphyria.
◆ You have diabetes.

Pregnancy Sodium valproate is not usually prescribed. It may cause abnormalities in the developing baby. If the drug is prescribed, extra folic acid supplements should also be taken. Discuss with your doctor.

Breast-feeding The drug passes into the breast milk, but at normal doses adverse effects on the baby are unlikely. Discuss with your doctor.

Infants and children Reduced dose necessary.

Over 60 Reduced dose may be necessary.

Driving and hazardous work Your underlying condition may make such activities inadvisable. Discuss with your doctor.

Alcohol Avoid. Alcohol may increase the sedative effects of this drug.

PROLONGED USE

This drug may cause liver damage, which is more likely in the first 6 months of use.

Monitoring Periodic blood tests of liver function and blood composition may be carried out.

Sotalol

Brand names Beta-Cardone, Sotacor
Used in the following combined preparations
None

QUICK REFERENCE

Drug group Beta blocker (p.30)
Overdose danger rating Medium
Dependence rating Low
Prescription needed Yes
Available as generic Yes

GENERAL INFORMATION

Sotalol is a non-cardioselective beta blocker used in preventing and treating ventricular and supraventricular arrhythmias (see p.34).

Sotalol has an additional anti-arrhythmic action compared to other beta blockers. The drug is, however, no longer prescribed for the other conditions for which beta blockers are prescribed. This is due to a serious side effect called "torsades de pointes", a kind of ventricular arrhythmia that is serious enough to produce symptoms and, rarely, death. Because of this risk, anyone taking sotalol will be carefully monitored.

INFORMATION FOR USERS

Your drug prescription is tailored for you. Do not alter dosage without checking with your doctor.
How taken Tablets, injection.
Frequency and timing of doses 2 x daily (tablets); 6-hourly intervals when necessary (injections).
Adult dosage range 80mg daily initially, increased at 2–3-day intervals to 160–320mg daily. Higher doses of 480–640mg under specialist supervision.
Onset of effect 30–60 minutes.
Duration of action 12 hours.
Diet advice None.
Storage Keep in a closed container in a cool, dry place out of reach of children. Protect from light.
Missed dose Take as soon as you remember. If your next dose is due within 3 hours, take a single dose now and skip the next.
Stopping the drug Do not stop taking the drug without consulting your doctor, who will supervise a gradual reduction in dosage.

Sudden withdrawal may lead to worsening of your condition.
Exceeding the dose An occasional unintentional extra dose is unlikely to be a cause for concern. Large overdoses, however, may cause wheezing, low blood pressure, slow heart rate, and heart arrhythmias; notify your doctor immediately.

POSSIBLE ADVERSE EFFECTS

Sotalol may cause lethargy, fatigue, dizziness, cold hands and feet, and nightmares or vivid dreams. A very fast heart rate with palpitations could be a symptom of torsades de pointes; if you experience this or suffer from dizzy spells or fainting, notify your doctor immediately. You should also consult your doctor if you develop either shortness of breath or wheezing.

INTERACTIONS

Phenothiazines, antidepressants, terfenadine, and erythromycin (IV) These drugs increase the risk of torsades de pointes with sotalol.
Verapamil and diltiazem Combining these calcium channel blockers with sotalol will have very adverse effects on heart function.
Anti-arrhythmics such as amiodarone, disopyramide, quinidine, lidocaine, and procainamide Taking any of these drugs together with sotalol may slow the heart rate and adversely affect heart function.
Calcium channel blockers These may cause low blood pressure, slow heartbeats, and heart failure if taken with sotalol.
Diuretics, amphotericin, corticosteroids, and some laxatives These drugs may lower blood potassium levels, increasing the risk of torsades de pointes.
Sympathomimetics such as epinephrine (adrenaline), norepinephrine (noradrenaline), and dobutamine There is a risk of severe high blood pressure if these drugs are taken with sotalol.

SPECIAL PRECAUTIONS

Be sure to tell your doctor if:
◆ You have liver or kidney problems.
◆ You have a breathing disorder such as asthma, bronchitis, or emphysema.
◆ You have heart failure.
◆ You have diabetes.

◆ You have poor circulation in the legs.
◆ You are taking other medications.

Pregnancy Not usually prescribed. May affect the developing baby. Discuss with your doctor.

Breast-feeding The drug passes into the breast milk and may affect the baby. Discuss with your doctor.

Infants and children Not prescribed.

Over 60 Reduced dose may be necessary.

Driving and hazardous work No problems expected.

Alcohol No special problems.

PROLONGED USE

Sotalol may be taken indefinitely for prevention of ventricular arrhythmias.

Monitoring Periodic blood tests are usually performed to monitor levels of potassium and magnesium. The electrocardiogram is usually monitored for signs of development of torsades de pointes.

Streptokinase

Brand names Streptase
Used in the following combined preparation
Varidase

QUICK REFERENCE

Drug group Drug that affects blood clotting (p.38)
Overdose danger rating Medium
Dependence rating Low
Prescription needed Yes
Available as generic Yes

GENERAL INFORMATION

Streptokinase, an enzyme produced by the streptococcus bacteria, is used in hospitals to dissolve the fibrin of blood clots, especially those in the arteries of the heart and lungs. It is also used on the clots formed in shunts during kidney dialysis.

A fast-acting thrombolytic drug (see p.40), streptokinase is most effective in dissolving newly formed clots. The drug is often released at the site of the clot via a catheter inserted into an artery. When administered in the early stages of a heart attack to dissolve a clot (thrombus) in the coronary arteries, it can reduce the amount of damage to heart mus-

cle. Because excessive bleeding is a common side effect, treatment is closely supervised.

Streptokinase is also used to treat wounds and ulcers in combination with another enzyme called streptodornase. For this use, powder is applied locally.

Streptokinase is a protein and can cause allergic reactions. Antihistamines may be given at the start of treatment to reduce this risk.

INFORMATION FOR USERS

The drug is only given under medical supervision and is not for self-administration.

How taken Powder, injection.

Frequency and timing of doses 1–2 x daily (powder); by a single injection or continuously over a period of 24–72 hours.

Dosage range Dosage is determined individually by the patient's condition and response.

Onset of effect As soon as streptokinase reaches the blood clot, it begins to dissolve within minutes. Most of the clot will be dissolved within a few hours.

Duration of action The effect disappears within a few minutes of the drug being stopped.

Diet advice None.

Storage Not applicable. This drug is not normally kept in the home.

Missed dose Not applicable. This drug is given only in hospital under close medical supervision.

Stopping the drug The drug is usually given for up to 3 days.

Exceeding the dose Overdosage is unlikely since treatment is carefully monitored.

POSSIBLE ADVERSE EFFECTS

Streptokinase is given under strict supervision and all adverse effects are closely monitored so that they can be quickly dealt with. Excessive bleeding is the most important adverse effect. Nausea or vomiting, rash or itching, fever, wheezing, and abnormal heart rhythms may also occur.

INTERACTIONS

Anticoagulants There is an increased risk of bleeding when these drugs are taken at the same time as streptokinase.

Antiplatelet drugs The risk of bleeding is increased if these drugs are given together with streptokinase.

SPECIAL PRECAUTIONS

Streptokinase is prescribed only under close medical supervision, usually only in life-threatening circumstances.

Pregnancy Not usually prescribed. If the drug is used during the first 18 weeks of pregnancy, there is a risk that the placenta may separate from the wall of the uterus.

Breast-feeding No evidence of risk.

Infants and children Reduced dose necessary.

Over 60 There is an increased likelihood of bleeding into the brain.

Driving and hazardous work Not applicable.

Alcohol Not applicable.

PROLONGED USE

Streptokinase is never used for the long term.

Further instructions Once you have had a dose, you will be given a card which you must keep with you at all times and present to any doctor in case further treatment is required. A second course of treatment would not normally be given within 6 months of the first.

Sucralfate

Brand name Antepsin
Used in the following combined preparations
None

QUICK REFERENCE

Drug group Ulcer-healing drug (p.43)
Overdose danger rating Low
Dependence rating Low
Prescription needed Yes
Available as generic Yes

GENERAL INFORMATION

Sucralfate, a drug that is partly derived from aluminium, is prescribed to treat gastric and duodenal ulcers. The drug does not neutralize stomach acid, but instead forms a barrier over the ulcerated area that protects it from attack by digestive juices, giving it time to heal.

If antacids are necessary during treatment to relieve pain, they should be taken at least half an hour before or after sucralfate.

There are a few reports of seriously ill patients developing bezoars (balls of indigestible material) in their stomachs while on sucralfate. In addition, the safety of the drug for long-term use has not yet been confirmed. Therefore, courses of more than 12 weeks are not recommended.

INFORMATION FOR USERS

Your drug prescription is tailored for you. Do not alter dosage without checking with your doctor.

How taken Tablets, liquid.

Frequency and timing of doses 2–4 x daily, 1 hour before each meal and at bedtime, at least 2 hours after food. The tablets may be dispersed in a little water before swallowing. Occasionally, up to 6 x daily.

Dosage range 4–8g daily.

Onset of effect Some improvement may be noted after one or two doses, but it takes a few weeks for an ulcer to heal.

Duration of action Up to 5 hours.

Diet advice Your doctor will advise if supplements are needed.

Storage Keep in a closed container in a cool, dry place out of reach of children.

Missed dose Do not make up the dose you missed. Take your next dose on your original schedule.

Stopping the drug Do not stop taking the drug without consulting your doctor; symptoms may recur.

Exceeding the dose An occasional unintentional extra dose is unlikely to be a cause for concern. But if you notice any unusual symptoms, or if a large overdose has been taken, notify your doctor.

POSSIBLE ADVERSE EFFECTS

Most people do not experience any adverse effects while they are taking sucralfate. The most common is constipation, which will diminish as your body adjusts to the drug. Some people may experience indigestion, nausea, diarrhoea, a dry mouth, dizziness, insomnia, and a rash or itching.

INTERACTIONS

General note Sucralfate may reduce the absorption and effect of a range of drugs, including ranitidine, digoxin, phenytoin, warfarin, levothyroxine, and antibacterials. Take these and other medications at least 30 minutes before or after sucralfate.

Antacids and other indigestion remedies These reduce the effectiveness of sucralfate and should be taken more than 30 minutes before or after sucralfate.

SPECIAL PRECAUTIONS

Be sure to tell your doctor if:
◆ You have a long-term kidney problem.
◆ You are taking other medications.
Pregnancy Safety in pregnancy not established. Discuss with your doctor.
Breast-feeding No evidence of risk.
Infants and children Not usually prescribed.
Over 60 No special problems.
Driving and hazardous work Usually no problems, but sucralfate may cause dizziness in some people.
Alcohol Avoid. Alcohol may counteract the beneficial effect of this drug.

PROLONGED USE

Sucralfate is not usually prescribed for periods longer than 12 weeks at a time. Prolonged use may lead to deficiency of vitamins A, D, E, and K.

Sulfasalazine

Brand name Salazopyrin, Sulazine EC, Ucine
Used in the following combined preparations
None

QUICK REFERENCE

Drug group Drug for inflammatory bowel disease (p.46) and antirheumatic drug (p.52)
Overdose danger rating Low
Dependence rating Low
Prescription needed Yes
Available as a generic Yes

GENERAL INFORMATION

Sulfasalazine, which is a chemical combination of a sulphonamide (see Antibacterial drugs, p.66) and a salicylate drug, is used to treat two inflammatory disorders affecting the bowel. One such disorder is ulcerative colitis, which affects mainly the large intestine; the other is Crohn's disease, which usually affects the small intestine. Sulfasalazine is also effective in the treatment of rheumatoid arthritis.

The drug may cause adverse effects such as nausea, loss of appetite, and general discomfort; these effects are more likely when higher doses are taken. It may also cause stomach irritation, but this problem may be avoided by changing to a specially coated tablet form of the drug. In addition, allergic reactions, such as fever and rash, may occur but may be avoided or minimized by low initial doses of the drug, followed by gradual increases. Maintenance of adequate fluid intake is important while taking sulfasalazine. In rare cases, men may temporarily become sterile.

INFORMATION FOR USERS

Your drug prescription is tailored for you. Do not alter dosage without checking with your doctor.
How taken Tablets, liquid, suppositories, enema.
Frequency and timing of doses 4 x daily after meals, taken with a glass of water (tablets); 2 x daily (suppositories); once daily, usually at bedtime (enema).
Adult dosage range *Crohn's disease/ulcerative colitis* 4–8g daily. *Rheumatoid arthritis* 500mg–3g daily.
Onset of effect Adverse effects may occur within a few days, but full beneficial effects may take 1–3 weeks, depending on the severity of the condition.
Duration of action Up to 24 hours.
Diet advice It is important to drink plenty of liquids (at least 1.5 litres a day) during treatment. Sulfasalazine may reduce the absorption of folic acid from the intestine, leading to a deficiency of this vitamin. To counteract the problem, you should eat plenty of green vegetables.
Storage Keep in a closed container in a cool, dry place out of reach of children.
Missed dose Take as soon as you remember. If your next dose is due within 2 hours, take a single dose now and skip the next.
Stopping the drug Do not stop taking the drug without consulting your doctor; symptoms may recur.
Exceeding the dose An occasional unintentional extra dose is unlikely to be a cause for concern. But if you notice any unusual symptoms, or if a large overdose has been taken, notify your doctor.

POSSIBLE ADVERSE EFFECTS

Adverse effects, including headache, malaise, loss of appetite, joint pain, and ringing in the ears, are common with high doses, but may disappear with a reduction in the dose. Symptoms such as nausea and vomiting may be helped by taking the drug with food. Orange or yellow discoloration of the urine is no cause for alarm. If you develop a fever or rash, or you experience bleeding or abnormal bruising, consult your doctor urgently.

INTERACTIONS

General note 1 Sulfasalazine may increase the effects of a variety of drugs, including oral anticoagulants, oral antidiabetics, anticonvulsants, and methotrexate.

General note 2 Sulfasalazine reduces the absorption and effect of some drugs, including digoxin, folic acid, and iron.

SPECIAL PRECAUTIONS

Be sure to tell your doctor if:
◆ You have long-term liver or kidney problems.
◆ You have glucose-6-phosphate dehydrogenase (G6PD) deficiency.
◆ You have a blood disorder.
◆ You suffer from porphyria.
◆ You know you are allergic to sulphonamides or aspirin.
◆ You wear soft contact lenses.
◆ You are taking other medications.

Pregnancy There is no evidence of risk to the developing baby, but folic acid supplements may be required. Discuss with your doctor.

Breast-feeding The drug passes into the breast milk and may affect the baby. Discuss with your doctor.

Infants and children Not recommended under 2 years. Reduced dose necessary for older children, according to bodyweight.

Over 60 No special problems.

Driving and hazardous work No special problems.

Alcohol No known problems.

PROLONGED USE

Blood disorders may occur with prolonged use of this drug. Maintenance dosage is usually continued indefinitely.

Monitoring Periodic tests of blood composition and liver function are usually required.

Sumatriptan

Brand name Imigran
Used in the following combined preparations
None

QUICK REFERENCE

Drug group Drug for migraine (p.20)
Overdose danger rating Medium
Dependence rating Low
Prescription needed Yes
Available as generic No

GENERAL INFORMATION

Sumatriptan is a highly effective drug for migraine that is usually given to people who fail to respond to analgesics such as aspirin and paracetamol. The drug relieves the symptoms of migraine by preventing the dilation of blood vessels in the brain, which causes the attack.

Sumatriptan is of considerable value in treating acute migraine attacks, whether or not they are preceded by an aura (physical warning signs of an attack), but is not meant to be taken regularly to prevent attacks. The drug is also used for the acute treatment of cluster headache (a form of migraine headache). It should be taken as soon as possible after the onset of an attack, although, unlike other drugs for migraine, it will be of benefit at whatever stage of the attack it is taken.

INFORMATION FOR USERS

Your drug prescription is tailored for you. Do not alter dosage without checking with your doctor.

How taken Tablets, injection, nasal spray.

Frequency and timing of doses Should be taken as soon as possible after the onset of an attack. However, it is equally effective at whatever stage it is taken. DO NOT take a second dose for the same attack. The tablets should be swallowed whole with water.

Adult dosage range *Tablets* 50–100mg per attack, up to a maximum of 300mg in 24 hours if another attack occurs. *Injection* 6mg per attack, up to a maximum of 12mg (two injections) in 24 hours if another attack occurs . *Nasal spray* 20mg per attack, up to a maximum of 40mg (2 puffs) in 24 hours if another attack occurs.

Onset of effect *Tablets* 30 minutes. *Injection* 10–15 minutes.

Duration of action *Tablets* The maximum effect occurs after 2–4 hours. *Injection* The maximum effect occurs after 1½–2 hours.

Diet advice None unless otherwise advised.

Storage Keep in a closed container in a cool, dry place out of reach of children. Protect from light.

Missed dose Not applicable, as it is taken only to treat a migraine attack.

Stopping the drug Taken only to treat a migraine attack.

Exceeding the dose An occasional unintentional extra tablet or injection is unlikely to cause problems. But if you notice any unusual symptoms, or if a large overdose has been taken, notify your doctor.

POSSIBLE ADVERSE EFFECTS

Adverse effects of sumatriptan include pain at the injection site; flushing; a hot, tingling feeling; dizziness; a feeling of heaviness or weakness; fatigue; and drowsiness. Many of the adverse effects will disappear after about 1 hour as your body becomes accustomed to the medicine. If the symptoms persist or are severe, contact your doctor. If you experience palpitations or chest pain, consult your doctor urgently.

INTERACTIONS

Antidepressants MAOIs and some other antidepressants, such as fluvoxamine, fluoxetine, paroxetine, and sertraline, increase the risk of adverse effects with sumatriptan.

Lithium Patients taking lithium should not take sumatriptan due to the high risk of adverse effects.

Ergotamine must be taken at least 6 hours after sumatriptan, and sumatriptan must be taken at least 24 hours after ergotamine.

SPECIAL PRECAUTIONS

Be sure to tell your doctor if:
◆ You have liver or kidney problems.
◆ You have heart problems.
◆ You have high blood pressure.
◆ You have had a heart attack.
◆ You have angina.
◆ You are allergic to some medicines.
◆ You are taking other medications.

Pregnancy Safety in pregnancy not established. Discuss with your doctor.

Breast-feeding Safety not established. Discuss with your doctor.

Infants and children Not recommended.

Over 60 Not recommended over 65 years.

Driving and hazardous work It is inadvisable to undertake such activities once a migraine attack appears to be developing.

Alcohol No special problems, but some drinks may provoke migraine in some people.

Surgery and general anaesthetics Notify your doctor or dentist if you have used sumatriptan within 48 hours prior to surgery.

PROLONGED USE

Sumatriptan should not be used continuously to prevent migraine but only to treat migraine attacks.

Tamoxifen

Brand names Nolvadex, Soltamox
Used in the following combined preparations
None

QUICK REFERENCE

Drug group Anticancer drug (p.96)
Overdose danger rating Low
Dependence rating Low
Prescription needed Yes
Available as generic Yes

GENERAL INFORMATION

Tamoxifen is an anti-oestrogen drug (oestrogen is a naturally occurring female sex hormone; see p.88). It is used for two conditions: infertility and breast cancer. When given as treatment for certain types of infertility, tamoxifen is taken only on certain days of the menstrual cycle. Used as an anticancer drug for breast cancer, it works against oestrogens. By latching on to cells that recognize these hormones, it can slow the growth of the tumour and even shrink it. It can also be used to prevent the recurrence of a breast cancer that has been surgically removed.

Because its effect is specific, tamoxifen has fewer adverse effects than most other drugs used for breast cancer.

INFORMATION FOR USERS

Your drug prescription is tailored for you. Do not alter dosage without checking with your doctor.
How taken Tablets, liquid.
Frequency and timing of doses 1–2 x daily.
Adult dosage range *Breast cancer* 20mg daily. *Infertility* 20–80mg daily.
Onset of effect Side effects may be felt within days; beneficial effects may take 4–10 weeks.
Duration of action Effects may be felt for several weeks after stopping the drug.
Diet advice None.
Storage Keep in a closed container in a cool, dry place out of reach of children. Protect from light.
Missed dose Take as soon as you remember. If your next dose is due within 2 hours, take a single dose now and skip the next.
Stopping the drug Do not stop taking the drug without consulting your doctor; stopping it may lead to worsening of your underlying condition.
Exceeding the dose An occasional unintentional extra dose is unlikely to be a cause for concern. But if you notice any unusual symptoms, or if a large overdose has been taken, notify your doctor.

POSSIBLE ADVERSE EFFECTS

Adverse effects are rarely serious with tamoxifen and do not usually require treatment to be stopped. Nausea, vomiting, and hot flushes are the most common reactions. Ankle swelling may also occur. There is a small risk of endometrial cancer (cancer of the uterine lining) developing; you should, therefore, notify your doctor of any symptoms, such as irregular vaginal bleeding or discharge, as soon as possible. If you experience bone or tumour pain, develop a rash or itching, or experience blurred vision or headache, consult your doctor.

INTERACTIONS

Anticoagulants People treated with anticoagulants such as warfarin usually need a lower dose of the anticoagulant.

SPECIAL PRECAUTIONS

Be sure to tell your doctor if:
◆ You have cataracts or poor eyesight.
◆ You suffer from porphyria.
◆ You are taking other medications.
Pregnancy Not usually prescribed. May have effects on the developing baby. Discuss with your doctor.
Breast-feeding Not usually prescribed. Discuss with your doctor.
Infants and children Not prescribed.
Over 60 No special problems.
Driving and hazardous work No special problems.
Alcohol No known problems.

PROLONGED USE

There is a small increase in the risk of endometrial cancer with long-term treatment. This is far outweighed by the benefits of treatment, however. There is a risk of damage to the eye with long-term, high-dose treatment.
Monitoring Eyesight may be tested periodically to detect any adverse effects.

Tamsulosin

Brand name Flomax MR
Used in the following combined preparations
None

QUICK REFERENCE

Drug group Drug for urinary disorders (p.112)
Overdose danger rating Medium
Dependence rating Low
Prescription needed Yes
Available as generic No

GENERAL INFORMATION

Tamsulosin is a selective alpha blocker drug
(see Vasodilators, p.30). It is used to treat urinary retention resulting from an enlarged
prostate gland – a condition known as benign prostatic hypertrophy, or BPH. As it
passes through the prostate, tamsulosin relaxes the muscle in the wall of the urethra,
thereby increasing the flow of urine.

To exclude other conditions with similar
symptoms, your doctor will arrange for you
to have a physical examination and a special
blood test, which may be repeated at intervals during treatment.

Like other alpha blockers, tamsulosin may
lower the blood pressure rapidly after the
first dose, causing dizziness or weakness. For
this reason, the first dose should be taken at
home so that, if these effects occur, you can
lie down until they have disappeared.

INFORMATION FOR USERS

Your drug prescription is tailored for you.
Do not alter dosage without checking with
your doctor.
How taken SR-capsules.
Frequency and timing of doses Once daily after
breakfast.
Adult dosage range 400mcg.
Onset of effect 1–2 hours.
Duration of action 24 hours.
Diet advice None.
Storage Keep in a closed container in a cool,
dry place out of reach of children.
Missed dose Taken as soon as you remember.
If your next dose is due within 4 hours, take
a single dose now and skip the next.
Stopping the drug Do not stop taking the drug
without consulting your doctor; stopping

tamsulosin suddenly may lead to a rise in
blood pressure.
Exceeding the dose An occasional unintentional extra dose is unlikely to cause problems. Large overdoses may produce sedation,
dizziness, low blood pressure and rapid
pulse; notify your doctor immediately.

POSSIBLE ADVERSE EFFECTS

Dizziness seems to be the most common
adverse effect of treatment with tamsulosin,
but this usually improves after the first few
doses. Other common adverse effects include
headache, drowsiness, ejaculatory problems,
and palpitations. Rarer effects include nausea and vomiting, diarrhoea, and constipation. If you develop a rash or itching,
consult your doctor.

INTERACTIONS

**Antidepressants, beta-blockers, calcium channel
blockers, diuretics, and thymoxamine** All of
these drugs are likely to increase the blood-
pressure-lowering effect of tamsulosin.

SPECIAL PRECAUTIONS

Be sure to tell your doctor if:
◆ You have had low blood pressure.
◆ You have liver or kidney problems.
◆ You have heart failure.
◆ You have a history of depression.
◆ You are taking an MAOI drug.
◆ You are taking antihypertensive drugs
(drugs for high blood pressure).
◆ You are taking other medications.
Pregnancy Not prescribed.
Breast-feeding Not prescribed.
Infants and children Not prescribed.
Over 60 No special problems.
Driving and hazardous work Avoid such activ-
ities until you have learned how tamsulosin
affects you because the drug can cause
drowsiness and dizziness.
Alcohol Avoid excessive amounts. Alcohol
can further lower blood pressure.
Surgery and general anaesthetics Treatment
with tamsulosin may need to be stopped before you have any surgery. Discuss this with
your doctor or dentist.

PROLONGED USE

No special problems.

Temazepam

Brand name None
Used in the following combined preparations
None

QUICK REFERENCE

Drug group Sleeping drug (p.11)
Overdose danger rating Medium
Dependence rating High
Prescription needed Yes
Available as generic Yes

GENERAL INFORMATION

Temazepam belongs to the benzodiazepine group of drugs, which are described more fully under Anti-anxiety drugs (see p.13).

Temazepam is used in the short-term treatment of insomnia. Because it is short-acting compared to some other benzodiazepines, it is less likely to cause drowsiness and/or lightheadedness the next day. For this reason, the drug is not usually effective in preventing early wakening, but hangover is less common than with other benzodiazepines.

Like other benzodiazepines, the drug can be habit-forming if taken regularly over a long period. Its effects also grow weaker with time. For these reasons, treatment is usually only continued for a few days at a time.

INFORMATION FOR USERS

Your drug prescription is tailored for you. Do not alter dosage without checking with your doctor.

How taken Tablets, capsules, liquid.
Frequency and timing of doses Once daily, 30 minutes before bedtime.
Adult dosage range 10–40mg.
Onset of effect 15–40 minutes, or longer.
Duration of action 6–8 hours.
Diet advice None.
Storage Keep in a closed container in a cool, dry place out of reach of children. Protect from light.
Missed dose If you fall asleep without having taken a dose and wake some hours later, do not take the missed dose. If necessary, return to your normal dose schedule the next night.
Stopping the drug If you have been taking the drug continuously for less than 2 weeks, it can be safely stopped as soon as you no longer need it. If you have been taking the drug for longer, consult your doctor, who may supervise a gradual reduction in dosage. Stopping the drug abruptly may lead to withdrawal symptoms.
Exceeding the dose An occasional unintentional extra dose is unlikely to be a cause for concern. Large overdoses, however, may cause unusual drowsiness; notify your doctor.

POSSIBLE ADVERSE EFFECTS

The principal adverse effects of this drug are related to its sedative and tranquillizing properties. They include dizziness, unsteadiness, daytime drowsiness, vivid dreams, nightmares, headache, and confusion. These effects normally diminish after the first few days of treatment.

INTERACTIONS

Sedatives All drugs that have a sedative effect on the central nervous system are likely to increase the sedative properties of temazepam. These drug types include other anti-anxiety drugs and sleeping drugs, opioid analgesics, antidepressants, antihistamines, and antipsychotics.

SPECIAL PRECAUTIONS

Be sure to tell your doctor if:
◆ You have severe respiratory disease.
◆ You suffer from porphyria.
◆ You suffer from depression.
◆ You have liver or kidney problems.
◆ You have myasthenia gravis.
◆ You have had problems with alcohol or drug abuse.
◆ You are taking other medications.
Pregnancy Safety in pregnancy not established. Discuss with your doctor.
Breast-feeding The drug passes into the breast milk, but at normal doses adverse effects on the baby are unlikely. Discuss with your doctor.
Infants and children Not recommended.
Over 60 Reduced dose may be necessary. Increased likelihood of adverse effects.
Driving and hazardous work Avoid such activities until you have learned how temazepam affects you because the drug can cause reduced alertness and slowed reactions.
Alcohol Avoid. Alcohol may increase the sedative effect of this drug.

PROLONGED USE

Regular use of temazepam over several weeks can lead to a reduction in its effect as the body adapts. The drug may also be habit-forming if taken for extended periods. It should not normally be used for longer than 1–2 weeks.

Tenecteplase

Brand name Metalyse
Used in the following combined preparations
None

QUICK REFERENCE

Drug group Drug that affects blood clotting (p.38)
Overdose danger rating Medium
Dependence rating Low
Prescription needed Yes
Available as generic No

GENERAL INFORMATION

Tenecteplase is a fibrinolytic or thrombolytic drug (see p.40). It dissolves clots (thrombi) in blood vessels by boosting the action of the enzyme plasmin in breaking up the strands of fibrin that hold the clot together.

Tenecteplase is licensed only for treatment of heart attacks. It is given by intravenous injection. The sooner this is done after the formation of the clot, the greater the success rate in clearing the clot from the coronary arteries in the heart, and reducing the damage to heart muscle. Fibrinolytics are usually given in hospitals, where all the resources needed for this kind of urgent action are held in readiness.

After the tenecteplase has been given, aspirin (see p.146) and heparin (see p.262) are used to maintain the anticoagulant effect and stop further clotting. Low-dose aspirin will usually be prescribed for the long term, and heparin will be given for a few days until the situation is stable.

Because tenecteplase activates the destruction of the body's fibrin (which causes clotting), the main side effect is bleeding, most often at the injection site.

INFORMATION FOR USERS

The drug is only given under medical supervision and is not for self-administration.

How taken Injection.
Frequency and timing of doses A single intravenous injection over 10 seconds.
Adult dosage range 30–50mg (6,000–10,000 units) depending on bodyweight.
Onset of effect The drug reaches and begins to dissolve the clot within minutes. Most of the clot will be gone within a few hours.
Duration of action 25–30 minutes.
Diet advice None.
Storage Not applicable. The drug is not normally kept in the home.
Missed dose Not applicable. The drug is given once, in urgent circumstances, in hospital.
Stopping the drug Not applicable.
Exceeding the dose Overdose is unlikely because dosage is carefully monitored.

POSSIBLE ADVERSE EFFECTS

Nausea and vomiting, bleeding, palpitations, chest pain, and fainting and dizziness are common adverse effects. In rare cases a rash, itching, or wheezing may develop. Because tenecteplase is only given under close medical supervision, most of these symptoms can be dealt with quickly. Tenecteplase is a protein, and can, therefore, produce allergic reactions. In all cases, seek medical advice.

INTERACTIONS

Anticoagulants and drugs affecting platelet function These drugs may increase the tendency towards bleeding.

SPECIAL PRECAUTIONS

Tenecteplase is prescribed only under close medical supervision, usually only under life-threatening circumstances.
Pregnancy Safety not established. The benefit of treatment must be weighed against the risks of bleeding and loss of the baby.
Breast-feeding Breast milk should be discarded for the first 24 hours after tenecteplase treatment, because it is not known whether the drug enters breast milk or is harmful.
Infants and children Reduced dose necessary.
Over 60 No known problems.
Driving and hazardous work Not applicable.
Alcohol Not applicable.

PROLONGED USE

Not applicable.

Terazosin

Brand names Hytrin, Hytrin BPH
Used in the following combined preparations
None

QUICK REFERENCE

Drug group Antihypertensive drug (p.36) and drug
for urinary disorders (p.112)
Overdose danger rating Medium
Dependence rating Low
Prescription needed Yes
Available as generic Yes

GENERAL INFORMATION

Terazosin belongs to a group of antihypertensive drugs known as alpha blockers. It is used to treat high blood pressure (hypertension), and works by relaxing the muscles in the blood vessel walls. Terazosin is also used to relieve the obstruction caused by an enlarged prostate (benign prostatic hypertrophy, or BPH); it acts by relaxing the muscle in the wall of the urethra, thereby improving the flow of urine.

Dizziness and fainting, especially on standing up, are common at the start of treatment with terazosin because the first dose may cause a marked drop in blood pressure. For this reason, the initial dose that is prescribed is usually low. To avoid experiencing these effects, it is advisable to take the drug just before going to bed.

INFORMATION FOR USERS

Your drug prescription is tailored for you. Do not alter dosage without checking with your doctor.
How taken Tablets.
Frequency and timing of doses Once daily.
Adult dosage range *Hypertension* 1mg at bedtime (starting dose), doubled after 7 days if necessary. Usual dosage range 2–10mg. *Benign prostatic hypertrophy* 1mg at bedtime (starting dose), doubled after 1–2 weeks if necessary. Usual dosage range 5–10mg.
Onset of effect *Hypertension* Within 3 hours. *Benign prostatic hypertrophy* Improvements in symptoms can occur as early as 2 weeks after starting treatment. Full beneficial effects may not, however, be felt for 4–6 weeks.

Duration of action 24 hours.
Diet advice None.
Storage Keep in a closed container in a cool, dry place out of the reach of children.
Missed dose Do not double up on a dose. Take the next dose at the usual time.
Stopping the drug Do not stop the drug without consulting your doctor. Stopping it may lead to an increase in blood pressure.
Exceeding the dose An occasional unintentional extra dose is unlikely to be a cause for concern. Large overdoses, however, may drop blood pressure and cause dizziness or fainting; notify your doctor.

POSSIBLE ADVERSE EFFECTS

Rarely, headaches occur with terazosin treatment. A common problem with the drug, however, is that it may cause dizziness or fainting when you stand up. Other common effects include palpitations, nausea, drowsiness, stuffy nose, blurred vision, and swelling of the ankles. If the symptoms are severe, seek medical advice.

INTERACTIONS

Anaesthetics, antidepressants, and hypotensive drugs These drugs may enhance the blood-pressure-lowering effect of terazosin.

SPECIAL PRECAUTIONS

Be sure to tell your doctor if:
◆ You are taking other medications.
Pregnancy Safety in pregnancy not established. Discuss with your doctor.
Breast-feeding Safety not established. Discuss with your doctor.
Infants and children Not recommended.
Over 60 No special problems.
Driving and hazardous work Avoid such activities until you have learned how terazosin affects you because the drug can cause dizziness, lightheadedness, or drowsiness.
Alcohol Avoid. Alcohol may increase some of the adverse effects of terazosin, such as drowsiness.
Surgery and general anaesthetics Terazosin may need to be stopped before you have any surgery. Discuss this with your doctor or dentist.

PROLONGED USE

No problems expected.

Terbinafine

Brand name Lamisil, Lamisil AT
Used in the following combined preparations
None

QUICK REFERENCE

Drug group Antifungal drug (p.76)
Overdose danger rating Low
Dependence rating Low
Prescription needed Yes (except for some skin preparations)
Available as generic No

GENERAL INFORMATION

Terbinafine is an antifungal drug used to treat fungal infections of the skin and nails. It is used particularly for tinea (ringworm), but is also used as a cream for candida (yeast) infections. Tinea infections may be cleared up in two to six weeks, but treatment of nail infections may take up to six months.

Terbinafine has largely replaced older antifungal drugs such as griseofulvin because it is more easily absorbed and is therefore more effective.

The drug commonly causes gastrointestinal problems, but these are generally mild. Rare adverse effects of treatment with terbinafine include jaundice and a severe rash, both of which should be reported to your doctor without delay.

INFORMATION FOR USERS

Your drug prescription is tailored for you. Do not alter dosage without checking with your doctor.
How taken Tablets, cream, skin spray.
Frequency and timing of doses Once daily (tablets); 1–2 x daily (cream).
Adult dosage range *Tinea infections* 250mg (tablets). *Candida infections* As directed (cream).
Onset of effect 1 hour.
Duration of action 24 hours.
Diet advice None.
Storage Keep in a closed container in a cool, dry place out of reach of children. Protect from light.
Missed dose Take the missed dose as soon as you remember. If your next dose is due within 4 hours, take a single dose now and skip the next one.

Stopping the drug Take the full course. Even if you feel better, the original infection may still be present and may recur if treatment is stopped too soon.
Exceeding the dose An occasional unintentional extra dose is unlikely to be a cause for concern. But if you notice any unusual symptoms, or if a large overdose has been taken, notify your doctor.

POSSIBLE ADVERSE EFFECTS

The adverse effects of terbinafine are generally mild and do not last long. They include nausea, indigestion, bloating, mild abdominal pain, diarrhoea, and headache. Some people may experience a disturbance or loss of taste, dizziness, "pins and needles", and muscle or joint pain.

If you develop jaundice, severe rash, a sore throat, or bruising and bleeding in the mouth, stop taking the drug and contact your doctor immediately.

INTERACTIONS

Oral contraceptives "Breakthrough" bleeding may occur when these drugs are taken with terbinafine.
Rifampicin This drug may reduce the blood level and effect of terbinafine.
Cimetidine This drug may increase the blood level of terbinafine.

SPECIAL PRECAUTIONS

Be sure to tell your doctor if:
◆ You have any long-term liver or kidney problems.
◆ You have psoriasis.
◆ You are taking other medications.
Pregnancy Safety in pregnancy not established. Discuss with your doctor.
Breast-feeding The drug passes into the breast milk and may affect the baby adversely. Discuss with your doctor.
Infants and children Safety not established. Discuss with your doctor.
Over 60 No special problems.
Driving and hazardous work No known problems.
Alcohol No known problems.

PROLONGED USE

No special problems.

Terbutaline

Brand names Bricanyl, Monovent
Used in the following combined preparations
None

QUICK REFERENCE

Drug group Bronchodilator (p.23)
Overdose danger rating Low
Dependence rating Low
Prescription needed Yes
Available as generic Yes

GENERAL INFORMATION

Terbutaline is a sympathomimetic broncho-dilator. It works by dilating (widening) the bronchioles (small airways in the lungs). The drug is used in treating and preventing bron-chospasm (constriction of the air passages) in asthma, chronic bronchitis, and emphysema. It also acts on the uterus and is used to delay premature labour.

Muscle tremor, especially of the hands, is common with terbutaline and usually disappears on reduction of the dose or with continued use as the body adapts to the drug. In common with the other sympathomimetic drugs, terbutaline may also produce nervousness and restlessness.

INFORMATION FOR USERS

Your drug prescription is tailored for you. Do not alter dosage without checking with your doctor.
How taken Tablets, liquid, injection, inhaler.
Frequency and timing of doses 3 x daily (tablets); as necessary (inhaler).
Dosage range *Adults* 7.5–15mg daily (tablets); up to 2mg daily (inhaler). *Children* Reduced dose according to age and weight.
Onset of effect Within a few minutes (inhaler); within 1–2 hours (tablets).
Duration of action 4–8 hours (tablets).
Diet advice None.
Storage Keep in a closed container in a cool, dry place out of reach of children. Protect from light. Do not puncture or burn aerosol containers.
Missed dose Do not take the missed dose. Take your next dose as usual.
Stopping the drug Do not stop without consulting your doctor; symptoms may recur.

Exceeding the dose An occasional unintentional extra dose is unlikely to be a cause for concern. But if you notice any unusual symptoms, or if a large overdose has been taken, notify your doctor.

POSSIBLE ADVERSE EFFECTS

Possible adverse effects include tremor, nervousness, anxiety, restlessness, muscle cramps, and nausea. These may be reduced by adjustment of the dosage. Palpitations and headache, resulting from stimulation of the heart and narrowing of the blood vessels, may occur but are rare. Nausea or vomiting and muscle cramps may also occur.

INTERACTIONS

Other sympathomimetics may add to the effects of terbutaline and vice versa, thereby increasing the risk of adverse effects.
MAOIs Terbutaline may interact with these drugs to cause a dangerous rise in blood pressure.
Beta blockers These may reduce the beneficial effects of terbutaline.

SPECIAL PRECAUTIONS

Be sure to tell your doctor if:
◆ You have heart problems.
◆ You have high blood pressure.
◆ You have diabetes.
◆ You have an overactive thyroid.
◆ You are taking other medications.
Pregnancy Safety in early pregnancy not established, although problems are unlikely with inhaled terbutaline. It is given by injection in late pregnancy to prevent premature labour. Discuss with your doctor.
Breast-feeding No problems expected with inhaled terbutaline.
Infants and children Reduced dose necessary.
Over 60 Reduced dose may be necessary. Increased likelihood of adverse effects.
Driving and hazardous work No problems expected.
Alcohol No special problems.

PROLONGED USE

Prolonged use may result in tolerance to terbutaline's effects. However, failure to respond to the drug may be the result of worsening asthma, requiring prompt medical attention.

Testosterone

Brand names Andropatch, Restandol, Sustanon, Virormone
Used in the following combined preparations
None

QUICK REFERENCE

Drug group Male sex hormone (p.87)
Overdose danger rating Low
Dependence rating Low
Prescription needed Yes
Available as generic Yes

GENERAL INFORMATION

Testosterone is a male sex hormone produced by the testes in males and, in small quantities, by the ovaries in females. It encourages bone and muscle growth in both sexes and stimulates sexual development in men.

The drug is used to initiate puberty in adolescent males if this has been delayed through deficiency of the natural hormone. It may help to increase fertility in men with either pituitary or testicular disorders. Rarely, testosterone is used to treat breast cancer.

Testosterone can interfere with growth or cause over-rapid sexual development in adolescents. High doses in women may cause deepening of the voice, excessive hair growth, or hair loss.

INFORMATION FOR USERS

Your drug prescription is tailored for you. Do not alter dosage without checking with your doctor.
How taken Capsules, injection, patch, implanted pellets.
Frequency and timing of doses 2 x daily (capsules); once every 3 weeks to 2 x weekly, depending on condition (injection); every 6 months (implant); once daily (patch).
Dosage range Varies with method of administration and the condition being treated.
Onset of effect 2–3 days.
Duration of action 1–2 days (capsules and patch); 1–3 weeks (injection); about 6 months (implant).
Diet advice None.
Storage Keep in a closed container in a cool, dry place out of reach of children. Protect from light.

Missed dose No cause for concern, but take as soon as you remember. If your next dose (by mouth) is due within 3 hours, take a single dose now and skip the next.
Stopping the drug Do not stop taking the drug without consulting your doctor.
Exceeding the dose An occasional unintentional extra dose is unlikely to be a cause for concern. But if you notice unusual symptoms, or if a large overdose was taken, notify your doctor.

POSSIBLE ADVERSE EFFECTS

Most of the more serious adverse effects are likely only with long-term treatment and may be helped by dosage reduction. Men may experience difficulty in passing urine and abnormal erection; women may experience unusual hair growth or hair loss, voice changes, and an enlarged clitoris. Fluid retention, leading to ankle swelling, may occur. If you develop jaundice, stop taking the drug and seek urgent medical advice.

INTERACTIONS

Anticoagulant drugs Testosterone may increase the effect of these drugs. Dosage of anticoagulants may need to be adjusted.
Antidiabetic agents As testosterone may lower the blood sugar, dosage of antidiabetic drugs and insulin may need to be reduced.

SPECIAL PRECAUTIONS

Be sure to tell your doctor if:
◆ You have long-term liver or kidney problems.
◆ You have heart problems.
◆ You have prostate trouble.
◆ You have high blood pressure.
◆ You have epilepsy or migraine headaches.
◆ You are taking other medications.
Pregnancy Not prescribed.
Breast-feeding Not prescribed.
Infants and children Not prescribed for infants and young children. Reduced dose necessary in adolescents.
Over 60 Rarely required. Increased risk of prostate problems in elderly men. Reduced dose may therefore be necessary.
Driving and hazardous work No special problems.
Alcohol No special problems.

PROLONGED USE

Prolonged use of this drug may lead to reduced growth in adolescents.

Monitoring Regular blood tests for the effects of testosterone treatment are required.

Tetracycline/Lymecycline

Brand names Economycin, Tetrachel, Tetralysal 300, Topicycline
Used in the following combined preparations
Deteclo

QUICK REFERENCE

Drug group Antibiotic (p.62)
Overdose danger rating Low
Dependence rating Low
Prescription needed Yes
Available as generic Yes

GENERAL INFORMATION

Tetracycline and lymecycline were once a very widely used group of antibiotics, but the development of strains of bacteria resistant to them has reduced their effectiveness in many types of infection. Tetracyclines are still used for chest infections due to chlamydia (for example, psittacosis) and mycoplasma microorganisms. Tetracycline and lymecycline are also used in non-specific urethritis and rarer conditions such as Q fever, cholera, Rocky Mountain spotted fever, and brucellosis.

Tetracycline drugs are also used to improve acne. They are given as long-term treatment, either by mouth or as a topical solution.

Common side effects are nausea, vomiting, and diarrhoea. Rashes may also occur. Tetracycline may discolour developing teeth if taken by children or by the mother during pregnancy. People with poor kidney function are not given tetracycline drugs because they can cause further deterioration.

INFORMATION FOR USERS

Your drug prescription is tailored for you. Do not alter dosage without checking with your doctor.

How taken Tablets, capsules, ointment, eye/ear ointment. To prevent irritation of the oesophagus, tablets should be taken with a full glass of water while standing.

Frequency and timing of doses *By mouth* 4 x daily, at least 1 hour before or 2 hours after meals (tetracycline); 2 x daily (lymecycline). Long-term treatment of acne may require only a single dose daily.
Skin preparations 1–3 times daily as directed.
Adult dosage range *Infections* 1–2g daily.
Acne 250mg–1g daily.
Onset of effect 4–12 hours. Improvement in acne may not be noticed for up to 4 weeks.
Duration of action Up to 6 hours.
Diet advice Avoid milk products for 1 hour before and 2 hours after taking the drug.
Storage Keep in a closed container in a cool, dry place out of reach of children.
Missed dose Take as soon as you remember. If your next dose is due within 2 hours, take a single dose now and skip the next.
Stopping the drug Take the full course. Even if you feel better, the original infection may still be present and may recur if treatment is stopped too soon.
Exceeding the dose An occasional unintentional extra dose is unlikely to be a cause for concern. But if you notice any unusual symptoms, or if a large overdose has been taken, notify your doctor.

POSSIBLE ADVERSE EFFECTS

Adverse effects are rare with ointment. Nausea, vomiting, or diarrhoea may occur with oral forms; rash, itching, and jaundice are rare. If headaches or visual disturbances occur, stop the drug and consult your doctor urgently.

INTERACTIONS

Iron This may reduce the effectiveness of tetracycline/lymecycline.
Oral anticoagulants Tetracycline/lymecycline may increase the action of these drugs.
Retinoids These may increase the adverse effects of tetracycline/lymecycline.
Oral contraceptives Tetracycline/lymecycline may reduce oral contraceptives' effectiveness.
Antacids and milk These interfere with the absorption of tetracycline/lymecycline and may reduce their effectiveness. Doses should be separated by 1–2 hours.

SPECIAL PRECAUTIONS

Be sure to tell your doctor if:
◆ You have long-term liver or kidney problems.

◆ You have previously suffered an allergic reaction to a tetracycline antibiotic.

◆ You have myasthenia gravis.

◆ You have systemic lupus erythematosus.

◆ You are taking other medications.

Pregnancy Not usually prescribed. May discolour the teeth and damage the bones of the developing baby. Discuss with your doctor.

Breast-feeding The drug passes into breast milk. It may damage the baby's bones and discolour the teeth. Discuss with your doctor.

Infants and children Not recommended under 12 years. Reduced dose necessary for older children. May discolour developing teeth.

Over 60 No special problems.

Driving and hazardous work No known problems.

Alcohol No known problems.

PROLONGED USE

No problems expected.

Theophylline/ Aminophylline

Brand names [theophylline] Nuelin, Slo-Phyllin, Uniphyllin; [aminophylline] Phyllocontin
Used in the following combined preparations
[theophylline] Do-Do Tablets, Franol

QUICK REFERENCE

Drug group Bronchodilator (p.23)
Overdose danger rating High
Dependence rating Low
Prescription needed No (except for injection)
Available as generic Yes

GENERAL INFORMATION

Theophylline (and aminophylline, which breaks down to theophylline in the body) is used to treat bronchospasm (constriction of the air passages) in patients suffering from asthma, bronchitis, and emphysema.

The drugs are usually taken continuously as a preventative but are also used to treat acute attacks. Slow-release formulations are effective for up to 12 hours. These may be prescribed twice daily, but are also useful as a single dose taken at night to prevent nighttime asthma and early morning wheezing.

Treatment with theophylline must be carefully monitored because the effective dose is very close to the toxic dose. Some adverse effects, such as indigestion, nausea, headache, and agitation, can be controlled by regulating the dosage and checking blood levels of the drug.

INFORMATION FOR USERS

Your drug prescription is tailored for you. Do not alter dosage without checking with your doctor.

How taken Tablets, SR-tablets, SR-capsules, liquid, injection.

Frequency and timing of doses
3–4 x daily (tablets, liquid); every 12 or 24 hours (SR-tablets/SR-capsules). The drug should be taken at the same time each day in relation to meals.

Dosage range *Adults* 375–1,000mg daily, depending on which product is used.

Onset of effect Within 30 minutes (by mouth); within 90 minutes SR-tablets/SR-capsules.

Duration of action Up to 8 hours (by mouth); 12–24 hours (SR-tablets/SR-capsules).

Diet advice None.

Storage Keep in a closed container in a cool, dry place out of reach of children.

Missed dose Take as soon as you remember. If your next dose is due within 2 hours, take half the dose now (short-acting preparations) or leave out the missed dose and take your next dose now (SR-preparations). Return to your normal dose schedule thereafter.

Stopping the drug Unless palpitations occur, do not stop taking the drug without consulting your doctor; stopping it may lead to worsening of the underlying condition.

OVERDOSE ACTION

Seek immediate medical advice in all cases. Take emergency action if chest pains, confusion, or loss of consciousness occur.

POSSIBLE ADVERSE EFFECTS

Most adverse effects of theophylline are related to dosage. These include effects related to the drug's action on the central nervous system, such as headache, agitation and insomnia. Nausea, vomiting, and diarrhoea may also occur. If you experience palpitations, stop taking the drug and seek urgent medical advice.

INTERACTIONS

General note Many drugs, such as erythromycin and cimetidine, increase the effect of theophylline. Conversely, other drugs (such as carbamazepine, phenytoin, and rifampicin) reduce its effect. Discuss with your doctor.

SPECIAL PRECAUTIONS

Be sure to consult your doctor or pharmacist before taking this drug if:
◆ You have a long-term liver problem.
◆ You have angina or an irregular heart beat.
◆ You have high blood pressure.
◆ You have epilepsy.
◆ You have hyperthyroidism.
◆ You have porphyria.
◆ You have stomach ulcers.
◆ You smoke.
◆ You are taking other medications.
Pregnancy Safety in pregnancy not established. Discuss with your doctor.
Breast-feeding The drug passes into the breast milk and may affect the baby. Discuss with your doctor.
Infants and children Reduced dose necessary according to age and weight.
Over 60 Reduced dose may be necessary.
Driving and hazardous work No known problems.
Alcohol Avoid excess alcohol as this may alter levels of the drug and may increase gastrointestinal symptoms.

PROLONGED USE

No problems expected.
Monitoring Periodic checks on blood levels of this drug are usually required.

Tibolone

Brand name Livial
Used in the following combined preparations
None

QUICK REFERENCE

Drug group Female sex hormone (p.88)
Overdose danger rating Low
Dependence rating Low
Prescription needed Yes
Available as generic No

GENERAL INFORMATION

Tibolone is a female sex hormone used to treat menopausal symptoms such as sweating, depressed mood, and decreased sex drive and is particularly effective in controlling hot flushes. It is usually only advised for short-term use.

Tibolone is taken continuously and, since it has both oestrogenic and progestogenic activity (unlike most other available types of HRT), the treatment does not require a cyclical course of progestogen to be taken as well.

Side effects are rare, and tibolone does not cause withdrawal bleeding in postmenopausal women. The drug is no longer recommended for treatment of osteoporosis or for long-term use (see Prolonged use, p.406).

INFORMATION FOR USERS

Your drug prescription is tailored for you. Do not alter dosage without checking with your doctor.
How taken Tablets.
Frequency and timing of doses Daily, preferably at the same time each day. Swallow the tablets whole – do not chew.
Adult dosage range 2.5mg daily.
Onset of effect A few weeks, but best results are obtained after at least 3 months.
Duration of action A few days.
Diet advice None.
Storage Keep in a closed container in a cool, dry place out of reach of children. Protect from light.
Missed dose Take as soon as you remember.
Stopping the drug Do not stop taking the drug without consulting your doctor; symptoms may recur.
Exceeding the dose An occasional unintentional extra dose is unlikely to be a cause for concern. Several tablets taken together may cause a stomach upset; notify your doctor.

POSSIBLE ADVERSE EFFECTS

Tibolone is well tolerated, and adverse effects are rare. They include weight gain, ankle swelling, dizziness, acne, headache, visual problems, stomach upset, and facial hair growth. If joint or muscle pain or acne occur, consult your doctor. Vaginal bleeding is more likely if less than one year has passed since your menopause. Therefore, the drug is not recommended if it is less than 12 months since your last period. If jaundice occurs, stop taking the drug and call your doctor immediately.

INTERACTIONS

Some anticonvulsants Phenytoin, phenobarbital, primidone, and carbamazepine can all accelerate the metabolism of tibolone, thereby decreasing its blood levels and effectiveness.

Rifampicin This drug can accelerate the metabolism of tibolone, decreasing its blood levels and effectiveness.

SPECIAL PRECAUTIONS

Be sure to tell your doctor if:
◆ You have long-term liver or kidney problems.
◆ You suffer from epilepsy or migraine.
◆ You have diabetes.
◆ You have a tumour.
◆ You have a history of cardiovascular or cerebrovascular disease.
◆ You have a high cholesterol level.
◆ You have vaginal bleeding.
◆ You have had a period within the last 12 months.
◆ You are taking other medications.

Pregnancy Not prescribed.

Breast-feeding Not prescribed.

Infants and children Not prescribed.

Over 60 No special problems.

Driving and hazardous work No problems expected.

Alcohol No known problems.

PROLONGED USE

Tibolone is no longer normally recommended for long-term use or for the treatment of osteoporosis due to the increased risk of disorders such as breast cancer, stroke, and thromboembolism.

Monitoring Periodic examination by your doctor is advised.

Timolol

Brand names Betim, Glau-opt, Nyogel, Timoptol
Used in the following combined preparations Cosopt, Moducren, Prestim, Xalacom

QUICK REFERENCE

Drug group Beta blocker (p.30) and drug for glaucoma (p.114)

Overdose danger rating High
Dependence rating Low
Prescription needed Yes
Available as generic Yes

GENERAL INFORMATION

Timolol is a beta blocker prescribed to treat hypertension (high blood pressure) and angina (pain due to narrowing of the coronary arteries). It may be given after a heart attack to prevent further damage to the heart muscle. When used to treat hypertension, timolol may also be given with a diuretic. The drug is also commonly administered as eye drops to people with certain types of glaucoma, and is occasionally given to prevent migraine (see p.20).

Timolol can cause breathing difficulties, especially in people suffering from asthma, chronic bronchitis, or emphysema. This problem is more likely to occur in people taking the drug in tablet form, although it can also occur in those using timolol eye drops. As with other beta blockers, timolol may mask the response of the body to low blood glucose; for that reason, it is prescribed with caution to diabetic people.

INFORMATION FOR USERS

Your drug prescription is tailored for you. Do not alter dosage without checking with your doctor.

How taken Tablets, eye drops.

Frequency and timing of doses 1–3 x daily.

Adult dosage range *Hypertension* 10–60mg daily (tablets). *Angina* 10–45mg daily (tablets). *After a heart attack* 10–20mg daily (tablets). *Migraine prevention* 10–20mg daily (tablets). *Glaucoma* 1 drop, 1–2 x daily (eye drops).

Onset of effect Within 30 minutes (by mouth/eye drops).

Duration of action Up to 24 hours.

Diet advice None.

Storage Keep in a closed container in a cool, dry place out of reach of children.

Missed dose Take as soon as you remember. If your next dose is due within 3 hours, take a single dose now and skip the next one.

Stopping the drug Do not stop taking the drug without consulting your doctor; stopping the drug may lead to worsening of the underlying condition.

OVERDOSE ACTION
Seek immediate medical advice in all cases of overdose by mouth. Take emergency action if breathing difficulties, palpitations, or loss of consciousness occur.

POSSIBLE ADVERSE EFFECTS
Lethargy, fatigue, headache, nightmares, vivid dreams, and cold hands or feet are common with timolol taken in tablet form. Occasionally, heart problems and asthma can be provoked or worsened. If breathlessness or wheezing occur, stop taking the drug and contact your doctor urgently. Blurred vision is common with eye drops; rarely, eye irritation and headache occur.

INTERACTIONS
Sympathomimetics These drugs, which are included in many cold and cough remedies, can cause a dangerous rise in blood pressure when taken with timolol.

Salbutamol, salmeterol, and other beta agonists These drugs have opposing effects to beta blockers, so timolol may reduce their effects.

SPECIAL PRECAUTIONS
Be sure to tell your doctor if:
◆ You have a lung disorder such as asthma, bronchitis, or emphysema.
◆ You have diabetes.
◆ You have myasthenia gravis.
◆ You have poor circulation.
◆ You have allergies.
◆ You are taking other medications.

Pregnancy Safety in pregnancy not established. Discuss with your doctor.

Breast-feeding The drug passes into the breast milk, but at normal doses adverse effects on the baby are unlikely. Discuss with your doctor.

Infants and children Not usually prescribed.

Over 60 Reduced dose may be necessary.

Driving and hazardous work Avoid such activities until you have learned how timolol affects you because the tablets may cause drowsiness and the eye drops may cause blurred vision.

Alcohol May enhance lowering of blood pressure; avoid excessive amounts.

Surgery and general anaesthetics Timolol by mouth may need to be stopped before you have a general anaesthetic. Discuss with your doctor or dentist before any surgery.

PROLONGED USE
No problems expected.

Tiotropium

Brand name Spiriva
Used in the following combined preparations None

QUICK REFERENCE
Drug group Bronchodilator (p.23)
Overdose danger rating Low
Dependence rating Low
Prescription needed Yes
Available as generic No

GENERAL INFORMATION
Tiotropium is an anticholinergic (see Autonomic nervous system, p.8) bronchodilator that relaxes the muscles surrounding the bronchioles (airways in the lungs). It is used in the maintenance treatment of reversible airway disorders, such as chronic bronchitis.

Tiotropium is long acting, but its effects are felt after only five minutes or so. It is not suitable for acute attacks of wheezing or in the emergency treatment of asthma. It is taken by inhalation, as a powder, and acts directly on the internal surface of the lungs, not via the blood.

INFORMATION FOR USERS
Your drug prescription is tailored for you. Do not alter dosage without checking with your doctor.

How taken Powder in capsules for inhaler.

Frequency and timing of doses Once daily, at the same time each day.

Adult dosage range 18mcg daily.

Onset of effect 5 minutes.

Duration of action 24 hours.

Diet advice None.

Storage Keep in a closed container in a cool, dry place out of reach of children.

Missed dose Take as soon as you remember. If your next dose is due within 8 hours, take a single dose now and skip the next.

Stopping the drug Do not stop without consulting your doctor; symptoms may recur.

Exceeding the dose An occasional unintentional extra dose is unlikely to cause problems. But if you have any unusual symptoms or a large overdose has been taken, notify your doctor.

POSSIBLE ADVERSE EFFECTS

Dry mouth, sore throat, and constipation are common. Rarer effects include a fast heart beat, palpitations, difficulty in passing urine, rash, and wheezing after inhalation. If eye pain or visual disturbances occur, stop taking the drug and seek medical advice. Contact your doctor immediately if you get the powder in your eyes, as it could trigger glaucoma.

INTERACTIONS

Atropine and ipratropium These drugs are likely to increase tiotropium's effects and toxicity.

SPECIAL PRECAUTIONS

Be sure to tell your doctor if:
◆ You are allergic to atropine or ipratropium.
◆ You have prostate problems.
◆ You have urinary retention.
◆ You have glaucoma.
◆ You have kidney problems.
◆ You are taking other medications.
Pregnancy Safety not established. Discuss with your doctor.
Breast-feeding Safety not established. Discuss with your doctor.
Infants and children Not recommended under 18 years.
Over 60 No known problems.
Driving and hazardous work No known problems.
Alcohol No known problems.
Protecting your eyes Avoid getting the powder in the eyes as it can trigger glaucoma or make existing glaucoma worse. If eye or vision problems develop, call your doctor immediately.

PROLONGED USE

No known problems.

Tolbutamide

Brand name None
Used in the following combined preparations
None

QUICK REFERENCE
Drug group Drug used in diabetes (p.82)
Overdose danger rating High
Dependence rating Low
Prescription needed Yes
Available as generic Yes

GENERAL INFORMATION

Tolbutamide is an antidiabetic agent that lowers blood glucose by stimulating insulin secretion from the pancreas. Taken by mouth, it is used to treat adult (maturity-onset, or Type 2) diabetes in which active insulin-secreting cells are still present. When these cells are absent, as in juvenile diabetes, it is ineffective. The drug is always given in conjunction with a special diabetic diet that limits carbohydrate intake.

Because tolbutamide is shorter acting than many other oral antidiabetics, it may help in the initial control of diabetes. It may also be prescribed to people with impaired kidney function because it is less likely to build up in the body and cause excessive lowering of blood glucose. As with other oral antidiabetics, tolbutamide may need to be replaced with insulin (see p.271) during serious illness, injury, or surgery, when diabetic control is lost.

INFORMATION FOR USERS

Your drug prescription is tailored for you. Do not alter dosage without checking with your doctor.
How taken Tablets.
Frequency and timing of doses Taken with meals either once daily in the morning or 2 x daily in the morning and evening.
Adult dosage range 500mg–2g daily.
Onset of effect Within 1 hour.
Duration of action 6–10 hours.
Diet advice A low-carbohydrate diet must be maintained for the drug to be fully effective. Follow the advice of your doctor.
Storage Keep in a closed container in a cool, dry place out of reach of children. Protect from light.
Missed dose Take as soon as you remember. If your next dose is due within 2 hours, take a single dose now and skip the next.
Stopping the drug Unless severe adverse effects occur (see below), do not stop taking the drug without consulting your doctor; stop-

ping the drug may lead to worsening of the underlying condition.

OVERDOSE ACTION

Seek immediate medical advice in all cases. If faintness, confusion, or headache occur, eat something sugary. Take emergency action if fits or loss of consciousness occur.

POSSIBLE ADVERSE EFFECTS

Serious effects are rare. Dizziness, sweating, weakness, and confusion are symptoms of low blood glucose. Headache or ringing in the ears, and nausea or vomiting may also occur. If jaundice, a rash, or itching occur, stop taking the drug and contact your doctor immediately.

INTERACTIONS

General note Many drugs, such as corticosteroids, oestrogens, diuretics, and rifampicin, can oppose tolbutamide's effects, raising blood glucose levels. Others increase the risk of low blood glucose. These include sulphonamides, warfarin, beta blockers, chloramphenicol, clofibrate, aspirin and other NSAIDs, some antibiotics and antifungals, and MAOIs.

SPECIAL PRECAUTIONS

Be sure to tell your doctor if:
◆ You have long-term liver or kidney problems.
◆ You are allergic to sulphonamides.
◆ You have thyroid problems.
◆ You have porphyria.
◆ You are taking other medications.

Pregnancy Not usually prescribed. May cause birth defects if taken in the first 3 months of pregnancy. Discuss with your doctor.

Breast-feeding The drug passes into the breast milk and may affect the baby. Discuss with your doctor.

Infants and children Not prescribed.

Over 60 Increased risk of low blood glucose. Reduced dose may therefore be necessary

Driving and hazardous work Usually no problem. Avoid these activities, however, if you have warning signs of low blood sugar.

Alcohol Keep consumption low. Alcohol may upset diabetic control.

Surgery and general anaesthetics Tell your doctor that you are diabetic before any surgery; insulin treatment may need to be substituted.

PROLONGED USE

No problems expected.

Monitoring Regular monitoring of urine and/or blood glucose is required.

Tolterodine

Brand name Detrusitol
Used in the following combined preparations
None

QUICK REFERENCE

Drug group Drug for urinary disorders (p.112)
Overdose danger rating Medium
Dependence rating Low
Prescription needed Yes
Available as generic No

GENERAL INFORMATION

Tolterodine is an anticholinergic (see Autonomic nervous system, p.8) and antispasmodic drug used to treat urinary frequency and incontinence in adults. It reduces the bladder's contractions, allowing it to expand and hold more. It also stops spasms and delays the desire to empty the bladder.

Tolterodine's usefulness is limited to some extent by its side effects, and dosage needs to be reduced in the elderly. Children are more susceptible than adults to its anticholinergic effects. The drug can also trigger glaucoma.

INFORMATION FOR USERS

Your drug prescription is tailored for you. Do not alter dosage without checking with your doctor.

How taken Tablets, SR-capsules.
Frequency and timing of doses 2 x daily.
Dosage range 4mg daily, reduced to 2mg daily, if necessary, to minimize side effects.
Onset of effect 1 hour.
Duration of action 12 hours.
Diet advice None.
Storage Keep in a closed container in a cool, dry place out of reach of children.
Missed dose Take as soon as you remember. If your next dose is due within 2 hours, take a single dose now and skip the next.
Stopping the drug Do not stop taking the drug without consulting your doctor; symptoms may recur.

Exceeding the dose An occasional unintentional extra dose is unlikely to cause problems. Large overdoses, however, may cause visual disturbances, urinary difficulties, hallucinations, convulsions, and breathing difficulties; notify your doctor.

POSSIBLE ADVERSE EFFECTS

Common side effects, such as dry mouth/eyes, digestive upset, constipation, or blurred vision, are due to the drug's anticholinergic action and may improve with time. Headache, drowsiness, and nervousness may also occur. If chest pain, confusion, or difficulty in passing urine occur, consult your doctor.

INTERACTIONS

General note All drugs that have an anticholinergic effect will have increased side effects when taken with tolterodine.

Domperidone and metoclopramide Tolterodine may decrease the effects of these drugs.

Erythromycin, clarithromycin, itraconazole, ketoconazole, and miconazole These drugs may increase blood levels of tolterodine.

SPECIAL PRECAUTIONS

Be sure to tell your doctor if:
◆ You have liver or kidney problems.
◆ You have thyroid problems.
◆ You have heart problems.
◆ You have porphyria.
◆ You have hiatus hernia.
◆ You suffer from prostate problems or urinary retention.
◆ You have ulcerative colitis.
◆ You have glaucoma.
◆ You have myasthenia gravis.
◆ You are taking other medications.

Pregnancy Safety in pregnancy not established. The drug may harm the developing baby. Discuss with your doctor.

Breast-feeding Safety not established. Discuss with your doctor.

Infants and children Not recommended. Safety not established.

Over 60 Reduced dose may be necessary.

Driving and hazardous work Avoid such activities until you have learned how tolterodine affects you because it can cause drowsiness, disorientation, and blurred vision.

Alcohol No special problems.

PROLONGED USE

No special problems. The effectiveness of the drug, and the continuing clinical need for it, are usually reviewed after 6 months.

Monitoring Periodic eye tests for glaucoma may be performed.

Tramadol

Brand names Dromadol, Tramake, Zamadol, Zydol
Used in the following combined preparations
None

QUICK REFERENCE

Drug group Analgesic (p.9)
Overdose danger rating High
Dependence rating Low
Prescription needed Yes
Available as generic Yes

GENERAL INFORMATION

Tramadol is a synthetic opioid analgesic, which is chemically similar to the body's natural opioids. It is used to prevent or treat moderately severe pain – for example, from injury, surgery, or cancer. The painkilling effect wears off after about 4 hours, but a slow-release (long-acting) form may give relief for up to 12 hours.

Tramadol can be habit-forming, and dependence may occur, but most people taking it for the short term do not become dependent and can stop taking it without difficulty. It is said to be less likely than older opioids to cause breathing problems and constipation.

INFORMATION FOR USERS

Your drug prescription is tailored for you. Do not alter dosage without checking with your doctor.

How taken Tablets, SR-tablets, soluble tablets, capsules, SR-capsules, injection, powder in sachets.

Frequency and timing of doses Usually 2 x daily (SR-preparations); up to 6 x daily (other preparations).

Adult dosage range Up to 400mg daily (by mouth); 600mg daily (injection).

Onset of effect 30–60 minutes (by mouth); 15–30 minutes (injection).

Duration of action 4 hours.

Diet advice None.

Storage Keep in a closed container in a cool, dry place out of reach of children.

Missed dose Take the dose as soon as you remember, and return to your normal schedule as soon as possible.

Stopping the drug If the reason for taking tramadol no longer exists, you may stop taking the drug and notify your doctor. If you have been taking it for a long time, you may experience withdrawal effects.

OVERDOSE ACTION

Seek immediate medical advice in all cases. Take emergency action if breathing difficulties, severe drowsiness, or loss of consciousness occur.

POSSIBLE ADVERSE EFFECTS

Adverse effects such as tiredness and drowsiness seem more common with tramadol than with some other opioids. Other effects include dry mouth, constipation, nausea, and vomiting. Dizziness and headaches are rare side effects. If you experience confusion or hallucinations, consult your doctor. If convulsions, wheezing, or breathlessness occur, stop taking the drug and seek urgent medical advice.

INTERACTIONS

Antidepressants Taken with tramadol, some of these may increase the risk of convulsions.

Carbamazepine This drug may reduce blood levels and effects of tramadol.

Sedatives All drugs that have a sedative effect are likely to increase the sedative effects of tramadol. These drugs include antidepressants, antipsychotics, antihistamines, and sleeping drugs.

SPECIAL PRECAUTIONS

Be sure to tell your doctor if:
◆ You have had a head injury.
◆ You have any long-term liver or kidney problems.
◆ You have heart or circulatory problems.
◆ You have a lung disorder such as asthma or bronchitis.
◆ You have thyroid disease.
◆ You have a history of epileptic fits.
◆ You are taking other medications.

Pregnancy Safety not established. Discuss with your doctor.

Breast-feeding The drug passes into the breast milk and may make the baby drowsy. Discuss with your doctor.

Infants and children Not recommended under 12 years.

Over 60 Reduced dose may be necessary.

Driving and hazardous work Avoid. Tramadol can cause drowsiness.

Alcohol Avoid. Alcohol increases the sedative effects of tramadol.

PROLONGED USE

Dependence may occur if tramadol is taken for long periods.

Triamterene

Brand name Dytac
Used in the following combined preparations
Dyazide (co-triamterzide), Dytide, Frusene, Kalspare, Triam-Co, TriamaxCo

QUICK REFERENCE

Drug group Diuretic (p.32)
Overdose danger rating Low
Dependence rating Low
Prescription needed Yes
Available as generic Yes (in combined products)

GENERAL INFORMATION

Triamterene belongs to the class of drugs known as potassium-sparing diuretics. In combination with thiazide or loop diuretics (see p.33), it is given for the treatment of hypertension. Triamterene, on its own or, more commonly, with a thiazide diuretic, may also be used to treat oedema (fluid retention) as a complication of heart failure, nephrotic syndrome, or cirrhosis of the liver.

Triamterene is fast acting; its effect on urine flow is apparent within two hours and may last for 12 hours. For this reason, the drug should be taken early in the day. As with other potassium-sparing diuretics, unusually high levels of potassium may build up in the blood if the kidneys are functioning abnormally. Therefore, triamterene is prescribed with caution to people with kidney failure.

INFORMATION FOR USERS

Your drug prescription is tailored for you. Do not alter dosage without checking with your doctor.

How taken Tablets.

Frequency and timing of doses 1–2 x daily after meals or on alternate days.

Adult dosage range 50–250mg daily.

Onset of effect Within 2 hours.

Duration of action 9–12 hours.

Diet advice Avoid foods that are high in potassium, such as dried fruit and salt substitutes,

Storage Keep in a closed container in a cool, dry place out of reach of children.

Missed dose Take as soon as you remember. However, if it is late in the day, do not take the missed dose, or you may need to get up at night to pass urine. Take the next scheduled dose as usual.

Stopping the drug Do not stop taking the drug without consulting your doctor; symptoms may recur.

Exceeding the dose An occasional unintentional extra dose is unlikely to be a cause for concern. But if you notice any unusual symptoms, or if a large overdose has been taken, notify your doctor.

POSSIBLE ADVERSE EFFECTS

Triamterene has few adverse effects; the main problem is the possibility of potassium being retained by the body, resulting in muscle weakness and numbness. Dry mouth, digestive disturbance, and headache may also occur. If you develop muscle weakness or a rash, consult your doctor. The drug may colour your urine blue, but this is not a cause for concern.

INTERACTIONS

Lithium Triamterene may increase the blood levels of lithium, leading to an increased risk of lithium toxicity.

NSAIDs These drugs, taken with triamterene, may increase the risk of raised blood levels of potassium.

ACE inhibitors These drugs increase the risk of raised levels of potassium in the blood with triamterene.

Ciclosporin This drug may increase levels of potassium with triamterene.

SPECIAL PRECAUTIONS

Be sure to tell your doctor if:

◆ You have any long-term liver or kidney problems.

◆ You have had kidney stones.

◆ You have gout.

◆ You are taking other medications.

Pregnancy Not usually prescribed. May produce a reduction in the blood supply to the developing baby. Discuss with your doctor.

Breast-feeding The drug passes into the breast milk and may affect the baby. It could also reduce your milk supply. Discuss with your doctor.

Infants and children Not usually prescribed. Reduced dose necessary.

Over 60 Increased likelihood of adverse effects, so reduced dose may be necessary.

Driving and hazardous work No special problems.

Alcohol No known problems.

PROLONGED USE

Serious problems are unlikely, but levels of salts such as sodium and potassium may occasionally become abnormal during prolonged use.

Monitoring Blood tests may be performed to check kidney function and the levels of body salts.

Trimethoprim

Brand names Monotrim, Trimopan
Used in the following combined preparations
Fectrim, Polytrim, Septrin

QUICK REFERENCE

Drug group Antibacterial drug (p.66)
Overdose danger rating Low
Dependence rating Low
Prescription needed Yes
Available as generic Yes

GENERAL INFORMATION

Trimethoprim is an antibacterial drug that became popular in the 1970s for preventing and treating infections of the urinary and respiratory tracts. This drug has been used for many years in combination with another antibacterial drug, sulfamethoxazole, in a preparation known as co-trimoxazole (see p.205). Trimethoprim has fewer adverse effects than co-trimoxazole, however, and is equally effective in treating many conditions. The drug can also be given by injection to treat severe infections.

Although the side effects of trimethoprim are not usually troublesome, tests to monitor blood composition are often advised when the drug is taken for prolonged periods.

INFORMATION FOR USERS

Your drug prescription is tailored for you. Do not alter dosage without checking with your doctor.

How taken Tablets, liquid, injection, eye ointment, eye drops.

Frequency and timing of doses 1–2 x daily.

Adult dosage range 300–400mg daily (treatment); 100–200mg daily (prevention).

Onset of effect 1–4 hours.

Duration of action Up to 24 hours.

Diet advice None.

Storage Keep in a closed container in a cool, dry place out of reach of children. Protect from light.

Missed dose Take as soon as you remember.

Stopping the drug Unless severe adverse effects occur (see below), take the full course. Even if you feel better, the original infection may still be present and symptoms may recur if treatment is stopped too soon.

Exceeding the dose An occasional unintentional extra dose is unlikely to be a cause for concern. But if you notice any unusual symptoms, or if a large overdose has been taken, notify your doctor.

POSSIBLE ADVERSE EFFECTS

Taken on its own, trimethoprim rarely causes adverse effects other than nausea. However, additional adverse effects may occur when trimethoprim is taken in combination with sulfamethoxazole (as co-trimoxazole). If you develop a rash or itching, a sore throat, fever, bruising, or bleeding, stop taking the drug and contact your doctor immediately.

INTERACTIONS

Cytotoxic drugs Trimethoprim increases the risk of blood problems if taken with azathio-prine or mercaptopurine. When it is taken with methotrexate, there is an increased risk of folate deficiency, which results in blood abnormalities.

Phenytoin When taken with trimethoprim, this drug may increase the risk of folate deficiency.

Warfarin Trimethoprim may increase the anticoagulant effect of warfarin.

Ciclosporin Trimethoprim increases the risk of this drug causing kidney damage.

Antimalarials containing pyrimethamine Drugs such as Fansidar or maloprim may increase the risk of folate deficiency, resulting in blood abnormalities, if they are taken with trimethoprim.

SPECIAL PRECAUTIONS

Be sure to tell your doctor if:
◆ You have long-term liver or kidney problems.
◆ You have a blood disorder.
◆ You have porphyria.
◆ You are taking other medications.

Pregnancy Safety in pregnancy not established. Discuss with your doctor.

Breast-feeding The drug passes into the breast milk, but at normal doses adverse effects on the baby are unlikely. Discuss with your doctor.

Infants and children Reduced dose necessary.

Over 60 Increased likelihood of adverse effects. Reduced dose may therefore be necessary.

Driving and hazardous work No known problems.

Alcohol No known problems.

PROLONGED USE

Long-term use of this drug may lead to folate deficiency, which, in turn, may lead to blood abnormalities. Folic acid supplements (see Vitamins, p.90) may be prescribed.

Monitoring Periodic blood tests to monitor blood composition are usually advised.

Venlafaxine

Brand name Efexor, Efexor XL
Used in the following combined preparations
None

QUICK REFERENCE

Drug group Antidepressant (p.14)
Overdose danger rating High
Dependence rating Low
Prescription needed Yes
Available as generic No

GENERAL INFORMATION

Venlafaxine is an antidepressant drug with a chemical structure unlike other types of antidepressant. It combines the therapeutic properties of selective serotonin reuptake inhibitors (SSRIs) and tricyclic antidepressants, without anticholinergic (see Autonomic nervous system, p.8) adverse effects. As with other antidepressants, venlafaxine elevates mood, controls sleep patterns, and restores interest in everyday activities.

Nausea, dizziness, drowsiness or insomnia, and restlessness are common. Weight loss may occur due to decreased appetite. At high doses, the drug can elevate blood pressure, which should be monitored during treatment.

INFORMATION FOR USERS

Your drug prescription is tailored for you. Do not alter dosage without checking with your doctor.
How taken Tablets, SR-capsules.
Frequency and timing of doses Twice daily (tablets); once daily (SR-capsules) with food.
Dosage range 75–150mg daily (outpatients); up to 375mg daily (severely depressed patients).
Onset of effect Can appear within days, although the full antidepressant effect may not be felt for 2–4 weeks or longer.
Duration of action About 8–12 hours; 24 hours for SR-tablets. Following prolonged treatment, antidepressant effects may persist for up to 6 weeks.
Diet advice None.
Storage Keep in the original container in a cool, dry place out of reach of children.
Missed dose Do not make up a missed dose; just take your next scheduled dose.

Stopping the drug Unless severe adverse effects occur (see below), do not stop taking the drug without consulting your doctor. Stopping the drug abruptly can cause withdrawal symptoms.

OVERDOSE ACTION

Seek immediate medical advice in all cases. Take emergency action if fits, slow or irregular pulse, or loss of consciousness occur.

POSSIBLE ADVERSE EFFECTS

The most common effects, some of which may wear off in a few days, are weakness, nausea, decreased appetite, restlessness, drowsiness, and dizziness. Anxiety, nervousness, tremor, insomnia, abnormal dreams, agitation, and confusion may also occur. If you have sexual dysfunction, itching, or a rash, stop taking the drug and consult your doctor.

INTERACTIONS

Sedatives All drugs that have a sedative effect are likely to increase the sedative effects of venlafaxine.
Antihypertensive drugs Venlafaxine may reduce the effectiveness of these drugs.
MAOIs Venlafaxine may interact with MAOIs to produce a dangerous rise in blood pressure. At least 14 days should elapse between stopping them and starting venlafaxine.

SPECIAL PRECAUTIONS

Be sure to tell your doctor if:
◆ You have had an adverse reaction to any other antidepressants.
◆ You have long-term liver or kidney problems.
◆ You have a heart problem or high blood pressure.
◆ You have had epileptic fits.
◆ You have had problems with alcohol or drug misuse/abuse.
◆ You are taking other medications.
Pregnancy Safety in pregnancy not established. Discuss with your doctor.
Breast-feeding Not recommended. Discuss with your doctor.
Infants and children Not recommended under 18 years.
Over 60 Reduced dose may be necessary. Increased likelihood of adverse effects.

Driving and hazardous work Avoid such activities until you have learned how venlafaxine affects you because the drug can cause dizziness, drowsiness, and blurred vision.
Alcohol Avoid. Alcohol may increase the sedative effects of this drug.

PROLONGED USE

Withdrawal symptoms may occur if the drug is not stopped gradually after prolonged use. However, these symptoms rarely last for more than 1–2 weeks.
Monitoring Blood pressure should be measured periodically if high doses of venlafaxine are prescribed.

Verapamil

Brand names Cordilox, Securon, Univer, Verapress, Vertab, Zolvera
Used in the following combined preparations None

QUICK REFERENCE

Drug group Anti-angina drug (p.35), anti-arrhythmic drug (p.33), and antihypertensive drug (p.36)
Overdose danger rating Medium
Dependence rating Low
Prescription needed Yes
Available as generic Yes

GENERAL INFORMATION

Verapamil belongs to a group of drugs called calcium channel blockers. These act by blocking the conduction of electrical signals in the muscles of the heart and blood vessels.

Verapamil is used in the treatment of hypertension, abnormal heart rhythms, and angina. It reduces the frequency of angina attacks; however, it does not work quickly enough to relieve pain during an attack. The drug increases the ability to tolerate physical exertion and, unlike some drugs, does not affect breathing, so it can be used safely by asthmatic people. Because of its effects on the heart, it is also given, as tablets or injections, for certain types of abnormal heart rhythm.

The drug is not usually given to people with low blood pressure, slow heart beat, or heart failure, because it may worsen these conditions. It may also cause constipation.

INFORMATION FOR USERS

Your drug prescription is tailored for you. Do not alter dosage without checking with your doctor.
How taken Tablets, SR-tablets, SR-capsules, liquid, injection.
Frequency and timing of doses 2–3 x daily (tablets, liquid); 1–2 x daily (SR-tablets).
Adult dosage range 120–480mg daily.
Onset of effect 1–2 hours (tablets); 2–3 minutes (injection).
Duration of action 6–8 hours. During prolonged treatment some beneficial effects may last for up to 12 hours. SR-tablets act for 12–24 hours.
Diet advice Avoid grapefruit juice, which may increase blood levels of verapamil.
Storage Keep in a closed container in a cool, dry place out of reach of children.
Missed dose Take as soon as you remember. If your next dose is due within 3 hours (tablets, liquid) or 8 hours (SR-tablets, SR-capsules), take a single dose now and skip the next.
Stopping the drug Do not stop taking the drug without consulting your doctor; symptoms may recur.
Exceeding the dose An occasional unintentional extra dose is unlikely to be a cause for concern. Large overdoses, however, may cause dizziness; notify your doctor.

POSSIBLE ADVERSE EFFECTS

Verapamil has fewer adverse effects than other calcium channel blockers but it can still cause a variety of minor symptoms, such as nausea, constipation, headache, and ankle swelling. Rarer adverse effects include flushing and dizziness; rarely, gynaecomastia (breast enlargement in males) and an increase in gum tissue may occur after long-term use. If you develop a rash, contact your doctor immediately.

INTERACTIONS

Beta blockers When verapamil is taken with these drugs, there is a slight risk of abnormal heart beat and heart failure.
Carbamazepine The effects of this drug may be enhanced by verapamil.
Ciclosporin The blood levels of this drug may be increased by verapamil and its dose may need to be reduced.

Antihypertensive drugs Blood pressure may be further lowered when these drugs are taken with verapamil.

Digoxin The effects of this drug may be increased if it is taken with verapamil. The dosage of digoxin may need to be reduced.

Grapefruit juice Grapefruit juice may increase the effects of verapamil and is best avoided.

SPECIAL PRECAUTIONS

Be sure to tell your doctor if:

◆ You have a long-term liver problem.
◆ You have heart failure.
◆ You have porphyria.
◆ You are taking other medications.

Pregnancy Not usually prescribed. May inhibit labour if taken during the later stages of pregnancy. Discuss with your doctor.

Breast-feeding The drug passes into the breast milk, but at normal doses adverse effects on the baby are unlikely. Discuss with your doctor.

Infants and children Usually given on specialist advice only. Reduced dose necessary.

Over 60 No special problems.

Driving and hazardous work Avoid such activities until you have learned how verapamil affects you because the drug can cause dizziness.

Alcohol Avoid heavy intake. Alcohol may further reduce blood pressure, causing dizziness or other symptoms.

Surgery and general anaesthetics Verapamil may need to be stopped before surgery. Discuss this with your doctor or dentist.

PROLONGED USE

No problems expected.

Warfarin

Brand name Marevan
Used in the following combined preparations
None

QUICK REFERENCE

Drug group Drug that affects blood clotting (p.38)
Overdose danger rating High
Dependence rating Low
Prescription needed Yes
Available as generic Yes

GENERAL INFORMATION

Warfarin is an anticoagulant drug (see p.39) used to prevent clots in blood vessels, mainly in areas where blood flow is slowest, particularly the leg and pelvic veins. Such clots can break off and travel through the bloodstream to the lungs, where they lodge to form a pulmonary embolism. The drug is also used for people with atrial fibrillation, or those who have had artificial heart valves fitted, to reduce the risk of clots forming in the heart; any clots could travel to the brain and cause a stroke.

A widely used oral anticoagulant drug, warfarin requires regular monitoring to ensure proper maintenance dosage. Because its full beneficial effects are not felt for 2 to 3 days, a faster-acting drug such as heparin (see p.262) is often used to complement the effects of warfarin at the start of treatment.

The most serious adverse effect of warfarin, as with all anticoagulants, is the risk of excessive bleeding, which is usually the result of excessive dosage.

INFORMATION FOR USERS

Your drug prescription is tailored for you. Do not alter dosage without checking with your doctor.
How taken Tablets.
Frequency and timing of doses Once daily, taken at the same time each day.
Dosage range *Starting dose* 10–15mg daily according to age and weight. *Maintenance dose* 1–9mg daily, as determined by blood tests.
Onset of effect Within 24–48 hours, with full effect after several days.
Duration of action 2–3 days.
Diet advice Major changes in diet may alter the anticoagulant effect of warfarin.

Storage Keep in a closed container in a cool, dry place out of reach of children. Protect from light.
Missed dose Take as soon as you remember. Take the following dose on your original schedule.
Stopping the drug Unless nausea, fever, or vomiting occur, do not stop taking the drug without consulting your doctor; stopping it may lead to worsening of the underlying condition.

OVERDOSE ACTION

Seek immediate medical advice in all cases.

POSSIBLE ADVERSE EFFECTS

Bleeding is the most common adverse effect of treatment with warfarin. Other, rarer, effects include abdominal pain, diarrhoea, rash, and hair loss; these should be discussed with your doctor. If you experience nausea or vomiting, bleeding or bruising, or develop a fever or jaundice, stop taking the drug and contact your doctor urgently.

INTERACTIONS

General note A wide variety of drugs – such as aspirin, barbiturates, oral contraceptives, cimetidine, diuretics, certain laxatives, antidepressants, and antibiotics – interact with warfarin, either by increasing or decreasing the anticlotting effect. Consult your pharmacist before using any over-the-counter medicines.

SPECIAL PRECAUTIONS

Be sure to tell your doctor if:
◆ You have long-term liver or kidney problems.
◆ You have high blood pressure.
◆ You have peptic ulcers.
◆ You bleed easily.
◆ You are taking other medications.

Pregnancy Not usually prescribed. If given in early pregnancy, the drug can cause malformations in the developing baby. Taken near the time of delivery, it may cause the mother to bleed excessively. Discuss with your doctor.
Breast-feeding The drug passes into the breast milk, but at normal doses adverse effects on the baby are unlikely. Discuss with your doctor.

Infants and children Reduced dose necessary.

Over 60 No special problems.

Driving and hazardous work Use caution when undertaking these activities. Even minor bumps can cause bad bruises and excessive bleeding.

Alcohol Avoid excessive amounts. Alcohol may increase the effects of this drug.

Surgery and general anaesthetics Warfarin may need to be stopped before surgery. Discuss with your doctor or dentist.

PROLONGED USE

No special problems.

Monitoring Regular blood tests are performed during treatment.

Zanamivir

Brand name Relenza
Used in the following combined preparations
None

QUICK REFERENCE
Drug group Antiviral drug (p.69)
Overdose danger rating Low
Dependence rating Low
Prescription needed Yes
Available as generic No

GENERAL INFORMATION

Zanamivir is a new type of antiviral drug used to treat influenza (flu), a virus that infects and multiplies in the lungs. The drug works by preventing the virus from multiplying.

Flu causes fever, chills, headache, and aches and pains. Other symptoms include a sore throat, cough, and nasal symptoms. Zanamivir, when taken by inhaler, helps to clear these symptoms and may shorten the duration of the illness. There is no benefit, however, if you do not have a fever. Therefore, treatment should begin as soon as possible, and certainly within 48 hours of the onset of symptoms. Zanamivir also reduces the risk of flu being passed on to others if it is taken by people in contact with the virus. Flu symptoms usually subside in 2 to 7 days, unless complications such as a chest infection occur.

Elderly people, and those with long-term illnesses such as chronic lung and heart disease, are at most risk of complications. Zanamivir should be used with caution by people with asthma because it may provoke wheezing requiring urgent use of a bronchodilator (see p.23).

INFORMATION FOR USERS

Your drug prescription is tailored for you. Do not alter dosage without checking with your doctor.
How taken Silver foil blisters of dry powder, to be taken by inhaler.
Frequency and timing of doses 2 x daily. Inhale the contents of the blisters one at a time.
Adult dosage range 20mg (4 x 5mg blisters) daily for 5 days.
Onset of effect Within 7 days.

Duration of action Up to 12 hours.
Diet advice None.
Storage Keep in a cool, dry place out of reach of children.
Missed dose Take as soon as you remember. If your next dose is due within 2 hours, take a single dose now and skip the next.
Stopping the drug Unless wheezing or breathlessness occur, do not stop without consulting your doctor; symptoms may recur.
Exceeding the dose An occasional unintentional dose is unlikely to cause problems. However, if you notice any unusual symptoms, or if a large overdose has been taken, notify your doctor.

POSSIBLE ADVERSE EFFECTS

Adverse effects are rare. Those that do occur, such as headache, sore throat, a cough, and nasal symptoms, are similar to the signs and symptoms of flu; they may sometimes be due to the virus rather than the drug. If wheezing or breathlessness develop, stop taking the drug and consult your doctor.

INTERACTIONS

Inhaled drugs (such as salbutamol and beclometasone) These should be inhaled just before zanamivir is administered.

SPECIAL PRECAUTIONS

Be sure to tell your doctor if:
◆ You have ever had an allergic reaction to zanamivir or lactose monohydrate.
◆ You have a long-term illness.
◆ You have a lung disease such as asthma.
◆ You have poor immunity to infections.
◆ You suffer from asthma.
◆ You are taking other medications.
Pregnancy Safety in pregnancy not established. Discuss with your doctor.
Breast-feeding Safety not established. Discuss with your doctor.
Infants and children Not recommended.
Over 60 No special problems.
Driving and hazardous work No known problems.
Alcohol No known problems.

PROLONGED USE

This drug should only be used for 5 days and is not prescribed for long-term use.

Zidovudine/Lamivudine

Brand name Retrovir (zidovudine); Epivir (lamivudine)
Used in the following combined preparation
Combivir

QUICK REFERENCE

Drug group Drug for HIV and AIDS (p.100)
Overdose danger rating Medium
Dependence rating Low
Prescription needed Yes
Available as generic No

GENERAL INFORMATION

Zidovudine and lamivudine belong to a class of drugs known as reverse transcriptase inhibitors and are used in the treatment of HIV infection. The two drugs are combined in one tablet, which is usually prescribed with another class of drug to treat HIV: either another reverse transcriptase inhibitor or a protease inhibitor. This combination of three drugs (known as combination antiretroviral therapy) is more effective at treating HIV than either a single or a double regime of drugs.

Although not a cure for HIV, combination antiretroviral therapy slows down production of the virus and, therefore, reduces the damage done to the immune system. The drugs need to be taken regularly and on a long-term basis to remain effective.

INFORMATION FOR USERS

Your drug prescription is tailored for you. Do not alter dosage without checking with your doctor.
How taken Tablets.
Frequency and timing of doses Every 12 hours.
Adult dosage range One tablet.
Onset of effect 1 hour.
Duration of action 12 hours.
Diet advice None.
Storage Keep in a tightly closed container in a cool, dry place out of reach of children.
Missed dose Take the missed dose as soon as you remember. If your next dose is due within 2 hours, take a single dose now and skip the next one. It is very important not to miss doses on a regular basis because this could lead to the development of drug-resistant HIV.

Stopping the drug Do not stop taking the drug without consulting your doctor; symptoms may recur.
Exceeding the dose An occasional unintentional extra dose is unlikely to cause problems. But if you notice any unusual symptoms, or if a large overdose has been taken, notify your doctor.

POSSIBLE ADVERSE EFFECTS

The most common adverse effects of zidovudine and lamivudine are nausea, vomiting, headache, and diarrhoea. Sometimes anaemia may develop with prolonged use; symptoms include pallor, fatigue, and shortness of breath. Sore throat and fever are less frequent effects, and result from a decreased number of white blood cells. If you experience numbness or unusual sensations, aching muscles, or skin discoloration, consult your doctor. In case of severe abdominal pain, seek urgent medical advice.

INTERACTIONS

General note A wide range of drugs may interact with zidovudine and lamivudine, causing either an increase in adverse effects or a reduction in the effect of the antiretroviral drugs. Check with your doctor or pharmacist before taking any new drugs, including those from dentists and supermarkets, and herbal medicines.

SPECIAL PRECAUTIONS

Be sure to tell your doctor if:
◆ You have long-term liver or kidney problems.
◆ You have other infections, such as hepatitis B or C.
◆ You are taking other medications.
Pregnancy Safety in pregnancy not established. If you are pregnant, or planning a pregnancy, discuss with your doctor.
Breast-feeding Safety not established. Breast-feeding by HIV-positive mothers is not recommended because the virus may be passed to the baby.
Infants and children Reduced dose necessary.
Over 60 Increased likelihood of adverse effects. Reduced dose may be necessary.
Driving and hazardous work No special problems.
Alcohol No known problems.

PROLONGED USE

There is an increased risk of serious blood disorders, such as anaemia, with long-term use of zidovudine and lamivudine.

Monitoring Regular blood checks will be carried out to monitor the drugs' effects on the virus and to look for signs of anaemia.

Zopiclone

Brand names Zileze, Zimovane
Used in the following combined preparations
None

QUICK REFERENCE

Drug group Sleeping drug (p.11)
Overdose danger rating Medium
Dependence rating Medium
Prescription needed Yes
Available as generic Yes

GENERAL INFORMATION

Zopiclone is a hypnotic (sleeping drug) used for the short-term treatment of insomnia. Sleep problems can take the form of difficulty in falling asleep or frequently waking at night and/or early in the morning. Hypnotics are given only when non-drug measures (such as avoiding caffeine) have proved ineffective.

Unlike benzodiazepines, zopiclone possesses no anti-anxiety properties, so it may be suited for insomnia that is not accompanied by anxiety – for example, insomnia that is due to international travel or a change in shift work routine.

Hypnotics are intended for occasional use only. Dependence can develop after as little as a week of continuous use. Some doctors may recommend taking the drug intermittently (for example, 3 times a week).

INFORMATION FOR USERS

Your drug prescription is tailored for you. Do not alter dosage without checking with your doctor.

How taken Tablets.
Frequency and timing of doses Once daily at bedtime when required.
Dosage range 3.75–7.5mg.
Onset of effect Within 30 minutes.
Duration of action 4–6 hours.

Diet advice None.
Storage Keep in a closed container in a cool, dry place out of reach of children. Protect from light.
Missed dose If you fall asleep without having taken a dose and wake some hours later, do not take the missed dose.
Stopping the drug If you have been taking the drug continuously for less than 1 week, it can be safely stopped as soon as you feel you no longer need it. However, if you have been taking the drug for longer, consult your doctor.
Exceeding the dose An occasional, unintentional extra dose is unlikely to cause problems. Large overdoses, however, may cause prolonged sleep, drowsiness, lethargy, and poor muscle coordination and reflexes; notify your doctor immediately.

POSSIBLE ADVERSE EFFECTS

The most common adverse effects are daytime drowsiness, which normally diminishes after the first few days of treatment, and a bitter taste in the mouth. Dizziness or weakness and nausea or diarrhoea are less common complications. Persistent morning drowsiness or impaired coordination are signs of excessive doses and you should consult your doctor. If you develop amnesia or confusion, or a rash, stop taking the drug and call your doctor without delay.

INTERACTIONS

Sedatives All drugs, including alcohol, that have a sedative effect on the central nervous system are likely to increase the sedative effects of zopiclone. These drug types include other sleeping drugs and anti-anxiety drugs, antihistamines, antidepressants, opioid analgesics, and antipsychotics.

SPECIAL PRECAUTIONS

Be sure to tell your doctor if:
◆ You have or have had any problems with alcohol or drug abuse.
◆ You have myasthenia gravis.
◆ You have had epileptic fits.
◆ You have liver or kidney problems.
◆ You are taking other medications.
Pregnancy Not recommended.
Breast-feeding Not recommended.
Infants and children Not recommended.

Over 60 Increased likelihood of adverse effects. Reduced dose may therefore be necessary.

Driving and hazardous work Avoid such activities until you have learned how zopiclone affects you as the drug can cause drowsiness, reduced alertness, and slowed reactions.

Alcohol Avoid excessive amounts. Alcohol increases the sedative effects of this drug.

PROLONGED USE

Zopiclone is intended for occasional use only. Continuous use of this, or any other, sleeping drug for as little as 1 week may result in dependence.

PART 3

DRUG FINDER
INDEX

This part of the book consists of a drug finder index, which helps you to find information on specific brand-named drugs and generic substances, as well as directing you to further information about them throughout the book.

DRUG FINDER INDEX

This section contains the names of approximately 2,500 individual drug products and substances. It provides a quick and easy reference for readers interested in finding out about a specific drug or medication, as well as directing the reader to information about them throughout the book. There is no need for you to know what group a drug belongs to, whether an item is a brand name or generic name, or whether it is a prescription or an over-the-counter drug; all types of drug and the major drug groups are listed.

WHAT IT CONTAINS

The entries are listed alphabetically and include all major generic drugs and many less widely used substances. A broad range of brand names, as well as many vitamins and minerals, are also included. This comprehensive selection reflects the wide diversity of products available for the treatment and prevention of disease. Inclusion of a drug or product does not imply BMA endorsement, nor does the exclusion of a particular drug or product indicate BMA disapproval.

HOW THE REFERENCES WORK

References are to the pages in Part 2, containing the drug profiles of each principal generic drug, and to the section in Part 1 that describes the relevant drug group, as appropriate. Some entries for generic drugs that do not have a full profile contain a brief description here.

A

abacavir a reverse transcriptase inhibitor drug for HIV/AIDS 100

abciximab an antiplatelet drug 39

Abelcet a brand name for amphotericin 143 (an antifungal drug 76)

Abidec a brand-named multivitamin 91

Abtrim a brand name for clotrimazole 196 (an antifungal drug 76)

acamprosate an alcohol abuse treatment 130

acarbose an oral antidiabetic 82

Accolate a brand name for zafirlukast (a leukotriene antagonist drug for asthma 24)

Accupro a brand name for quinapril (an ACE inhibitor vasodilator 31)

Accuretic a brand name for quinapril (an ACE inhibitor vasdilator 31) with hydrochlorothiazide 263 (a diuretic 32)

acebutolol a beta blocker 30

aceclofenac a non-steroidal anti-inflammatory drug 50

ACE inhibitors a group of vasodilators 31 and antihypertensive drugs 36

acemetacin a non-steroidal anti-inflammatory drug 50

acenocoumarol an anticoagulant drug 38

Acepril a brand name for captopril 168 (an ACE inhibitor 31)

acetazolamide a carbonic anhydrase inhibitor diuretic 32 and drug for glaucoma 114

acetomenaphthone a vitamin K substance used with nicotinic acid to treat chilblains

acetylcholine a neurotransmitter that stimulates the parasympathetic nervous system 9 and is used as a miotic drug for glaucoma 114

acetylcholinesterase inhibitors a group of drugs for dementia 19

acetylcysteine a mucolytic drug for coughs 27

Acezide a brand name for captopril 168 (an ACE inhibitor 31) with hydrochlorothiazide 263 (a thiazide diuretic 32)

aciclovir 131 (an antiviral 69)

Acid-Eze a brand name for cimetidine 183 (an H_2 blocker anti-ulcer drug 43)

Aci-Jel a brand name for acetic acid (an antiseptic)

acipimox a lipid-lowering drug 37

Acitak a brand name for cimetidine 183 (an H_2 blocker anti-ulcer drug 43)

acitretin a drug for psoriasis 124

aclarubicin an anticancer drug 96

Acnecide a brand name for benzoyl peroxide 156 (a drug used to treat acne 123)

acne, drugs used to treat 123

Acnisal a brand name for salicylic acid (a keratolytic used to treat acne 123)

Acoflam a brand name for diclofenac 212 (an NSAID 50)

acrivastine an antihistamine 58

Actal a brand-named antacid containing alexitol (an antacid 42)

Acticin a brand name for tretinoin (a drug used to treat acne 123)

Actifed Compound a brand name for dextromethorphan (an opioid drug for coughs 27) with pseudoephedrine (a decongestant 26) and triprolidine (an antihistamine 58)

Actifed Expectorant a brand name for guaifenesin (an expectorant drug for coughs 27) with pseudoephedrine (a decongestant 26) and triprolidine (an antihistamine 58)

Actilyse a brand name for alteplase (a thrombolytic drug that affects blood clotting 38)

Actinac a brand-named drug used to treat acne 123 containing chloramphenicol 175, hydrocortisone 264, allantoin, butoxyethyl nicotinate, and sulphur

actinomycin D another name for dactinomycin (an anticancer drug 96)

Actiq a brand name for fentanyl (an opioid analgesic 9)

activated charcoal a substance used in the emergency treatment of poisoning

Actonel a brand name for risedronate (a drug for bone disorders 56)

Actonorm a brand-named drug containing atropine 150 (an anticholinergic and mydriatic drug affecting the pupil 116), various minerals 93, and peppermint oil

Acular a brand name for ketorolac (an NSAID analgesic 9)

Acupan a brand name for nefopam (a non-opioid analgesic 9)

Adalat a brand name for nifedipine 330 (a calcium channel blocker vasodilator 31, anti-angina drug 35, and antihypertensive 36)

Adalat Retard a brand name for nifedipine 330 (a calcium channel blocker vasodilator 31, anti-angina drug 35, and antihypertensive 36)

adapalene a retinoid drug to treat acne 123

Adcortyl a brand name for triamcinolone (a corticosteroid 80)

Adenocor a brand name for adenosine (an anti-arrhythmic drug 33)

adenosine an anti-arrhythmic drug 33

Adgyn-Combi, -Estro, -Medro brand names for oestrogen/progestogen (a female sex hormone replacement 88)

Adipine MR a brand name for nifedipine 330 (a calcium channel blocker vasodilator 31, anti-angina drug 35, and antihypertensive 36)

Adizem-SR, Adizem-XL a brand name for diltiazem 217 (a calcium channel blocker vasodilator 31)

adrenaline see **epinephrine**

AeroBec a brand name for beclometasone 154 (a corticosteroid 80)

Aerocrom a brand name for sodium cromoglicate 386 (an anti-allergy drug 60) with salbutamol 379 (a bronchodilator drug 23)

Aerodiol a brand name for estradiol 238 (a female sex hormone replacement 88)

Aerolin a brand name for salbutamol 379 (a sympathomimetic bronchodilator drug 23)

Aerrane a brand name for isoflurane (a general anaesthetic)

Afrazine a brand name for oxymetazoline (a topical decongestant 26)

Agenerase a brand name for amprenavir (a protease inhibitor drug for HIV/AIDS 100)

Aggrastat a brand name for tirofiban (an antiplatelet drug that affects blood clotting 38)

Ailax a brand name for co-danthramer (a stimulant laxative 45)

Airomir a brand name for salbutamol 379 (a sympathomimetic bronchodilator drug 23)

Akineton a brand name for biperiden (an anticholinergic for parkinsonism 18)

Aknemin a brand name for minocycline 318 (a tetracycline antibiotic 62)

albendazole an anthelmintic drug 78

alclometasone a topical corticosteroid 120

Alcobon a brand name for flucytosine (an antifungal drug 76)

Aldactide a brand name for co-flumactone (a combined diuretic 32 with hydroflumethiazide and spironolactone)

Aldactone a brand name for spironolactone (a potassium-sparing diuretic 32)

Aldara a brand name for imiquimod (a drug to treat warts)

aldesleukin an anticancer drug 96

Aldomet a brand name for methyldopa 313 (an antihypertensive 36)

alemtuzumab a monoclonal antibody (an immunosuppressant drug 99)

alendronate 132 a drug for bone disorders 124

alexitol an antacid 42

alfacalcidol vitamin D (a vitamin 90)

AlfaD a brand name for alfacalcidol (a vitamin 90)

alfentanil an anaesthetic

alfuzosin an alpha blocker drug used for prostate (urinary) disorders 112

Algesal a brand name for diethylamine salicylate (a rubefacient, which warms the skin to relieve muscle pain)

Algicon a brand name for aluminium hydroxide 136, magnesium carbonate, and potassium bicarbonate (all antacids 42) with magnesium alginate (an alginate 133)

alginates 133 substances extracted from brown seaweed used to protect stomach and oesophagus from acid reflux (antacids 42)

Algisite M a brand-named alginate 133

Amix a brand name for amoxicillin 142 (a penicillin antibiotic 62)

amlodipine 141 a calcium channel blocker vasodilator 31 used as an anti-angina drug 35 and antihypertensive drug 36

Ammonaps a brand name for sodium phenylbutyrate (a drug for metabolic disorders)

ammonium chloride a drug that increases urine acidity to treat urinary disorders 112, speeds excretion of poisons, and is an expectorant drug to treat coughs 27

amobarbital a barbiturate sleeping drug 11

Amoram a brand name for amoxicillin 142 (a penicillin antibiotic 62)

amorolfine an antifungal drug 76

amoxapine a tricyclic antidepressant 14

amoxicillin 142 (a penicillin antibiotic 62)

Amoxil a brand name for amoxicillin 142 (a penicillin antibiotic 62)

Amphocil a brand name for amphotericin 143 (an antifungal drug 76)

amphotericin 143 an antifungal drug 76

ampicillin a penicillin antibiotic 62

amprenavir a protease inhibitor drug for HIV/AIDS 100

amsacrine an anticancer drug 96

Amsidine a brand name for amsacrine (an anticancer drug 96)

amylase a pancreatic enzyme preparation for pancreatic disorders 49

Amytal a brand name for amobarbital (a barbiturate sleeping drug 11)

Anabact a brand name for metronidazole 316 (an antibacterial 66 and antiprotozoal 73)

anabolic steroids 88 (male sex hormones 87)

Anacal a brand-named preparation for haemorrhoids 47) containing heparinoid

Anadin a brand-named analgesic 9 containing aspirin 146 and caffeine

Anadin 500 a brand-named analgesic 9 containing aspirin 146 and caffeine

Anadin Cold Control a brand-named cold cure 27 containing paracetamol 341, caffeine, and phenylephrine (a decongestant 26)

Anadin Extra a brand-named analgesic 9 containing aspirin 146, paracetamol 341, and caffeine

Anadin Paracetamol a brand-named analgesic 9 containing aspirin 146 and paracetamol 341

anaesthetics , local 11 drugs used as analgesics 9, in antipruritics 118, in labour 110, and in rectal and anal disorders 47)

Anaflex a brand name for polynoxylin (an antifungal drug 76 and antibacterial drug 66)

Anafranil, Anafranil SR brand names for clomipramine 193 (a tricyclic antidepressant 14)

Ana-Guard a brand name for epinephrine (adrenaline) 233

analgesics painkillers 9 (used in labour 110)

anakinra a drug for rheumatoid arthritis 119

Anapen a brand name for epinephrine (adrenaline) 233

anastrozole 144 a hormonal anticancer drug 96

Anbesol a brand-named liquid for mouth ulcers and teething pain, with lidocaine (a local anaesthetic 11), cetylpyridinium, and chlorocresol (both topical antiseptics)

Ancotil a brand name for flucytosine (an antifungal drug 76)

Andrews Antacid a brand name for calcium carbonate and magnesium carbonate (both antacids 42)

Androcur a brand name for cyproterone acetate (an anti-androgen; male sex hormones 87)

androgens male sex hormones 87

Andropatch a brand name for testosterone 402 (a male sex hormone 87)

Anectine a brand name for suxamethonium (a muscle relaxant used in general anaesthesia)

Anethaine a brand name for tetracaine (a local anaesthetic; analgesics 9)

Anexate a brand name for flumazenil (an antidote for benzodiazepine overdose)

Angettes a brand-named antiplatelet drug that affects blood clotting 38, with aspirin 146

Angilol a brand name for propranolol 399 (a beta blocker 99)

Angiopine a brand name for nifedipine 330 (a calcium channel blocker vasodilator 31, anti-angina drug 35, and antihypertensive 36)

Angiopine MR a brand name for nifedipine 330 (a calcium channel blocker vasodilator 31, anti-angina drug 35, and antihypertensive drug 36)

angiotensin II blockers a group of vasodilators 31

Angiozem a brand name for diltiazem 217 (a calcium channel blocker vasodilator 31, anti-angina drug 35, and antihypertensive 36)

Angitak a brand name for isosorbide dinitrate 277 (an anti-angina drug 35)

Angitil SR a brand name for diltiazem 217 (a calcium channel blocker vasodilator 31, anti-angina drug 35, and antihypertensive 36)

Anhydrol Forte a brand name for aluminium chloride (an antiperspirant)

Anodesyn a brand-named preparation for haemorrhoids 47 with allantoin (a topical wound treatment), lidocaine (a local anaesthetic 11), and ephedrine 232

argipressin synthetic vasopressin for diabetes insipidus 85)

Aricept a brand name for donepezil 221 (a drug for Alzheimer's disease)

Aridil a brand name for amiloride 137 with furosemide 251 (both diuretics 32)

Arimidex a brand name for anastrozole (a drug for breast cancer)

Arixtra a brand name for fondaparinux (an injected anticoagulant 38)

Aromasin a brand name for exemestane (a drug for breast cancer)

Arpicolin a brand name for procyclidine 356 (an anticholinergic for parkinsonism 18)

Arret a brand name for loperamide 294 (an opioid antidiarrhoeal drug 44)

Artelac SDU a brand name for hypromellose (an ingredient of artificial tears)

artemether with lumefantrine an antimalarial drug 75

artesunate an antimalarial drug 75

Arthrofen a brand name for ibuprofen 267 (an analgesic 9 and non-steroidal anti-inflammatory drug 50)

Arthrosin a brand name for naproxen 326 (a non-steroidal anti-inflammatory drug 50 and drug for gout 53)

Arthrotec a brand-named antirheumatic drug 52 containing diclofenac 212 with misoprostol 321

Arthroxen a brand name for naproxen 326 (a non-steroidal anti-inflammatory drug 50 and drug for gout 53)

articaine a local anaesthetic 11

artificial tear preparations eye drops that keep the eyes moist in the same way as tears

Arythmol a brand name for propafenone (an anti-arrhythmic 33)

Asacol a brand name for mesalazine 308 (a drug for inflammatory bowel disease 46)

Asasantin a brand name for aspirin 146 with dipyridamole 218 (an antiplatelet drug that affects blood clotting 38)

Ascabiol a brand name for benzyl benzoate (a drug to treat skin parasites 122)

ascorbic acid vitamin C (a vitamin 90)

Asendis a brand name for amoxapine (a tricyclic antidepressant 14)

Aserbine a brand-named product for wound cleaning

Asilone a brand name for a combined antacid 42 with aluminium hydroxide 136 and magnesium oxide (both antacids), and dimeticone (an antifoaming agent)

Asmabec a brand name for beclometasone 154 (a corticosteroid 80)

Asmasal a brand name for salbutamol 379 (a sympathomimetic bronchodilator drug 23)

asparaginase a drug for leukaemia

Aspav a brand-named analgesic 9 containing aspirin 146 and papaveretum (an opioid)

aspirin 146 a non-opioid analgesic 9 and antiplatelet drug that affects blood clotting 38

Aspro Clear a brand name for soluble aspirin 146 (a non-opioid analgesic 9)

AS Saliva Orthana a brand name for artificial saliva

asthma, drugs for 24

AT 10 a brand name for dihydrotachysterol (vitamin D, 90)

Atarax a brand name for hydroxyzine (an anti-anxiety drug 13)

Atenix a brand name for atenolol 147 (a beta blocker 30)

atenolol 147 a beta blocker 30

Ativan a brand name for lorazepam (a benzodiazepine anti-anxiety drug 13 and sleeping drug 11)

atorvastatin 149 a lipid-lowering drug 37

atosiban a uterine muscle relaxant used in labour 110

atovaquone an antiprotozoal drug 73 and (with proguanil) antimalarial drug 75

atracurium a drug used to relax the muscles in general anaesthesia

atropine 150 an anticholinergic drug for irritable bowel syndrome 45 and a mydriatic drug affecting the pupil 116

Atrovent a brand name for ipratropium bromide 274 (an anticholinergic bronchodilator drug 23)

Audax a brand-named analgesic drug for ear disorders 117 containing choline salicylate

Audicort a brand-named anti-infectiveear preparation 117 with benzocaine, neomycin, and triamcinolone (a corticosteroid 80)

Augmentin a brand name for co-amoxiclav (a combined product containing amoxicillin 142, a penicillin antibiotic 62, with clavulanic acid, a substance that increases the effectiveness of amoxicillin)

auranofin a gold-based antirheumatic drug 52

Aureocort a brand name for chlortetracycline (a tetracycline antibiotic 62) with triamcinolone (a corticosteroid 80)

Aureomycin a brand name for chlortetracycline (a tetracycline antibiotic 62)

aurothiomalate see **sodium aurothiomalate**

Avandia a brand name for rosiglitazone 377 (an oral rug used in diabetes 82)

Avloclor a brand name for chloroquine 177 (an antimalarial drug 75 and antirheumatic drug 52)

Avomine a brand name for promethazine 360 (an antihistamine 58 and anti-emetic 21)

Avonex a brand name for interferon beta 272 (a drug for multiple sclerosis)

Axid a brand name for nizatidine (an H_2 blocker anti-ulcer drug 43)

Axsain a brand name for capsaicin (a rubefacient, which warms the skin to relieve muscle pain)

Azactam a brand name for aztreonam (an antibiotic 62)

Azamune a brand name for azathioprine 151 (an antirheumatic drug 52, anticancer drug 96, and immunosuppressant drug 99)

azapropazone a non-steroidal anti-inflammatory drug 50

azatadine an antihistamine 58

azathioprine 151 an antirheumatic drug 52, anti-cancer drug 96, and immunosuppressant 99

azelaic acid an antibacterial drug for acne 123

azelastine a topical preparation for allergic conjunctivitis

azidothymidine zidovudine 450 (an antiretroviral drug for HIV infection and AIDS 160)

azithromycin a macrolide antibiotic 130

Azopt a brand name for brinzolamide (a carbonic anhydrase inhibitor drug for glaucoma 114)

AZT see **zidovudine**

aztreonam an antibiotic 62

B

bacitracin an anti-infective skin preparation 120

baclofen 153 a muscle relaxant 54

Baclospas a brand of baclofen 153 (a muscle relaxant 54)

Bactrim a brand name for co-trimoxazole 205 (a combined antibacterial 66 product containing trimethoprim 412 and sulfamethoxazole)

Bactroban a brand name for mupirocin (an anti-infective skin preparation 120)

Balgifen a brand name for baclofen 153 (a muscle relaxant 54)

balsalazide a drug for inflammatory bowel disease 46

Bambec a brand name for bambuterol (a sympathomimetic bronchodilator drug 23)

bambuterol a sympathomimetic bronchodilator 23

Baratol a brand name for indoramin 270 (an alpha blocker antihypertensive drug 36 and drug for urinary disorders 112)

barbiturates a type of sleeping drug 11

basiliximab an immunosuppressant 99

Baxan a brand name for cefadroxil (a cephalosporin antibiotic 62)

Bazuka a brand-named preparation for verrucas with salicylic acid (a keratolytic 123) and lactic acid (a substance that enhances the effect of salicylic acid)

becaplermin a drug for healing skin ulcers

Beclazone a brand name for beclometasone 154 (a corticosteroid 80)

Becloforte a brand name for beclometasone 154 (a corticosteroid 80)

beclometasone 154 a corticosteroid 80

Becodisks a brand of beclometasone 154 (a corticosteroid 80)

Beconase a brand name for beclometasone 154 (a corticosteroid 80)

Becotide a brand name for beclometasone 154 (a corticosteroid 80)

Becotide Rotacaps a brand name for 154 (a corticosteroid 80)

Bedranol SR a brand name for propranolol 361 (a beta blocker 30)

Beechams Pills a brand name for aloin (a stimulant laxative 45)

Beechams Powders a brand name for paracetamol 341 (a non-opioid analgesic 9) with pseudoephedrine (a decongestant 26)

Beechams Powders Capsules a brand name for paracetamol 341 (a non-opioid analgesic 9) with phenylephrine (a decongestant 26) and caffeine

Benadryl a brand name for cetirizine 154 (an antihistamine 58)

bendroflumethiazide 155 a thiazide diuretic 32

Benoral a brand name for benorilate (a non-steroidal anti-inflammatory drug 50)

benorilate a non-steroidal anti-inflammatory drug 50

benperidol an antipsychotic 15

Benquil a brand name for benperidol (an antipsychotic 15)

benserazide a drug used to enhance effect of levodopa 286 (a drug for parkinsonism 18)

Benylin a brand name for diphenhydramine (an antihistamine 58) with menthol and, in some preparations, codeine 198 (an opioid analgesic 9)

benzalkonium chloride a skin antiseptic 120

Benzamycin a brand name for erythromycin 235 (a macrolide antibiotic 62) and benzoyl peroxide 156 (a drug used to treat acne 123)

benzatropine a drug for parkinsonism 18

benzocaine a local anaesthetic 11

benzodiazepines a type of sleeping drug 11 and anti-anxiety drug 13

benzoin tincture a resin used in inhalations for sinusitis and as a decongestant 26

benzoyl peroxide 156 a drug to treat acne 123 and topical antifungal drug 76

benzthiazide a thiazide diuretic 32

benzydamine an analgesic 9 used in mouthwash and throat spray

benzyl benzoate a drug for skin parasites 122

benzylpenicillin a penicillin antibiotic 62

beractant a drug to mature the lungs of premature babies

Berkatens a brand name for verapamil 415 (a calcium channel blocker vasodilator 31, anti-arrhythmic drug 33, anti-angina drug 35, and antihypertensive drug 36)

Beta-Adalat a brand name for nifedipine 330 (a calcium channel blocker vasodilator 31, anti-angina drug 35, and antihypertensive drug 36)

beta blockers 30

Betacap a brand name for betamethasone 158 (a corticosteroid 80)

Beta-Cardone a brand name for sotalol 389 (a beta blocker 30)

betacarotene vitamin A (a vitamin 90 and food additive)

Betadine a brand name for povidone iodine (an anti-infective skin preparation 120)

Betaferon a brand name for interferon beta 272 (a drug for multiple sclerosis)

Betagan a brand name for levobunolol (a beta blocker 30 and drug for glaucoma 114)

betahistine 157 an anti-emetic drug 21 for Ménière's disease

Betaloc a brand name for metoprolol 315 (a beta blocker 30)

betamethasone 158 a corticosteroid 80

Beta-Prograne a brand name for propranolol 361 (a beta blocker 30)

betaxolol a beta blocker 30 also used in glaucoma 114

bethanechol a parasympathomimetic 9 for urinary retention 113) and paralytic ileus

Betim a brand name for timolol 406 (a beta blocker 30 and drug for glaucoma 114)

Betnelan a brand name for betamethasone 158 (a corticosteroid 80)

Betnesol a brand name for betamethasone 158 (a corticosteroid 80)

Betnesol-N a brand name for betamethasone 158 (a corticosteroid 80) with neomycin (an aminoglycoside antibiotic 62)

Betnovate a brand name for betamethasone 158 (a corticosteroid 80)

Betnovate-C a brand name for betamethasone 158 (a corticosteroid 80) with clioquinol (an anti-infective drug for ear disorders 117)

Betnovate-N a brand name for betamethasone 158 (a corticosteroid 80) with neomycin (an aminoglycoside antibiotic 62)

Betoptic a brand-named drug for glaucoma 114 containing betaxolol (a beta blocker 30)

Bettamousse a brand name for betamethasone 158 (a corticosteroid 80)

bexarotene an anticancer drug 96

bezafibrate 159 a lipid-lowering drug 37

Bezalip a brand name for bezafibrate 159 (a lipid-lowering drug 37)

Bezalip-Mono a brand name for bezafibrate 159 (a lipid-lowering drug 37)

bicalutamide a hormonal anticancer drug 96

BiCNU a brand name for carmustine (an anticancer drug 96)

bimatoprost a drug for glaucoma 114

BiNovum a brand-named oral contraceptive 105 containing ethinylestradiol 240 and norethisterone 332 (both female sex hormones 88)

Bioplex a brand-named drug for mouth ulcers containing carbenoxolone (an anti-ulcer drug 43)

Bioral a brand-named drug for mouth ulcers containing carbenoxolone (an anti-ulcer drug 43)

Biorphen a brand name for orphenadrine 338 (an anticholinergic drug for parkinsonism 18)

biotin a vitamin 90

biperiden an anticholinergic drug for parkinsonism 18

bisacodyl a stimulant laxative 45

Bismag a brand name for sodium bicarbonate 385 with magnesium carbonate (both antacids 42)

bismuth a metallic compound used as an anti-ulcer drug 43 and for haemorrhoids 47

BiSoDol a brand name for sodium bicarbonate 385 with calcium carbonate and magnesium carbonate (all antacids 42)

bisoprolol a beta blocker 30

Blemix a brand name for minocycline 318 (a tetracycline antibiotic 62)

bleomycin a cytotoxic antibiotic for cancer 96

blood clotting, drugs that affect 38

Bocasan a brand-named mouthwash with sodium perborate (an antimicrobial agent)

Bondronat a brand name for ibandronic acid (a drug for bone disorders 56)

bone disorders, drugs for 56

Bonefos a brand name for sodium clodronate for high blood calcium in cancer patients

Bonjela a brand name for choline salicylate (a drug similar to aspirin 146)

Bonjela pastilles brand-named pastilles for mouth ulcers containing lidocaine (a local anaesthetic 11 and aminacrine (an anti-infective skin preparation 120)

Boots Avert a brand name for aciclovir 131, an antiviral drug 69

Boots Diareze a brand name for loperamide 294 (an antidiarrhoeal drug 44)

Boots Hayfever and Allergy Relief All Day a brand name for loratadine 297 (an antihistamine 58)

Boots Nicotine Gum a brand name for nicotine 329 given as a drug for relief of smoking withdrawal symptoms

Boots Nicotine Inhalator a brand name for nicotine 329 given as a drug for relief of smoking withdrawal symptoms

Boots NRT Patch a brand name for nicotine 329 given as a drug for relief of smoking withdrawal symptoms

bosentan a drug for pulmonary arterial hypertension

Botox a brand name for botulinum toxin 160 (a muscle relaxant 54)

botulinum toxin 160 a muscle relaxant 54

Bradosol a brand name for benzalkonium chloride (anti-infective skin preparation 120)

Brasivol a brand-named abrasive paste for acne 123

bretylium tosilate an anti-arrhythmic 33

Brevibloc a brand name for esmolol (a beta blocker 30)

Brevinor a brand-named oral contraceptive 105 containing ethinylestradiol 240 and norethisterone 332 (both female sex hormones 88)

Brevoxyl a brand name for benzoyl peroxide (a drug for acne 123)

Brexidol a brand name for piroxicam 350 (a non-steroidal anti-inflammatory drug 50)

Bricanyl a brand name for terbutaline 401 (a sympathomimetic bronchodilator drug 23 and uterine muscle relaxant used in labour 110)

brimonidine a sympathomimetic drug for glaucoma 114

brinzolamide a carbonic anhydrase inhibitor drug for glaucoma 114

Britlofex a brand name for lofexidine (a drug to treat opioid withdrawal symptoms)

Broflex a brand name for trihexyphenidyl (a drug for parkinsonism 18)

Brolene a brand name for propamidine isethionate (an antibacterial) for eye infections

bromocriptine 161 (a pituitary agent 85 and drug for parkinsonism 18)

brompheniramine an antihistamine 58

bronchodilators 23

Brufen, Brufen Retard brand names for ibuprofen 267 (a non-steroidal anti-inflammatory drug 50)

Buccastem a brand name for prochlorperazine 355 (an anti-emetic 21)

buclizine an antihistamine 58 and anti-emetic 21 used for motion sickness

Budenofalk a brand name for budesonide 163 (a corticosteroid 80)

budesonide 163 a corticosteroid 80

bulk-forming agents antidiarrhoeal drugs 44 and laxatives 45

bumetanide 164 a loop diuretic 32

bupivacaine a long-lasting local anaesthetic 11 used in labour 110

buprenorphine an opioid analgesic 9

bupropion 165 a nicotine withdrawal aid

Burinex a brand name for bumetanide 164 (a loop diuretic 32)

Burinex-A a brand name for bumetanide 164 with amiloride 137 (both diuretics 32)

Burinex-K a brand name for bumetanide 164 (a loop diuretic 32) with potassium

BurnEze a brand name for benzocaine (a local anaesthetic 11

Buscopan a brand name for hyoscine 265 (an antispasmodic antidiarrhoeal drug 44 and drug for irritable bowel syndrome 45)

buserelin a drug for menstrual disorders 104

Buspar a brand name for buspirone (an anti-anxiety drug 13)

buspirone an anti-anxiety drug 13

busulfan an alkylating anticancer drug for certain leukaemias 96

Butacote a brand name for phenylbutazone (a non-steroidal anti-inflammatory drug 50)

butobarbital a barbiturate sleeping drug 11

butoxyethyl nicotinate a vasodilator 31

butylcyanoacrylate a tissue and skin adhesive for closing wounds

butyrophenones a group of antipsychotic drugs 15 and anti-emetics 21

C

Cabaser a brand name for cabergoline (a drug to reduce prolactin levels (drugs to treat pituitary disorders 85) and to treat Parkinson's disease 18)

cabergoline a drug to treat pituitary disorders 85 and to treat Parkinson's disease 18

Cacit a brand name for calcium carbonate (a drug for bone disorder 56)

Caelyx a brand name for doxorubicin 226 (a cytotoxic anticancer drug 96)

Cafergot a brand name for ergotamine 234 (a drug for migraine 20) with caffeine

caffeine a nervous system stimulant 19 in coffee, tea, and cola, also in some analgesics 9

Caladryl a brand name for diphenhydramine (an antihistamine 58) with calamine lotion (an antipruritic 118)

calamine an antipruritic 118 containing zinc carbonate, used to soothe irritated skin

Calceos a brand name for ergocalciferol (vitamin D, a vitamin 90)

Calcicard CR a brand name for diltiazem 217 (a calcium channel blocker vasodilator 31, anti-angina drug 35, and antihypertensive drug 36)

calciferol vitamin D (a vitamin 90)

Calcijex a brand name for calcitriol (a vitamin 90)

Calciparine a brand name for heparin 262 (an anticoagulant drug 38)

calcipotriol 167 a drug for psoriasis 124

calcitonin a drug for bone disorders 56

calcitonin (salmon) a drug for bone disorders 56

calcitriol vitamin D (a vitamin 90)

calcium a mineral 93

calcium carbonate a calcium salt (a mineral 93) used as an antacid 42

calcium channel blockers vasodilators 31 used as anti-arrhythmics 33, anti-angina drugs 35, and antihypertensive drugs 36

calcium folinate folinic acid salt used to reduce side effects of methotrexate 311

calcium resonium a brand name for calcium polystyrene sulphonate (a drug to remove excess potassium from the blood)

Calcort a brand name for deflazacort (a corticosteroid 80)

Calgel a brand-named teething gel containing lidocaine (a local anaesthetic 11 and cetylpyridinium (an oral antiseptic)

Calimal a brand name for chlorphenamine 178 (an antihistamine 58)

Calmurid HC a brand-named treatment for eczema 125 containing hydrocortisone 264 with lactic acid and urea (to soften the skin)

Calpol a brand name for paracetamol 341 (a non-opioid analgesic 9)

Calsynar a brand name for calcitonin (salmon) (a drug for bone disorders 56)

CAM a brand name for ephedrine 232 (a sympathomimetic bronchodilator drug 23)

Camcolit a brand name for lithium 292 (an antimanic drug 16)

camphor a topical antipruritic 118

Campral EC a brand name for acamprosate 130 (an alcohol abuse treatment)

Campto a brand name for irinotecan (an anticancer drug 96

candesartan an angiotensin II blocker vasodilator 31

Candiden a brand name for clotrimazole 196 (an antifungal drug 76)

Canesten a brand name for clotrimazole 196 (an antifungal drug 76)

Canesten HC a brand name for clotrimazole 196 (an antifungal drug 76) with hydrocortisone 264 (a corticosteroid 80)

Capasal a brand name for a coal tar shampoo for dandruff 126 and psoriasis 124

Capastat a brand name for capreomycin (an antituberculous drug 67)

capecitabine an antimetabolite anticancer drug 96

Caplenal a brand name for allopurinol 133 (a drug for gout 53)

Capoten a brand name for captopril 168 (an ACE inhibitor vasodilator 31)

Capozide a brand name for captopril 168 (an ACE inhibitor vasodilator 31) with hydrochlorothiazide 263 (a thiazide diuretic 32)

capreomycin an antituberculous drug 67

Caprin a brand name for aspirin 146 (a non-opioid analgesic 9 and antiplatelet drug that affects blood clotting 38)

capsaicin a rubefacient, which warms the skin to relieve muscle pain

Capto-co a brand name for captopril 168 (an ACE inhibitor vasodilator 31) with hydrochlorothiazide 263 (a thiazide diuretic 32)

captopril 168 an ACE inhibitor vasodilator 31

Carace a brand name for lisinopril 291 (an ACE inhibitor vasodilator 31)

Carace Plus a brand-named preparation for high blood pressure 36 containing lisinopril 291 and hydrochlorothiazide 263

carbachol a miotic drug for glaucoma 114 and parasympathomimetic drug for urinary retention 112

Carbagen a brand name for carbamazepine 169 (an anticonvulsant drug 16 and antimanic drug 16)

Carbalax a brand name for sodium acid phosphate (a laxative 45) with sodium bicarbonate 385 (an antacid 42)

carbamazepine 169 an anticonvulsant 16 and antimanic drug 16

carbaryl 170 an antiparasitic 122 for head lice

Carbellon a brand-named indigestion remedy with magnesium hydroxide 299 (an antacid 42 and laxative 45), charcoal (an adsorbent), and peppermint oil (an antispasmodic 45)

carbenoxolone an anti-ulcer drug 43

carbidopa a substance that enhances the effect of levodopa 286 (a drug for parkinsonism 18)

Cetrotide a brand name for cetrorelix (a drug for infertility 109)

cetylpyridinium an oral antiseptic

Chemydur a brand name for isosorbide mononitrate 277 (a nitrate vasodilator 31 anti-angina drug 35)

Chimax a brand name for flutamide 249 (an anticancer drug 96)

Chloractil a brand name for chlorpromazine 180 (a phenothiazine antipsychotic 15 and anti-emetic 21)

chloral hydrate a sleeping drug 11

chlorambucil an anticancer drug 96 used for chronic lymphocytic leukaemia and lymphatic and ovarian cancers, and as an immuno-suppressant 99 for rheumatoid arthritis 52

chloramphenicol 175 an antibiotic 62

chlordiazepoxide 176 a benzodiazepine anti-anxiety drug 13

chlorhexidine a skin antiseptic (anti-infective skin preparations 120)

chlormethine previoiusly known as mustine, a drug for Hodgkin's disease 96)

Chloromycetin a brand name for chloramphenicol 175 (an antibiotic 62)

chloroquine 177 an antimalarial drug 75 and antirheumatic drug 52

chloroxylenol a skin antiseptic (anti-infective skin preparations 120)

chlorphenamine 178 an antihistamine 58

chlorpromazine 180 a phenothiazine antipsychotic 15 and anti-emetic 21

chlorpropamide a sulphonylurea drug used in diabetes 82

chlortalidone a thiazide diuretic 32

chlortetracycline a tetracycline antibiotic 62

choline salicylate a drug similar to aspirin 146, used in analgesic mouth gels and ear drops

Choragon a brand name for chorionic gonadotrophin 181 (a drug for infertility 109)

choriogonadotropin alfa a drug for infertility 109

chorionic gonadotrophin 181 a drug for infertility 109

chromium a mineral 93

Cicatrin a brand name for bacitracin (an anti-infective skin preparation 120) with neomycin (an antibiotic 62)

ciclosporin 182 an immunosuppressant 99

cidofovir an antiviral 69 for cytomegalovirus in people with AIDS

Cidomycin a brand name for gentamicin 254 (an aminoglycoside antibiotic 62)

cilastatin an enzyme inhibitor used to make imipenem (an antibiotic 62) more effective

cilazapril an ACE inhibitor vasodilator 31

Cilest a brand-named oral contraceptive 105 containing ethinylestradiol 240 and norgestimate (a progestogen)

cilostazol a vasodilator 31

Ciloxan a brand name for ciprofloxacin 186 (a quinolone antibacterial 66)

cimetidine 183 an H_2 blocker anti-ulcer drug 43

Cinaziere a brand name for cinnarizine 184 (an antihistamine anti-emetic 21)

cinchocaine a local anaesthetic 11

cinnarizine 184 an antihistamine anti-emetic 21

Cipralex a brand name for escitalopram (an antidepressant 14)

Cipramil a brand name for citalopram 188 (an antidepressant 14)

ciprofibrate 185 a lipid-lowering drug 37

ciprofloxacin 186 a quinolone antibacterial 66

Ciproxin a brand name for ciprofloxacin 186 (an antibacterial 66)

cisatracurium a drug used to relax the muscles in general anaesthesia

cisplatin 187 an anticancer drug 96

citalopram 188 an antidepressant 14

Citanest a brand name for prilocaine (a local anaesthetic 11

Citramag a brand name for magnesium citrate (an osmotic laxative 45)

cladribine an anticancer drug 96

Claforan a brand name for cefotaxime (a cephalosporin antibiotic 62)

clarithromycin 190 a macrolide antibiotic 62

Clarityn a brand name for loratadine 297 (an antihistamine 58)

Clarityn Allergy a brand name for loratadine 297 (an antihistamine 58)

clavulanic acid a substance given with amoxicillin 142 (a penicillin antibiotic 62) to make it more effective

clemastine an antihistamine 58

Clexane a brand name for enoxaparin, a low molecular weight heparin 262, an anticoagulant drug 38)

Climagest a brand-named preparation for HRT 89 containing estradiol 236 and norethisterone 332 (both female sex hormones 88)

Climaval a brand-named preparation for menopause (female sex hormones 88) with estradiol 236

Climesse a brand-named preparation for HRT 89 containing estradiol 236 and norethisterone 332 (both female sex hormones 88)

clindamycin a lincosamide antibiotic 62

Clinitar a brand name for coal tar (a substance used to treat psoriasis 124 and dandruff 126)

Cogentin a brand name for benzatropine (an anticholinergic drug for parkinsonism 18)

Colazide a brand name for balsalazide (an aminosalicylate drug for inflammatory bowel disease 46)

colchicine 199 a drug for gout 53

cold cream an antipruritic 118

colecalciferol vitamin D (a vitamin 90)

Colestid a brand name for colestipol (a lipid-lowering drug 37)

colestipol a lipid-lowering drug 37

colestyramine 200 a lipid-lowering drug 37

colfosceril palmitate a drug to mature the lungs of premature babies

Colifoam a brand name for hydrocortisone 264 (a corticosteroid 80)

colistimethate the injection form of colistin (an antibiotic 62)

colistin an antibiotic 62

collodion a substance that dries to form a sticky film, protecting broken skin 120

Colofac a brand name for mebeverine 301 (an antispasmodic drug for irritable bowel syndrome 45)

Colomycin a brand name for colistin (an antibiotic 62)

Colpermin a brand name for peppermint oil (a substance used to relieve indigestion and an antispasmodic for irritable bowel syndrome 45)

co-magaldrox a combined product containing aluminium hydroxide 136 with magnesium hydroxide 299 (both antacids 42)

Combivent a brand-named inhaler containing salbutamol 379 and ipratropium bromide 274 (both bronchodilators 23)

Combivir a brand-named preparation containing zidovudine/lamivudine 420 (drugs for HIV/AIDS 100)

co-methiamol a combined product containing paracetamol 341 and methionine (an antidote to paracetamol poisoning)

Compound W a brand-named preparation for warts, containing salicylic acid (a keratolytic 123)

Comtess a brand name for entacapone (a drug for parkinsonism 18)

Concavit a brand-named multivitamin (vitamins 90)

Concerta XL a brand name for methylphenidate (a drug used for attention deficit hyperactivity disorder)

Condyline a brand name for podophyllotoxin (a topical treatment for genital warts)

conjugated oestrogens 201 female sex hormones 88

Conotrane a brand name for benzalkonium chloride with a dimeticone base (anti-infective skin preparations 120)

Contac 400 a brand name for chlorphenamine 178 (an antihistamine 58) with phenylpropanolamine 347 (a decongestant 26)

Convulex a brand name for sodium valproate 387 (an anticonvulsant 16)

Copaxone a brand name for glatiramer (a drug for multiple sclerosis)

co-phenotrope a combined product containing diphenoxylate with atropine 150 (both antidiarrhoeal drugs 44)

copper a mineral 93

co-prenozide a combined product containing oxprenolol (a beta blocker 30) with cyclopenthiazide (a thiazide diuretic 32)

co-proxamol 204 a combined product containing dextropropoxyphene (an opioid) and paracetamol 341 (both analgesics 9)

Coracten a brand name for nifedipine 330 (a calcium channel blocker vasodilator 31, anti-angina drug 35, and antihypertensive 36)

Cordarone X a brand name for amiodarone 138 (an anti-arrhythmic drug 33)

Cordilox a brand name for verapamil 415 (a calcium channel blocker vasodilator 31, anti-arrhythmic drug 33, anti-angina drug 35, and antihypertensive drug 36)

Corgard a brand name for nadolol (a beta blocker 30)

Corgaretic a brand name for bendroflumethiazide 155 (a thiazide diuretic 32) with nadolol (a beta blocker 30)

Corlan a brand name for hydrocortisone 264 (a corticosteroid 80)

Coroday MR a brand name for nifedipine 330 (a calcium channel blocker vasodilator 31, anti-angina drug 35, and antihypertensive drug 36)

Coro-Nitro a brand name for glyceryl trinitrate 257 (an anti-angina drug 35)

Corsodyl a brand-named mouthwash and oral gel containing chlorhexidine (an oral antiseptic)

corticosteroids 80 (as allergy treatments 60; bronchodilators 23; in ear disorders 117; and in inflammatory bowel disease 46)

corticosteroids, topical 120

corticotrophin a pituitary hormone 85

cortisol an old name for hydrocortisone 264

cortisone a corticosteroid 80

Cosalgesic a brand name for co-proxamol 204 (an opioid analgesic 9)

co-simalcite a antacid product 42 containing hydrotalcite with dimeticone (an antifoaming agent)

CosmoFer a brand name for iron dextran (an iron compound: minerals 93)

Cosopt a brand-named preparation containing dorzolamide 222 and timolol 406 (both drugs for glaucoma 114)

Cosuric a brand name for allopurinol 133 (a drug for gout 53)

co-tenidone a combined product containing atenolol 147 (a beta blocker 30) with chlortalidone (a thiazide diuretic 32)

co-triamterzide a combined product containing hydrochlorothiazide 263 with triamterene 411 (both diuretics 32)

co-trimoxazole 205 a combined sulphonamide antibacterial drug containing trimethoprim 412 and sulfamethoxazole

Covermark a brand name for a masking cream for skin disfigurement

Coversyl a brand name for perindopril 343 (an ACE inhibitor vasodilator 31)

Coversyl Plus a brand name for perindopril 343 (an ACE inhibitor vasodilator 31) with indapamide 269 (a thiazide-like diuretic 32)

cox-2 inhibitors a type of non-steroidal anti-inflammatory drug 50

Cozaar a brand name for losartan 297 (an angiotensin II blocker vasodilator 31)

Cozaar-Comp a brand-named preparation containing losartan 297 (an angiotensin II blocker vasodilator 31) and hydrochlorothiazide 263 (a diuretic 32)

Cream of Magnesia a brand name for magnesium hydroxide 299 (an antacid 42 and laxative 45)

Cremalgin a brand name for a topical preparation for muscular pain relief containing glycol salicylate, methyl nicotinate, and capsicum oleoresin

Creon a brand name for pancreatin (a preparation of pancreatic enzymes 49)

Crinone a brand name for progesterone (a female sex hormone 88)

crisantaspase an anticancer drug 96

Crixivan a brand name for indinavir (a protease inhibitor drug for HIV/AIDS 100)

Cromogen a brand name for sodium cromoglicate 386 (an anti-allergy drug 60)

crotamiton an antipruritic 118 and antiparasitic drug 122 for scabies

Crystacide a brand name for hydrogen peroxide cream (an anti-infective skin preparation 120)

Crystapen a brand name for penicillin G (a penicillin antibiotic 62)

Cuplex a brand-named wart preparation containing copper acetate, lactic acid, and salicylic acid (a keratolytic 123)

Cuprofen a brand name for ibuprofen 267 (a non-steroidal anti-inflammatory drug 50)

Curatoderm a brand name for tacalcitol (a drug for psoriasis 124)

Curosurf a brand name for poractant alfa (a drug to mature the lungs of premature babies)

Cutivate a brand name for fluticasone 250 (a corticosteroid 80)

cyanocobalamin vitamin B12 (a vitamin 90)

Cyclimorph a brand name for morphine 323 (an opioid analgesic 9) with cyclizine (an antihistamine anti-emetic 21)

cyclizine an antihistamine 58 used as an anti-emetic 9021

Cyclogest a brand name for progesterone (a female sex hormone 88)

cyclopenthiazide a thiazide diuretic 32

cyclopentolate an anticholinergic mydriatic drug affecting the pupil 116

cyclophosphamide 206 an anticancer drug 96

Cyclo-Progynova a brand name for estradiol 238 with levonorgestrel 289 (both female sex hormones 88)

cycloserine an antibiotic antituberculous drug 67

Cyklokapron a brand name for tranexamic acid (an antifibrinolytic drug that affects blood clotting 38 and drug for menstrual disorders 104)

Cymalon a brand-named preparation for cystitis with sodium bicarbonate 385, citric acid, sodium citrate, and sodium carbonate

Cymevene a brand name for ganciclovir (an antiviral drug 69)

cyproheptadine an antihistamine 58 used to treat allergies and migraine 20

Cyprostat a brand name for cyproterone acetate (male sex hormones 87) used for acne 123 and cancer of the prostate 96

cyproterone acetate a synthetic male sex hormone 87 used for acne 123, cancer of the prostate 96, and male sexual disorders

Cystagon a brand name for mercaptamine (a drug used for a metabolic disorder)

Cysticide a brand name for praziquantel (an anthelmintic 78)

Cystoleve a brand name for sodium citrate (a drug for urinary disorders 112)

Cystopurin a brand name for potassium citrate (a drug for urinary disorders 112)

Cystrin a brand name for oxybutynin 339 (an anticholinergic and antispasmodic drug for urinary disorders 112)

cytarabine a drug for leukaemia 96

cytokines a type of anticancer drug 96

Cytotec a brand name for misoprostol 321 (an anti-ulcer drug 43)

cytotoxic drugs a type of anticancer drug 96

D

dacarbazine a drug for malignant melanoma and cancer of soft tissues 96

daclizumab an immunosuppressant 99

dactinomycin a cytotoxic antibiotic for cancer 96

Daktacort a brand name for hydrocortisone 264 (a corticosteroid 80) with miconazole 318 (an antifungal drug 76)

Daktarin a brand name for miconazole 318 (an antifungal drug 76)

Daktarin Gold a brand name for ketoconazole 280 (an antifungal drug 76)

Dalacin C a brand name for clindamycin (a lincosamide antibiotic 62)

dalfopristin an antibiotic 62

Dalivit a brand-named multivitamin 90

Dalmane a brand name for flurazepam (a benzodiazepine sleeping drug 11)

dalteparin a low molecular weight heparin 262 (an anticoagulant drug 38)

danaparoid an anticoagulant 38

danazol 208 a drug for menstrual disorders 104

dandruff, drugs for 126

Danol a brand name for danazol 208 (a drug for menstrual disorders 104)

Dantrium a brand name for dantrolene (a muscle relaxant 54)

dantrolene a muscle relaxant 54

dantron a stimulant laxative 45

Daonil a brand name for glibenclamide 255 (an oral drug used in diabetes 82)

dapsone an antibacterial drug 66

Daraprim a brand name for pyrimethamine 364 (an antimalarial 75)

darbepoetin alfa a drug for anaemia

daunorubicin a cytotoxic antibiotic (an anticancer drug 96)

DaunoXome a brand name for daunorubicin (an anticancer drug 96)

Day Nurse a brand name for dextromethorphan (an opioid cough suppressant 27) with paracetamol 341 (a non-opioid analgesic 9) and phenylpropanolamine 347 (a decongestant 26)

DDAVP a brand name for desmopressin 209 (a pituitary hormone 85 for diabetes insipidus)

Decadron a brand name for dexamethasone 210 (a corticosteroid 80)

Deca-Durabolin a brand name for nandrolone, an anabolic steroid 88

De-capeptyl SR a brand name for triptorelin (an anticancer drug 96)

decongestants 26 used in ear disorders 117

DEET another name for diethyltoluamide (a mosquito repellent)

deferiprone a drug used to remove excess iron from the blood in thalassaemia

deflazacort a corticosteroid 80

Delfen a brand name for nonoxinol '9' (a spermicidal agent)

Deltacortril Enteric a brand name for prednisolone 354 (a corticosteroid 80)

Deltastab a brand name for prednisolone 354 (a corticosteroid 80)

demeclocycline a tetracycline antibiotic 62

dementia, drugs for 19

Demix a brand of doxycycline 227 (a tetracycline antibiotic 62)

Demser a brand name for metirosine, a drug for phaeochromocytoma (adrenal gland tumour)

De-Nol a brand name for bismuth (a metallic substance used as an anti-ulcer drug 43)

Dentomycin a brand name for minocycline 318 (a tetracycline antibiotic 62)

Depakote a brand name for valproic acid (a drug for mania 16)

Depixol a brand name for flupentixol 248 (an antipsychotic drug 15 and antidepressant 14)

Depo-Medrone a brand name for methyl-prednisolone (a corticosteroid 80)

Deponit a brand name for glyceryl trinitrate 257 (an anti-angina drug 35)

Depo-Provera a brand name for medroxy-progesterone 301 (a female sex hormone 88)

Dequacaine a brand name for benzocaine (a local anaesthetic 11) with dequalinium (an oral antibacterial antiseptic)

Dequadin a brand name for dequalinium (an oral antibacterial antiseptic)

dequalinium an antibacterial antiseptic used for mouth infections

Derbac-M a brand-named shampoo containing malathion 300 (a drug for skin parasites 122)

Dermablend a brand name for a masking cream for skin disfigurement

Dermabond a brand name for octylcyanoacrylate (a skin adhesive)

Dermacolor a brand name for a masking cream for skin disfigurement

Dermacort a brand-named hydrocortisone cream 264 (topical corticosteroids 120)

Dermestril a brand name for estradiol 238, used for HRT 89

Dermidex Cream a brand-named cream for skin irritation containing chlorobutanol, lidocaine, cetrimide, and alcloxa

Dermovate a brand name for clobetasol 191 (a topical corticosteroid 120)

Dermovate-NN a brand name for nystatin 333 (an antifungal drug 76) with clobetasol 191 (a topical corticosteroid 120) and neomycin (an aminoglycoside antibiotic 62)

Deseril a brand name for methysergide (a drug to prevent migraine 20)

Desferal a brand name for desferrioxamine (an antidote for iron overdose)

desferrioxamine an antidote for iron overdose

desflurane a general anaesthetic

desirudin an injected anticoagulant 38

desloratadine an antihistamine 58

desmopressin 209 a pituitary hormone 85 used for diabetes insipidus

Desmospray a brand name for desmopressin 209 (a pituitary hormone 85 used for diabetes insipidus)

Desmotabs a brand name for desmopressin 209 (a pituitary hormone 85 used for diabetes insipidus)

desogestrel a progestogen oral contraceptive 105

desoximetasone a topical corticosteroid 120

Destolit a brand name for ursodeoxycholic acid (a drug for gallstones 48)

Deteclo a brand name for tetracycline 403 with chlortetracycline and demeclocycline (all tetracycline antibiotics 62)

Detrunorm a brand name for propiverine (a drug for urinary frequency 112)

Detrusitol a brand name for tolterodine 409 (an anticholinergic and antispasmodic drug for urinary disorders 112

Dettol a brand-named liquid skin antiseptic (anti-infective skin preparations 120) containing chloroxylenol

dexamethasone 210 a corticosteroid 80

Dexa-Rhinaspray a brand name for dexamethasone 210 (a corticosteroid 80) with neomycin (an aminoglycoside antibiotic 62) and tramazoline (a decongestant 26)

dexketoprofen a non-steroidal anti-inflammatory drug 50

dextromethorphan an opioid drug for coughs 27

dextromoramide an opioid analgesic 9

dextropropoxyphene an opioid analgesic 9

DF 118 Forte a brand name for dihydrocodeine 216 (an opioid analgesic 9)

DHC Continus a brand name for dihydrocodeine 216 (an opioid analgesic 9)

Diabetamide a brand name for glibenclamide 255 (an oral drug used in diabetes 82)

diabetes, drugs used in 82

DIAGLYK a brand name for gliclazide 256 (an oral drug used in diabetes 82)

Dialar a brand of diazepam 211 (a benzodiazepine anti-anxiety drug 13, muscle relaxant 54, and anticonvulsant 66)

Diamicron a brand name for gliclazide 256 (an oral drug used in diabetes 82)

Diamicron MR a brand name for gliclazide 256 (an oral drug used in diabetes 82)

diamorphine an opioid analgesic 9

Diamox a brand name for acetazolamide (a carbonic anhydrase inhibitor diuretic 32 and drug for glaucoma 114)

Dianette a brand name for co-cyprindiol (a drug for acne 181)

Diarphen a brand name for diphenoxylate (an opioid) with atropine 150 (both antidiarrhoeal drugs 44)

Diasorb a brand name for loperamide 294 (an antidiarrhoeal drug 44)

Diazemuls a brand name for diazepam 211 (a benzodiazepine anti-anxiety drug 13, muscle relaxant 54, and anticonvulsant 16)

diazepam 211 a benzodiazepine anti-anxiety drug 13, muscle relaxant 54, and anticonvulsant 16

diazoxide an antihypertensive 36 also used for hypoglycaemia 82

Dibenyline a brand name for phenoxybenzamine, a drug for phaeochromocytoma (adrenal gland tumour)

dibromopropamidine an antibacterial agent (anti-infective skin preparations 120)

diclofenac 212 a non-steroidal anti-inflammatory drug 50

Dicloflex a brand name for diclofenac 212 (a non-steroidal anti-inflammatory drug 50)

Diclomax Retard a brand name for diclofenac 212 (a non-steroidal anti-inflammatory 50)

Diclomax SR a brand name for diclofenac 212 (a non-steroidal anti-inflammatory drug 50)

dicobalt edetate an antidote for cyanide poisoning

Diconal a brand name for dipipanone (an opioid analgesic 9)

dicycloverine 214 an antispasmodic drug for irritable bowel syndrome 45

Dicynene a brand name for etamsylate (an antifibrinolytic to promote blood clotting 38)

didanosine a reverse transcriptase inhibitor drug for HIV/AIDS 100

Didronel a brand name for etidronate 241 (a drug for bone disorders 56)

Didronel PMO a brand name for etidronate 241 (a drug for bone disorders 56) with calcium carbonate

diethylamine salicylate a rubefacient, which warms the skin to relieve muscle pain

diethylcarbamazine an anthelmintic 78

diethylstilbestrol a female sex hormone 88

diethyltoluamide (DEET) a mosquito repellent

Differin a brand name for adapalene (a retinoid drug used to treat acne 123)

Difflam a brand name for benzydamine (an analgesic 9 used in mouthwashes and throat sprays)

Diflucan a brand name for fluconazole 245 (an antifungal drug 76)

diflucortolone a topical corticosteroid 120

diflunisal a non-steroidal anti-inflammatory 50

Digibind an antidote for digoxin 215 overdose

digitalis drugs 29 used as anti-arrhythmics 33

digitoxin a digitalis drug 29

digoxin 215 (a digitalis drug 29)

dihydrocodeine 216 an opioid analgesic 9

dihydrotachysterol vitamin D (a vitamin 90)

Dijex a brand-named antacid 42 containing aluminium and magnesium

Dilcardia SR a brand name for diltiazem 217 (a calcium channel blocker vasodilator 31, anti-angina drug 35, and antihypertensive drug 36)

diloxanide furoate an antiprotozoal 73 for amoebic dysentery

diltiazem 217 a calcium channel blocker vasodilator 31, anti-angina drug 35, and antihypertensive 36

Dilzem a brand name for diltiazem 217 (a calcium channel blocker vasodilator 31, anti-angina drug 35, and antihypertensive 36)

dimercaprol an antidote for heavy metal poisoning

dimethyl sulfoxide a drug used to treat bladder inflammation

dimeticone a silicone-based substance used in barrier creams (anti-infective skin preparations 120) and as an antifoaming agent (antacids 42)

Dimetriose a brand name for gestrinone (a drug for menstrual disorders 104)

Dimotane a brand name for brompheniramine (an antihistamine 58)

Dimotapp a brand name for phenylephrine with phenylpropanolamine 347 (both decongestants 26) and brompheniramine (an antihistamine 58)

dinoprostone a prostaglandin used to terminate pregnancy 110

Diocalm a brand-named antidiarrhoeal drug 44 containing attapulgite and morphine 323

Diocalm Ultra a brand name for loperamide 294 (an antidiarrhoeal drug 44)

Diocaps a brand name for loperamide 294 (an antidiarrhoeal drug 44)

Dioctyl a brand name for docusate sodium (a stimulant laxative 45)

Dioderm a brand name for hydrocortisone 264 (a corticosteroid 80)

Dioralyte a brand name for rehydration salts containing sodium bicarbonate 385, glucose, potassium chloride, and sodium chloride

Diovan a brand name for valsartan (an angiotensin II blocker vasodilator 31)

Dipentum a brand name for olsalazine (a drug for inflammatory bowel disease 46)

diphenhydramine an antihistamine 58, anti-emetic 21, and antipruritic 118

diphenoxylate an opioid antidiarrhoeal 44

diphenylpyraline an antihistamine 58

dipipanone an opioid analgesic 9

dipivefrine a sympathomimetic drug for glaucoma 114

Diprobase a brand-named emollient (softening) skin preparation

Diprosalic a brand-named skin preparation with betamethasone 151 (a corticosteroid 80) and salicylic acid (a keratolytic 123)

Diprosone a brand name for betamethasone 151 (a corticosteroid 80)

dipyridamole 218 (an antiplatelet drug that affects blood clotting 38)

Dirythmin SA a brand name for disopyramide (an anti-arrhythmic 33)

Disipal a brand name for orphenadrine 338 (a drug for parkinsonism 18)

disopyramide an anti-arrhythmic 33

Disprin a brand name for soluble aspirin 146 (a non-opioid analgesic 9)

Disprin Extra a brand-named soluble analgesic drug 9 containing aspirin 146 and paracetamol 341

Disprol a brand name for paracetamol 341 (a non-opioid analgesic 9)

Distaclor a brand name for cefaclor (a cephalosporin antibiotic 62)

Distaclor MR a brand name for cefaclor (a cephalosporin antibiotic 62)

Distalgesic a brand name for co-proxamol 204 (an opioid analgesic 9)

Distamine a brand name for penicillamine (an antirheumatic drug 52)

distigmine a parasympathomimetic for urinary retention 112 and myasthenia gravis 55

disulfiram an alcohol abuse deterrent 219

dithranol a drug for psoriasis 124

Dithrocream a brand name for dithranol (a drug for psoriasis 124)

Ditropan a brand name for oxybutynin 339 (an anticholinergic and antispasmodic for urinary disorders 112)

Diurexan a brand name for xipamide (a thiazide diuretic 32)

Dytac a brand name for triamterene 411 (a potassium-sparing diuretic 32)

Dytide a brand name for benzthiazide with triamterene 411 (both diuretics 32)

E

Ear disorders, drugs for 117

Earex a brand-named drug for ear wax removal

Ebixa a brand name for memantidine, a drug used to treat Alzheimer's disease

Ebufac a brand name for ibuprofen 267 (a non-steroidal anti-inflammatory drug 50)

Econacort a brand name for econazole (an antifungal drug 76) with hydrocortisone 264 (a corticosteroid 80)

econazole an antifungal drug 76

Economycin a brand name for tetracycline 403 (an antibiotic 62)

Ecopace a brand name for captopril 168 (an ACE inhibitor vasodilator 31)

Ecostatin a brand name for econazole (an antifungal drug 76)

ecothiopate a drug for glaucoma 114

eczema, treatments for 125

Ednyt a brand name for enalapril 231 (an ACE inhibitor vasodilator 31 and antihypertensive drug 36)

Edronax a brand name for reboxetine (an antidepressant 14)

edrophonium a drug for diagnosis of myasthenia gravis 55

Efalith a brand-named ointment for dermatitis 126) containing lithium succinate and zinc sulphate

efavirenz a reverse transcriptase inhibitor drug for HIV/AIDS 100

Efcortelan a brand name for hydrocortisone 264 (a corticosteroid 80)

Efcortesol a brand name for hydrocortisone 264 (a corticosteroid 80)

Efexor a brand name for venlafaxine 414 (an antidepressant 14)

Efexor XL a brand name for venlafaxine 414 (an antidepressant 14)

Effercitrate a brand name for potassium (a mineral 93)

Efudix a brand name for fluorouracil (an anticancer drug 96)

Elantan a brand name for isosorbide mononitrate 277 (a nitrate vasodilator 31 and anti-angina drug 35)

Elavil a brand name for amitriptyline 140 (a tricyclic antidepressant 14)

Eldepryl a brand name for selegiline (a drug for parkinsonism 18)

Eldisine a brand name for vindesine (an anticancer drug 96)

Electrolade brand-named oral rehydration salts with potassium(minerals 93), sodium chloride, sodium bicarbonate 385, and glucose

eletriptan a drug for migraine 20

Elidel cream a brand name for pimecrolimus (an anti-inflammatory drug for eczema 125)

Elleste Duet a brand-named preparation for HRT 89 containing estradiol 238 and norethisterone 332 (both female sex hormones 88)

Elleste Solo a brand name for estradiol 238, an oestrogen (female sex hormones 88)

Elocon a brand name for mometasone 322 (a topical corticosteroid 120)

Eloxatin a brand name for oxaliplatin (an anticancer drug 96)

Eltroxin a brand name for levothyroxine 290 (a drug for thyroid disorders 84)

Eludril a brand name for chlorhexidine (anti-infective skin preparations 120)

Elyzol a brand name for metronidazole 316 (an antibacterial 66 and antiprotozoal 73)

Emadine a brand name for emedastine (an antihistamine 58)

Emcor a brand name for bisoprolol (a beta blocker 30)

emedastine an antihistamine 58

Emeside a brand name for ethosuximide (an anticonvulsant 16)

Emflex a brand name for acemetacin (a non-steroidal anti-inflammatory drug 50)

Emla a brand-named local anaesthetic (analgesics 9) with lidocaine and prilocaine

emollients, in antipruritic preparations 118 and treatments for eczema 125

Enacard a brand name for enalapril 231 (an ACE inhibitor vasodilator 31 and antihypertensive 36)

enalapril 231 an ACE inhibitor vasodilator 31 and antihypertensive 36

Enbrel brand name for etanercept (an immunosuppressant 99 and antirheumatic 52)

enbucrilate a tissue and skin adhesive for closing wounds

En-De-Kay a brand name for fluoride (a mineral 93)

Endoxana a brand name for cyclophosphamide 206 (an anticancer drug 96)

enflurane a general anaesthetic

ENO's a brand-named antacid 42 containing sodium bicarbonate 385, sodium carbonate, and citric acid

etynodiol a progestogen female sex hormone 88

Eucardic a brand name for carvedilol (a beta blocker 30)

Eudemine a brand name for diazoxide (an antihypertensive 36 used to treat hypoglycaemia in diabetes 82)

Euglucon a brand name for glibenclamide 255 (an oral drug used in diabetes 82)

Eugynon-30 a brand-named oral contraceptive 105 containing ethinylestradiol 240 and levonorgestrel 289

Eumovate a brand name for clobetasone (a topical corticosteroid 120)

Eurax a brand name for crotamiton (an antipruritic 118)

Eurax-Hydrocortisone a brand name for hydrocortisone 264 (a corticosteroid 80) with crotamiton (an antipruritic 118)

Evista a brand name for raloxifene 369 (a drug for bone disorders 56)

Evorel a brand name for estradiol 238, an oestrogen (female sex hormones 88)

Exelderm a brand name for sulconazole (an antifungal drug 76)

Exelon a brand name for rivastigmine 376 (a drug for dementia 19 used in Alzheimer's disease)

exemestane an anti-breast cancer drug 96

Ex-Lax a brand name for senna (a stimulant laxative 45)

Exocin a brand name for ofloxacin (a quinolone antibacterial drug 66)

Exorex a brand name for coal tar lotion (for psoriasis 124 and eczema 125)

Expulin a brand-named cough preparation 27 containing chlorphenamine 178, menthol, pholcodine, and pseudoephedrine

Exterol brand-named ear drops for wax removal containing urea (a softening agent)

F

factor VIIa a blood extract to promote blood clotting 38

factor VIII a blood extract to promote blood clotting 38

factor IX a blood extract to promote blood clotting 38

famciclovir an antiviral 69

famotidine an H_2 blocker anti-ulcer drug 43

Famvir a brand name for famciclovir (an antiviral 69)

Fansidar a brand-named antimalarial 75 containing pyrimethamine 364 and sulfadoxine

Fareston a brand name for toremifene (an anticancer drug 96)

Farlutal a brand name for medroxyprogesterone 301 (a female sex hormone 88)

Fasigyn a brand name for tinidazole (an antibacterial drug 66)

Faverin a brand name for fluvoxamine (an SSRI antidepressant 14)

Fectrim a brand name for co-trimoxazole 205 (a sulphonamide antibacterial containing trimethoprim 412 and sulfamethoxazole)

Fefol a brand name for folic acid (a vitamin 90) with iron (a mineral 93)

felbinac a non-steroidal anti-inflammatory 50

Feldene a brand name for piroxicam 350 (a non-steroidal anti-inflammatory drug 50 and drug for gout 53)

felodipine a calcium channel blocker vasodilator 31

felypressin a vasoconstrictor used in dentistry

female sex hormones 88

Femapak a brand-named preparation for menopause (female sex hormones 88) with estradiol 238 and dydrogesterone 228

Femara a brand name for letrozole (an anticancer drug 96)

Fematrix a brand name for estradiol 238, an oestrogen (female sex hormones 88)

Feminax a brand-named analgesic for dysmenorrhoea 104) containing paracetamol 341, codeine 198, hyoscine 265, and caffeine

Femodene a brand-named oral contraceptive 105 containing ethinylestradiol 240 and gestodene (a progestogen)

Femodette a brand-named oral contraceptive 105 containing ethinylestradiol 240 and gestodene (a progestogen)

Femoston a brand-named preparation for menopause (female sex hormones 88) with estradiol 238 and dydrogesterone 228

FemSeven a brand name for estradiol 238, an oestrogen (female sex hormones 88)

Femseven Conti a brand name for estradiol 238 with levonorgestrel 289 (both female sex hormones 88) used for HRT 89

Femulen a brand-named oral contraceptive 105 containing etynodiol (a progestogen)

Fenbid a brand name for ibuprofen 267 (a non-steroidal anti-inflammatory drug 50)

fenbufen a non-steroidal anti-inflammatory 50

fenofibrate a lipid-lowering drug 37

Fenoket a brand name for ketoprofen 281 (a non-steroidal anti-inflammatory drug 50)

fenoprofen a non-steroidal anti-inflammatory drug 50

Fenopron a brand name for fenoprofen (a non-steroidal anti-inflammatory drug 50)

fenoterol a sympathomimetic bronchodilator drug 23

fentanyl an opioid analgesic 9 used in general anaesthesia and labour 110

Fentazin a brand name for perphenazine (an antipsychotic 15 and anti-emetic 21)

fenticonazole an antifungal drug 76

Feospan a brand name for iron (a mineral 93)

Ferfolic SV a brand name for folic acid (a vitamin 90) and ferrous gluconate, a form of iron (a mineral 93)

ferric ammonium citrate iron (a mineral 93)

Ferriprox a brand name for deferiprone (used to treat iron overload)

Ferrograd a brand name for iron (a mineral 93)

Ferrograd C a brand name for iron (a mineral 93) with vitamin C (a vitamin 90)

Ferrograd Folic a brand name for folic acid (a vitamin 90) with iron (a mineral 93)

ferrous fumarate iron (a mineral 93)

ferrous gluconate iron (a mineral 93)

ferrous glycine sulphate iron (a mineral 93)

ferrous sulphate iron (a mineral 93)

Fersaday a brand name for iron (a mineral 93)

Fersamal a brand name for iron (a mineral 93)

fexofenadine an antihistamine 58

fibrates a group of lipid-lowering drugs 37

Fibro-vein a brand name for sodium tetradecyl sulphate (a drug for varicose veins)

Filair a brand name for beclometasone 154 (a corticosteroid 80)

filgrastim 243 a blood cell growth stimulant

finasteride 244 an anti-androgen drug (male sex hormone 87) for benign prostatic hypertrophy 112 and hair loss 127

Flagyl a brand name for metronidazole 316 (an antibacterial 66 and antiprotozoal 73)

Flamazine a brand name for silver sulfadiazine (an antibacterial skin preparation 120)

flavoxate an antispasmodic drug for urinary disorders 112

flecainide an anti-arrhythmic 33

Flexin Continus a brand name for indometacin (a non-steroidal anti-inflammatory drug 50)

Flixonase a brand name for fluticasone 250 (a corticosteroid 80)

Flixotide a brand name for fluticasone 250 (a corticosteroid 80)

Flomax MR a brand name for tamsulosin 396, an alpha blocker for prostate (urinary) disorders 112

Florinef a brand name for fludrocortisone (a corticosteroid 80)

Floxapen a brand name for flucloxacillin 244 (a penicillin antibiotic 62)

Flu-Amp a brand name for co-fluampicil (a combined penicillin antibiotic 62 containing flucloxacillin 244 with ampicillin)

Fluanxol a brand name for flupentixol 248 (an antipsychotic 15 also used to treat depression 14)

Fluclomix a brand name for flucloxacillin 244 (a penicillin antibiotic 62)

flucloxacillin 244 a penicillin antibiotic 62

fluconazole 245 an antifungal drug 76

flucytosine an antifungal drug 76

fludarabine an anticancer drug 96

fludrocortisone a corticosteroid 80

fludroxycortide a topical corticosteroid 120

flumazenil an antidote for benzodiazepine overdose

flumetasone a corticosteroid 80

flunisolide a corticosteroid 80

flunitrazepam a benzodiazepine sleeping drug 11

fluocinolone a topical corticosteroid 120

fluocinonide a topical corticosteroid 120

fluocortolone a topical corticosteroid 120

Fluor-a-day a brand name for fluoride (a mineral 93)

fluorescein a drug used to stain the eye before examination

fluoride a mineral 93

Fluorigard a brand name for fluoride (a mineral 93)

fluorometholone a corticosteroid 80 for eye disorders

fluorouracil an anticancer drug 96

fluoxetine 246 an SSRI antidepressant 14

flupentixol 248 an antipsychotic 15 also used in depression 14

fluphenazine an antipsychotic 15 also used in depression 14

flurazepam a benzodiazepine sleeping drug 11

flurbiprofen a non-steroidal anti-inflammatory drug 50

flutamide 249 an anticancer drug 96 for prostate cancer

fluticasone 250 a corticosteroid 80

fluvastatin a lipid-lowering drug 37

fluvoxamine an SSRI antidepressant 14

FML a brand name for fluorometholone (a corticosteroid 80 for eye disorders)

folate sodium folic acid (a vitamin 90)

folic acid a vitamin 90

folinic acid a vitamin 90

follicle-stimulating hormone (FSH) a natural hormone for infertility 109

follitropin alfa a drug for infertility 109

follitropin beta a drug for infertility 109

fomepizole antidote for ethylene glycol or methanol poisoning

fomivirsen an antiviral 69

fondaparinux an injected anticoagulant drug 38)

Foradil a brand name for formoterol (a sympathomimetic bronchodilator drug 23)

Forcaltonin a brand name for calcitonin (salmon) (a drug for bone disorders 56)

formoterol a sympathomimetic bronchodilator drug 23

Fortipine LA a brand name for nifedipine 330 (a calcium channel blocker vasodilator 31, anti-angina drug 35, and antihypertensive 36)

Fortovase a brand name for saquinavir (a protease inhibitor drug for HIV/AIDS 100)

Fortral a brand name for pentazocine (an opioid analgesic 9)

Fortum a brand name for ceftazidime (a cephalosporin antibiotic 62)

Fosamax a brand name for alendronate 132 (a drug for bone disorders 56)

Fosamax Once Weekly a brand name for alendronate 132 (a drug for bone disorders 56)

foscarnet an antiviral drug 69

Foscavir a brand name for foscarnet (an antiviral 69)

fosinopril an ACE inhibitor vasodilator 31

fosphenytoin 348 an anticonvulsant 16

Fragmin a brand name for dalteparin, a low molecular weight heparin 262: an anticoagulant drug 38)

framycetin a topical aminoglycoside antibiotic for ear, eye, and skin infections (anti-infective skin preparations 120)

frangula a mild stimulant laxative 45

Franol a brand-named bronchodilator drug 23 containing ephedrine 232 and theophylline 404

Frisium a brand name for clobazam (a benzodiazepine anti-anxiety drug 13)

Froben a brand name for flurbiprofen (a non-steroidal anti-inflammatory drug 50)

Froop a brand name for furosemide 251 (a loop diuretic 32)

Fru-Co a brand name for co-amilofruse (a combined diuretic product 32 containing amiloride 137 with furosemide 251)

Frumil LS a brand name for co-amilofruse (a combined diuretic product 32 containing amiloride 137 with furosemide 251)

Frusene a brand name for furosemide 251 with triamterene 411 (both diuretics 32)

Frusol a brand name for furosemide 251 (a loop diuretic 32)

FSH follicle-stimulating hormone (a natural hormone for infertility 109)

Fucibet a brand name for betamethasone 158 (a corticosteroid 80) with fusidic acid (an antibiotic 62)

Fucidin a brand name for fusidic acid (an antibiotic 62)

Fucidin H a brand name for fusidic acid (an antibiotic 62) and hydrocortisone 264 (a corticosteroid 80)

Fucithalmic a brand name for fusidic acid (an antibiotic 62)

Full Marks a brand name for phenothrin (a topical drug to treat skin parasites 122)

Fungilin a brand name for amphotericin 143 (an antifungal drug 76)

Fungizone a brand name for amphotericin 143 (an antifungal drug 76)

Furadantin a brand name for nitrofurantoin (an antibacterial 66)

furosemide 251 a loop diuretic 32

fusafungine a topical antibacterial 120

fusidic acid a topical antibiotic 120

Fybogel a brand name for ispaghula (a bulk-forming laxative 45 and antidiarrhoeal 44)

Fybogel-Mebeverine a brand name for ispaghula (a bulk-forming antidiarrhoeal agent 44) with mebeverine 301 (an antispasmodic for irritable bowel syndrome 45)

G

gabapentin an anticonvulsant 16

Gabitril a brand name for tiagabine (an anticonvulsant 16)

galantamine a drug for dementia 19

Galcodine a brand name for codeine 198 (an opioid cough suppressant 27)

Galenamet a brand name for amoxicillin 142 (a penicillin antibiotic 62)

Galenamox a brand name for amoxicillin 142 (a penicillin antibiotic 62)

Galenphol a brand name for pholcodine (an opioid cough suppressant 27)

Galfer a brand name for iron (a mineral 93)

Galfer FA a brand name for folic acid (a vitamin 90) with iron (a mineral 93)

gallamine a drug used to relax the muscles in general anaesthesia

gallstones, drug treatment for 48

Galpseud a brand name for pseudoephedrine (a decongestant 26)

Galpseud Plus a brand name for chlorphenamine 178 (an antihistamine 58) with pseudoephedrine (a decongestant 26)

Gamanil a brand name for lofepramine 293 (a tricyclic antidepressant 14)

gamma globulin an immune globulin (vaccines and immunization 70)

gamolenic acid an extract of evening primrose

ganciclovir an antiviral drug 69

Ganda a brand-named preparation for glaucoma 114 containing epinephrine 233 and guanethidine

ganirelix a drug for treatment of infertility 109

Garamycin a brand name for gentamicin 254 (an aminoglycoside antibiotic 62)

Gardenal a brand name for phenobarbital 345 (a barbiturate anticonvulsant 16)

Gastrobid Continus a brand name for metoclopramide 314 (a gastrointestinal motility regulator and anti-emetic 21)

Gastrocote a brand-named antacid 42 containing aluminium hydroxide 136, sodium bicarbonate 385, magnesium trisilicate, and alginic acid

Gastroflux a brand name for metoclopramide 314 (a gastrointestinal motility regulator and anti-emetic 21)

Gaviscon a brand-named antacid 42 containing aluminium hydroxide 136, sodium bicarbonate 385, magnesium trisilicate, and alginic acid

gemcitabine an anticancer drug 96

gemeprost a prostaglandin drug used in labour 110

gemfibrozil a lipid-lowering drug 37

Gemzar a brand name for gemcitabine (an anticancer drug 96)

Genotropin a brand name for somatropin, synthetic growth hormone (pituitary hormones 85)

gentamicin 254 an aminoglycoside antibiotic 62

gentian mixture, acid/alkaline an appetite stimulant

Genticin a brand name for gentamicin 254 (an aminoglycoside antibiotic 62)

Gentisone HC a brand name for gentamicin 254 (an aminoglycoside antibiotic 62) with hydrocortisone 264 (a corticosteroid 80)

gestodene a progestogen female sex hormone 88 and oral contraceptive 105

Gestone a brand name for progesterone (a female sex hormone 88)

gestonorone a progestogen (female sex hormones 88)

gestrinone a drug for menstrual disorders 104

Glandosane a brand name for artificial saliva

glatiramer a drug for multiple sclerosis

glaucoma, drugs for 114

Glau-opt a brand name for timolol 406 (a beta blocker 30 and drug for glaucoma 114)

glibenclamide 255 an oral drug used in diabetes 82

Glibenese a brand name for glipizide (an oral drug used in diabetes 82)

gliclazide 256 an oral drug used in diabetes 82

glimepiride an oral drug used in diabetes 82

glipizide an oral drug used in diabetes 82

gliquidone an oral drug used in diabetes 82

GlucaGen a brand name for glucagon (a drug for hypoglycaemia used in diabetes 82)

glucagon a pancreatic hormone for hypoglycaemia 82

Glucobay a brand name for acarbose (an oral drug used in diabetes 82)

Glucophage a brand name for metformin 309 (an oral drug used in diabetes 82)

Glurenorm a brand name for gliquidone (an oral drug used in diabetes 82)

glutaraldehyde a topical preparation for warts

Glutarol a brand name for glutaraldehyde (a topical wart preparation)

glycerol a drug used to reduce pressure in the eye in glaucoma 114 and an ingredient in cough mixtures 27, skin preparations 120, laxative suppositories 45, and ear-wax softeners

glyceryl trinitrate 257 an anti-angina drug 35

glycopyrronium bromide an anticholinergic used in general anaesthesia

Glypressin a brand name for terlipressin, a drug similar to vasopressin (a pituitary hormone 85), used to stop bleeding

Glytrin a brand name for glyceryl trinitrate 257 (an anti-angina drug 35)

gold a metal used medically for rheumatoid arthritis 52

gold-based drugs a group of antirheumatic drugs 52

Golden Eye a brand name for propamidine isetionate (an antibacterial 66 for eye infections)

gonadorelin a drug for infertility 109

gonadotrophin, human chorionic 181 a drug for infertility 109

Gopten a brand name for trandolapril (an ACE inhibitor vasodilator 31)

goserelin 259 an anticancer drug 96, also used for menstrual disorders 104 and infertility 109

gout, drugs for 53

gramicidin a topical aminoglycoside antibiotic 120 for eye, ear, and skin infections

Graneodin a brand name for gramicidin (anti-infective skin preparations 120) with neomycin (both aminoglycoside antibiotics 62)

granisetron an anti-emetic 21

Granocyte a brand name for lenograstim (a blood growth stimulant)

Gregoderm a brand name for hydrocortisone 264 (a corticosteroid 80) with nystatin 333 (an antifungal 76), neomycin (an aminoglycoside antibiotic 62), and polymyxin B (a topical antibiotic 120)

griseofulvin an antifungal drug 76

Grisovin a brand name for griseofulvin (an antifungal drug 76)

growth-factor inhibitors anticancer drugs 96

growth hormone somatropin (pituitary hormones 85)

GTN 300mcg a brand name for glyceryl trinitrate 257 (an anti-angina drug 35)

guaifenesin an expectorant to treat coughs 27

guanethidine an antihypertensive 36

Guarem a brand name for guar gum (used to control blood glucose levels in diabetes 82)

guar gum a drug used to control blood glucose levels in diabetes 82

Gyno-Daktarin a brand name for miconazole 318 (an antifungal drug 76)

Gynol II a brand name for nonoxinol '9' (a spermicidal agent)

Gyno-Pevaryl a brand name for econazole (an antifungal drug 76)

H

H₂ blockers a group of anti-ulcer drugs 43

Haelan a brand name for fludroxycortide (a topical corticosteroid 120)

haem arginate a drug to treat porphyria

hair loss, drugs for 127

Halciderm Topical a brand name for halcinonide (a topical corticosteroid 120)

halcinonide a topical corticosteroid 120

Haldol a brand name for haloperidol 261 (a butyrophenone antipsychotic 15)

Half Sinemet CR a brand name for co-careldopa (a drug for parkinsonism 18)

halibut liver oil a natural fish oil rich in vitamin A and vitamin D (both vitamins 90)

haloperidol 261 a butyrophenone antipsychotic drug 15

halothane a gas used to induce general anaesthesia

Halycitrol a brand name for vitamin A with vitamin D (both vitamins 90)

hamamelis an astringent in rectal preparations 47)

Harmogen a brand name for estropipate, a drug for hormone replacement therapy (female sex hormones 88)

Hay-Crom a brand name for sodium cromoglicate 386 (an anti-allergy drug 8)

Haymine a brand name for chlorphenamine 178 (an antihistamine 58) with ephedrine 232 (a bronchodilator drug 23 and decongestant 26)

HCG human chorionic gonadotrophin 181 (a drug for infertility 109)

Hedex a brand name for paracetamol 341 (a non-opioid analgesic 9)

Hedex Extra a brand name for paracetamol 341 (a non-opioid analgesic 9) with caffeine

Heliclear a brand name anti-ulcer product 43 containing lansoprazole 284 (a proton pump inhibitor) with amoxicillin 142 and clarithromycin 190 (both antibiotics)

Hemabate a brand name for carboprost, a drug to control bleeding after childbirth 110

Heminevrin a brand name for clomethiazole (a non-benzodiazepine, non-barbiturate sleeping drug 11)

heparin 262 an anticoagulant drug 38

heparinoid a topical treatment for skin inflammation

Herceptin a brand name for trastuzumab (an anticancer drug 96)

Herpetad a brand name for aciclovir 131 (an antiviral drug 69)

Herpid a brand name for idoxuridine (an antiviral drug 69)

hexachlorophene a skin antiseptic (anti-infective skin preparations 120)

hexamine another name for methenamine, a drug for urinary tract infections 112

hexetidine an antiseptic mouthwash

Hexopal a brand name for nicotinic acid (a vasodilator 31)

Hibitane a brand name for chlorhexidine (anti-infective skin preparations 120)

Hioxyl a brand name for hydrogen peroxide (an antiseptic mouthwash)

Hiprex a brand name for hexamine (a drug for urinary tract infections 112)

Hirudoid a brand name for heparinoid (a topical treatment for skin inflammation)

Histalix a brand-named cough preparation 27 containing diphenhydramine, ammonium chloride, and menthol

Histoacryl a brand name for enbucrilate (a tissue adhesive)

Hivid a brand name for zalcitabine (a reverse transcriptase inhibitor drug for HIV/AIDS 100)

HIV and AIDS, drugs for 100

homatropine a mydriatic affecting the pupil 116

Honvan a brand name for fosfestrol (a female sex hormone 88 and anticancer drug 96)

hormones female sex hormones 88, male sex hormones 87, as anticancer treatment 96, in diabetes 82, for infertility 109, in menstrual disorders 104, in pituitary disorders 85, in adrenal gland disorders (corticosteroids) 80, in thyroid disorders 84, in oral contraceptives 104, and for acne 123

Hormonin a brand name for estradiol 238 (a female sex hormone 88)

HRT see female sex hormones 88

Humalog a brand name for insulin lispro 271 (a drug used in diabetes 82)

Human Actrapid a brand name for insulin 271 (a drug used in diabetes 82)

Human chorionic gonadotrophin see chorionic gonadotrophin 181

Human Insulatard a brand name for insulin 271 (a drug used in diabetes 82)

human menopausal gonadotrophins also known as menotrophin, a drug for infertility 109

Human Mixtard a brand name for insulin 271 (a drug used in diabetes 82)

Human Monotard a brand name for insulin 271 (a drug used in diabetes 82)

Human Ultratard a brand name for insulin 271 (a drug used in diabetes 82)

Human Velosulin a brand name for insulin 271 (a drug used in diabetes 82)

Humatrope a brand name for somatropin, synthetic growth hormone (a pituitary hormone 85)

Humulin a brand name for insulin 271 (a drug used in diabetes 82)

Hyalase a brand name for hyaluronidase (which helps injections to penetrate tissues)

hyaluronidase an enzyme that helps injections to penetrate tissues

Hycamtin a brand name for topotecan (an anticancer drug 96)

Hydergine a brand name for co-dergocrine mesylate (a vasodilator 31 used to improve blood flow to the brain in senile dementia)

hydralazine a vasodilator 31

Hydrea a brand name for hydroxycarbamide (an anticancer drug 96)

hydrochlorothiazide 263 a thiazide diuretic 32

hydrocortisone 264 a corticosteroid 80 and antipruritic 118

Hydrocortistab a brand name for hydrocortisone 264 (a corticosteroid 80)

Hydrocortone a brand name for hydrocortisone 264 (a corticosteroid 80)

hydroflumethiazide a thiazide diuretic 32

hydrogen peroxide antiseptic mouthwash

hydromorphone an opioid analgesic 9

hydrotalcite an antacid 42

hydroxocobalamin vitamin B12 (a vitamin 90)

hydroxyapatite a drug for bone disorders 56

hydroxycarbamide a drug for chronic myeloid leukaemia 96

hydroxychloroquine an antimalarial 75 and antirheumatic drug 52

hydroxyprogesterone a progestogen (female sex hormones 88) used to prevent miscarriage

hydroxyzine an anti-anxiety drug 13

Hygroton a brand name for chlortalidone (a thiazide diuretic 32)

hyoscine 265 an antidiarrhoeal drug 44, drug for irritable bowel syndrome 45, and drug affecting the pupil 116

Hypnovel a brand name for midazolam (a benzodiazepine drug used as premedication)

Hypotears a brand name for polyvinyl alcohol (artificial tears)

Hypovase a brand name for prazosin (an alpha blocker antihypertensive 36)

hypromellose an ingredient of artificial tear preparations

Hypurin a brand name for insulin 271 (a drug used in diabetes 82)

Hytrin a brand name for terazosin (an alpha blocker antihypertensive 36)

Hytrin BPH a brand name for terazosin (an alpha blocker antihypertensive 36)

I

ibandronic acid a drug for bone disorders 56

Ibugel a brand name for ibuprofen 267 (a non-steroidal anti-inflammatory drug 50)

Ibuleve a brand name for ibuprofen 267 (a non-steroidal anti-inflammatory drug 50)

ibuprofen 267 a non-opioid analgesic 9 and non-steroidal anti-inflammatory drug 50

Ibuspray a brand name for ibuprofen 267 (a non-steroidal anti-inflammatory drug 50)

ichthammol a substance in skin preparations for eczema 125

idarubicin a cytotoxic anticancer drug 96

idoxuridine an antiviral 69

ifosfamide an anticancer drug 96

Ikorel a brand name for nicorandil (a potassium channel activator anti-angina drug 35)

Ilube brand-named eye drops containing acetylcysteine (a mucolytic) with hypromellose (used in artificial tear preparations)

imatinib an anticancer drug 96

Imazin XL a brand name for aspirin 146 with isosorbide mononitrate 277 (for prevention of angina and heart attacks)

Imdur a brand name for isosorbide mononitrate 277 (a nitrate vasodilator 31 and anti-angina drug 35)

imidapril an ACE inhibitor vasdilator 31

imiglucerase an enzyme for replacement therapy

Imigran a brand name for sumatriptan 393 (a drug for migraine 20)

imipenem an antibiotic 62

imipramine 268 a tricyclic antidepressant 14 and drug for urinary disorders 112

imiquimod a drug to treat warts

Immukin a brand name for interferon gamma 272 (an antiviral 69)

immunoglobulin a preparation injected to prevent infectious diseases (vaccines and immunization 70)

Immunoprin a brand name for azathioprine 151 (an antirheumatic 52 and immunosuppressant drug 99)

immunosuppressant drugs 99 (used as anti-rheumatic drugs 52 and in inflammatory bowel disease 46)

Imodium a brand name for loperamide 294 (an opioid antidiarrhoeal drug 44)

Implanon a brand name for etonorgestrel, a progestogen (female sex hormones 88)

Imunovir a brand name for inosine pranobex (an antiviral drug 69)

Imuran a brand name for azathioprine 151 (an antirheumatic 52 and immunosuppressant drug 99)

indapamide 269 a thiazide-like diuretic 32 and antihypertensive drug 36

Inderal a brand name for propranolol 361 (a beta blocker 30)

Inderal-LA a brand name for propranolol 361 (a beta blocker 30)

Inderetic a brand name for bendroflumethiazide 155 (a thiazide diuretic 32) with propranolol 361 (a beta blocker 30)

Inderex a brand name for bendroflumethiazide 155 (a thiazide diuretic 32) with propranolol 361 (a beta blocker 30)

Indermil a brand name for enbucrilate (a tissue adhesive)

indinavir a protease inhibitor drug for HIV/AIDS 100

Indivina a brand name for estradiol 238 with medroxyprogesterone 301 (both female sex hormones 88) used as HRT

Indocid a brand name for indometacin (an NSAID 50 and drug for gout 53)

Indocid-R a brand name for indometacin (a non-steroidal anti-inflammatory drug 50 and drug for gout 53)

Indolar a brand name for indometacin, a non-steroidal anti-inflammatory drug 50 and drug for gout 53

indometacin a non-steroidal anti-inflammatory drug 50 and drug for gout 53

Indomod a brand name for indometacin (a non-steroidal anti-inflammatory drug 50 and drug for gout 53)

indoramin 270 an alpha blocker antihypertensive 36 and drug for urinary disorders 112

Infacol a brand name for dimeticone, an antifoaming agent (antacids 42)

Infadrops a brand name for paracetamol 341 (a non-opioid analgesic 9)

infertility, drugs for 109

inflammatory bowel disease drugs for 46

Inflexal V a brand name for influenza vaccine (vaccines and immunization 70)

infliximab a drug for Crohn's disease 46) and rheumatoid arthritis 52

Innohep a brand name for tinzaparin (a low molecular weight heparin 262 used as an anticoagulant 38)

Innovace a brand name for enalapril 231 (an ACE inhibitor vasodilator 31 and antihypertensive 36)

Innozide a brand name for enalapril 231 (an ACE inhibitor vasodilator 31 and antihypertensive 36)

inosine pranobex an antiviral 69

inositol a vitamin B preparation related to nicotinic acid (vitamins 90)

Inoven a brand name for ibuprofen 267 (an analgesic 9 and non-steroidal anti-inflammatory drug 50)

Insulatard a brand name for insulin 271 (a drug used in diabetes 82)

insulin 271 a drug used in diabetes 82

insulin aspart a type of insulin 271 (a drug used in diabetes 82)

insulin glargine a type of insulin 271 (a drug used in diabetes 82)

insulin lispro a type of insulin 271 (a drug used in diabetes 82)

Insuman a brand name for insulin (human) 271 (a drug used in diabetes 82)

Intal a brand name for sodium cromoglicate 386 (an anti-allergy drug 60)

integrilin a brand name for eptifibatide (a drug for prevention of heart attacks)

interferon 272 an antiviral drug 69 and anticancer drug 96

Intralgin a brand-named topical gel for muscle strains and sprains

Intron-A a brand name for interferon 272 (an antiviral 69 and anticancer drug 96)

Invanz a brand name for ertapenem (an antibiotic 62)

Invirase a brand name for saquinavir (a protease inhibitor drug for HIV/AIDS 100)

iodine a mineral 93

Iopidine a brand name for apraclonidine (a sympathomimetic drug for glaucoma 114)

ipecacuanha a drug used to induce vomiting in drug overdose and poisoning, also used as an expectorant 27

Ipocol a brand name for mesalazine 308 (a drug for inflammatory bowel disease 46)

ipratropium bromide 274 an anticholinergic bronchodilator drug 23

irbesartan 275 an angiotensin II blocker vasodilator 31

irinotecan an anticancer drug 96

iron a mineral 93

irritable bowel syndrome, drugs for 45

Ismelin a brand name for guanethidine (an antihypertensive drug 36 also used for glaucoma 114)

Ismo a brand name for isosorbide mononitrate 277 (a nitrate vasodilator 31 and anti-angina drug 35)

isocarboxazid an MAOI antidepressant 14

isoflurane a general anaesthetic

Isogel a brand name for ispaghula (a laxative 45 and antidiarrhoeal drug 44)

Isoket a brand name for isosorbide dinitrate 277 (a nitrate vasodilator 31 and anti-angina drug 35)

isometheptene mucate a drug for migraine 20

Isomide CR a brand name for disopyramide (an anti-arrhythmic 33)

isoniazid 276 an antituberculous drug 67

isophane insulin a type of insulin 271 (a drug used in diabetes 82)

isoprenaline a bronchodilator drug 23

Isopto Alkaline brand-named eye drops with hypromellose (used in artificial tear preparations)

Isopto Atropine brand-named eye drops with atropine 150 (an anticholinergic mydriatic affecting the pupil 116) and hypromellose (used in artificial tear preparations)

Isopto Plain brand-named eye drops with hypromellose (used in artificial tear preparations)

Isordil a brand name for isosorbide dinitrate 277 (a nitrate vasodilator 31 and anti-angina drug 35)

isosorbide dinitrate 277 (a nitrate vasodilator 31 and anti-angina drug 35)

isosorbide mononitrate 277 (a nitrate vasodilator 31 and anti-angina drug 35)

Isotard a brand name for isosorbide mononitrate 277 (a nitrate vasodilator 31 and anti-angina drug 35)

Isotrate a brand name for isosorbide mononitrate 277 (a nitrate vasodilator 31 and anti-angina drug 35)

isotretinoin 278 (a drug for acne 123)

Isotrex a brand name for isotretinoin 278 (a drug for acne 123)

Isotrexin a brand-named drug for acne 123 with isotretinoin 278 and erythromycin 235

ispaghula a bulk-forming laxative 45 and agent for diarrhoea 44

isradipine a calcium channel blocker vasodilator 31

Istin a brand name for amlodipine 141 (a calcium channel blocker vasodilator 31)

itraconazole an antifungal drug 76

ivermectin an anthelmintic drug 78

J

Jectofer a brand name for iron (a mineral 93)

Joy-rides a brand name for hyoscine 265 (an anti-emetic 21 for motion sickness)

K

Kaletra a brand name for lopinavir with ritonavir (both protease inhibitor drugs for HIV/AIDS 100)

Kalspare a brand name for triamterene 411 with chlortalidone (both diuretics 32)

Kalten a brand name for amiloride 137 with hydrochlorothiazide 265 (both diuretics 32) and atenolol 147 (a beta blocker 30)

Kaltostat a wound dressing with alginates 133

Kamillosan a brand-named ointment containing camomile used for treating nappy rash, sore nipples, and chapped skin

Kaodene a brand name for codeine 198 with kaolin (both antidiarrhoeal drugs 44)

kaolin an adsorbent antidiarrhoeal drug 44

Kapake a brand name for codeine 198 (an opioid analgesic 9) and paracetamol 341 (a non-opioid analgesic 9)

Kaplon a brand name for captopril 168 (an ACE inhibitor vasodilator 31)

Karvol a brand name for menthol (a decongestant inhalant)

Kay-Cee-L a brand name for potassium (a mineral 93)

Kefadim a brand name for ceftazidime (a cephalosporin antibiotic 62)

Kefadol a brand name for cefamandole (a cephalosporin antibiotic 62)

Keflex a brand name for cefalexin 172 (a cephalosporin antibiotic 62)

Kefzol a brand name for cefazolin (a cephalosporin antibiotic 62)

Kemadrin a brand name for procyclidine 356 (a drug for parkinsonism 18)

Kemicetine a brand name for chloramphenicol 175 (an antibiotic 62)

Kenalog a brand name for triamcinolone (a corticosteroid 80)

Keppra a brand name for levetiracetam (an anticonvulsant 16)

Keral a brand name for dexketoprofen (a non-steroidal anti-inflammatory drug 50)

Kerlone a brand name for betaxolol (a beta blocker 30)

ketamine a drug used to induce general anaesthesia

Ketek a brand name for telithromycin (an antibiotic 62)

Ketocid a brand name for ketoprofen 281 (a non-steroidal anti-inflammatory drug 50)

ketoconazole 280 an antifungal drug 76

ketoprofen 281 a non-steroidal anti-inflammatory drug 50

ketorolac a non-steroidal anti-inflammatory drug 50 used as an analgesic 9

ketotifen a drug similar to sodium cromoglicate 386 for allergies and asthma 24

Ketovail a brand name for ketoprofen 281 (a non-steroidal anti-inflammatory drug 50)

Ketovite a brand-named vitamin supplement (vitamins 90)

Ketozip XL a brand name for ketoprofen 281 (a non-steroidal anti-inflammatory drug 50)

Kineret a brand name for anakinra (an antirheumatic drug 52)

Klaricid a brand name for clarithromycin 190 (a macrolide antibiotic 62)

Klaricid XL a brand name for clarithromycin 190 (a macrolide antibiotic 62)

Klean-prep a brand-named osmotic laxative 45

Kliofem a brand-named product for HRT 89 containing estradiol 238 and norethisterone 332 (both female sex hormones 88)

Kliovance a brand-named product for HRT 89 with estradiol 238 and norethisterone 332 (both female sex hormones 88)

Kloref a brand-named potassium supplement (a mineral 93)

Kolanticon a brand name for aluminium hydroxide 136 and magnesium oxide (both antacids 42) with dicycloverine 214 (an antispasmodic 45) and dimeticone (an antifoaming agent)

Konakion a brand name for phytomenadione (vitamin K; vitamins 90)

Kwells a brand name for hyoscine 265 used as an anti-emetic 21 for motion sickness

Kytril a brand name for granisetron (an anti-emetic 21)

L

labetalol a beta blocker 30

Labosept brand-named throat pastilles with dequalinium (an antibacterial antiseptic for mouth and throat infections)

labour, drugs used in 110

lacidipine a calcium channel blocker vasodilator 31

Lacri-Lube a brand-named ointment for dry eyes

lactic acid an ingredient in wart preparations, emollients (skin-softening agents), and pessaries

Lactugal a brand name for lactulose 283 (an osmotic laxative 45)

lactulose 283 an osmotic laxative 45

Ladropen a brand name for flucloxacillin 244 (a penicillin antibiotic 62)

Lamictal a brand name for lamotrigine 283 (an anticonvulsant 16)

Lamisil a brand name for terbinafine 400 (an antifungal drug 76)

lamivudine a reverse transcriptase inhibitor drug for HIV/AIDS 100

lamotrigine 283 an anticonvulsant 16

Lamprene a brand name for clofazimine (a drug for Hansen's disease (leprosy) 67)

Lanoxin a brand name for digoxin 215 (a digitalis drug 29)

Lanoxin-PG a brand name for digoxin 215 (a digitalis drug 29)

lanreotide an anticancer drug for pituitary disorders 85

lansoprazole 284 a proton pump inhibitor anti-ulcer drug 43

Lantus a brand name for insulin glargine, a type of insulin 271 (a drug for diabetes 82)

Lanvis a brand name for tioguanine (an anticancer drug 96)

Larafen a brand name for ketoprofen 281 (a non-steroidal anti-inflammatory drug 50)

Largactil a brand name for chlorpromazine 180 (an antipsychotic 15 and anti-emetic 21)

Lariam a brand name for mefloquine 304 (an antimalarial drug 75)

Lasikal a brand name for furosemide 251 (a loop diuretic 32) with potassium (a mineral 93)

Lasilactone a brand name for furosemide 251 with spironolactone (both diuretics 32)

Lasix a brand name for furosemide 251 (a loop diuretic 32)

Lasonil a brand name for heparinoid (a topical treatment for skin inflammation)

Lasoride a brand name for amiloride 137 (a potassium-sparing diuretic 32) with furosemide 251 (a loop diuretic 32 and antihypertensive 36)

Lassar's Paste a drug for psoriasis 124 with dithranol, zinc oxide, and salicylic acid (a keratolytic 123)

latanoprost 285 a drug for glaucoma 114

laxatives 45

Laxoberal a brand name for sodium picosulfate (a stimulant laxative 45)

Ledclair a brand name for sodium calcium edetate (an antidote for lead and heavy metal poisoning)

Lederfen a brand name for fenbufen (a non-steroidal anti-inflammatory drug 50)

Lederfolin a brand name for folinic acid (a vitamin 90)

Ledermycin a brand name for demeclocycline (a tetracycline antibiotic 62)

leflunomide an antirheumatic drug 52

Lemsip a brand name for paracetamol 341 (a non-opioid analgesic 9) with phenylephrine (a decongestant 26), chlorphenamine 178 (an antihistamine 58), and caffeine

lenograstim a blood growth stimulant

lepirudin an anticoagulant drug 38

lercanidipine a calcium channel blocker vasodilator 31

Lescol a brand name for fluvastatin (a lipid-lowering drug 37)

Lescol XL a brand name for fluvastatin (a lipid-lowering drug 37)

letrozole an anticancer drug 96

Leucomax a brand name for molgramostim (a blood growth stimulant)

Leukeran a brand name for chlorambucil (an anticancer drug 96)

leukotriene antagonists a group of drugs for asthma 24 and treatments for allergy 58

leuprorelin a drug for menstrual disorders 104

levamisole an anthelmintic drug 78

levetiracetam an anticonvulsant drug 16

levobunolol a beta blocker 30 and drug for glaucoma 114

levobupivacaine a local anaesthetic 11

levocabastine a topical antihistamine 58

levocetirizine an antihistamine 58

levodopa 286 a drug for parkinsonism 18

levofloxacin 288 a quinolone antibacterial 66

levomepromazine an antipsychotic drug 15

Levonelle-2 brand named postcoital contraception 109 containing levonorgestrel 289 (a female sex hormone 88 and oral contraceptive 105)

levonorgestrel 289 a female sex hormone 88 and oral contraceptive 105

levothyroxine 290 a thyroid hormone 84)

Librium a brand name for chlordiazepoxide 176 (a benzodiazepine anti-anxiety drug 13)

lidocaine a local anaesthetic 11, anti-arrhythmic 33, and antipruritic 118

Li-liquid a brand name for lithium 292 (an antimanic drug 16)

lincosamides a group of antibiotics 62

linezolid an antibiotic 62

Lioresal a brand name for baclofen 153 (a muscle relaxant 54)

liothyronine a thyroid hormone 84

Lipantil a brand name for fenofibrate (a lipid-lowering drug 37)

lipase a pancreatic enzyme preparation for pancreatic disorders 49

lipid-lowering drugs 37

Lipitor a brand name for atorvastatin 149 (a lipid-lowering drug 37)

Liposic a brand-named artificial tear preparation

Lipostat a brand name for pravastatin 353 (a lipid-lowering drug 37)

liquid paraffin a lubricating agent used as a laxative 45 and in artificial tear preparations

Liquifilm Tears brand-named eye drops containing polyvinyl acetate (artificial tears)

liquorice a substance for peptic ulcers 43

lisinopril 291 an ACE inhibitor vasodilator 31

Liskonum a brand name for lithium 292 (an antimanic drug 16)

lisuride a drug for parkinsonism 18

lithium 292 an antimanic drug 16

Lithonate a brand name for lithium 292 (an antimanic drug 16)

Livial a brand name for tibolone 405 (a female sex hormone 88)

Livostin a brand name for levocabastine (an antihistamine 58)

Locabiotal a brand name for fusafungine (a topical antibacterial 120)

local anaesthetics see analgesics 9

Loceryl a brand name for amorolfine (an antifungal drug 76)

Locoid a brand name for hydrocortisone 264 (a corticosteroid 80)

Locorten-Vioform a brand name for clioquinol (an anti-infective skin preparation 120) with flumetasone (a corticosteroid 80)

Lodine a brand name for etodolac (a non-steroidal anti-inflammatory drug 50)

Iodoxamide a topical treatment for allergic conjunctivitis

Loestrin 20 a brand-named oral contraceptive 105 containing ethinylestradiol 240 and norethisterone 332 (both female sex hormones 88)

lofepramine 293 a tricyclic antidepressant 14

lofexidine a drug to treat opioid withdrawal symptoms

Logynon a brand-named oral contraceptive 105 containing ethinylestradiol 240 and levonorgestrel 289

Logynon ED a brand-named oral contraceptive 105 containing ethinylestradiol 240 and levonorgestrel 289

Lomexin a brand name for fenticonazole (an antifungal drug 76)

Lomotil a brand-named antidiarrhoeal 44 with atropine 150 and diphenoxylate (an opioid)

lomustine an alkylating agent for Hodgkin's disease 96

Loniten a brand name for minoxidil 320 (a vasodilator 31 and antihypertensive 36)

loop diuretics a group of diuretic drugs 32

LoperaGen a brand name for loperamide 294 (an opioid antidiarrhoeal 44)

loperamide 294 an opioid antidiarrhoeal 44

Lopid a brand name for gemfibrozil (a lipid-lowering drug 37)

Lopinavir with ritonavir a combination of two protease inhibitor drugs for HIV/AIDS 100

loprazolam a benzodiazepine sleeping drug 11

Lopresor a brand name for metoprolol 315 (a cardioselective beta blocker 30)

Lopresor SR a brand name for metoprolol 315 (a cardioselective beta blocker 30)

loratadine 297 an antihistamine 58

lorazepam a benzodiazepine anti-anxiety drug 13 and sleeping drug 11

lormetazepam a benzodiazepine sleeping drug 11

lornoxicam a non-steroidal anti-inflammatory 50

losartan 297 an angiotensin II blocker vasodilator 31 and antihypertensive 36

Losec a brand name for omeprazole 336 (an anti-ulcer drug 43)

Lotriderm a brand-named product containing betamethasone 158 (a corticosteroid 80) and clotrimazole 196 (an antifungal 76)

Luborant a brand name for artificial saliva

Ludiomil a brand name for maprotiline (an antidepressant 14)

Lugol's solution an iodine liquid for overactive thyroid gland 84

lumefantrine see **artemether with lumefantrine**

Lustral a brand name for sertraline 381 (an SSRI antidepressant 14)

luteinizing hormone a drug for infertility 109

lutropin alfa a drug for infertility 109

Lyclear a brand name for permethrin 344 (a drug to treat skin parasites 122)

lymecycline a tetracycline antibiotic 62

Lysovir a brand name for amantadine (an antiviral drug used for influenza 69)

M

Maalox a brand-named antacid 42 containing aluminium hydroxide 136 and magnesium hydroxide 299

Maalox Plus a brand-named antacid 42 with aluminium hydroxide 136, magnesium hydroxide 299, and dimeticone

Mabcampath a brand name for alemtuzumab (an anticancer drug 96)

Mabthera a brand name for rituximab (an anticancer drug 96)

Macrobid a brand name for nitrofurantoin (an antibacterial 66)

Macrodantin a brand name for nitrofurantoin (an antibacterial 66)

Madopar a brand name for co-beneldopa (a drug for parkinsonism 18)

Magnapen a brand name for ampicillin with flucloxacillin 244 (penicillin antibiotics 62)

magnesium a mineral 93

magnesium alginate an antifoaming agent 42

magnesium carbonate an antacid 42

magnesium citrate an osmotic laxative 45

magnesium compounds a type of antacid 42

magnesium hydroxide 299 (an antacid 42 and osmotic laxative 45)

magnesium oxide an antacid 42

magnesium sulphate an osmotic laxative 45

magnesium trisilicate an antacid 42

Malarone a brand-named antimalarial 75 containing proguanil with atovaquone 358

malathion 300 an antiparasitic drug 122 for head lice and scabies

male sex hormones 87

Manerix a brand name for moclobemide (a reversible MAOI antidepressant 14)

Manevac a brand name for ispaghula (a bulk-forming agent) with senna (both laxatives 45)

mannitol an osmotic diuretic 32

MAOIs see **monoamine oxidase inhibitors**

maprotiline an antidepressant 14

Marcain a brand name for bupivacaine (a local anaesthetic used in labour 110)

Marevan a brand name for warfarin 417, an anticoagulant drug 38

Marvelon a brand-named oral contraceptive 105 with ethinylestradiol 240 and desogestrel

Maxalt a brand name for rizatriptan (a drug for migraine 20)

Maxepa a brand name for concentrated fish oils (used to lower triglyceride levels in the blood 37)

Maxidex a brand name for dexamethasone 210 (a corticosteroid 80) with hypromellose (used in artificial tear preparations)

Maxitrol a brand name for dexamethasone 210 (a corticosteroid 80) with hypromellose (used in artificial tear preparations) and neomycin and polymyxin B (both antibiotics 62)

Maxolon a brand name for metoclopramide 314 (a gastrointestinal motility regulator and anti-emetic 21)

Maxtrex a brand name for methotrexate 311 (an antimetabolite anticancer drug 96)

MCR-50 a brand name for isosorbide mononitrate 277 (a nitrate vasodilator 31 and anti-angina drug 35)

MCT Oil a drug used to treat cystic fibrosis

mebendazole an anthelmintic 78

mebeverine 301 an antispasmodic for irritable bowel syndrome 45

meclozine an antihistamine 58 used for travel sickness (anti-emetics 21)

mecysteine a mucolytic for coughs 27

Medijel a brand name for an analgesic mouth gel containing lidocaine (a local anaesthetic 9) and aminacrine (a skin antiseptic 120)

Medinex a brand name for diphenhydramine (an antihistamine 58)

Medinol a brand name for paracetamol 381 (a non-opioid analgesic 80)

Medised a brand name for paracetamol 341 (a non-opioid analgesic 9) with promethazine 360 (an antihistamine 58 and anti-emetic 21)

Medrone a brand name for methylprednisolone (a corticosteroid 80)

medroxyprogesterone 301 a female sex hormone 88 and anticancer drug 96

mefenamic acid 302 a non-steroidal anti-inflammatory drug 50

mefloquine 304 an antimalarial drug 75

Mefoxin a brand name for cefoxitin (a cephalosporin antibiotic 62)

Megace a brand name for megestrol 305 (a female sex hormone 88 and anticancer drug 96)

megestrol 305 a female sex hormone 88 and anticancer drug 96

melatonin a hormone made by the pineal gland to regulate the sleep–wake cycle; synthetic forms are thought to relieve insomnia

Melgisorb a wound dressing with alginates 133

Melleril a brand name for thioridazine (a phenothiazine antipsychotic 15)

meloxicam 306 a non-steroidal anti-inflammatory drug 50 and analgesic 9

melphalan an alkylating agent for multiple myeloma 96

memantidine an NMDA receptor antagonist used to treat Alzheimer's disease

menadiol vitamin K (a vitamin 90)

Menorest a brand name for estradiol 238, an oestrogen (female sex hormones 88)

menotrophin also called human menopausal gonadotrophins, a drug for infertility 109

menthol an alcohol from mint oils used as an inhalation and topical antipruritic 118

mepacrine an antiprotozoal 73 for giardiasis

mepivacaine a local anaesthetic 11

meprobamate an anti-anxiety drug 13

meptazinol an opioid analgesic 9

Meptid a brand name for meptazinol (an opioid analgesic 9)

mepyramine a topical antihistamine used in skin cream (antipruritics 118)

Merbentyl a brand name for dicycloverine 214 (a drug for irritable bowel syndrome 45)

mercaptamine a drug used for metabolic disorders

mercaptopurine 307 an anticancer drug 96

Mercilon a brand-named oral contraceptive 105 containing ethinylestradiol 240 and desogestrel (a progestogen)

Merional a brand name for menotrophin (a drug for infertility 109)

Merocaine Lozenges brand-named lozenges for sore throat and minor mouth infections, with benzocaine, a local anaesthetic 11 and cetylpyridinium (an antiseptic)

Merocets a brand name for cetylpyridinium (an antiseptic)

meropenem an antibiotic 62

mesalazine 308 a drug for ulcerative colitis (an inflammatory bowel disease 46)

mesna a drug used to protect the urinary tract from damage caused by some anticancer drugs 96

mesterolone a male sex hormone 87

Mestinon a brand name for pyridostigmine 363 (a drug for myasthenia gravis 55)

mestranol an oestrogen (female sex hormones 88) and oral contraceptive 105

metaraminol a drug used to treat hypotension (low blood pressure)

Metenix-5 a brand name for metolazone (a thiazide-like diuretic 32)

metformin 309 a drug used in diabetes 82

methadone 310 an opioid used to treat heroin dependence and as an analgesic 9

Methadose a brand name for methadone 310 (an opioid used to treat heroin dependence and as an analgesic 9)

Metharose a brand name for methadone 310 (an opioid used to treat heroin dependence and as an analgesic 9)

methenamine a drug for urinary tract infections 112

Methex a brand name for methadone 310 (an opioid used to treat heroin dependence and as an analgesic 9)

methionine an antidote for poisoning with paracetamol 341

methocarbamol a muscle relaxant 54

methotrexate 311 an antimetabolite anticancer drug 96

methylcellulose 312 (a laxative 45, antidiarrhoeal 44, and artificial tear preparation)

methyldopa 313 an antihypertensive 36

methylphenidate a drug used to treat hyperactivity in children

methylprednisolone a corticosteroid 80

methyl salicylate a topical analgesic 9 for muscle and joint pain

methysergide a drug to prevent migraine 20

metipranolol a beta blocker 30 used for glaucoma 114

metirosine a drug for phaeochromocytoma (tumour of the adrenal glands)

metoclopramide 314 a gastrointestinal motility regulator and anti-emetic 21

metolazone a thiazide-like diuretic 32

Metopirone a brand name for metyrapone (a diuretic used to reduce fluid retention in Cushing's disease)

metoprolol 315 a beta blocker 30

Metosyn a brand name for fluocinonide (a topical corticosteroid 120)

Metrodin a brand name for urofollitropin (a drug for infertility 109)

Metrogel a brand name for topical metronidazole 316 (an antibacterial 66)

Metrolyl a brand name for metronidazole 316 (an antibacterial 66 and antiprotozoal 73)

metronidazole 316 an antibacterial drug 66 and antiprotozoal drug 73

Metrotop a brand name for topical metronidazole 316 (an antibacterial 66)

metyrapone a diuretic used to reduce fluid retention in Cushing's disease

mexiletine an anti-arrhythmic 33

Mexitil a brand name for mexiletine (an anti-arrhythmic 33)

mianserin an antidepressant 14

Micardis Plus a brand-named antihypertensive 36 with telmisartan (an angiotensin II blocker vasodilator 31) and hydrochlorothiazide 263 (a thiazide diuretic 32)

miconazole 318 an antifungal drug 76

Microgynon 30 a brand-named oral contraceptive 105 with ethinylestradiol 240 and levonorgestrel 289

Micronor a brand-named oral contraceptive 105 containing norethisterone 332 (both female sex hormones 88)

Microval a brand-named oral contraceptive 105 containing levonorgestrel 289

Mictral a brand-named drug for urinary tract infections 112 containing nalidixic acid (an antibacterial 66) and sodium bicarbonate 385

midazolam a benzodiazepine used as premedication

Midrid a brand-named drug for migraine 20 containing paracetamol 341 and isometheptene mucate

Mifegyne a brand name for mifepristone (a drug used during labour 110)

mifepristone a drug used during labour 110

migraine, drugs used for 20

Migraleve a brand-named drug for migraine 20 with codeine 198, paracetamol 341, and buclizine (an antihistamine anti-emetic 21)

MigraMax a brand-named analgesic for migraine 20 containing aspirin 146 and metoclopramide 314 (an anti-emetic 21)

Migril a brand-named drug for migraine 20 with ergotamine 234, caffeine, and cyclizine

Milk of Magnesia a brand name for magnesium hydroxide 299 (an antacid 42 and osmotic laxative 45)

Milpar a brand-named laxative 45 containing magnesium hydroxide 299 and liquid paraffin

milrinone a drug used for its vasodilator 31 effects to treat heart failure

minerals 93

Minihep a brand name for heparin 262, an anticoagulant drug 38)

Min-I-Jet Adrenaline a brand name for epinephrine 233

Minims Atropine a brand name for atropine 150 (a mydriatic drug affecting the pupil 116)

Minims Chloramphenicol a brand name for chloramphenicol 175 (an antibiotic 62)

Minims Cyclopentolate a brand name for cyclopentolate (a mydriatic drug affecting the pupil 116)

Minims Gentamicin a brand name for gentamicin 254 (an aminoglycoside antibiotic 62)

Minims Phenylephrine a brand name for phenylephrine (a decongestant 26)

Minims Pilocarpine a brand name for pilocarpine 349 (a miotic for glaucoma 114)

Minims Prednisolone a brand name for prednisolone 354 (a corticosteroid 80)

Minitran a brand name for glyceryl trinitrate 257 (an anti-angina drug 35)

Minocin a brand name for minocycline 318 (a tetracycline antibiotic 62)

minocycline 318 (a tetracycline antibiotic 62)

Minodiab a brand name for glipizide (an oral drug used in diabetes 82)

minoxidil 320 a vasodilator 31 used as an antihypertensive 36 and as a treatment for hair loss 127

Mintec a brand name for peppermint oil (a substance for irritable bowel syndrome 45)

Mintezol a brand name for tiabendazole (an anthelmintic 78)

Minulet a brand-named oral contraceptive 105 containing ethinylestradiol 240 and gestodene (a progestogen)

miotics a group of drugs for glaucoma 114 and drugs affecting the pupil 116

Mirapexin a brand name for pramipexole (a drug for parkinsonism 18)

Mirena a brand-named intrauterine contraceptive device containing levonorgestrel 289 (a female sex hormone 88)

mirtazapine an antidepressant 14

misoprostol 321 an anti-ulcer drug 43

Mistamine a brand name for mizolastine (an antihistamine 58)

mitobronitol an anticancer drug 96

mitomycin a cytotoxic antibiotic for breast and stomach cancer 96

mitoxantrone an anticancer drug 96

mivacurium a drug used to relax muscles during general anaesthesia

Mixtard a brand name for insulin 271 (a drug used in diabetes 82)

mizolastine an antihistamine 58

Mizollen a brand name for mizolastine (an antihistamine 58)

Mobic a brand name for meloxicam 306 (a non-steroidal anti-inflammatory drug 50 and analgesic 9)

Mobiflex a brand name for tenoxicam (a non-steroidal anti-inflammatory dug 50)

moclobemide a reversible MAOI antidepressant drug 14

modafinil a drug for narcolepsy (nervous system stimulants 19)

Modalim a brand name for ciprofibrate (a lipid-lowering drug 37)

Modecate a brand name for fluphenazine (an antipsychotic 15)

Modisal XL a brand name for isosorbide mononitrate 277 (a nitrate vasodilator 31 and anti-angina drug 35)

Moditen a brand name for fluphenazine (an antipsychotic 15)

Modrasone a brand name for alclometasone (a topical corticosteroid 120)

Modrenal a brand name for trilostane, an adrenal antagonist used for Cushing's syndrome (an adrenal disorder) and for breast cancer 96

Moducren a brand-named antihypertensive 36 containing amiloride 137 and hydrochlorothiazide 263 (both diuretics), and timolol 406 (a beta blocker 30)

Moduret-25 a brand name for amiloride 137 with hydrochlorothiazide 263 (both diuretics 32)

Moduretic a brand name for amiloride 137 with hydrochlorothiazide 263 (both diuretics 32)

moexipril an ACE inhibitor vasodilator 31

Mogadon a brand name for nitrazepam 331 (a benzodiazepine sleeping drug 11)

molgramostim a blood growth stimulant

Molipaxin a brand name for trazodone (an antidepressant 14)

molybdenum a mineral 93 required in minute amounts in the diet, but poisonous if ingested in large quantities

mometasone 322 a topical corticosteroid 120

Monit a brand name for isosorbide mononitrate 277 (a nitrate vasodilator 31 and anti-angina drug 35)

Monoamine oxidase inhibitors (MAOIs) a group of antidepressants 14

Mono-Cedocard a brand name for isosorbide mononitrate 277 (a nitrate vasodilator 31 and anti-angina drug 35)

Monoclate-P a brand name for factor VIII, a blood extract used to promote blood clotting 38

monoclonal antibodies a group of anticancer drugs 96

Monocor a brand name for bisoprolol (a beta blocker 30)

Monomax a brand name for isosorbide mononitrate 277 (a nitrate vasodilator 31 and anti-angina drug 35)

Monoparin, Monoparin CA brand names for heparin 262 (an anticoagulant drug 38)

Monotrim a brand name for trimethoprim 412 (an antibacterial 66)

Monovent a brand name for terbutaline 401 (a sympathomimetic bronchodilator drug 23 and drug for premature labour 110)

Monozide 10 a brand name for bisoprolol (a beta blocker 30) with hydrochlorothiazide 263 (a thiazide diuretic 32)

Monphytol a brand-named antifungal drug 76 for athlete's foot

montelukast 323 a leukotriene antagonist for asthma 24 and allergy 60

moracizine an anti-arrhythmic agent 33

Morcap SR a brand name for morphine 323 (an opioid analgesic 9)

morphine 323 an opioid analgesic 9

Motens a brand name for lacidipine (a calcium channel blocker vasodilator 31)

Motifene a brand name for diclofenac 212 (a non-steroidal anti-inflammatory drug 50)

Motilium a brand name for domperidone 220 (an anti-emetic 21)

Motipress a brand name for fluphenazine (an antipsychotic 15) with nortriptyline (a tricyclic antidepressant 14)

Motival a brand name for fluphenazine (an antipsychotic 15) with nortriptyline (a tricyclic antidepressant 14)

Motrin a brand name for ibuprofen 267 (a non-steroidal anti-inflammatory drug 50)

Movelat a brand-named topical preparation containing mucopolysaccharide and salicylic acid

Movicol a brand-named osmotic laxative 45 containing sodium bicarbonate 385, sodium chloride, and potassium chloride

moxisylyte a drug used to reduce pupil size after examination 116 and as a vasodilator 31 to improve blood supply to the limbs

moxonidine 325 a centrally acting antihypertensive drug 36

MST Continus a brand name for morphine 323 (an opioid analgesic 9)

Mucodyne a brand name for carbocisteine (a mucolytic drug for coughs 27)

Mucogel a brand-named antacid 42 containing aluminium hydroxide 136 and magnesium hydroxide 299

Mu-Cron Tablets a brand name for phenylpropanolamine 347 (a decongestant 26) with paracetamol 341 (a non-opioid analgesic 9)

Multiparin a brand name for heparin 262 (an anticoagulant drug 38)

mupirocin an anti-infective skin preparation 120 for skin and nose infections

MUSE a brand name for alprostadil 135 (a prostaglandin and drug for impotence 109)

MXL a brand name for morphine sulphate 323 (an opioid analgesic 9)

myasthenia gravis, drugs used for 55

Mycil a brand name for clotrimazole 196 (an antifungal drug 76)

Mycobutin a brand name for rifabutin (an antituberculous drug 67)

mycophenolate mofetil an immunosuppressant drug 99

Mycota a brand name for undecanoate acid (an antifungal drug 76)

Mydriacyl a brand name for tropicamide (a mydriatic drug affecting the pupil 116)

Mydrilate a brand name for cyclopentolate (a mydriatic drug affecting the pupil 116)

Myelobromol a brand name for mitobronitol (an anticancer drug 96)

Myleran a brand name for busulphan (an alkylating anticancer drug 96)

Myocet a brand name for doxorubicin 226 (a cytotoxic anticancer drug 96)

Myocrisin a brand name for sodium aurothiomalate (an antirheumatic drug 52)

Myotonine a brand name for bethanechol (a parasympathomimetic drug for urinary retention 112)

Mysoline a brand name for primidone (an anticonvulsant 16)

N

nabilone an anti-emetic 21 derived from marijuana and used for nausea and vomiting induced by anticancer drugs 96

nabumetone a non-steroidal anti-inflammatory drug 50

nadolol a beta blocker 30

nafarelin a drug for menstrual disorders 104

naftidrofuryl 326 a vasodilator 31

nalbuphine an opioid analgesic 9

Nalcrom a brand name for sodium cromoglicate 386 (an anti-allergy drug 60)

nalidixic acid a quinolone antibacterial 66

Nalorex a brand name for naltrexone (a drug for opioid withdrawal)

naloxone an antidote for opioid poisoning

naltrexone a drug for opioid withdrawal

nandrolone an anabolic steroid 88

Napratec a brand named antirheumatic drug 52 containing naproxen 326 (a non-steroidal anti-inflammatory drug 50 and drug for gout 53) and misoprostol 321 (an anti-ulcer drug 43)

Naprosyn a brand name for naproxen 326 (an NSAID 50 and drug for gout 53)

naproxen 326 a non-steroidal anti-inflammatory drug 50 and drug for gout 53

Naramig a brand name for naratriptan (a 5HT$_1$ agonist drug for migraine 20)

naratriptan a 5HT$_1$ agonist drug for migraine 20

Narcan a brand name for naloxone (an antidote for opioid poisoning)

Nardil a brand name for phenelzine (an MAOI antidepressant 14)

Naropin a brand name for ropivacaine (a local anaesthetic 9)

Naseptin a brand name for chlorhexidine (a skin antiseptic 120) with neomycin (an aminoglycoside antibiotic 62)

Nasobec a brand name for beclometasone 154 (a corticosteroid 80)

Nasonex a brand name for mometasone 322 (a topical corticosteroid 120)

nateglinide a drug used in diabetes 82

Natrilix a brand name for indapamide 269 (a thiazide-like diuretic 32 and antihypertensive drug 36)

Navelbine a brand name for vinorelbine (an anticancer drug 96)

Navidrex a brand name for cyclopenthiazide (a thiazide diuretic 32)

Navispare a brand name for cyclopenthiazide with amiloride 137 (both diuretics 32)

Navoban a brand name for tropisetron (an anti-emetic 21)

Nebcin a brand name for tobramycin (an aminoglycoside antibiotic 62)

Nebilet a brand name for nebivolol (a beta blocker 30 and antihypertensive 36)

nebivolol a beta blocker 30 and antihypertensive 36

nedocromil a drug similar to sodium cromoglicate 386, used to prevent asthma attacks 24

nefopam a non-opioid analgesic 9

Negram a brand name for nalidixic acid (a quinolone antibacterial 66)

nelfinavir a protease inhibitor drug for HIV/AIDS 100

NeoClarityn a brand name for desloratadine (an antihistamine 58)

Neogest a brand name for norgestrel (a female sex hormone 88)

Neo-Mercazole a brand name for carbimazole 179 (an antithyroid drug 84)

neomycin an aminoglycoside antibiotic 62 also used in ear drops 117

Neo-NaClex a brand name for bendroflumethiazide 155 (a thiazide diuretic 32)

Neo-NaClex-K a brand name for bendroflumethiazide 155 (a thiazide diuretic 32) with potassium (a mineral 91)

Neoral a brand name for ciclosporin 182 (an immunosuppressant 99)

NeoRecormon a brand name for erythropoietin 237 (a kidney hormone)

Neosporin a brand name for gramicidin with neomycin and polymyxin B (all antibiotics 62)

neostigmine a drug for myasthenia gravis 55

Neotigason a brand name for acitretin (a drug for psoriasis 124)

Nerisone a brand name for diflucortolone (a topical corticosteroid 120)

Netillin a brand name for netilmicin (an aminoglycoside antibiotic 62)

netilmicin an aminoglycoside antibiotic 62

Neulactil a brand name for pericyazine (an antipsychotic 15)

Neupogen a brand name for filgrastim 243 (a blood growth stimulant)

Neurontin a brand name for gabapentin 253 (an anticonvulsant 16)

nevirapine a reverse transcriptase inhibitor drug for HIV/AIDS 100

Nexium a brand name for esomeprazole (an anti-ulcer drug 43)

niacin a B vitamin (vitamins 90)

nicardipine a calcium channel blocker vasodilator 31

niclosamide an anthelmintic drug 78 for tapeworms

nicorandil 328 an anti-angina drug 35

Nicorette a brand name for nicotine 329 given to relieve smoking withdrawal symptoms

nicotinamide a B vitamin (vitamins 90)

nicotine 329 a substance given as a drug to relieve smoking withdrawal symptoms

Nicotinell a brand name for nicotine 329 given to relieve smoking withdrawal symptoms

nicotinic acid a vitamin 90, also called niacin; a vasodilator 31; and a lipid-lowering drug 37

nicotinyl alcohol tartrate niacin (a vitamin 90)

nifedipine 330 a calcium channel blocker vasodilator 31, anti-angina drug 35, and antihypertensive 36

Nifedipress MR a brand name for nifedipine 330 (a calcium channel blocker vasodilator 31, anti-angina drug 35, and antihypertensive 36

Niferex a brand name for iron (a mineral 93)

Night Nurse a brand-named cold remedy containing paracetamol 341 (a non-opioid analgesic 9) with promethazine 360 (an antihistamine 58 and anti-emetic 21)

nikethamide a respiratory stimulant

nimodipine a calcium channel blocker vasodilator 31

Nindaxa a brand name for indapamide 269 (a thiazide-like diuretic 32 and antihypertensive 36)

Nipent a brand name for pentostatin (an anticancer drug 96)

NiQuitin CQ a brand name for nicotine 329 used to relieve smoking withdrawal symptoms

Nirolex for Chesty Coughs an expectorant drug for coughs 27 containing guaiphenesin

Nirolex Lozenges a cough suppressant 27 containing dextromethorphan and menthol

nisoldipine a calcium channel blocker vasodilator 31, anti-angina drug 35, and antihypertensive drug 36

nitrates a group of vasodilators 31 used as anti-angina drugs 35

nitrazepam 331 a benzodiazepine sleeping drug 11

Nitrocine a brand name for glyceryl trinitrate 257 (an anti-angina drug 35)

Nitro-Dur a brand name for glyceryl trinitrate 257 (an anti-angina drug 35)

nitrofurantoin an antibacterial 66 for urinary disorders 112

Nitrolingual a brand name for glyceryl trinitrate 257 (an anti-angina drug 35)

Nitronal a brand name for glyceryl trinitrate 257 (an anti-angina drug 35)

nitroprusside antihypertensive 36

nitrous oxide anaesthetic gas

Nivaquine a brand name for chloroquine 177 (an antimalarial 75 and antirheumatic 52)

Nivemycin a brand name for neomycin (an aminoglycoside antibiotic 62)

nizatidine an H_2 blocker anti-ulcer drug 43

Nizoral a brand name for ketoconazole 280 (an antifungal drug 76)

Nocutil a brand name for desmopressin 209 (a synthetic pituitary hormone 85 used for diabetes insipidus)

Nolvadex a brand name for tamoxifen 395 (an anticancer drug 96)

Nolvadex Forte a brand name for tamoxifen 395 (an anticancer drug 96)

non-opoid analgesics 9

nonoxinol '9' a spermicidal agent

nonacog alfa a synthetic form of factor IX to promote blood clotting 38

Non-steroidal anti-inflammatory drugs (NSAIDs) 50 (analgesics 9, drugs for menstrual disorders 104, and antirheumatic drugs 52)

Nootropil a brand name for piracetam (an anticonvulsant 16)

noradrenaline see **norepinephrine**

Norditropin a brand name for somatropin (a synthetic pituitary hormone 85)

norepinephrine also known as noradrenaline (a drug similar to epinephrine 233 used to raise blood pressure in shock)

norethisterone 332 a progestogen female sex hormone 88 and oral contraceptive 105

norfloxacin a quinolone antibacterial 66

Norgalax a brand name for docusate sodium (a stimulant laxative 45)

norgestimate an oral contraceptive 105

Norgeston a brand-named oral contraceptive 105 containing levonorgestrel 289

norgestrel a progestogen female sex hormone 88

Noriday a brand-named oral contraceptive 105 containing norethisterone 332 (a female sex hormone 88)

Norimin a brand-named oral contraceptive 105 containing ethinylestradiol 240 and norethisterone 332 (both female sex hormones 88)

Norimode a brand name for loperamide 294 (an opioid antidiarrhoeal drug 44)

Norinyl a brand-named oral contraceptive 105 containing norethisterone 332 and mestranol (both female sex hormones 88)

Norinyl-1 a brand-named oral contraceptive 105 containing norethisterone 332 and mestranol (both female sex hormones 88)

Noristerat a brand-named injectable contraceptive containing norethisterone 332 (a female sex hormone 88)

Noritate a brand name for metronidazole 316 (an antibacterial 66 and antiprotozoal 73)

Normacol Plus a brand name for frangula with sterculia (both laxatives 45)

Normaloe a brand name for loperamide 294 (an opioid antidiarrhoeal drug 44)

Normax a brand name for dantron and docusate (both laxatives 45)

Normosang a brand name for haem arginate (a drug to treat porphyria)

Norprolac a brand name for quinagolide (a drug to reduce prolactin levels and for pituitary disorders 85)

nortriptyline a tricyclic antidepressant 14

Norvir a brand name for ritonavir (a protease inhibitor drug for HIV/AIDS 100)

NovoNorm a brand name for repaglinide 372 (an oral drug used in diabetes 82)

NovoRapid a brand name for insulin aspart, a type of insulin 271 (a drug for diabetes 82)

Nozinan a brand name for methotrimeprazine (an antipsychotic 15)

NSAIDs see **Non-steroidal anti-inflammatory drugs**

Nubain a brand name for nalbuphine (an opioid analgesic 9)

Nuelin a brand name for theophylline 404 (a xanthine bronchodilator drug 23)

Nulacin a brand-named antacid 42 containing calcium carbonate, magnesium carbonate, magnesium trisilicate, and magnesium oxide

Nupercainal a brand name for cinchocaine, a local anaesthetic 11

Nurofen a brand name for ibuprofen 267 (a non-steroidal anti-inflammatory drug 50 and analgesic 9)

Nurofen Plus a brand name for ibuprofen 267 (a non-steroidal anti-inflammatory drug 50) with codeine 198 (an opioid analgesic 9)

Nu-Seals Aspirin a brand name for aspirin 146, a non-opioid analgesic 9 and antiplatelet drug 38

Nutraplus a brand name for urea (an emollient and hydrating agent for skin)

nutrition 90

Nutrizym GR a brand name for pancreatin (a preparation of pancreatic enzymes 49)

Nuvelle a brand name for estradiol 238 and levonorgestrel 289 (female sex hormones 88)

Nycopren a brand name for naproxen 326 (a non-steroidal anti-inflammatory drug 50 and drug for gout 53)

Nylax with senna a brand-named stimulant laxative 45 containing senna

Nyogel a brand name for timolol 406 (a beta blocker 30 and drug for glaucoma 114)

Nystaform a brand name for nystatin 333 (an antifungal drug 76) with chlorhexidine (a skin antiseptic 120)

Nystaform-HC a brand name for hydrocortisone 264 (a corticosteroid 80) with nystatin 333 (an antifungal drug 76) and chlorhexidine (a skin antiseptic 120)

Nystamont a brand name for nystatin 333 (an antifungal drug 76)

Nystan a brand name for nystatin 333 (an antifungal drug 76)

nystatin 333 an antifungal drug 76

Nytol a brand-named preparation for sleep disturbance containing diphenhydramine (an antihistamine 58)

O

Occlusal a brand name for salicylic acid (a keratolytic 123 wart remover)

octocog alfa synthetic form of factor VIII to promote blood clotting 38

octoxinol a spermicidal agent

octreotide a synthetic pituitary hormone 85 used to relieve symptoms of cancer of the pancreas 96

octylcyanoacrylate a tissue adhesive

Ocufen a brand name for flurbiprofen (a non-steroidal anti-inflammatory drug 50)

Odrik a brand name for trandolapril (an ACE inhibitor vasodilator 31)

Oestrogel a brand name for estradiol 238, an oestrogen (female sex hormones 88)

oestrogen a female sex hormone 88

ofloxacin a quinolone antibacterial 66

Oilatum Emollient a brand-named bath additive containing liquid paraffin for dry skin

Oilatum Gel a brand name for a shower gel containing liquid paraffin for dry skin

olanzapine 335 an antipsychotic drug 15

Olbetam a brand name for acipimox (a lipid-lowering drug 37)

olsalazine an aminosalicylate drug for inflammatory bowel disease 46

Omacor a brand name for omega 3 acid ethyl esters (a lipid-lowering drug 37)

omega 3 acid ethyl esters a lipid-lowering drug 37

omega 3 marine triglycerides a lipid-lowering drug 37

omeprazole 336 an anti-ulcer drug 43

Oncovin a brand name for vincristine (an anticancer drug 96)

ondansetron 337 an anti-emetic 21

One-Alpha a brand name for alfacalcidol, vitamin D (vitamins 90)

Opilon a brand name for moxisylyte (a vasodilator 31)

opioids drugs used as analgesics 9, as antidiarrhoeals 44, as cough suppressants 27, and in labour 110

opium morphine 323 (an opioid analgesic 9)

Oprisine a brand name for azathioprine 151 (an antirheumatic 52 and immunosuppressant drug 99)

Opticrom a brand name for sodium cromoglicate 386 (an anti-allergy drug 60)

Optrex Eye Lotion a brand-named preparation containing witch hazel (an astringent)

Orabase a brand-named ointment to protect the skin or mouth from damage

oral contraceptives 105

Oraldene a brand-named antiseptic mouthwash containing hexetidine

Oramorph a brand name for morphine 323 (an opioid analgesic 9)

Orap a brand name for pimozide (an antipsychotic 15)

orciprenaline a sympathomimetic drug for asthma 24

Orelox a brand name for cefpodoxime (a cephalosporin antibiotic 62)

Organan a brand name for danaparoid, an anticoagulant drug 38

Orimeten a brand name for aminoglutethimide (an anticancer drug 96)

Orlept a brand name for sodium valproate 387 (an anticonvulsant 16)

orlistat 337 an anti-obesity drug

Orovite a brand-named multivitamin 90

orphenadrine 338 an anticholinergic muscle relaxant 54 and drug for parkinsonism 18

Ortho-Creme a brand name for nonoxinol '9' (a spermicidal agent)

Orthoforms a brand name for nonoxinol '9' (a spermicidal agent)

Ortho-Gynest a brand name for estriol, an oestrogen (female sex hormones 88)

Orudis a brand name for ketoprofen 281 (a non-steroidal anti-inflammatory drug 50)

Oruvail a brand name for ketoprofen 281 (a non-steroidal anti-inflammatory drug 50)

oseltamivir an antiviral drug 69 for influenza

osmotic diuretics 32

osmotic laxatives 45

Ossopan a brand name for hydroxyapatite (a calcium supplement to treat bone disorders 56)

Ostram a brand name for calcium phosphate (a mineral 93)

Otomize a brand name for dexamethasone 210 (a corticosteroid 80) with neomycin (an aminoglycoside antibiotic 62)

Otosporin a brand name for hydrocortisone 264 (a corticosteroid 80) with neomycin and polymyxin B (both antibiotics 62)

Otrivine a brand name for xylometazoline (a decongestant 26)

Otrivine-Antistin brand-named eye drops containing antazoline (an antihistamine 58) with xylometazoline (a decongestant 26)

Ovestin a brand name for estriol, an oestrogen (female sex hormones 88)

Ovex a brand name for mebendazole (an anthelmintic 78)

Ovranette a brand-named oral contraceptive 105 containing ethinylestradiol 240 and levonorgestrel 289

Ovysmen a brand-named oral contraceptive 105 containing ethinylestradiol 240 and norethisterone 332 (both female sex hormones 88)

oxaliplatin an anticancer drug 96

oxazepam a benzodiazepine anti-anxiety drug 13

oxcarbazepine an anticonvulsant 16

oxerutin a drug used to treat peripheral vascular disease

oxitropium an anticholinergic bronchodilator 23

Oxivent a brand name for oxitropium (an anticholinergic bronchodilator drug 23)

oxprenolol a beta blocker 30

oxybenzone an ingredient in sunscreens 128

oxybuprocaine a local anaesthetic 11

oxybutynin 339 an anticholinergic and antispasmodic for urinary disorders 112

oxycodone an opioid analgesic 9

oxymetazoline a topical decongestant 26 also used for ear disorders 117

Oxymycin a brand name for oxytetracycline (a tetracycline antibiotic 62)

oxytetracycline a tetracycline antibiotic 62

oxytocin a drug used in labour 110

P

Pacifene a brand name for ibuprofen 267 (an analgesic 9 and non-steroidal anti-inflammatory drug 50)

paclitaxel an anticancer drug 96

Painkillers see **Analgesics**

Paldesic a brand name for paracetamol 341 (a non-opioid analgesic 9)

Palfium a brand name for dextromoramide (an opioid analgesic 9)

palivizumab an antiviral drug 69

Palladone a brand name for hydromorphone (an opioid analgesic 9)

Paludrine a brand name for proguanil 358 (an antimalarial drug 75)

pamidronate a drug for bone disorders 56

Panadeine a brand name for paracetamol 341 (a non-opioid analgesic 9) with codeine 198

Panadol a brand name for paracetamol 341 (a non-opioid analgesic 9)

Panadol Extra a brand name for paracetamol 341 (a non-opioid analgesic 9) with caffeine

Panadol Ultra a brand name for paracetamol 341 with codeine 198 (both analgesics 9)

Panaleve a brand name for paracetamol 341 (a non-opioid analgesic 9)

Pancrease a brand name for pancreatin (a pancreatic enzyme preparation for pancreatic disorders 49)

pancreatin a pancreatic enzyme preparation for pancreatic disorders 49

Pancrex a brand name for pancreatin (a pancreatic enzyme preparation for pancreatic disorders 49)

pancuronium a muscle relaxant 54 used during general anaesthesia

Panoxyl a brand name for benzoyl peroxide 156 (a drug to treat acne 123)

panthenol pantothenic acid (a vitamin 90)

pantoprazole a proton pump inhibitor anti-ulcer drug 43

pantothenic acid a B vitamin (vitamins 90)

papaveretum an opioid analgesic 9

papaverine a muscle relaxant 54

Papulex a brand name for nicotinamide (a drug used to treat acne 123)

paracetamol 341 a non-opioid analgesic 9

Paracodol a brand-named analgesic 9 containing codeine 198 and paracetamol 341

Paradote a brand-named analgesic 9 containing paracetamol 341 and methionine (an antidote for paracetamol poisoning)

Parake a brand-named analgesic 9 containing codeine 198 and paracetamol 341

paraldehyde an anticonvulsant 16 used for status epilepticus

Paramax a brand-named migraine drug 20 containing paracetamol 341 and metoclopramide 314

Paramol a brand name for paracetamol 341 with dihydrocodeine 216 (both analgesics 9)

Paraplatin a brand name for carboplatin (an anticancer drug 96)

Parasympathomimetics drugs used for urinary disorders 112 and myasthenia gravis 55

parecoxib an analgesic 9 and non-steroidal anti-inflammatory drug 50

Pariet a brand name for rabeprazole (a proton pump inhibitor anti-ulcer drug 43)

parkinsonism, drugs for 18

Parlodel a brand name for bromocriptine 161 (a pituitary agent 85 and drug for parkinsonism 18)

Parnate a brand name for tranylcypromine (an MAOI antidepressant 14)

paromomycin an antiprotozoal 73

Paroven a brand name for oxerutin (a vasodilator 31 used to treat peripheral vascular disease)

paroxetine 342 an SSRI antidepressant 14

Parvolex a brand name for acetylcysteine (an antidote for paracetamol overdosage)

Pavacol-D a brand name for pholcodine (an opioid cough suppressant 27)

Pegasys a brand name for peginterferon alfa (an antiviral 69 used to treat hepatitis C)

peginterferon alfa an antiviral 69 used to treat hepatitis C

PegIntron a brand name for peginterferon alfa (an antiviral 69 used to treat hepatitis C)

Penbritin a brand name for ampicillin (a penicillin antibiotic 62)

penciclovir an antiviral drug 69

penicillamine an antirheumatic drug 52

penicillin antibiotics 62

penicillin G see benzylpenicillin (a penicillin antibiotic 62)

penicillin V see phenoxymethylpenicillin 346 (a penicillin antibiotic 62)

Pentacarinat a brand name for pentamidine (an antiprotozoal drug 73)

pentamidine an antiprotozoal 73

Pentasa a brand name for mesalazine 308 (a drug for inflammatory bowel disease 46)

pentazocine an opioid analgesic 9

pentostatin an anticancer drug 96

pentoxifylline a vasodilator 31 used to improve blood flow to the limbs in peripheral vascular disease

Pepcid a brand name for famotidine (an H_2 blocker anti-ulcer drug 43)

peppermint oil a substance for indigestion and bowel spasm in irritable bowel syndrome 45

Peptimax a brand name for cimetidine 183 (an H_2 blocker anti-ulcer drug 43)

Pepto-Bismol a brand-named preparation for diarrhoea 44 and upset stomach, containing bismuth

Percutol a brand name for glyceryl trinitrate 257 (an anti-angina drug 35)

Perdix a brand name for moexipril (an ACE inhibitor vasodilator 31)

Perfan a brand name for enoximone (a drug for heart failure)

pergolide a drug for parkinsonism 18

Periactin a brand name for cyproheptadine (an antihistamine 58 used to stimulate appetite)

pericyazine an antipsychotic 15

Perinal a brand-named spray for haemorrhoids 47 with hydrocortisone 264 (a corticosteroid 80) and lidocaine (a local anaesthetic 9)

perindopril 343 an ACE inhibitor vasodilator 31

permethrin 344 a topical antiparasitic 122

Peroxyl a brand of hydrogen peroxide antiseptic mouthwash

perphenazine an antipsychotic 15 and anti-emetic 21

Persantin a brand name for dipyridamole 218, an antiplatelet drug 38

Peru balsam an antiseptic 120 for haemorrhoids 47

pethidine an opioid analgesic 9 and drug used in labour 110

Pevaryl a brand name for econazole (an antifungal drug 76)

phenelzine an MAOI antidepressant 14

Phenergan a brand name for promethazine 360 (an antihistamine 58 and anti-emetic 21)

phenindione an oral anticoagulant drug 38

phenobarbital 345 a barbiturate anticonvulsant drug 16

phenol an antiseptic used in throat lozenges and sprays

phenothiazines a group of antipsychotic drugs 15 and anti-emetics 21

phenothrin a topical antiparasitic drug for head and pubic lice 122

phenoxybenzamine a drug for phaeochromo-cytoma (adrenal gland tumour)

phenoxymethylpenicillin 346 a penicillin antibiotic 62

Phensic a brand-named analgesic 9 containing aspirin 146 and caffeine

phentermine an appetite suppressant

phenylbutazone a non-steroidal anti-inflammatory drug 50

phenylephrine a decongestant 26

phenylpropanolamine 347 (a decongestant 26)

phenytoin 348 (an anticonvulsant 16)

Phimetin a brand name for cimetidine 183 (an H_2 blocker anti-ulcer drug 43)

Phiso-Med a brand name for chlorhexidine, a skin antiseptic 120

pholcodine an opioid cough suppressant 27

phosphorus a mineral 93

Phyllocontin Continus a brand name for aminophylline 404 (a xanthine bronchodilator 23)

Physeptone a brand name for methadone 310 (an opioid used to treat heroin addiction and as an analgesic 9)

Physiotens a brand name for moxonidine 325 (a centrally acting antihypertensive 36)

Phytex a brand-named antifungal drug 76 containing salicylic acid (a keratolytic 123)

phytomenadione vitamin K (a vitamin 90)

Picolax a brand name for sodium picosulfate and magnesium citrate (both laxatives 45)

pilocarpine 349 a miotic drug for glaucoma 114

Pilogel a brand name for pilocarpine 349 (a miotic drug for glaucoma 114)

pimecrolimus an anti-inflammatory drug for eczema 125

pimozide an antipsychotic 15

pindolol a beta blocker 30

pioglitazone an oral drug used in diabetes 82

piperacillin a penicillin antibiotic 62

piperazine an anthelmintic 78

piperonal a head lice repellent

pipotiazine palmitate an antipsychotic 15

piracetam an anticonvulsant 16

pirenzepine an anticholinergic drug for peptic ulcers 43

Piriteze a brand name for cetirizine (an antihistamine 58)

Piriton a brand name for chlorphenamine 178 (an antihistamine 58)

piroxicam 350 (a non-steroidal anti-inflammatory drug 50 and drug for gout 53)

Pirozip a brand name for piroxicam 350 (a non-steroidal anti-inflammatory drug 50 and drug for gout 53)

pituitary disorders, drugs for 85

pivmecillinam an antibiotic 62

pizotifen 352 a drug for migraine 20

Plaquenil a brand name for hydroxychloroquine (an antimalarial drug 75 and antirheumatic drug 52)

Plavix a brand name for clopidogrel 195 (an antiplatelet drug 38)

Plendil a brand name for felodipine (a calcium channel blocker vasodilator 31)

Pletal a brand name for cilostazol (a vasodilator 31)

podophyllin a topical treatment for genital warts

podophyllotoxin a topical treatment for genital warts

podophyllum a topical treatment for warts

poloxamer a stimulant laxative 45

Polyfax a brand name for bacitracin with polymyxin B (both antibiotics 62)

polymyxin B an antibiotic 62

polynoxylin an antifungal drug 76 and antibacterial drug 66

polystyrene sulphonate a drug to remove excess potassium from the blood

Polytar a brand name for coal tar (a substance used to treat eczema 125, psoriasis 124, and dandruff 126)

Polytrim a brand-named antibacterial drug 66 containing trimethoprim 412 and polymyxin B

polyvinyl alcohol an ingredient of artificial tear preparations

Ponstan a brand name for mefenamic acid 302 (a non-steroidal anti-inflammatory drug 50)

Poractant alfa a drug to mature the lungs of premature babies

porfimer an anticancer drug 96

Pork Insulatard a brand name for insulin 271 (a drug used in diabetes 82)

Pork Mixtard a brand name for insulin 271 (a drug used in diabetes 82)

Posalfilin a brand name for podophyllum with salicylic acid (both drugs for warts)

postcoital contraception see **oral contraceptives**

potassium a mineral 93

potassium bicarbonate an antacid 42

potassium channel openers a group of vasodilators 31 and anti-angina drugs 35

potassium chloride a potassium salt (minerals 93) used in oral rehydration therapy

potassium citrate a drug for cystitis 112

potassium clavulanate a preparation of clavulanic acid (a substance given with amoxicillin 142 to make it more effective)

potassium hydroxyquinolone sulphate an antibacterial, antifungal, and deodorant skin preparation 120 and treatment for acne 123

potassium iodide a drug used to treat an overactive thyroid before surgery 84

potassium permanganate a skin antiseptic (anti-infective skin preparations 120)

potassium-sparing diuretics 32

povidone-iodine a skin antiseptic (anti-infective skin preparations 120)

Powergel a brand name for ketoprofen 281 (a non-steroidal anti-inflammatory drug 50)

Pragmatar a brand-named preparation for eczema 125, psoriasis 124, and dandruff 126 containing coal tar, salicylic acid, and sulphur

pralidoxime mesylate an antidote for organophosphorus poisoning

pramipexole a drug for parkinsonism 18

pramocaine a local anaesthetic 11

Pralenal a brand name for enalapril 231 (an ACE inhibitor vasodilator 31 and antihypertensive 36)

pravastatin 353 a lipid-lowering drug 37

Praxilene a brand name for naftidrofuryl 326 (a vasodilator 31)

praziquantel an anthelmintic 78 for tapeworms

prazosin an alpha blocker used as an antihypertensive 36 and to relieve urinary obstruction 112

Predenema a brand name for prednisolone 354 (a corticosteroid 80)

Predfoam a brand name for prednisolone 354 (a corticosteroid 80)

Pred Forte a brand name for prednisolone 354 (a corticosteroid 80)

prednisolone 354 a corticosteroid 80

Predsol a brand name for prednisolone 354 (a corticosteroid 80)

Predsol-N a brand name for prednisolone 354 (a corticosteroid 80) with neomycin (an aminoglycoside antibiotic 62)

Pregaday a brand name for folic acid (a vitamin 90) with iron (a mineral 93)

Pregnyl a brand name for human chorionic gonadotrophin 181 (a drug for infertility 109)

Premarin a brand name for conjugated oestrogens 201 (a female sex hormone 88)

Premique a brand-named preparation for menopause (female sex hormones 88) containing conjugated oestrogens 201 with medroxyprogesterone 301

Prempak-C a brand-named drug containing conjugated oestrogens 201 and norgestrel (a progestogen) (female sex hormones 88) used as HRT

Prepadine a brand name for dosulepin 223 (a tricyclic antidepressant 14)

Prescal a brand name for isradipine (a calcium channel blocker vasodilator 31)

Preservex a brand name for aceclofenac (a non-steroidal anti-inflammatory drug 50)

Prestim a brand name for bendroflumethiazide 155 (a thiazide diuretic 32) with timolol 406 (a beta blocker 30)

Priadel a brand name for lithium 292 (an antimanic drug 16)

prilocaine a local anaesthetic 11

Primacor a brand name for milrinone (a drug used for its vasodilator 31 effects to treat heart failure)

primaquine an antimalarial drug 75 and antiprotozoal drug 73

Primaxin a brand name for imipenem (an antibiotic 62) with cilastatin (a substance used to make imipenem more effective)

primidone an anticonvulsant drug 16

Primolut N a brand name for norethisterone 332 (a female sex hormone 88)

Primoteston Depot a brand name for testosterone 402 (a male sex hormone 87)

Primperan a brand name for metoclopramide 314 (a gastrointestinal motility regulator and anti-emetic 21)

Prioderm a brand name for malathion 300 (a drug to treat skin parasites 122)

Pripsen a brand name for piperazine (an anthelmintic drug 78) with senna (a stimulant laxative 45)

Pro-Banthine a brand name for propantheline (an anticholinergic antispasmodic drug for irritable bowel syndrome 45 and urinary incontinence 112)

probenecid a uricosuric for gout 53

procainamide an anti-arrhythmic drug 33

procaine a local anaesthetic 11

procaine benzylpenicillin a penicillin antibiotic drug 62

procarbazine a drug for lymphatic cancers and small-cell cancer of the lung 96

prochlorperazine 355 a phenothiazine anti-emetic 21 and antipsychotic 15

Proctofoam HC a brand-named preparation for haemorrhoids 47 containing hydrocortisone 264 (a corticosteroid 80) with pramocaine, a local anaesthetic 11

Proctosedyl a brand-named preparation for haemorrhoids 47 containing hydrocortisone 264 (a corticosteroid 80) with cinchocaine (a local anaesthetic 11)

procyclidine 356 an anticholinergic drug for parkinsonism 18

Pro-Epanutin a brand name for fosphenytoin 348 (an anticonvulsant drug 16)

Profasi a brand name for chorionic gonadotrophin 181 (a drug for infertility 109)

Proflex a brand name for ibuprofen 267 (a non-steroidal anti-inflammatory drug 50)

progesterone a female sex hormone 88

Prograf a brand name for tacrolimus (an immunosuppressant 99)

proguanil with atovaquone 358 an antimalarial drug 75

Progynova a brand name for estradiol 238, an oestrogen female sex hormone 88

Progynova TS a brand name for estradiol 238 (an oestrogen female sex hormone 88

Proluton Depot a brand name for hydroxyprogesterone (a progestogen 88 used to prevent miscarriage)

promazine 359 a phenothiazine antipsychotic 15

promethazine 360 an antihistamine 58 and anti-emetic 21

Propaderm a brand name for beclometasone 154 (a corticosteroid 80)

propafenone an anti-arrhythmic drug 33

Propain a brand-named analgesic 9 containing codeine 198, diphenhydramine, paracetamol 341, and caffeine

propamidine isetionate an antibacterial drug 66 for eye infections

propantheline an anticholinergic antispasmodic drug for irritable bowel syndrome 45 and urinary incontinence 112

Propecia a brand name for finasteride 244 (a drug for benign prostatic hypertrophy 112 and hair loss 127)

Propine a brand name for dipivefrine (a sympathomimetic drug for glaucoma 114)

propiverine a drug for urinary frequency 112

Pro-Plus a brand name for caffeine

propofol an anaesthetic agent

propranolol 361 a beta blocker 30 and anti-anxiety drug 13

propylthiouracil 362 an antithyroid drug 84

Proscar a brand name for finasteride 244 (a drug for benign prostatic hypertrophy 112 and hair loss 127)

Prostap SR a brand name for leuprorelin (a drug for menstrual disorders 104)

Prostin VR a brand name for alprostadil 135 (a prostaglandin and drug for impotence 109)

protamine an antidote for heparin 262

protease a pancreatic enzyme preparation for pancreatic disorders 49

protease inhibitors a group of drugs used to treat HIV/AIDS 100

Prothiaden a brand name for dosulepin 223 (a tricyclic antidepressant 14)

protirelin a test of thyroid function

Protium a brand name for pantoprazole (a proton pump inhibitor ulcer-healing drug 43)

Proton pump inhibitors a group of anti-ulcer drugs 43

Provera a brand name for medroxyprogesterone 301 (a female sex hormone 88)

Provigil a brand name for modafinil (a nervous system stimulant drug 19 for narcolepsy)

Pro-Viron a brand name for mesterolone (a male sex hormone 87)

proxymetacaine a local anaesthetic 11

Prozac a brand name for fluoxetine 246 (an SSRI antidepressant 14)

Proziere a brand name for prochlorperazine 355 (a phenothiazine anti-emetic 21)

pseudoephedrine a decongestant 26

psoriasis, drugs for 124

Psorin a brand-named drug for psoriasis 124 containing dithranol, coal tar, and salicylic acid (a keratolytic 123)

Pulmicort a brand name for budesonide 163 (a corticosteroid 80)

Pulmozyme a brand name for dornase alfa (a drug for cystic fibrosis)

pumactant a drug to mature the lungs of premature babies

Pupils, drugs affecting 116

Puri-Nethol a brand name for mercaptopurine 307 (an anticancer drug 96)

Pylorid a brand name for ranitidine bismuth citrate (an anti-ulcer drug 43)

Pyralvex an anti-inflammatory drug for mouth ulcers

pyrazinamide an antituberculous drug 67

pyridostigmine 363 a drug for myasthenia gravis 55

pyridoxine a B vitamin (vitamins 90)

pyrimethamine 364 an antimalarial drug 75

pyrithione zinc an antimicrobial drug for dandruff 126

Pyrogastrone a brand-named preparation for indigestion containing aluminium hydroxide 136, magnesium trisilicate, and sodium bicarbonate 385 (all antacids 42), carbenoxolone (an anti-ulcer drug 43), and alginic acid (an antifoaming agent)

Q

Quellada M a brand name for malathion 300 (a drug to treat skin parasites 122)

Questran a brand name for colestyramine 200 (a lipid-lowering drug 37)

quetiapine 366 an antipsychotic drug 15

quinagolide a drug to reduce prolactin levels and for pituitary disorders 85

quinapril an ACE inhibitor vasodilator 31

quinidine an anti-arrhythmic drug 33

quinine 367 an antimalarial drug 75 and muscle relaxant 54

Quinocort a brand name for hydrocortisone 264 (a corticosteroid 80) with potassium hydroxyquinoline sulphate (an anti-infective skin preparation 120)

Quinoderm a brand-named preparation for acne 123 containing benzoyl peroxide 156 and potassium hydroxyquinoline sulphate (an anti-infective skin preparation 120)

quinolones a group of antibacterial drugs 66

Quinoped a brand-named antifungal drug 76 containing benzoyl peroxide 156 and potassium hydroxyquinoline sulphate (an anti-infective skin preparation 120)

quinupristin an antibiotic 62

Qvar a brand name for beclometasone 154 (a corticosteroid 80)

R

rabeprazole a proton pump inhibitor anti-ulcer drug 43

RadianB a brand-named topical gel containing ibuprofen 267 (a non-opioid analgesic 9 and non-steroidal anti-inflammatory drug 50

raloxifene 369 a drug used to treat osteoporosis 56

raltitrexed an anticancer drug 96

ramipril 370 an ACE inhibitor vasodilator 31 and antihypertensive 36

Ranitic a brand name for ranitidine 371 (an H$_2$ blocker anti-ulcer drug 43)

ranitidine 371 an H$_2$ blocker anti-ulcer drug 43

ranitidine bismuth citrate an anti-ulcer drug 43

Rantec a brand name for ranitidine 371 (an H$_2$ blocker anti-ulcer drug 43)

Rapilysin a brand name for reteplase, a thrombolytic drug 38

Rapitil a brand name for nedocromil (a drug similar to sodium cromoglicate 386, used to prevent asthma attacks 24)

Rappell a brand name for piperonal (a head lice repellent)

rasburicase a drug for gout 53

razoxane a cytotoxic anticancer drug 96

Rebif a brand name for interferon beta 272 (a drug for multiple sclerosis)

reboxetine an antidepressant 14

Redoxon a brand name for vitamin C (a vitamin 90)

Reductil a brand name for sibutramine 382 (an appetite suppressant and nervous system stimulant 19)

Refludan a brand name for lepirudin, an anticoagulant drug 38

Refolinon a brand name for folinic acid (a vitamin 90)

Regaine a brand name for minoxidil 320 used for hair loss 127

Regranex a brand name for becaplermin, a drug for healing skin ulcers

Regulan a brand name for ispaghula (a bulk-forming agent used as a laxative 45)

Regulose a brand of lactulose 283 (an osmotic laxative 45)

Rehidrat a brand name for oral rehydration salts containing potassium, sodium chloride, sodium bicarbonate 385, and glucose

Relaxit a brand-named lubricant laxative 45

Relenza a brand name for zanamivir, an antiviral drug 69

Relifex a brand name for nabumetone (a non-steroidal anti-inflammatory drug 50)

Remedeine a brand name for paracetamol 341 (a non-opioid analgesic 9) with dihydrocodeine 216 (an opioid analgesic 9)

remifentanil a drug used in anaesthesia

Remnos a brand name for nitrazepam 331 (a benzodiazepine sleeping drug 11)

Rennie Digestif a brand-named antacid 42 containing calcium carbonate with magnesium carbonate

Rennie Duo a brand-named antacid 42 containing calcium carbonate with magnesium carbonate and sodium alginate

repaglinide 372 an oral drug for diabetes 82

Requip a brand name for ropinirole (drug for parkinsonism 87)

Resolve a brand-named analgesic 9 and antacid 42 with paracetamol 341, sodium bicarbonate 385, potassium bicarbonate, calcium carbonate, citric acid, and vitamin C

Resonium A a brand name for sodium polystyrene sulphonate (a drug to remove excess potassium from the blood)

resorcinol a keratolytic mainly for acne 123

Respiratory stimulants nervous system stimulants 19

Respontin a brand name for ipratropium bromide 274 (an anticholinergic bronchodilator drug 23)

Restandol a brand name for testosterone 402 (a male sex hormone 87)

reteplase a thrombolytic drug 38

Retin-A a brand name for tretinoin (a drug for acne 123)

retinoic acid vitamin A (a vitamin 90)

retinoids vitamin A (a vitamin 90)

retinol vitamin A (a vitamin 90)

Retinova a brand name for tretinoin (a drug for acne 123)

Retrovir a brand name for zidovudine 420 (a reverse transcriptase inhibitor drug for HIV/AIDS 100)

Revanil a brand name for lisuride (a drug for parkinsonism 18)

reverse transcriptase inhibitors a group of drugs for HIV/AIDS 100

reviparin a type of heparin 262, an anticoagulant drug 38

Rheumacin LA a brand name for indometacin (a non-steroidal anti-inflammatory drug 50 and drug for gout 53)

Rheumox a brand name for azapropazone (a non-steroidal anti-inflammatory drug 50)

Rhinocort a brand name for budesonide 163 (a corticosteroid 80)

Rhinolast a brand name for azelastine (an antihistamine 58)

Rhumalgan a brand name for diclofenac 212 (a non-steroidal anti-inflammatory drug 50)

Riamet a brand name for artemether with lumefantrine (both antimalarial drugs 75)

ribavirin an antiviral 69 used for certain lung infections in infants and children

riboflavin a vitamin 90

Ridaura a brand name for auranofin (an antirheumatic drug 52)

Rideril a brand name for thioridazine (a phenothiazine antipsychotic 15)

rifabutin an antituberculous drug 67

Rifadin a brand name for rifampicin 373 (an antituberculous drug 67)

rifampicin 373 an antituberculous drug 67

Rifater a brand name for isoniazid 276 with rifampicin 373 and pyrazinamide (all antituberculous drugs 67)

Rifinah a brand name for isoniazid 276 with rifampicin 373 (antituberculous drugs 67)

Rilutek a brand name for riluzole (a glutamate inhibitor used to help patients with some forms of motor neurone disease)

riluzole a glutamate inhibitor used to help patients with some forms of motor neurone disease

Rimactane a brand name for rifampicin 373 (an antituberculous drug 67)

Rimactazid a brand name for isoniazid 276 with rifampicin 373 (both antituberculous drugs 67)

Rimapam a brand name for diazepam 211 (a benzodiazepine anti-anxiety drug 13, muscle relaxant 54, and anticonvulsant 16)

Rimapurinol a brand name for allopurinol 133 (a drug for gout 53)

rimexolone a corticosteroid 80

Rimoxallin a brand name for amoxicillin 142 (a penicillin antibiotic 62)

Rimso-50 a brand name for dimethyl sulfoxide (a drug for urinary infection 112)

Rinatec a brand name for ipratropium bromide 274 (an anticholinergic bronchodilator drug 23)

risedronate a drug for bone disorders 56

Risperdal a brand name for risperidone 374 (an antipsychotic 15)

risperidone 374 an antipsychotic 15

Ritalin a brand name for methylphenidate (a drug for hyperactivity)

ritodrine a drug used in labour 110

ritonavir a protease inhibitor drug for HIV/AIDS 100

rituximab an anticancer drug 96

rivastigmine 376 a drug for dementia 19 used in Alzheimer's disease

Rivotril a brand name for clonazepam 194 (a benzodiazepine anticonvulsant 16)

rizatriptan a drug for migraine 20

Roaccutane a brand name for isotretinoin 278 (a drug for acne 123)

Robaxin a brand name for methocarbamol (a muscle relaxant 54)

Robinul a brand name for glycopyrronium bromide (a drug used in general anaesthesia)

Robinul-Neostigmine a brand name for neostigmine (a drug for myasthenia gravis 55)

Robitussin Dry Cough a brand name for guaifenesin (an expectorant for coughs 27)

Rocaltrol a brand name for calcitriol: vitamin D (a vitamin 90)

rocuronium a drug to relax the muscles during general anaesthesia

Roferon-A a brand name for interferon 272 (an antiviral 69 and anticancer drug 96)

Rohypnol a brand name for flunitrazepam (a benzodiazepine sleeping drug 11)

Rommix a brand name for erythromycin 235 (a macrolide antibiotic 62)

ropinirole a drug for parkinsonism 18

ropivacaine a local anaesthetic 11

rosiglitazone 377 an oral drug for diabetes 82

Roter a brand-named antacid 42 containing sodium bicarbonate 385, magnesium carbonate, frangula, and bismuth

Rowachol a brand-named preparation of essential oils for gallstones 48

Rowatinex a brand-named preparation to dissolve kidney stones and to treat kidney infections

Rozex a brand name for metronidazole 316 (an antibacterial 66)

Rusyde a brand name for furosemide 251 (a loop diuretic 32)

Rynacrom a brand name for sodium cromoglicate 386 (an anti-allergy drug 60)

Rynacrom Compound a brand name for sodium cromoglicate 386 (an anti-allergy drug 60) with xylometazoline (a decongestant 26)

Rythmodan a brand name for disopyramide (an anti-arrhythmic drug 33)

S

Sabril a brand name for vigabatrin (an anticonvulsant 16)

Saizen a brand name for somatropin, synthetic growth hormone for pituitary disorders 85

Salactol a brand-named wart preparation with salicylic acid , lactic acid, and collodion

Salagen a brand name for pilocarpine 349 (a miotic drug for glaucoma 114)

Salamol a brand name for salbutamol 379 (a sympathomimetic bronchodilator drug 23)

Salatac a brand-named wart preparation with salicylic acid, lactic acid, and collodion

Salazopyrin a brand name for sulfasalazine 392 (a drug for inflammatory bowel disease 46 and an antirheumatic drug 52)

Salbulin a brand name for salbutamol 379 (a sympathomimetic bronchodilator drug 23)

salbutamol 379 a sympathomimetic broncho-dilator 23 and drug used in labour 110

salicylic acid a keratolytic for acne 123, dandruff 126, psoriasis 124, and warts

Saliveze a brand name for artificial saliva

Salivix a brand name for artificial saliva

salmeterol 380 a sympathomimetic bronchodilator drug 23

Salofalk a brand name for mesalazine 308 (a drug for inflammatory bowel disease 46)

Salzone a brand name for paracetamol 341 (a non-opioid analgesic 9)

Sandimmun a brand name for ciclosporin 182 (an immunosuppressant 99)

Sandocal a brand name for calcium (a mineral 93)

Sando-K a brand name for potassium (a mineral 93)

Sandostatin a brand name for octreotide (a synthetic pituitary hormone 85 used to relieve symptoms of pancreatic cancer 96)

Sanomigran a brand name for pizotifen 352 (a drug for migraine 20)

saquinavir a protease inhibitor drug for HIV/AIDS 100

Savlon a brand name for chlorhexidine with cetrimide (both skin antiseptics 120)

Scheriproct a brand name for prednisolone 354 (a corticosteroid 80) with cinchocaine, a local anaesthetic 11

Scopoderm TTS a brand-named anti-emetic 21 containing hyoscine 265

Sea-Legs a brand name for meclozine (an anti-histamine 58 used for motion sickness 21)

Seasorb a wound dressing with alginates 133

Secadrex a brand name for hydrochlorothiazide 263 (a thiazide diuretic 32) with acebutolol (a beta blocker 30)

secobarbital a barbiturate sleeping drug 11

Seconal Sodium a brand name for secobarbital (a barbiturate sleeping drug 11)

Sectral a brand name for acebutolol (a beta blocker 30)

Securon a brand name for verapamil 415 (a calcium channel blocker vasodilator 31, anti-arrhythmic drug 33, anti-angina drug 35, and antihypertensive drug 36)

Securon SR a brand name for verapamil 415 (a calcium channel blocker vasodilator 31, anti-arrhythmic drug 33, anti-angina drug 35, and antihypertensive drug 36)

Selective serotonin re-uptake inhibitors (SSRIs) a group of antidepressants 14

selegiline a drug for severe parkinsonism 18

selenium a mineral 93

selenium sulphide a substance to treat skin inflammation and dandruff 126

Selsun a brand-named dandruff shampoo 126 containing selenium sulphide

Semi-Daonil a brand name for glibenclamide 255 (an oral drug used in diabetes 82)

senna a stimulant laxative 45

Senokot a brand name for senna (a stimulant laxative 45)

Septanest a brand name for articaine, a local anaesthetic 11

Septrin a brand name for co-trimoxazole 205 (a sulphonamide antibacterial 66)

Serc a brand name for betahistine 157, a drug for Ménière's disease (anti-emetics 21)

Serenace a brand name for haloperidol 261 (a butyrophenone antipsychotic 15)

Seretide a brand name for fluticasone 250 (a corticosteroid 80)

Serevent a brand name for salmeterol 380 (a sympathomimetic bronchodilator drug 23)

sermorelin a drug for growth disorders

Seroquel a brand name for quetiapine 366 (an antipsychotic drug 15)

Seroxat a brand name for paroxetine 342 (an SSRI antidepressant 14)

sertindole an antipsychotic 15

Sominex a brand-named sleeping drug 11 with promethazine 360 (an antihistamine 58)

Somnite a brand name for nitrazepam 331 (a benzodiazepine sleeping drug 11)

Sonata a brand name for zaleplon (a sleeping drug 11)

Soneryl a brand name for butobarbital (a barbiturate sleeping drug 11)

Soothelip a brand name for aciclovir, an antiviral 69

sorbitol a sweetener used in diabetic foods, and included in skin creams as a moisturizer

Sorbsan a wound dressing with alginates 133

Sotacor a brand name for sotalol 389 (a beta blocker 30)

sotalol 389 a beta blocker 30

Spasmonal a brand name for alverine (an anti-spasmodic for irritable bowel syndrome 45)

Spasmonal Fibre a brand name for sterculia (a bulk-forming laxative 45) with alverine (an antispasmodic for irritable bowel syndrome 45)

Spectraban a brand name for aminobenzoic acid with padimate-O (both sunscreens 127)

Spiriva a brand name for tiotropium 407 (an anticholinergic bronchodilator drug 23)

spironolactone a potassium-sparing diuretic 32

Spirospare a brand name for spironolactone (a potassium-sparing diuretic 32)

Sporanox a brand name for itraconazole (an antifungal drug 76)

Sprilon a brand-named skin preparation 120 containing dimeticone and zinc oxide

SSRIs see selective serotonin re-uptake inhibitors

Staril a brand name for fosinopril (an ACE inhibitor vasodilator 31)

statins a group of lipid-lowering drugs 37

stavudine a reverse transcriptase inhibitor drug for HIV/AIDS 100

Stelazine a brand name for trifluoperazine (a phenothiazine antipsychotic 15 and anti-emetic 21)

Stemetil a brand name for prochlorperazine 355 (a phenothiazine anti-emetic 21 and antipsychotic 15)

sterculia a bulk-forming agent used as an antidiarrhoeal drug 44 and laxative 45

steroids see corticosteroids 80, corticosteroids for rheumatic disorders 53, male sex hormones 87, and topical corticosteroids 120

Ster-Zac a brand name for triclosan (an anti-infective skin preparation 120)

Stesolid a brand name for diazepam 211 (a benzodiazepine anti-anxiety drug 13, muscle relaxant 54, and anticonvulsant drug 16)

Stiedex a brand name for desoxymetasone (a topical corticosteroid 120)

Stiemycin a brand name for erythromycin 235 (a macrolide antibiotic 62)

Stilnoct a brand name for zolpidem (a sleeping drug 11)

stimulant laxatives 45

St John's Wort a herbal antidepressant that interacts with many other drugs

Strepsils a brand-named preparation for mouth and throat infections containing amylmetacresol and dichlorobenzyl alcohol

Streptase a brand name for streptokinase 390, a thrombolytic drug 38

streptokinase 390 a thrombolytic drug 38)

streptomycin an antituberculous drug 67 and aminoglycoside antibiotic 62

Stromba a brand name for stanozolol (an anabolic steroid 88)

Stugeron a brand name for cinnarizine 184 (an antihistamine anti-emetic 21)

sucralfate 391 an anti-ulcer drug 43

Sudafed a brand name for pseudoephedrine (a decongestant 26)

Sudafed-Co a brand name for paracetamol 341 (a non-opioid analgesic 9) with pseudoephedrine (a decongestant 26

Sudafed expectorant a brand name for guaifenesin (an expectorant for coughs 27) with pseudoephedrine (a decongestant 26)

Sudocrem a brand-named skin preparation containing benzyl benzoate and zinc oxide

Sulazine EC a brand name for sulfasalazine 392 (a drug for inflammatory bowel disease 46 and an antirheumatic drug 52)

sulconazole an antifungal drug 76

Suleo-M a brand name for malathion 300 (a drug to treat skin parasites 122)

sulfacetamide a sulphonamide antibacterial 66

sulfadiazine a sulphonamide antibacterial 66

sulfadoxine a drug used with pyrimethamine 364 for malaria 75

sulfamethoxazole a sulphonamide antibacterial 66 combined with trimethoprim in co-trimoxazole 205

sulfasalazine 392 a drug for inflammatory bowel disease 46 and an antirheumatic 52

sulfathiazole a sulphonamide antibacterial 66

sulfinpyrazone a drug to prevent attacks of gout 53

sulindac a non-steroidal anti-inflammatory 50

sulphonamides a group of antibacterials 66

sulphonylureas a group of oral drugs used in diabetes 82

sulphur a topical antibacterial and antifungal for acne 123 and dandruff 126

sulpiride 139 an antipsychotic 15

Sulpitil a brand name for sulpiride 139 (an antipsychotic 15)

sumatriptan 393 a drug for migraine 20

Suprane a brand name for desflurane (a general anaesthetic)

Suprax a brand name for cefixime (a cephalosporin antibiotic 62)

Suprecur a brand name for buserelin (a drug for menstrual disorders 104)

Suprefact a brand name for buserelin (a drug for menstrual disorders 104)

Surgam a brand name for tiaprofenic acid (a non-steroidal anti-inflammatory drug 50)

Surmontil a brand name for trimipramine (a tricyclic antidepressant 14)

Suscard a brand name for glyceryl trinitrate 257 (an anti-angina drug 35)

Sustac a brand name for glyceryl trinitrate 257 (an anti-angina drug 35)

Sustanon a brand name for testosterone 402 (a male sex hormone 87)

Sustiva a brand name for efavirenz (a reverse transcriptase inhibitor drug HIV/AIDS 100)

suxamethonium a muscle relaxant used in general anaesthesia

Symbicort a brand name for budesonide 163 (a corticosteroid 80)

Symmetrel a brand name for amantadine (an antiviral 69 and drug for parkinsonism 18)

sympathomimetic drugs bronchodilators 23, drugs for asthma 24, decongestants 26, drugs for glaucoma 114, drugs affecting the pupil 116, and drugs for urinary disorders 112

Synacthen a brand name for tetracosactide (a drug used to assess adrenal gland function)

Synagis a brand name for palivizumab, an antiviral drug 69

Synalar a brand name for fluocinolone (a topical corticosteroid 120)

Synalar C a brand name for fluocinolone (a topical corticosteroid 120) with clioquinol (an anti-infective skin preparation 120)

Synalar N a brand name for fluocinolone (a topical corticosteroid 120) with neomycin (an aminoglycoside antibiotic 62)

Synarel a brand name for nafarelin (a drug for menstrual disorders 104)

Syndol a brand name for codeine 198 and paracetamol 341 (both analgesics 9), with caffeine and doxylamine (an antihistamine 58)

Synercid a brand-named preparation containing quinupristin and dalfopristin (both antibiotics 62)

Synflex a brand name for naproxen 326 (a non-steroidal anti-inflammatory drug 50 and drug for gout 53)

Synphase a brand-named oral contraceptive 105 containing ethinylestradiol 240 and norethisterone 332 (both female sex hormones 88)

Syntaris a brand name for flunisolide (a corticosteroid 80)

Syntocinon a brand name for oxytocin (a drug used in labour 110)

Syntometrine a brand name for ergometrine with oxytocin (drugs used in labour 110)

Syprol a brand name for propranolol 361 (a beta blocker 30)

Syscor MR a brand name for nisoldipine (a calcium channel blocker vasodilator 31, anti-angina drug 35, and antihypertensive drug 36)

Sytron a brand name for sodium feredetate (iron, a mineral 93)

T

tacalcitol a drug for psoriasis 124

tacrolimus an immunosuppressant 99

Tagamet a brand name for cimetidine 183 (an H_2 blocker anti-ulcer drug 43)

Tambocor a brand name for flecainide (an anti-arrhythmic 33)

Tamiflu a brand name for oseltamivir (an antiviral drug 69 for influenza 69)

Tamofen a brand name for tamoxifen 395 (an anticancer drug 96)

tamoxifen 395 an anticancer drug 96

Tampovagan a brand name for diethylstilbestrol (a female sex hormone 88) with lactic acid

tamsulosin 396 an alpha blocker drug for prostate disorders 112

Tanatril a brand name for imidapril (an ACE inhibitor vasodilator 31)

Targocid a brand name for teicoplanin (an antibiotic 62)

Targretin a brand name for bexarotene (an anticancer drug 96)

Tarivid a brand name for ofloxacin (a quinolone antibacterial 66)

Tavanic a brand name for levofloxacin 288 (a quinolone antibacterial 66)

Tavegil a brand name for clemastine (an antihistamine 126)

taxanes a group of anticancer drugs 96

Taxol a brand name for paclitaxel (an anticancer drug 96)

Taxotere a brand name for docetaxel (an anticancer drug 96)

tazarotene a drug for psoriasis 124

Tazocin a brand name for piperacillin (a penicillin antibiotic 62) with tazobactam (which increases the effectiveness of piperacillin)

TCAs see **tricyclic antidepressants**

TCP a brand-named skin antiseptic 120 with phenol, chlorophenol, and 2-iodophenol

Tears Naturale a brand-named artificial tear preparation containing hypromellose

tegafur an anticancer drug 96

Tegretol a brand name for carbamazepine 169 (an anticonvulsant 16)

teicoplanin an antibiotic 62

Telfast a brand name for fexofenadine (an antihistamine 58)

telithromycin a macrolide antibiotic 62

telmisartan an angiotensin II blocker vasodilator 31 and antihypertensive drug 36

temazepam 397 a benzodiazepine sleeping drug 11

Temgesic a brand name for buprenorphine (an opioid analgesic 9)

Temodal a brand name for temozolomide (an anticancer drug 96)

temozolomide an anticancer drug 96

Tenchlor a brand name for atenolol 147 (a beta blocker 30) with chlortalidone (a thiazide diuretic 32)

tenecteplase 398 a thrombolytic drug 38

Tenif a brand name for atenolol 147 (a beta blocker 30) with nifedipine 330 (a calcium channel blocker vasodilator 31, anti-angina drug 35, and antihypertensive 36)

Tenkicin a brand name for phenoxymethyl-penicillin 346 (a penicillin antibiotic 62)

Tenkorex a brand name for cefalexin 172 (a cephalosporin antibiotic 62)

tenofovir disoproxil a reverse transcriptase inhibitor drug for HIV/AIDS 100

Tenoret-50 a brand name for atenolol 147 (a beta blocker 30) with chlortalidone (a thiazide diuretic 32)

Tenoretic a brand name for atenolol 147 (a beta blocker 30) with chlortalidone (a thiazide diuretic 32)

Tenormin a brand name for atenolol 147 (a beta blocker 30)

tenoxicam a non-steroidal anti-inflammatory 50

Tensipine MR a brand name for nifedipine 330 (a calcium channel blocker anti-angina drug 35)

Tensium a brand name for diazepam 211 (a benzodiazepine anti-anxiety drug 13 and muscle relaxant 54)

Tensopril a brand name for captopril 168 (an ACE inhibitor vasodilator 31 and antihypertensive 36)

Teoptic a brand name for carteolol (a beta blocker 30 used for glaucoma 114)

terazosin an alpha blocker antihypertensive 36

terbinafine 400 an antifungal drug 76

terbutaline 401 a sympathomimetic bronchodilator drug 23 and uterine muscle relaxant drug used in labour 110

terfenadine an antihistamine 58

Teril Retard a brand name for carbamazepine 169 (an anticonvulsant drug 16 and antipsychotic 15)

terlipressin a drug similar to vasopressin (a pituitary hormone 85) used to stop bleeding

Terra-Cortril a brand name for hydrocortisone 264 (a corticosteroid 80) with oxytetracycline (a tetracycline antibiotic 62)

Terra-Cortril Nystatin a brand name for hydrocortisone 264 (a corticosteroid 80) with nystatin 333 (an antifungal 76) and oxytetracycline (a tetracycline antibiotic 62)

Tertroxin a brand name for liothyronine (a hormone for thyroid disorders 84)

testosterone 402 a male sex hormone 87

tetrabenazine a drug for tremor

tetracaine a local anaesthetic 11

tetracosactide a drug similar to corticotropin (a pituitary hormone 85), used to assess adrenal gland function

tetracycline 403 an antibiotic 62 and antimalarial drug 75

Tetralysal 300 a brand name for lymecycline 403 (a tetracycline antibiotic 62)

T-Gel a brand name for coal tar (an agent for dandruff 126 and psoriasis 124)

thalidomide a drug for Hansen's disease 67

Theo-Dur a brand name for theophylline 404 (a xanthine bronchodilator drug 23)

theophylline 404 a xanthine bronchodilator 23

thiamine a vitamin 90

thiazides a group of diuretic drugs 32

thiopental a fast-acting barbiturate used to induce general anaesthesia

thioridazine a phenothiazine antipsychotic 15

thiotepa an anticancer drug 96

thrombolytic drugs a group of drugs that affect blood clotting 38

thyroid hormones drugs for thyroid disorders 84

tiabendazole an anthelmintic drug 78

tiagabine an anticonvulsant drug 16

tiaprofenic acid a non-steroidal anti-inflammatory drug 50

tibolone 405 a female sex hormone 88

ticarcillin a penicillin antibiotic 62

Ticlid a brand name for ticlopidine (an antiplatelet drug 38)

ticlopidine an antiplatelet drug 38

Tilade a brand name for nedocromil (a drug for asthma 24)

Tildiem a brand name for diltiazem 217 (a calcium channel blocker anti-angina drug 35)

Tiloryth a brand name for erythromycin 235 (a macrolide antibiotic 62)

tiludronic acid a drug for bone disorders 56

Timentin a brand name for ticarcillin (a penicillin antibiotic 62) with clavulanic acid (which increases the effectiveness of ticarcillin)

Timodine a brand name for hydrocortisone 264 (a corticosteroid 80) with nystatin 333 (an antifungal 76), benzalkonium chloride (an antiseptic), and dimeticone (a base for skin preparations 120)

timolol 406 a beta blocker 30 and drug for glaucoma 114

Timonil Retard a brand name for carbamazepine 169 (an anticonvulsant 16 and antipsychotic drug 15)

Timoptol a brand name for timolol 406 (a beta blocker 30 and drug for glaucoma 114)

Timpron a brand name for naproxen 326 (a non-steroidal anti-inflammatory drug 50 and drug for gout 53)

Tinaderm-M a brand name for nystatin 333 with tolnaftate (both antifungals 76)

tinidazole an antibacterial drug 66 and antiprotozoal drug 73

tinzaparin a type of heparin 262, an anticoagulant drug 38

tioconazole an antifungal drug 76

tioguanine an antimetabolite for acute leukaemia 96

tiotropium 407 an anticholinergic bronchodilator drug 23

tirofiban a drug that prevents heart attacks

tissue plasminogen activator see alteplase

Titralac a brand name for calcium carbonate (used to reduce blood phosphate levels) and glycine

Tixylix a brand name for promethazine 360 (an antihistamine 58) with pholcodine (an opioid cough suppressant 27)

Tixylix Cough and Cold a brand-named cough suppressant 27 and decongestant 26 with chlorphenamine 178, pseudoephedrine, and pholcodine

tizanidine a muscle relaxant 54

tobramycin an aminoglycoside antibiotic 62

tocopherol vitamin E (a vitamin 90)

tocopheryl vitamin E (a vitamin 90)

Tofranil a brand name for imipramine 268 (a tricyclic antidepressant 14)

tolbutamide 408 a drug used in diabetes 82

tolfenamic acid drug for migraine 20

tolnaftate an antifungal drug 76

tolterodine 409 an anticholinergic and antispasmodic for urinary disorders 112

Topal a brand-named antacid 42 containing aluminium hydroxide 136, magnesium carbonate, and alginic acid

Topamax a brand name for topiramate (an anticonvulsant 16)

topical corticosteroids 120

Topicycline a brand name for tetracycline 403 (an antibiotic 62)

topiramate an anticonvulsant 16

topotecan an anticancer drug 96

Toradol a brand name for ketorolac (a non-steroidal anti-inflammatory drug 50 used as an analgesic 9)

torasemide a loop diuretic 32

Torem a brand name for torasemide (a loop diuretic 32)

toremifene an anticancer drug 96

Totaretic a brand name for atenolol 147 (a beta blocker 30) with chlortalidone (a thiazide diuretic 32)

Tracleer a brand name for bosentan (a drug for pulmonary hypertension)

tramadol 410 a synthetic opioid analgesic 9

Tramake a brand name for tramadol 410 (a synthetic opioid analgesic 9)

tramazoline a nasal decongestant 26

Tramil 500 a brand name for paracetamol 341 (a non-opioid analgesic 9)

Trandate a brand name for labetalol (a beta blocker 30)

trandolapril an ACE inhibitor vasodilator 31

tranexamic acid an antifibrinolytic drug used to promote blood clotting 38)

Transiderm-Nitro a brand name for glyceryl trinitrate 257 (an anti-angina drug 35)

Transvasin a topical treatment for muscle aches and sprains

Tranxene a brand name for clorazepate (a benzodiazepine anti-anxiety drug 13)

tranylcypromine an MAOI antidepressant 14

Trasicor a brand name for oxprenolol (a beta blocker 30)

Trasidrex a brand name for cyclopenthiazide (a thiazide diuretic 32) with oxprenolol (a beta blocker 30)

trastuzumab a type of anticancer drug 96

Travatan a brand name for travoprost (a drug for glaucoma 114)

travoprost a drug for glaucoma 114

Traxam a brand name for felbinac (a non-steroidal anti-inflammatory drug 50)

trazodone an antidepressant 14

Trental a brand name for pentoxifylline (a vasodilator 31)

treosulfan a drug for ovarian cancer 96

tretinoin a drug for acne 123

Tri-Adcortyl a brand name for nystatin 333 (an antifungal 76) with gramicidin and neomycin (both aminoglycoside antibiotics 62) and triamcinolone (a corticosteroid 80)

Triadene a brand-named oral contraceptive 105 containing ethinylestradiol 240 and gestodene (a progestogen)

TriamaxCo a brand-named diuretic 32 containing triamterene 411 and hydrochlorothiazide 263

triamcinolone a corticosteroid 80 also used for ear disorders 117

Triam-Co a brand name for hydrochlorothiazide 263 with triamterene 411 (both diuretics 32)

triamterene 411 a potassium-sparing diuretic 32

Triapin a brand-named preparation with felodipine and ramipril (both vasodilators 31)

triclofos a non-benzodiazepine, non-barbiturate sleeping drug 11

triclosan an anti-infective skin preparation 120

tricyclic antidepressants a group of antidepressant drugs 14

Tridestra a brand-named preparation for menopause (female sex hormones 88) with estradiol 238 and medroxyprogesterone 301

trientine drug used for Wilson's disease

trifluoperazine a phenothiazine antipsychotic 15 and an anti-emetic 21

Trifyba a brand name for a bulk-forming laxative 45 containing bran

trihexyphenidyl a drug for parkinsonism 18

tri-iodothyronine see **liothyronine**

trilostane an adrenal antagonist used for Cushing's syndrome (an adrenal disorder) and breast cancer 96

tremetaphan camsylate a drug used to lower blood pressure below normal in surgery

trimethoprim 412 an antibacterial 66

Tri-Minulet a brand-named oral contraceptive 105 containing ethinylestradiol 240 and gestodene (a progestogen)

trimipramine a tricyclic antidepressant 14

Trimopan a brand name for trimethoprim 412 (an antibacterial 66)

Trimovate a brand name for clobetasone (a topical corticosteroid 120) with nystatin 333 (an antifungal 76) and oxytetracycline (a tetracycline antibiotic 62)

Trinordiol a brand-named oral contraceptive 105 containing ethinylestradiol 240 and levonorgestrel 289

TriNovum a brand-named oral contraceptive 105 containing ethinylestradiol 240 with norethisterone 332 (both female sex hormones 88)

tripotassium dicitratobismuthate a bismuth compound used to treat peptic ulcer 43

triprolidine an antihistamine 58

Triptafen a brand name for amitriptyline 140 (a tricyclic antidepressant 14) with perphenazine (an antipsychotic 15)

triptorelin an anticancer drug 96

Trisequens a brand name for estradiol 238 and estriol (female sex hormones 88)

trisodium edetate a drug to remove excess calcium from the blood

Tritace a brand name for ramipril 370 (an ACE inhibitor vasodilator 31 and antihypertensive drug 36)

Trizivir a brand name for abacavir (a reverse transcriptase inhibitor drug for HIV/AIDS 100)

Tropergen a brand name for diphenoxylate (an opioid antidiarrhoeal 44) and atropine 150

tropicamide a mydriatic drug affecting the pupil 116

tropisetron an anti-emetic 21

Tropium a brand name for chlordiazepoxide 176 (a benzodiazepine anti-anxiety drug 13)

tropsium an anticholinergic drug for urinary disorders 112

Trosyl a brand name for tioconazole (an antifungal drug 76)

Trusopt a brand name for dorzolamide 222 (a drug for glaucoma 114)

tryptophan an antidepressant 14

Tuinal a brand name for amobarbital with secobarbital (both barbiturate sleeping drugs 11)

Tylex a brand-named analgesic 9 containing codeine 198 and paracetamol 341

Tyrozets a brand name for benzocaine, a local anaesthetic 11 with tyrothricin (an antibiotic 62)

U

Ubretid a brand name for distigmine (a parasympathomimetic for urinary retention 112 and myasthenia gravis 55)

Ucerax a brand name for hydroxyzine (an anti-anxiety drug 13)

Uftoral a brand name for tegafur (an anticancer drug 96) with uracil (to prolong the drug's effects)

Ultec a brand name for cimetidine 183 (an H_2 blocker anti-ulcer drug 43)

Ultiva a brand name for remifentanil (a drug used in anaesthesia)

Ultralanum Plain a brand name for fluocortolone (a topical corticosteroid 120)

Ultraproct a brand name for fluocortolone (a topical corticosteroid 120) with cinchocaine, a local anaesthetic 11

undecenoic acid an antifungal drug 76

Uniflu with Gregovite C a brand-named cough remedy with codeine 198 (an opioid analgesic 9 and cough suppressant 27), diphenhydramine (an antihistamine 58), paracetamol 341 (a non-opioid analgesic 9), phenylephrine (a decongestant 26), and caffeine

Uniphyllin Continus a brand name for theophylline 404 (a xanthine bronchodilator drug 23)

Uniroid HC a brand name for hydrocortisone 264 (a corticosteroid 80) with cinchocaine, a local anaesthetic 11

Univer a brand name for verapamil 415 (a calcium channel blocker vasodilator 31, anti-angina drug 35, anti-arrhythmic drug 33, and antihypertensive drug 36)

Uprima a brand name for apomorphine 145 (a drug for parkinsonism 18 and impotence 109)

urea an emollient and moisturizer for dry skin and to soften ear wax

Uriben a brand name for nalidixic acid (a quinolone antibacterial 66)

Urispas a brand name for flavoxate (an anti-spasmodic drug for urinary disorders 112)

urofollitropin a drug for infertility 109

Uromitexan a brand name for mesna (used to protect the urinary tract from damage caused by some anticancer drugs 96)

ursodeoxycholic acid a drug for gallstones 48

Ursofalk a brand name for ursodeoxycholic acid (a drug for gallstones 48)

Utinor a brand name for norfloxacin (a quinolone antibacterial 66)

Utovlan a brand name for norethisterone 332 (a female sex hormone 88)

V

Vagifem a brand name for estradiol 238 (a female sex hormone 88)

Vaginyl a brand name for metronidazole 316 (an antibacterial 66 and antiprotozoal 73)

valaciclovir an antiviral drug 69

Valclair a brand name for diazepam 211 (a benzodiazepine anti-anxiety drug 13, muscle relaxant 54, and anticonvulsant 16)

Valderma Cream a brand-named cream for minor skin problems containing potassium hydroxyquinoline sulphate (an antibacterial and antifungal), and chlorocresol

valganciclovir an antiviral drug 69 for cytomegalovirus

Vallergan a brand name for trimeprazine (an antihistamine 58)

Valoid a brand name for cyclizine, an anti-emetic drug 21

valproate an anticonvulsant 16

valproic acid an anticonvulsant 16

valsartan an angiotensin II blocker vasodilator 31

Valtrex a brand name for valaciclovir, an antiviral drug 69

Vancocin a brand name for vancomycin, an antibiotic 62 for serious infections

vancomycin an antibiotic 62 for serious infections

Vaqta a brand-named vaccine against viral hepatitis (vaccines and immunization 70)

Varidase a brand-named preparation for leg ulcers, containing streptokinase 390 (a thrombolytic drug) and streptodornase (a fibrinolytic enzyme)

Varilrix a brand name for varicella-zoster vaccine (vaccines and immunization 70)

Vascace a brand name for cilazapril, an ACE inhibitor vasodilator 31

Vaseline Petroleum Jelly an ointment used to treat dry skin

vasodilator drugs 31

Vasogen a brand-named barrier cream (anti-infective skin preparations 120) containing calamine, dimeticone and zinc oxide

vasopressin a pituitary hormone for diabetes insipidus 85

Vectavir a brand name for penciclovir, an antiviral 69

vecuronium a muscle relaxant used in general anaesthesia

Veganin a brand-named analgesic 9 with aspirin 146, paracetamol 341, and codeine 198

Veil a brand-named preparation to hide scars

Velbe a brand name for vinblastine, an anticancer drug 96

Velosef a brand name for cefradine, a cephalosporin antibiotic 62

Velosulin a brand name for insulin 271 (a drug used in diabetes 82)

venlafaxine 414 an antidepressant 14

DRUG FINDER INDEX

Venofer a brand-named iron supplement (minerals 93)

Ventmax SR a brand name for salbutamol 379 (a sympathomimetic bronchodilator drug 23)

Ventodisks a brand name for salbutamol 379 (a sympathomimetic bronchodilator drug 23)

Ventolin a brand name for salbutamol 379 (a sympathomimetic bronchodilator drug 23)

Vepesid a brand name for etoposide (an anticancer drug 96)

Veracur a brand name for formaldehyde (a substance for warts)

verapamil 415 a calcium channel blocker vasodilator 31, anti-arrhythmic drug 33, anti-angina drug 35, and antihypertensive drug 36

Verapress MR a brand name for verapamil 415 (a calcium channel blocker vasodilator 31, anti-arrhythmic drug 33, anti-angina drug 35, and antihypertensive 36)

Vermox a brand name for mebendazole (an anthelmintic 78)

Verrugon a brand name for salicylic acid (a keratolytic for warts)

Vesagex a brand-named antiseptic skin preparation 120 containing cetrimide

Vesanoid a brand name for tretinoin (a drug for acne 123)

Vexol a brand name for rimexolone, a corticosteroid 80

Viagra a brand name for sildenafil 383 (a drug for impotence 109)

Viazem XL a brand name for diltiazem 217 (a calcium channel blocker vasodilator 31 and antihypertensive 36)

Vibramycin, Vibramycin-D brand names for doxycycline 227 (a tetracycline antibiotic 62)

Vicks Medinite a brand-named cold remedy containing paracetamol 341 (a non-opioid analgesic 9), dextromethorphan (an opioid cough suppressant 27), and pseudoephedrine (a decongestant 26)

Videne a brand name for povidone-iodine (an antiseptic skin preparation 120)

Videx a brand name for didanosine (a reverse transcriptase inhibitor drug for HIV/AIDS 100)

vigabatrin an anticonvulsant 16

Vigam a brand name for human normal immunoglobulin injection

Vigranon B a brand name for vitamin B complex

vinblastine an anticancer drug 96

vincristine an anticancer drug 96

vindesine an anticancer drug 96

vinorelbine an anticancer drug 96

Vioform-Hydrocortisone a brand name for hydrocortisone 264 (a corticosteroid 80) with clioquinol (an antimicrobial skin preparation 120)

Viracept a brand name for nelfinavir (a protease inhibitor drug for HIV/AIDS 100)

Viraferon a brand name for interferon alfa 272 (an antiviral 69 used to treat viral hepatitis)

ViraferonPeg a brand name for peginterferon alfa (an antiviral drug 69 used to treat hepatitis C)

Viramune a brand name for nevirapine (a reverse transcriptase inhibitor drug for HIV/AIDS 100)

Virasorb a brand name for aciclovir 131 (an antiviral drug 69)

Virazid a brand name for tribavirin (an antiviral 69)

Viread a brand name for tenofovir disoproxil (a reverse transcriptase inhibitor drug for HIV/AIDS 100)

Viridal, Viridal Duo brand names for alprostadil 135 (a prostaglandin used in the treatment of impotence 109)

Virormone a brand name for testosterone 402 (a male sex hormone 87)

Virovir a brand name for aciclovir 131 (an antiviral drug 69)

Visclair a brand name for mecysteine (a mucolytic for coughs 27)

Viscotears a brand-named artificial tear preparation

Viskaldix a brand name for pindolol (a beta blocker 30) with clopamide (a thiazide diuretic 32)

Visken a brand name for pindolol (a beta blocker 30)

Vista-Methasone a brand name for betamethasone 158 (a corticosteroid 80)

Vistide a brand name for cidofovir (an antiviral 69 used for cytomegalovirus infections in AIDS 100)

vitamin A a vitamin 90

vitamin B Complex vitamins 90

vitamin B1 a vitamin 90 also called thiamine

vitamin B2 a vitamin 90 also called riboflavin

vitamin B6 a vitamin 90 also called pyridoxine

vitamin B12 a vitamin 90 also called hydroxocobalamin

vitamin C a vitamin 90 also called ascorbic acid

vitamin D a vitamin 90

vitamin E a vitamin 90

vitamin K a vitamin 90

vitamins 90

Vividrin a brand name for sodium cromoglicate 386 (an anti-allergy drug 60)